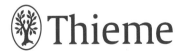

Reviews from Medical Students and Residents

- *"I think that the greatest strengths of the chapters are manifold. First, the succinctness of the text as a whole is impressive. Often, textbooks are worried about not covering material in adequate detail and are thus rather verbose. However, as a reader this can be overwhelming and hard to pick out the important points needed for understanding clinical management and preparing oneself for the USMLE Step 2/3 examinations. Second, I believe the use of tables is very beneficial in these chapters. It allows the reader to easily compare and contrast differing pathologies, and seeing important differences in presentations, labs, etc.; as these tend to be the highly tested nuances one must know for USMLE exams. Also, by the time most students take USMLE Step 2/3, they are quite familiar with the various pathologies, but a study resource that quickly covers basics while also highlighting the important differences between disease presentations and treatments. Lastly, the use of numerous figures/treatment algorithms and integration of those figures into the text are very well done in these chapters." "I appreciate the layout of this material, the authors' ability to boil down vast amounts of information into easy-to-understand, easy-to-find tables, and the addition of clinical case scenarios throughout."*

- *"These are excellent chapters that are clearly geared toward preparing medical students for the USMLE Steps 2 and 3 examinations. Important and highly tested points are emphasized, pathologies are easy to compare and contrast, and a clear emphasis on diagnostic workup and appropriate treatment is evident. This would be an excellent resource for medical students during their clinical years."*

- *"I think this is a great balance between step up to medicine and more simplistic books like Master the Boards."*

- *"The charts/tables provide very concise but very thorough information, key to any test prep publication."*

- *"The tables are phenomenal; essentially, the entire book is made up of tables."*

- *"I really liked how there is an image for everything to help clarify the disease or show what it looks like with imaging. I really like the graphs for all of the information. It makes it really easy to keep it organized."*

- *"I really enjoy the readability of the chapter and how the layout looks. The use of images to reinforce concepts is important too. There were many images on my exams and knowing what to look for is helpful. I like the shortened phrases (MCC, MC, NSIM, NSIDx) because these are the exact questions that are asked and it is helpful to see that from the get-go."*

- *"The tables are excellent. They are concise and contain the necessary information for a student studying for USMLE Step 2/3. Most importantly, they allow a student to quickly compare and contrast a number of similar presenting or similar pathophysiological diseases. This is how the test questions are written, and so it makes sense to studying accordingly."*

- *"The chapter is condensed down to tables with a lot of information, which is extremely helpful. It is easy to use when looking up for information on the wards in an easy-to-find fashion. The tables with differential diagnosis lay out the presentation and management, and compare the disease to other similar disease processes."*

Thieme Review for the USMLE: A WIN for Step 2 and 3 CK

Manoj Gurung, MD
Academic Hospitalist, Kent Hospital;
Assistant Professor
Department of Medicine
Warren Alpert Medical School of Brown University
Rhode Island, USA

Yayra Musabek, MD
Academic Hospitalist, Kent Hospital;
Assistant Professor
Department of Medicine
Warren Alpert Medical School of Brown University
Rhode Island, USA

560 illustrations

Thieme
New York • Stuttgart • Delhi • Rio de Janeiro

Library of Congress Cataloging-in-Publication Data
is available from the publisher

Important note: Medicine is an ever-changing science undergoing continual development. Research and clinical experience are continually expanding our knowledge, in particular our knowledge of proper treatment and drug therapy. Insofar as this book mentions any dosage or application, readers may rest assured that the authors, editors, and publishers have made every effort to ensure that such references are in accordance with **the state of knowledge at the time of production of the book.**

Nevertheless, this does not involve, imply, or express any guarantee or responsibility on the part of the publishers in respect to any dosage instructions and forms of applications stated in the book. **Every user is requested to examine carefully** the manufacturers' leaflets accompanying each drug and to check, if necessary in consultation with a physician or specialist, whether the dosage schedules mentioned therein or the contraindications stated by the manufacturers differ from the statements made in the present book. Such examination is particularly important with drugs that are either rarely used or have been newly released on the market. Every dosage schedule or every form of application used is entirely at the user's own risk and responsibility. The authors and publishers request every user to report to the publishers any discrepancies or inaccuracies noticed. If errors in this work are found after publication, errata will be posted at www.thieme.com on the product description page.

Some of the product names, patents, and registered designs referred to in this book are in fact registered trademarks or proprietary names even though specific reference to this fact is not always made in the text. Therefore, the appearance of a name without designation as proprietary is not to be construed as a representation by the publisher that it is in the public domain.

Thieme Medical Publishers, Inc.
333 Seventh Avenue, 18th Floor
New York, NY 10001, USA
www.thieme.com
+1 800 782 3488, customerservice@thieme.com

Cover design: Thieme Publishing Group
Typesetting by Thomson Digital, India

Printed in Germany by Beltz Grafische Betriebe, Bad Langensalza

ISBN 978-1-62623-925-8

87654

Also available as an e-book:
eISBN 978-1-62623-926-5

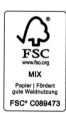

Contents

Contents

Preface

Dear Reader,

Thank you so much for purchasing this book. We are confident that this book will help you to achieve your goal of acing the exam and also benefit you throughout your entire medical career, from residency through clinical practice.

Before starting residency in the US, you need to complete the following steps (www.usmle.org):

"He who studies medicine without books sails an uncharted sea, but he who studies medicine without patients does not go to sea at all."

William Osler

USMLE Step 1	Testing centers worldwide
USMLE Step 2 CK	
USMLE Step 2 CS	There are only six testing centers in the US.
	Students need to get the result of Step 2 CS before applying for residency programs. Please look at their results schedule.
Apply to residency programs through ERAS • Interview season is late October to early February	Would recommend reading the book called "How doctors think" by J. Groopman; it serves as a great conversation subject in interviews and also helps you answer a common interview question about medical errors that you might have made or witnessed.
Step 3	Step 3 can be taken before or during residency. Most US graduates take it during residency, but if you are an international graduate, would strongly recommend getting step 3 results prior to starting residency, so that you can apply for an H1B visa, rather than J-1 visa, which does make a significant difference.

How to use our book?

The best way to use the book is to read a chapter two to three times, internalize key elements, and only then to try using Qbanks (USMLE World, Kaplan, NBME). In this book you will find multiple practice questions. Also, each algorithm and table in this book is a great tool to quiz yourself on the next step in management, the likely diagnosis, etc. Additionally, we have built the following for you.

"PRADIS"–a community of USMLE students to practice questions and discuss in forums

The authors have created a free app (www.pradis.us, "pradis" app), where you can practice with questions and discuss in reddit-like forums. The unique feature of this app is that the questions/discussion forums are indexed as per the pages of our book. E.g., read the first page, then practice questions or discuss topics related to the first page. You can also give back to the community by creating questions or flashcards. Note that these questions will be officially vetted, and higher quality questions are upvoted.

Manoj Gurung, MD
Yayra Musabek, MD

Dedication and Acknowledgments

Yayra would like to thank her parents, Guzal and Bakhram Musabekov, and her brother, Sarvar Musabekov, for their love, unwavering support, and wisdom.

Manoj would like to thank his parents, Dev Singh Gurung and Chenga Bhuti Gurung, for always being inspirational, nurturing, and caring; brother Santosh for being the elder in every way possible, and brother Saroj, for his constant encouragement.

And, to our children, Akbar and Maya, from newborns to grown up children who give us unlimited joy; who gave us the foresight required for the fortitude to finish this book; a daily reminder that every redwood tree started with a seed, every book started with the first page.

During our residency we were very fortunate to meet many amazing mentors and truly inspiring people. We especially would like to thank:

- Dr. Paul Bernstein for teaching us "how to learn".
- Dr. Richard Sterns for teaching us the magic of clinical thinking and for the most interesting professor rounds.
- Dr. Christopher Henderson for being the greatest teacher and friend.
- Dr. Mysore Seetharaman for showing us the beauty of algorithmic thinking in medicine.

We would also like to thank our acquisitions editor at Thieme, Delia DeTurris for believing in us and giving us the opportunity to publish this book; Prakash Naorem and his team in India for working diligently to complete this book in time, and lastly to everyone at Thieme publication for welcoming us into the family.

Manoj Gurung, MD
Yayra Musabek, MD

A Note on Board Questions

- A classic board question includes patient history, physical examination findings, and diagnostic or laboratory test results.
- The first cognitive step in most of the clinical questions is to identify the diagnosis. Be careful as some questions might have a "red herring", a detail that tries to derail us. For example, let's say a long vignette that sounds like a case of **Hodgkin lymphoma**, but the patient also has "**bilateral hilar lymphadenopathy.**" Then immediately you are taken off guard. You remember that sarcoidosis classically has "bilateral hilar lymphadenopathy" and on top of that it can have some common features of **Hodgkin lymphoma**!

So, what do we do?

- Find more than one supporting clue for your diagnosis. Relying on a single bit of information to make the diagnosis will often make you vulnerable to the "**red herring**", the detail that was supposed to distract you.

Another example: A vignette that looks like *N. meningitides* (petechial purpurae, neutrophilic predominance in spinal fluid), but there is an additional information that "the patient had just gone on a camping trip", which would make us think otherwise of *Lyme meningitis*. This isn't just an exam question, the presence of confounders is common in our daily lives.

"As any doctor can tell you, the most crucial step toward healing is having the right diagnosis. If the disease is precisely identified, a good resolution is far more likely. Conversely, a bad diagnosis usually means a bad outcome, no matter how skilled the physician."

Andrew Weil (American scientist)

- Some individual features of the diseases are so specific (only found in that disease) that you wouldn't have to think otherwise:
  - ➤ Positive anti-GBM antibody has to be Goodpasture syndrome, nothing else.
  - ➤ Positive anti-dsDNA is specific for SLE. Remember, ANA is a frequent "red-herring".

Clinical Case Scenarios

A 78-year-old immigrant from Haiti comes to the office complaining of myriad symptoms. He often has headaches and feels dizzy. He also has some recent onset visual problems. For the last several days, he has been feeling weak and numb in his feet. He lives with his son and isn't happy with the way his son treats him; however, he denies physical abuse. His past medical history is unremarkable. His vital signs are stable. Physical examination reveals multiple bruises on his body and sensory deficits in his feet, and bilateral ankle-reflex is absent. He has generalized lymphadenopathy and hepatosplenomegaly. Fundoscopy shows dilated, segmented, and tortuous retinal veins.
His lab report:

- WBC: 9,300 mm^3
- Hemoglobin: 8.9 g/dL
- Platelets: 90,000/mm^3
- Sodium: 142 mEq/L
- Potassium: 3.8 mEq/L
- Blood urea nitrogen: 22 mg/dL
- Creatinine: 0.9 mg/dL
- Glucose: 120 mg/dL

Serum electrophoresis and immunofixation reveal an IgM spike and very high levels of IgM. Which of the following is the most likely diagnosis?

(A) Multiple myeloma
(B) Chronic myeloid leukemia
(C) Hodgkin's disease

(D) Elderly abuse

(E) Heavy chain disease

(F) Chronic lymphocytic leukemia

(G) Mixed cryoglobulinemia

(H) Waldenstrom's macroglobulinemia

(I) Non-Hodgkin lymphoma

To tackle a lengthy question like this, a good strategy is to see the last part of the question and the answer choices. The last line reads "serum electrophoresis reveals IgM spike and high IgM levels." This is pathognomonic of Waldenstrom's macroglobulinemia. After this revelation, a seemingly complicated clinical case scenario (CCS) falls becomes clear. The whole scenario is of hyperviscosity syndrome.

Red herrings in this question are:

- Immigrant from Haiti—could lead you to think about a diagnosis like tuberculosis.
- He complains that his son isn't treating him well and he has multiple bruises—would lead you to think about elderly abuse. Note senile purpura is fairly common.
- Ankle-reflexes are absent bilaterally—elderly patients may have absent ankle or knee reflex.
- Positive ANA—would lead you to think in the lines of autoimmune disorder like SLE, but elderly patients can have positive ANA without any underlying disease.

A note on next step in management (NSIM)/next step in diagnosis (NSIDx)

Next Step In Management (NSIM), or "what you are supposed to do next" is a commonly asked question format: It can be either a treatment or a test. Next step in diagnosis (NSIDx) is test only. As these formats are so often asked, it is economical to abbreviate them in this book.

To answer these questions, know the following principles:

- Note that noninvasive tests or treatments are usually NSIDx/NSIM, whereas the invasive tests or treatments are usually the best SIDx/best SIM.

Example: In patients more than 50 years of age with iron deficiency anemia, what is the NSIM and the best SIM?

NSIM is a fecal occult blood test. The best SIM would be colonoscopy.

- Know the ABC's (or CAB) of emergency management; it's always the best **NSIM**.

Example:

A long CCS that goes like this: A 25-year-old female with ....

(!Remember the approach to a long CCS - look at the last line and the answer choices).

- If you see "secure 2 peripheral IV lines" or "give IV normal saline" in the answer choices, then even if the CCS might be of 1000 different conditions, **immediately** look at the blood pressure (BP) and heart rate in the question. If BP is low and the heart rate is high, choose either of the above options; you can't go wrong!

About the Authors

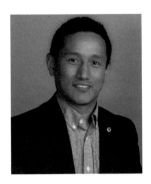

Manoj Gurung, MD
@:drmanojgrg

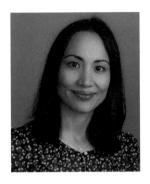

Yayra Musabek, MD
@:YayraMusabek

The authors were born, raised, and started their medical career in different parts of the world. Yayra graduated from the Tashkent Medical Academy in Uzbekistan; Manoj is from Nepal, and graduated from Tianjin Medical University in China. They met during their postgraduate training in Rochester General Hospital in Rochester, NY. Currently, they work as academic hospitalists at Kent hospital, Warwick, Rhode Island, and also serve as assistant professors at Warren Alpert Medical School of Brown University, Rhode Island. With their shared interest in teaching and passion for medicine, they decided to embark on an arduous but rewarding journey of writing what they hope is an ideal book for you.

1. Preventive Medicine

*"Treatment **without prevention is simply unsustainable.**"*
—Bill Gates

1.1 Types of Prevention

Primary prevention	⇒	Strategies to prevent the disease from occurring (e.g., vaccination)
Secondary prevention	⇒	Strategies for early detection of the disease (e.g., screening tests)—see the following table
Tertiary prevention	⇒	Strategies to prevent disease transmission or complications (e.g., contact isolation in hospitals). See the following table

1.2 General Screening Recommendations in Adults

Start screening at the following age	Patient group	Screen for	Testing modality	Frequency
—	• All patients who have risk factors for sexually transmitted disease (STD)[a] • All females aged < 25 years who are sexually active	Chlamydia trachomatis and gonorrhea	Nucleic acid detection method (urine or genital swabs)	Depends on presence of risk factors[a]
15	All patients	Human immunodeficiency virus (HIV)	Combination HIV-1/2 immuoassay (this detects both HIV antigen and antibody)	
20	Only in patients with risk factors for dyslipidemia (see the "Dyslipidemia" section below)	Dyslipidemia	Lipid profile	At regular intervals
21	All females	Cervical cancer	Pap smear test	See Ob/Gyn chapter for further details
35	All males	Dyslipidemia	Lipid profile	At regular intervals
45	All females	Dyslipidemia	Lipid profile	At regular intervals
	All patients	**Diabetes** • Start screening earlier if there are additional risk factors	Fasting blood glucose or HbA1C	At regular intervals
50	All females	Breast cancer[b]	Mammography	Every 1–2 years
	All patients	Colon cancer[c]	Colonoscopy (test of choice for screening)	Every 10 years
	Only in patients with family history of prostate cancer	Prostate cancer	Digital rectal examination and prostate-specific antigen (PSA)	At regular intervals
55	All patients with ≥ 30 pack-year smoking history[d]	Lung cancer	Low dose chest CT scan	Every 1 year • Stop screening at 80, or 15 years after smoking cessation
60	Female patients with risk factors for osteoporosis[e]	Osteoporosis	DEXA scan (dual-energy X-ray absorptiometry scan)	At regular intervals
65	All female patients	Osteoporosis		At regular intervals
	Male patients with significant smoking history	Abdominal aortic aneurysm	Abdominal ultrasound (!)	Once

⚠ **Caution**

(!) *Do not* choose CT scan.

[a] **Risk factors for STD:** men who have sex with men, contact with sex workers, illicit drug use, a new partner in the last 3 months, incarceration, and previous history of STD. Also, consider screening for other STDs - HIV, HBV, HCV, and syphilis.

[b] At age 40, all women can be offered screening mammography. At age 50, all women should begin screening.

[c] Patients with family history of colon cancer in any first-degree relative before age 60, or in two or more first-degree relatives at any age should begin screening at age 40, or 10 years before the youngest case in the family, whichever comes earlier. See Chapter 9, Gastroenterology, colon cancer section for further details.

[d] How to calculate pack-years? Multiply the number of packs of cigarettes smoked per day by the number of years the person has smoked. For example, smoking 1 packet per day for 30 years is equal to 1 x 30 = 30 pack-year smoking history.

[e] **Risk factors for osteoporosis:** family history, smoking, alcohol abuse, chronic steroid use, chronic anticonvulsant use, low body weight, and previous history of pathological fractures.

In a nutshell

- Patient's age is very important for screening purposes.
  - Is chlamydia screening recommended for a 27-year-old sexually active female patient with no risk factors? The answer is *no*.
  - What if the patient's age was 24? The answer is *yes*.
- Generally, preventive screening is stopped at the age of 70 to 80 years, or if life expectancy is less than 10 years.
- Do not screen a patient just because he/she requests it. Know the indications above.

Additional screening

All adults should be screened for depression, alcohol misuse, hypertension, obesity, and smoking at regular intervals.

Smoking cessation: patients who want to quit smoking, nicotine replacement therapy is recommended; use combination of nicotine patch plus gum, inhaler, or lozenges. Bupropion or varenicline (which decreases the urge to smoke) can also be considered.[1]

1.3 Preventive Management of Dyslipidemia

Start screening for dyslipidemia from 20 years of age, if patient has any of the following risk factor:
- Diabetes mellitus.
- Family history of dyslipidemia.
- Multiple risk factors for atherosclerotic cardiovascular disease (ASCVD) (e.g., smoking and hypertension).
- Family history of coronary artery disease (CAD) in a male relative < 50 years or female relative < 60 years—termed as premature CAD.
- Obese patient.

If none of the above is present, begin screening for dyslipidemia at the age of 35 years in male and 45 years in females.

When to initiate statin therapy ?

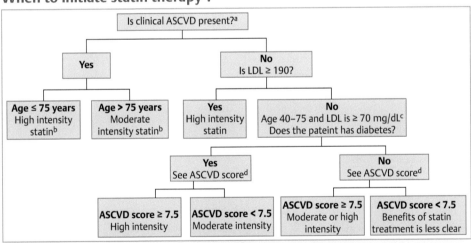

[a] If patient has any of following medical history, it is defined as Clinical ASCVD
- Cerebrovascular disease—history of ischemic stroke or transient ischemic attack.
- Peripheral vascular disease—history of claudication or vascular procedure.
- CAD—history of stable angina, acute coronary syndrome, or cardiovascular procedures.

[b] *The boards will not ask you what is high- or moderate-intensity dose for each statin (Just FYI- high intensity dose of atorvastatin is 40–80 mg).*

[c] Benefits of statin therapy may be less clear in the following patients: age < 45 or > 75, or with low-density lipoprotein (LDL) levels of <70 mg/dL.

[d] ASCVD score is a composite number calculated using following risk factors: age, gender, hypertension (controlled or uncontrolled), diabetes mellitus, race, cigarette smoking, and high-density lipoprotein. A 10-year risk score is used for dyslipidemia management. (The boards will not ask you to calculate ASCVD score, or what conditions are factored in 10-year ASCVD risk-score will be provided in the question itself).

[1] Varenicline is associated with higher rates of cardiovascular events. Avoid this in patients with cardiac conditions. Also, both varenicline and bupropion comes with black-box warning of increased risk of suicide. Consider this risk in patients with psychiatric conditions.

 MRS

The magic number is 75. Age cutoff is 75 and ASCVD score cutoff is 7.5.

Clinical Case Scenarios

Let us try some clinical case scenarios (CCS) using the above-mentioned guidelines: what is the next step in management (NSIM) regarding statin therapy in each of the following CCS?

1. A 60-year-old male has history of intermittent claudication. Total LDL is 100 mg/dL. What intensity of statin therapy is recommended?

2. What if the patient's age was 76?

3. A 65-year-old male is diagnosed with type 2 diabetes mellitus. Total LDL is 90 mg/dL. ASCVD score is 7.5.

4. What if the patient in question 3 had an ASCVD of 6.5?

5. A 39-year-old male with no history of clinical ASCVD and no history of diabetes has an LDL of 140 mg/dL.

1.4 Statin Therapy

Mechanism of action: statins (atorvastatin, simvastatin, pravastatin, etc.) are very good drugs to lower the LDL levels. They work by inhibiting HMG-CoA (hydroxymethylglutaryl-coenzyme A) reductase enzyme, the rate-limiting enzyme for biosynthesis of cholesterol. They have also been shown to stabilize atherosclerotic plaques.

Side effects

	Presentation	Management
Myopathy[b]	Generalized muscle pain ± increase in serum creatine kinase level	Discontinue statin and check thyroid-stimulating hormone (TSH)[a]
Hepatotoxicity[b]	↑ ALT/AST (alanine aminotransferase/aspartate aminotransferase) ± jaundice	If patient develops ALT elevation > 3 times the upper limit of normal, NSIM is to lower the statin dose or change medication

[a] There's increased incidence of myopathy with associated conditions like hypothyroidism and coadministration of fibrates.

[b] Check TSH and LFTs (liver function tests) prior to initiating statins

1.5 Adult Vaccination[2]

[2] Vaccination is one of the greatest achievements of modern medicine. All patients should receive specific vaccination in a timely fashion.

Vaccine	Indications
Influenza	All patients ≥ 6 months of age should receive yearly flu vaccine
Tetanus diphtheria (TD)	Every 10 years
Tetanus diphtheria and acellular pertussis (TDaP)	• All adults ≥ 19 years of age should receive TDaP vaccine once • TDaP must be given during each pregnancy • Health care workers and adults who have close contact with infants (<12 months of age) should receive one-time booster of TDaP regardless of the timing of the last booster • When TDaP is given, it becomes a substitute for TD

Vaccine	Indications
Human papilloma virus (9-valent)	All male patients **11–21** years of age
	All female patients **11–26** years of age
	In males who have sex with males, vaccination can be given up until 26 years of age
	Two to three doses are given
Measles, mumps, rubella (MMR)	All adults without documented vaccination or immunity; once is enough
	Booster dose is recommended in health care workers, college students and after exposure
Meningococcal	Adolescents, persons living in dormitories, HIV, and asplenia
Varicella	See pneumococcal vaccine section for further details.
Recombinant zoster for prevention of shingles[a]	Adults aged ≥ 50 (given twice)
Pneumococcal vaccine	All healthy adults aged ≥ 65. (*See pneumococcal vaccine section for further details.*)
Hepatitis A	Chronic liver disease and risk factors for STD
Hepatitis B	Chronic liver disease and risk factors for STD
	Additional indications would include health care workers, household contacts of a patient with hepatitis B, patients with end-stage renal disease, diabetics who are <60 years old, and anyone who requests this vaccination

[a] This is a new recombinant zoster vaccine. Unlike varicella vaccine, there is no need to determine the history of chicken pox, shingles, or to check antibodies.

1.5.1 Influenza Vaccine

In the United States, flu vaccine is administered annually from October to May, which is the flu season.

There are two common forms of flu vaccine—intramuscular inactivated vaccine (IIV) and live-attenuated intranasal vaccine (LAIV). There is no specific preference between the two, but know that LAIV is not recommended in the following situations:

- Age < 2 or ≥ 50 years.
- Children < 5 years of age with asthma.
- Patients with chronic lung, heart, liver, kidney, or hematologic issues.
- Patients with severe immunosuppression or pregnancy (because this is a live vaccine).

1.5.2 Influenza Vaccination in Patients with Egg Allergy

- Recombinant influenza vaccine (RIV) does not use eggs for its manufacturing process. It can be considered for egg-allergic patients ≥ 18 years of age.
- If RIV is not available or if the recipient's age is <18, most egg-allergic patients can safely receive IIV, even if egg reaction was anaphylaxis or severe, as most studies have demonstrated its safety.
- LAIV is generally not used in this setting because there is not much data available.

MRS

There is 11 in papi**ll**oma.

MRS

Oh, **M**y **G**od! It is the flu season! OMG = from **O**ctober to **M**ay, **G**ive flu vaccine.

Live Vaccines

- Adult live vaccines are herpes zoster or varicella, intranasal influenza, and MMR.
- Pediatric live vaccines are chicken pox, rotavirus, influenza-live attenuated type, MMR, *and e for epidemic typhus.*

These live vaccines are contraindicated in pregnancy and severe immunosuppression (e.g., patients with HIV and CD4 count of <200, hematologic/solid tumors, active chemotherapy, congenital immunodeficiency, and on long-term immunosuppressive therapy).

1.6 Pneumococcal Vaccination

There are two types of vaccine for reducing risk of infection with pneumococcus (*Streptococcus pneumoniae*).

PCV13 = pneumococcal conjugate vaccine—13 serotypes	PPSV23 = pneumococcal polysaccharide streptococcal vaccine—23 serotypes
Since this is a protein vaccine, it is processed by B cells and presented to T cells, thus inciting a T-cell-dependent B-cell response. This incites a longer-term immunity	This is a polysaccharide vaccine, and as polysaccharides cannot elicit a T-cell immunity, it is a T-cell independent B-cell response vaccine

- Usually, PCV13 is given before PPSV23 and a minimal interval must be maintained between the two vaccines. Both vaccines should not be given during the same visit
- All adult patients should receive only one-time dose of PCV13, regardless of their risk for pneumococcal infection

Note: The following recommendation guidelines is as per United States Advisory Committee on Immunization Practices (ACIP).

MRS

- PCV13 is given only once in a lifetime, whatever the underlying risk maybe.
- PPSV23 can be given twice or thrice in a patient's lifetime, depending on the risk factors.
- PCV13 is given before PPSV23, numerical order of 13 that comes before 23.

Risk of pneumococcal infection		Vaccination schedule
High risk	• Functional asplenia (e.g., in sickle cell disease patients) or postsplenectomy • Any immunocompromising condition (patients on chronic immunosuppressive therapy, HIV, any form of generalized malignancy, etc.) • Advanced kidney disease • Nephrotic syndrome	**First time:** PCV13 followed by PPSV23 **Second time:** revaccination with PPVS23 after 5 years **Third time:** PPSV23 at age of 65 or 5 years after the second dose, whichever is later; a minimum of 5-year interval must be maintained. For example, if patient gets 2nd dose of PPSV23 at 59, he gets the 3rd dose at 65: If 2nd dose was at 62 years, 3rd dose will be at 67. Note: If 1st round of PCV13+PPSV23 or 2nd dose of PPSV23 was at the age of 65 years or older, no further vaccination.[a]
Intermediate risk	• Presence of cochlear implant • Cerebrospinal fluid (CSF) leak	**First time:** PCV13 followed by PPSV23 **Second time:** they receive a booster dose of PPSV23 at the age of 65 or 5 years after the first dose, whichever is later; a minimum of 5-year interval must be maintained.
Low-intermediate risk	• Current cigarette smoking • Alcohol abuse • Chronic heart, lung, or liver disease • Diabetes mellitus	**First time:** PPSV23 alone **Second time:** PCV13 followed by PPSV23, at the age of 65 or 5 years after the first dose, whichever is later; a minimum of 5-year interval must be maintained.
Average risk	Healthy adults aged ≥ 65	PCV13; then PPSV23 at the next visit

[a] Whatever the underlying condition, patients aged ≥ 65 years receive this vaccine only once.

🔍 Clinical Case Scenarios

Now let us try some CCS using above-mentioned guidelines. The following patients come to your clinic for a routine visit:

6. A 65-year-old male with diabetes mellitus: he received PPSV23 vaccine 3 years ago. What is the NSIM regarding pneumococcal vaccination?

7. A 67-year-old male with nephrotic syndrome: he received PCV13 followed by PPSV23 at the age of 65. What is the NSIM regarding pneumococcal vaccination?

8. A 60-year-old female with diabetes mellitus: she received pneumococcal vaccine at the age of 55. What is the NSIM regarding pneumococcal vaccination?

9. A 35-year-old male with cystic fibrosis is here for a routine visit in the month of July: he received PPSV23 and TDaP 2 years ago. His last TD shot was 13 years ago. What vaccines should the patient receive during this visit?

10. A 35-year-old male with nephrotic syndrome: he received PPSV23 10 years ago. What is the NSIM regarding pneumococcal vaccination?

11. A 35-year-old male with diabetes mellitus is here for a routine visit in the month of November for the first time. He has not had vaccination as an adult. What vaccination is recommended during this visit?

12. A 47-year-old female has a history of hypertension, hypercholesterolemia, and myocardial infarction: her last checkup was 7 years ago and all her vaccinations are up-to-date. She asks about pneumococcal vaccine as she has not received one yet. What is the NSIM?

13. A perfectly healthy 62-year-old female is here for a routine visit in the month of December. Her last visit to a doctor was 5 years ago and her last DT shot was 10 years ago. What vaccines should she receive during this visit?

1.7 Asplenia

Patients with surgical splenectomy or functional asplenia (in sickle cell disease/hemoglobinopathies) should receive the following vaccinations against encapsulated organisms:

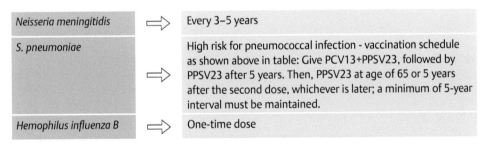

Neisseria meningitidis	⇒	Every 3–5 years
S. pneumoniae	⇒	High risk for pneumococcal infection - vaccination schedule as shown above in table: Give PCV13+PPSV23, followed by PPSV23 after 5 years. Then, PPSV23 at age of 65 or 5 years after the second dose, whichever is later; a minimum of 5-year interval must be maintained.
Hemophilus influenza B	⇒	One-time dose

In case of elective splenectomy, the above-mentioned vaccines should be given 2 weeks prior to the surgery. In emergent splenectomy cases, wait at least 2 weeks after the surgery.

1.8 Rabies

Background:

It is a preventable, deadly, neurodestructive viral infection acquired from a bite of an infected rabid animal.

Presentation:

Patient may present with fever and nonspecific symptoms that rapidly progress to severe neurologic symptoms, such as paresis, spasms of swallowing muscles precipitated by the sight or sound of water, and encephalitis. Severe convulsions and delirium ensue eventually leading to coma and death. The disease is almost universally fatal and most patients die within 1 to 2 weeks.[3]

[3] *As the incubation period can be as long as 3 months, board question might not give you a history of exposure or animal bite. In fact, children and/or mentally disabled or intoxicated people might not be able to provide you that history.*
Sometimes, board question might hint on it saying, "patient loves exploring caves (exposure to bats)."

Post-exposure prophylaxis for rabies prevention. When is it indicated? Is it active immunization (rabies vaccine), passive immunization (rabies immunoglobulin), or both?

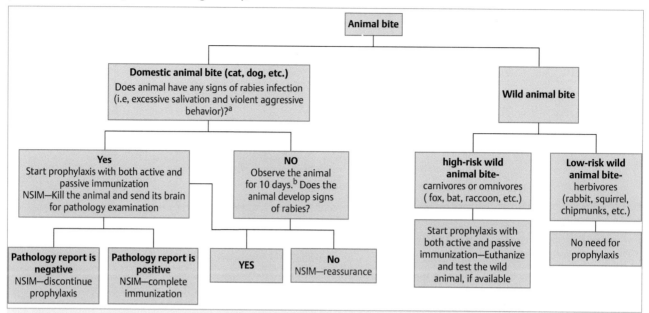

[a]If domestic animal is unavailable (e.g., the animal is nowhere to be found), start and complete prophylaxis.

[b]If the bite is in the face or the neck region, or if it is an extremely bad bite (particularly if it is unprovoked), consider giving both active and passive immunization immediately. Given the proximity of the injury site to the central nervous system, there is higher risk of early-onset rabies.

Clinical Case Scenarios

14   A wild bat is found in the same room with an unattended child or sleeping adult. There is no evidence of bite on physical examination. What is the NSIM regarding rabies prophylaxis?

Tetanus prevention with wounds

History of tetanus immunization	Clean, minor wounds	All other wounds[b]
Never vaccinated, unknown vaccination status, or <3 doses of vaccine in the past	TDaP[a]	TDaP[a] + TIG[c]
≥3 doses of vaccine	TD[d], only if last dose was ≥ 10 years ago	TD[d], only if last dose was ≥ 5 years ago

[a]Remember that all significant bite injuries (from human, dog, cat, raccoon, etc.) should get prophylaxis for *Pasteurella multocida*. Drug of choice is amoxicillin + clavulanate. It also covers anaerobes in oral cavity.

[a]Loss of mark—do not choose TD. (Technically, TD can be given; however, if patient has never been vaccinated, TDaP is preferable.)

[b]High risk for tetanus are wounds contaminated with dirt, soil or saliva (animal/human bite[a]), deep wounds, avulsions, burns, frostbite and crush injury.

[c]TIG—tetanus immunoglobulin (passive immunization).

[d]TD is recommended over tetanus toxoid alone; unless patient has severe allergic reaction diphtheria component.

15. A 24-year-old male presents with a human bite. His vaccination history is unknown. What is the NSIM regarding tetanus prevention?

16. A 24-year-old male presents with a clean wound. He had TD 7 years ago. What is the NSIM, regarding tetanus prevention?

17. What if patient in question 2 had a deep puncture wound?

1.9 Travel Medicine

- Most travelers should be up-to-date on routine vaccinations.
- All travelers to the developed world (e.g., North America and European countries) usually require no specific travel vaccination.

1.9.1 Prophylaxis for Hepatitis A

- **All travelers to the developing world should get hepatitis A vaccine.**
- Patients who are older than 40 years of age, are immunocompromised, or have chronic liver disease **and** who are traveling to hepatitis A endemic area **within 2 weeks** should be given both active and passive immunization (hepatitis A vaccine + immunoglobulin)[6]. Infants < 6 months of age should only receive Hep A immunoglobulin.

1.9.2 Malaria Prophylaxis

- Malaria is mostly endemic in hot, humid equatorial regions (see map area between the dotted lines).
- Let us look at three areas on the world map: the southern regions of Asian continent, sub-Saharan African continent, and the upper region of South America. Malaria in these areas have high incidence of chloroquine resistance, and hence mefloquine (DOC), doxycycline, or atovaquone-proguanil (MAD) are used for malaria prophylaxis.
- When traveling to "other" hot and humid regions where malaria is endemic, chloroquine is used for chemoprophylaxis.

 MRS

We become **MAD** when malaria is resistant to chloroquine.

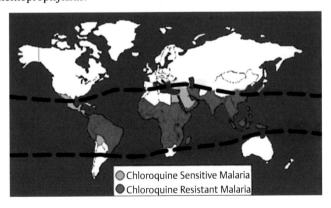

Chloroquine Sensitive Malaria
Chloroquine Resistant Malaria

Contraindications:

- Mefloquine is contraindicated in patients with cardiac conduction abnormalities and active depression.
- In pregnant patients, primaquine, atovaquone-proguanil, and doxycycline are contraindicated. Use chloroquine or mefloquine.

Note: *Traveling to only certain parts Mexico might require malaria prophylaxis, but popular tourist destinations in Mexico do not.*

1.9.3 Others

- **Yellow fever vaccination:** tourists traveling to most regions of South America and Central Africa are recommended to get this vaccination.
- **N. meningitidis vaccination:** tourists traveling for pilgrimage to Mecca in Saudi Arabia are legally mandated to have this vaccine. It is also indicated when traveling to sub-Saharan Africa.

What about prophylaxis against other diseases (e.g., typhoid, cholera)? It all depends on where our patient is going, what diseases are endemic in that area, and what their travel schedule and purposes are. Such information should be researched properly before traveling. Fortunately, these esoteric issues will not be asked on the boards.

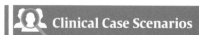 **Clinical Case Scenarios**

18. A 25-year-old female pregnant patient plans to travel to Nepal after 1 month, which patient reports cannot be deferred. She is going to a specific region of Nepal in the lower plains where malaria is endemic. What traveler's prophylaxis should she receive?

Answers

1. High-intensity statin therapy.
2. Moderate-intensity therapy.
3. High-intensity statin therapy.
4. Moderate-intensity statin therapy.
5. Benefits of statin may be less clear.
6. After 2 years, he gets revaccination with PCV13 followed by PPSV23.
7. Revaccination is not recommended for those who received their first-round of vaccination at or after the age of 65.
8. Pneumococcal vaccination to be given at the age of 65.
9. No vaccine is required during this visit. TDaP is a substitute for TD: he will need a TD shot 10 years after TDaP was given. Flu vaccine is usually given from October through May. Regarding pneumococcal vaccine, he will need PCV13 followed by PPSV23 at the age of 65.
10. He should receive PCV13 during this visit and a follow-up visit should be scheduled to administer PPSV23.
11. PPSV23, TDaP, and flu shot.
12. No vaccination is needed during this visit. Remember the difference between diabetes and other chronic diseases such as hypertension; patients with diabetes mellitus have higher risk of severe infections.
13. She gets TD booster dose, flu shot, and herpes zoster vaccine.
14. Start prophylaxis immediately and test the bat if available. Note, recent evidence suggests that transmission of rabies can occur from seemingly unimportant or unrecognized bite from bats.
15. TDaP and TIG.
16. Reassurance.
17. Administer TD.
18. It is a MAD chloroquine-resistant area; mefloquine is given. Also, consider active immunization against hepatitis A.

2. Endocrinology

*"It is not stress that kills **Addison, it is the absence of reaction to it.**"*

2.1 Disorders of the Anterior Pituitary Gland (Adenohypophysis)

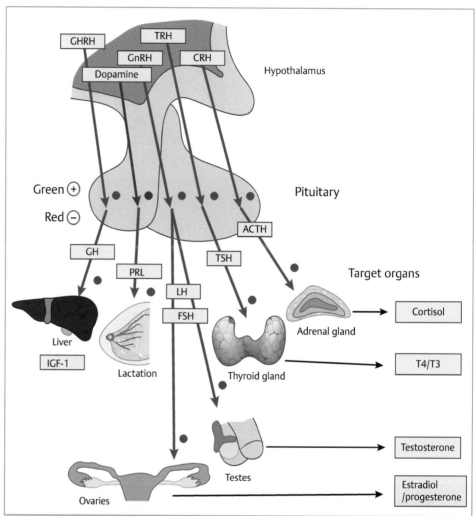

Abbreviations: GHRH, growth hormone releasing hormone; GH, growth hormone; IGF-1, insulin-like growth factor-1; Prl, prolactin; ACTH, adrenocorticotropic hormone; FSH, follicle-stimulating hormone; GH, growth hormone; GnRH, gonadotropin-releasing hormone; LH, luteinizing hormone; TSH, thyroid-stimulating hormone.

Hormone secreted by anterior pituitary gland	Pituitary adenoma producing the hormone in excess is called the following	Presentation
Prolactin	Lactotroph adenoma	Galactorrhea/amenorrhea syndrome
Growth hormone	Somatotroph adenoma	Acromegaly/gigantism
Adrenocorticotrophic hormone	Corticotroph adenoma	Cushing's disease
Thyroid-stimulating hormone	Thyrotroph adenoma	Secondary hyperthyroidism

2.1.1 Common Features of All Pituitary Adenomas

- As pituitary gland is near to the optic chiasm, pituitary adenomas cause compressive visual field defects, which primarily involve the temporal fields causing **bitemporal hemianopsia[1]**
- Large adenoma can compress surrounding pituitary tissue, causing pressure atrophy and **hypopituitarism.** This leads to sequential loss of anterior pituitary hormones. **G**rowth

[1] Think of a person always hitting the car on the side, but not on the front or the back of the car.

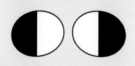

 MRS

GTA, my favorite video-game (**G**rand **T**heft **A**uto)

hormone (GH) and **g**onadotrophin-releasing hormones (GnRHs) are affected earlier in the disease course, followed by thyroid-stimulating hormone (**T**SH) and adrenocorticotropic hormone (**ACT**H).

- Children commonly present with stunted growth due to early development of GH deficiency.
- In adults, deficiency of GnRHs (luteinizing hormone [LH] and follicle-stimulating hormone [FSH] deficiency) is more problematic. Men commonly present with impotence and women with amenorrhea.
- An adenoma can be functioning (secreting a hormone in excess, as above) or nonfunctioning.
- A large functioning pituitary adenoma can present with signs of excess of one of the pituitary hormones and deficiency of other pituitary hormones. For example, a large somatotroph adenoma can present with acromegaly and central hypothyroidism/ hypocortisolemia.

2.1.2 Prolactinoma (Lactotroph Adenoma)

Background: Benign tumor that autonomously secretes prolactin hormone. It is the most common tumor of the pituitary gland.

Pathophysiology/presentation: Excessive secretion of prolactin stimulates mammary glands and also decreases GnRH secretion, causing hypogonadism (decreased LH/FSH production) and the following clinical effects

Females	• Galactorrhea
	• Development of low estrogen/progesterone state and its complications, such as osteoporosis, oligomenorrhea/amenorrhea, etc.
Males	• Loss of libido and impotence
	• Gynecomastia +/– galactorrhea

Presentation scenarios

- CCS: 40-year-old female presents with milky breast discharge and oligomenorrhea.
- CCS: 55-year-old male presents with decreased libido and impotence. Physical exam reveals visual defects primarily involving bitemporal visual fields.

Work-up: First SIM is to check serum prolactin level and rule out the following conditions that can increase prolactin secretion.

Pregnancy	Order qualitative beta-human chorionic gonadotropin test
Hypothyroidism	Check TSH level
Medication side effect	Dopamine directly inhibits prolactin secretion. So, medication that either block dopamine receptors (e.g., metoclopramide, typical antipsychotics) or deplete dopamine (α-methyldopa) can increase prolactin secretion

If the above conditions are ruled out and serum prolactin level is high, NSIDx is MRI of the pituitary gland.[2]

Treatment

Treatment is indicated in any degree of hypogonadism (e.g., amenorrhea) or in patients with bothersome galactorrhea.[3]

- Treatment of choice is pharmacologic. Use cabergoline, which has fewer side effects than bromocriptine. (Dopamine agonist decrease prolactin hormone secretion and shrink tumor size.)
- Surgical treatment (removal of adenoma) is done when patients fail to respond to medical management. Note that even in patients with significant neurologic symptoms, medical treatment should be tried first.
- Radiotherapy is considered when medical and surgical treatments fail.

[2] If a mass is seen in the pituitary area, also evaluate for hypersecretion of other pituitary hormones.

[3] In postmenopausal women with no visual defects, regular monitoring with MRI and prolactin levels may be done.

> ### 👥 Clinical Case Scenarios
>
> A 35-year-old male presents with gynecomastia and decreased libido. He also gives hx of longstanding issues with constipation and cold intolerance. Exam reveals mild decrease in bitemporal visual acuity. He is found to have low TSH and high serum prolactin level. MRI shows pituitary enlargement.
>
> 1. What is the likely dx?
>
> 2. What will be the dx if the patient had elevated TSH instead, along with high serum prolactin level? (Low-yield question; a little bit harder to answer).

2.1.3 Acromegaly and Gigantism

Etiology: Excess GH (Growth Hormone) secretion occurs most commonly from a tumor in the pituitary gland. Other rare causes are ectopic GH or GH-releasing hormone secretion from cancers.

Presentation

When excess GH secretion occurs in:	It results in:
Children	**Gigantism:** occurs when growth plates have not fused
Adults	**Acromegaly:** occurs when the growth plates have already fused. • Presents with bony and soft tissue overgrowth—enlargement of hands and feet, coarsening of facial features, thickening of skin folds, and enlargement of mandible (protruded jaws) • Most of the internal organs are also enlarged • Other associated findings are hypertension (HTN), impaired glucose tolerance, diabetes mellitus, entrapment neuropathy (e.g., carpal tunnel syndrome), and osteoarthritis • <u>Most common cause of death</u> is cardiovascular disease

Workup

*   First SIDx: measure insulin-like growth factor-1 (IGF-1) level aka somatomedin. Somatomedin (IGF-1) is a substance secreted by liver in response to GH. This is a great surrogate marker for GH level.
*   If IGF-1 level is elevated, NSIDx is glucose suppression test. GH levels are measured before and after patient ingests 100 g of glucose. Normally, glucose load should suppress GH secretion. Nonsuppressible GH level confirms diagnosis of autonomous GH secretion.
*   NSIDx is brain MRI to locate the tumor.

Treatment

*   Treatment of choice is surgical (transsphenoidal resection of pituitary adenoma).
*   Medical treatment is indicated in patients who are at high risk for surgery or when surgical therapy fails. Use somatostatin analogues (octreotide or lanreotide) +/– cabergoline, a dopamine agonist (both inhibit GH release). If still not controlled, use pegvisomant—a somatomedin antagonist that blocks somatomedin (GH) receptors.
*   Radiotherapy is considered when medical and surgical treatments fail.

In a nutshell

Management steps for various pituitary adenomas

Pituitary adenoma	Tests to be performed in the following order	Treatment (given in order of preference)
Prolactinoma	Thyroid-stimulating hormone, pregnancy test, and serum prolactin level[1] → MRI brain	Medical therapy → surgery → radiotherapy
Acromegaly	Insulin–like growth factor-1 levels[1] → oral glucose load test → MRI brain	Surgery → medical therapy → radiotherapy

In all endocrinology cases, when excess hormone secretion is suspected, first step in management is to check the hormone level. Imaging studies are done only after laboratory confirmation of high hormone levels.

Cushing's disease will be discussed in adrenal section of this chapter.

2.1.4 Hypopituitarism

Pathophysiology: Various pathologic processes can involve the pituitary gland and cause hypopituitarism—autoimmune, infectious, trauma, tumor compression, metastasis, infiltrative (sarcoidosis and hemochromatosis), postsurgical removal of pituitary adenoma, etc. Additional causative scenarios include the following.

Pituitary gland can be affected by	Which may occur in the following situations
Ischemic necrosis	Postpartum pituitary necrosis aka Sheehan's syndrome: CCS - patient with hx of severe postpartum bleeding now presents with inability to lactate
Inflammation	Postpartum pituitary hypophysitis (autoimmune destruction of pituitary gland)
Pressure atrophy	Craniopharyngioma[4] or pituitary macroadenoma: patients usually have bitemporal visual field defects

[4]**Craniopharyngioma**
- It is a benign tumor, derived from embryonic tissue (Rathke's pouch), which occurs most commonly in children but can present in any age group (even in people in 50–60s).
- It can present similarly to a nonfunctioning pituitary adenoma with features of pressure atrophy and visual deficits.
- Central nervous system imaging may reveal calcified mass around pituitary fossa or just above it.
- Treatment is surgical removal.

Hormone involved	Clinical features of deficiency	NSIDx (Next step in dx)
LH & FSH	• Females: decreased libido, oligomenorrhea/amenorrhea and anovulation (infertility) • Males: impotence, decreased libido, loss of hair, etc.	Serum LH & FSH

GH	• Children: delayed height development
	• Adults: nonspecific symptoms, such as fatigue and reduced muscle mass
		NSIDx is IGF-1 level
		• If low, dx is made.
		• If equivocal, NSIDx is to do provocative testing- measure serum growth hormone after administration of any of the following-
		  - Arginine+growth hormone releasing hormone (GHRH), or
		  - Arginine+L-DOPA, or
		  - glucagon injection, or
		  - macimorelin, a ghrelin agonist[a]

TSH	Features of hypothyroidism	TSH
ACTH	Fatigue, decreased appetite, weight loss, etc.	Serum cortisol, ACTH, and cosyntropin[b] stimulation test

[a] Insulin-induced hypoglycemia was used as a provocative method in the past, but it can be a very uncomfortable experience for the patient, so it is no longer used.

[b] Cosyntropin is a recombinant ACTH.

Abbreviations: ACTH, adrenocorticotropic hormone; FSH, follicle-stimulating hormone; GH, growth hormone; GnRH, gonadotropin-releasing hormone; IGF-1, insulin–like growth factor-1; LH, luteinizing hormone; TSH, thyroid-stimulating hormone.

Treatment

Hormone replacement. Replace cortisol before replacing thyroid hormone. If thyroid hormone is replaced before cortisol, this will increase the requirements for cortisone and precipitate a hypoadrenal crisis.

2.1.5 Pituitary Apoplexy

Background: Patients with large pituitary adenoma can develop pituitary apoplexy, an acute clinical syndrome caused by either hemorrhage and/or infarction of the pituitary gland.

Presentation: Hemorrhagic form usually presents with sudden severe headache ("thunderclap" headache) +/− signs of meningism. Look for rapidly worsening visual deficits (due to pressure on optic chiasm).

This may be followed by symptoms due to essential hormone deficiency. Predominant feature is hypotension due to acute adrenal insufficiency.

Management: It is a medical emergency. NSIM is IV fluids and IV hydrocortisone.

2.1.6 Posterior Pituitary Lobe (aka Neurohypophysis)

- Posterior pituitary secretes antidiuretic hormone (ADH aka **vasopressin**) and oxytocin.[5]
- ADH promotes reabsorption of free water from the kidneys and maintains serum sodium concentration and plasma osmolarity.
- Increased ADH secretion leads to increased total body water resulting in decreased serum Na+ concentration.[6]

[5] Oxytocin hormone is discussed further in Obstetrics chapter. ADH will be discussed in this chapter.

[6] $SerumNa^+ = \dfrac{Total\ body\ Na^+}{Total\ body\ water}$

2.2 Disorders of Sodium Hemostasis and Antidiuretic Hormone of Posterior Pituitary Gland

2.2.1 Diabetes Insipidus

Pathophysiology: Diabetes insipidus (DI) is either due to deficiency of ADH or resistance to ADH effect. This results in excretion of excessive amount of diluted urine by kidneys, resulting in loss of free water. The resulting polyuria is usually accompanied with compensatory polydipsia.

[7] Similar in etiology to hypopituitarism above

Central DI is due to absolute ADH deficiency	Various pathologic processes that can affect the posterior pituitary and cause central DI are: autoimmune, infectious, trauma, tumor compression, metastasis, infiltrative (sarcoidosis and hemochromatosis), postsurgical removal of pituitary adenoma, etc.[7]
Nephrogenic DI is due to kidneys' resistance to ADH	The causes of nephrogenic DI can be many: medications (e.g. lithium, amphotericin B), sarcoidosis, amyloidosis, polycystic kidney disease, hypercalcemia, hypokalemia, etc.

[8] Clinical features of hypo/ and hypernatremia are somewhat similar: headache, lethargy, coma, and eventually seizures can develop.

Presentation: Usually patients with polyuria have intact thirst mechanism, so if they lose 20 L of water, they will drink 20 L of water continuously replenishing the free water loss. In situations where thirst mechanism is impaired (sedatives, altered mental state) or if there is a problem with access to water (long car ride, incarceration), patients can become acutely ill, dehydrated, and may develop acute hypernatremia.[8]

Differential diagnosis of diabetes insipidus

Psychogenic polydipsia	⟹	Primary excessive intake of water (polydipsia followed by polyuria)
Drug-induced polydipsia	⟹	Any drug that blocks muscarinic receptors can lead to decreased salivation and dry mouth, making patients feel the need to drink a lot of water (e.g., tricyclic antidepressants induced polydipsia)
Uncontrolled diabetes	⟹	Glucose-induced diuresis (polyuria) and compensatory polydipsia

Work-up: NSIDx is serial measurements of urinary and plasma osmolarity (after water deprivation, followed by ADH administration) as shown below.

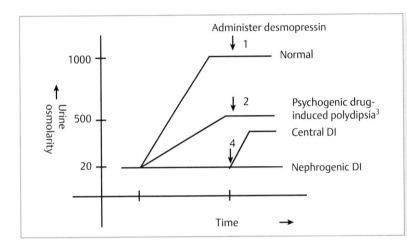

Fig. 2.3

[1,2] Exogenous ADH will not have effect, as ADH is already working at maximum after water deprivation.

[3] In psychogenic or drug-induced polydipsia the concentrating ability of kidneys gets impaired. It may take days, after normalizing water intake, for the concentrating ability of kidneys to come back to normal.

[4] To differentiate nephrogenic DI from central DI, administer desmopressin (an ADH analogue). More than 50% increase in urine osmolarity after desmopressin indicates ADH deficiency (central DI).

Table representation of the graph above

Plasma osmolarity	Urine osmolarity	What happens to urine osmolarity after giving desmopressin	Diagnosis
Low	Low	No change	Psychogenic or drug-induced polydipsia[a]
↑	Low[b]	No change	Nephrogenic DI
		↑	Central DI

[a]In psychogenic/drug-induced polydipsia, both plasma osmolarity and urine osmolarity is low.

[b]Low urine osmolarity despite high plasma osmolarity points towards DI.

Abbreviation: DI, diabetes insipidus.

Management of central/nephrogenic DI:

- Address the underlying cause.
- First step in treatment is to decrease solute intake (low salt and protein diet). This decreases polyuria. (In DI, the kidneys lose the ability to concentrate urine. With fixed urine osmolarity, urine output is primarily determined by amount of solute intake and solute content in urine.)
- Second step is to use hydrochlorothiazide (HCTZ) in patients with persistent polyuria. (Diuretics induce a state of partial volume depletion, which increases proximal sodium and water absorption, leading to less delivery of water to distal ADH-sensitive areas.)
- Desmopressin is used for central DI, if decreased solute/protein intake and/or HCTZ treatment fails to control polyuria, or if symptoms are severe.
- Nonsteroidal anti-inflammatory drugs (NSAIDs) (e.g., indomethacin), which increase renal concentrating ability, can also be used as an adjunct.
- For lithium-induced DI, amiloride is the drug of choice.

In a nutshell

Likely cause of polyuria + polydipsia in various settings

Polyuria + polydipsia +.... ↓	Likely diagnosis (dx)
Polyphagia	Uncontrolled diabetes mellitus (glucose-induced diuresis)
Fatigue + muscle weakness	Hypokalemia-induced nephrogenic DI
Constipation+ abdominal pain	Hypercalcemia-induced nephrogenic DI
Isolated	Diabetes insipidus or psychogenic/drug-induced polydipsia

2.2.2 Hypernatremia

Etiology

- Free water loss due to diabetes insipidus.
- Hypotonic fluid loss without water replacement[9]
- Fluid loss from skin, due to burns or excessive sweating (fever, vigorous exercise, hot weather, etc.).
- Fluid loss from gastrointestinal tract, due to osmotic diarrhea (e.g., lactulose ingestion) and diarrhea in infants. (Note: In adults, diarrheal fluid is isotonic.)
- Fluid loss from kidneys, due to osmotic diuresis (e.g., diabetic ketoacidosis [DKA], hyperosmolar nonketotic coma [HONK], or drugs such as mannitol).

Management

- First step is to look for coexistent volume depletion.
- If blood pressure is low (systolic BP ≤ 90 mmHg) and/or heart rate is high (> 90–100 beats per minute), 1st SIM is IV normal saline.
- If euvolemic, use IV hypotonic fluids such as 5% dextrose solution in water or if coexistent mild volume depletion is present, use 5% dextrose half normal saline.
- The rate of correction of chronic hypernatremia should not exceed > 10 to 12 mEq/L per day, otherwise **cerebral edema** may develop. For acute hypernatremia of less than 48 hours' duration, more aggressive correction can be done (1–2 mEq/L correction per hour).

[9]Absence of water replacement typically occurs in patients with advanced age, dementia, and mental retardation, because these patients have decreased or diminished thirst response mechanism.

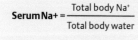

$$Serum\,Na+ = \frac{Total\,body\,Na^+}{Total\,body\,water}$$

2.2.3 Hyponatremia

First step is to find out if serum sodium is truly low: Is it true or is it pseudohyponatremia?

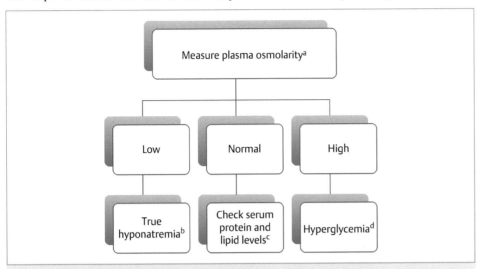

^aDo direct lab measurement of osmolarity, which might be different from calculated plasma osmolarity.[10]

^bIn true hyponatremia, measured plasma osmolarity should be low.

^cHypertriglyceridemia and hyperproteinemia can cause a decrease in measured serum Na⁺ level (pseudohyponatremia) with no change in directly measured plasma osmolarity. This is an artefactual issue.

^dHigh serum glucose level decreases measured serum Na⁺ level (pseudohyponatremia) and increases plasma osmolarity.[11]

[10]FYI: Calculated plasma osmolarity = 2 × serum Na⁺ (if BUN and glucose have normal values).

[11]In hyperglycemia, for every 100 mg/dL rise in blood glucose above 100 mg/dL, measured serum Na⁺ decreases by 1.6 mEq/L.
For example, electrolyte panel shows glucose level of 804 mg/dL and serum Na⁺ of 125 mEq/L. Corrected true serum Na⁺ = 7 × 1.6 + 125 = 136.2 mEq/L.
Explanation: 7 is because glucose is elevated 700 mg/dL above 100 mg/dL in this case.
Note: This situation is very common in DKA or HONK patients.

True Hyponatremia

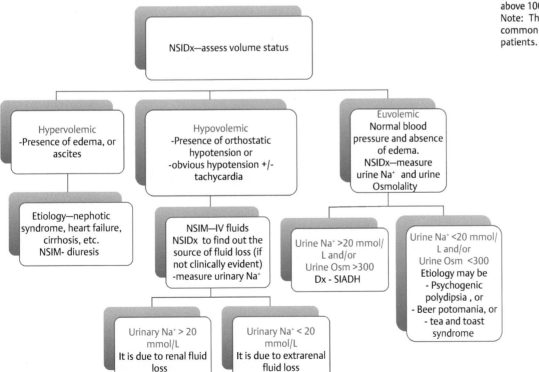

[12]In hypervolemic and hypovolemic states there is a compensatory increase in aldosterone and ADH secretion. Aldosterone reabsorbs isotonic fluid, but ADH reabsorbs hypotonic fluid (water). It is due to ADH that hyponatremia occurs.

[13]Look for clues such as dry mouth, elevated heart rate, low BP, orthostatic hypotension, Creatinine elevation, elevated bicarbonate, etc. that suggest hypovolemia

[14]Patients with hx of hyponatremia should not be on thiazide-like diuretics.

Hypervolemic Hyponatremia[12]

In these conditions, development of hyponatremia is a poor prognostic sign. Level of hyponatremia parallels the severity of the underlying condition. Treatment includes restriction of sodium/water intake and diuretics.

Hypovolemic Hyponatremia[13]

Measure urine Na^+ level to differentiate renal fluid loss from extrarenal fluid loss (if source of fluid loss is not clinically evident).

Urinary Na^+ > 20 mmol/L= renal fluid loss	• **Diuretics** (prescribed or surreptitiously ingested): thiazide-like diuretics are common perpetrators (e.g., HCTZ, metolazone)[14] • **Salt-losing nephropathies,** for example, Fanconi syndrome, or acute tubular necrosis (diuretic phase)
Urinary Na^+ < 20 mmol/L = extrarenal fluid loss	Patients develop hyponatremia due to compensatory increase in ADH/aldosterone secretion generally with increased free water intake • **GI losses** (diarrhea, vomiting, etc.) • **Skin losses** (burns, toxic epidermal necrolysis, etc.) • **Addison's disease** (loss of aldosterone and cortisol hormone)

Euvolemic hyponatremia

Urine Na^+ > 20 and/or urine osmolarity > 300	Despite hyponatremia and low serum osmolarity, kidneys are still inappropriately concentrating urine • MCC is syndrome of inappropriate secretion of ADH (SIADH) • **Hypothyroidism** (mechanism not completely understood)
Urine Na^+ < 20 and/or urine osmolarity < 300	• **Psychogenic polydipsia:** hx of drinking > 15–20 L of water per day • **Beer potomania** is due to significant intake of beer. Beer is poor in solutes and sodium, but high in calories, thus it suppresses hunger and reduces intake of other foods (and solute) • **Tea and toast diet:** some patients (particularly elderly) who have poor social support may resort to eating only simple foods like breads, crackers and water, which do not need to be cooked, but have very low salt content

Management of true hyponatremia

MRS

Remember the numbers 120 and 130 for degree of hyponatremia.

Severity (normal serum Na^+ is 135–145 mEq/L)	NSIM along with free water restriction and treatment of underlying cause ↓
130–135 mEq/L	Free water restriction only
121 to < 130 mEq/L with mild symptoms (mild confusion, fatigue, gait disturbance, nausea, vomiting, etc.)	Directed toward underlying etiology: • If hypovolemic—normal saline • In SIADH—salt tablets (1st step), +/− loop diuretics (induces ADH resistance) +/− vaptans[a] • In hypervolemic states—diuretics (such as Lasix), +/− vaptans[a]
≤ 120 mEq/L **and/or** severe symptoms (e.g., severe confusion, coma, seizures, respiratory arrest)	Hypertonic saline[b] +/− desmopressin to prevent rapid correction of sodium[c]

[a]Vasopressin receptor antagonist (tolvaptan, conivaptan, mozavaptan, etc.) can be used adjunctively in SIADH and hypervolemic states.

[b]Hypertonic saline is also indicated in acute symptomatic hyponatremia that develops within 24 hours (even if symptoms are only mild).

[c]Rate of sodium correction should not be faster than 0.5–1 mEq/L per hour. Rapid overcorrection may result in central pontine myelinolysis (osmotic demyelination), which usually presents with focal neurological deficits like the ones seen in pontine hemorrhage or infarction (severe cases might present with quadriplegic locked-in-syndrome). (See Chapter 10, Neurology for further details).

2.2.4 Syndrome of Inappropriate Secretion of ADH

Etiology: SIADH can be caused by multiple processes, such as trauma, infection, malignancy (especially in lung or brain, e.g., lung injury, head injury, pneumonia, encephalitis, small cell cancer) and medications.[MRS-1] Important association to remember is small-cell lung cancer.

Pathophysiology Excessive ADH secretion leads to excessive free water reabsorption and **hyponatremia**.

Treatment: Its treatment is directed toward underlying condition and also depends upon the severity of hyponatremia and symptoms (see table for management of true hyponatremia). Demeclocycline (ADH receptor blocker) is not commonly used nowadays because of increased risk of nephrotoxicity and high cost.

 MRS

[MRS-1] Drugs that can stimulate secretion of ADH (**Tip:** most of the drugs start with "**C**")

Antidiabetic	**C**hlorpropamide.
Antidyslipidemic	**C**lofibrate.
Anticancer	vin**C**ristine and vinblastine.
Anti-immune	**C**yclophosphamide.
Antipsychotic	**C**arbamazepine

Antidepressants SSRIs (**C**italopram, **s**ertraline, etc.), Tricyclic antidepressants

 In a nutshell

How to find out the cause of hyponatremia?

First step is to look at volume status	Urine Na+ (mmol/L)	Urine osmolarity	Dx
Hypovolemic	< 20	Elevated	Extrarenal fluid loss
	> 20		Renal fluid loss
Euvolemic	> 20	Elevated	Syndrome of inappropriate antidiuretic hormone secretion
	< 20	Low	Psychogenic polydipsia, beer potomania, or tea and toast diet

Clinical Case Scenarios

3. A 45-year-old female has serum sodium of 112 mEq/L and altered mental status. What is the NSIM?

2.3 Disorders of Calcium Hemostasis and Parathyroid Gland

2.3.1 Basics of Calcium (Ca²⁺) Metabolism

- Total serum calcium = bound calcium + free calcium.
- **Bound form:** Calcium is a positively charged ion which binds to albumin and other negatively charged compounds (e.g., citrate⁻, PO_4^-, SO_4^-).
- **Free form** is the one that is biologically active and closely regulated by parathyroid hormone (PTH).
- The two hormones that regulate calcium are PTH and Vitamin D.

PTH	Vitamin D
• Secreted by the parathyroid glands and works on kidneys and bones	Requires hydroxylation in liver and kidney to become biologically active
• Signals osteoblasts to activate osteoclasts. Osteoclasts then start dissolving bone, thereby decreasing bone density and in the process release more calcium and phosphorus into the blood	Signals the intestinal epithelial cells to increase absorption of both calcium and phosphate
• Signals the kidneys to increase reabsorption of Ca²⁺ and excretion of PO_4^-	

PTH	Vitamin D
Final effect is ↑ Ca^{2+} and decreased PO_4^{-1}	Final effect is ↑ Ca^{2+} and ↑ PO_4^{-1}

If calcium and phosphorus are in opposite directions, think PTH related and if they are both in same direction, think vitamin D related.

Patients with hypoalbuminemia (due to liver cirrhosis, protein-losing enteropathy, malnutrition, etc.) can have the following issue with calcium mechanics:
- Decreased total calcium but normal free Ca^{2+} level. These patients are asymptomatic.
Standard chem-7 or basal metabolic profile (BMP) tests measure total calcium. Hence if serum albumin is low, the calcium needs to be corrected with the help of a formula using serum albumin. We don't need to know this formula for boards.
A case of masked hypercalcemia:
I had once taken care of a patient, who didn't have a primary care doctor, who presented with fatigue. Complete metabolic profile revealed high normal calcium level and very low serum albumin. Corrected calcium value was found to be more than 14. She ended up having a diagnosis of severe acute hypercalcemia due to parathyroid adenoma. Hypoalbuminemia was probably a result of severe malnutrition due to hypercalcemia associated gastrointestinal symptoms.

2.3.2 Disorders of Calcium Metabolism

For the tables below, cover the diagnosis column (right most column) and try to explain mechanism of calcium disorder. Again, let us reiterate an important point—If calcium and phosphorus are in opposite directions, think PTH related; if they are both in same direction, think vitamin D related.

Hypercalcemia

Ca^{2+}	PO_4^-	PTH	Vitamin D	Diagnosis
↑	Low	↑ /or high N[a]	N or low[b]	NSIDx is 24-hour urinary calcium. • Elevated urinary Ca^{2+} = primary hyperparathyroidism (parathyroid adenoma or hyperplasia) • Low urinary Ca^{2+} = familial hypocalciuric hypercalcemia (discussed later in section of primary hyperparathyroidism)
↑	Low	**Low**	N or low[b]	PTH-related peptide (PTHrP) secreted from cancer cells (squamous cell cancer of lung, breast cancer, etc.). This peptide works just like PTH[c].
↑	↑	**Low**	↑	• Overproduction of calcitriol (vitamin D) from lymphomas or Granulomas (e.g., in sarcoidosis or generalized granulomatous infection) (glucocorticoids are effective in this form of hypercalcemia) • Excessive vitamin D intake
↑	N or ↑	**Low**	N	Consider causes that increase bone resorption—prolonged immobility[d], multiple myeloma, hyperthyroidism. (Look for elevated alkaline phosphatase)

[a]In hypercalcemia, PTH should be low if feedback mechanism is intact.
[b]Due to negative feedback from hypercalcemia.
[c]**Hypercalcemia** of **malignancy** can be due to PTHrP secretion (typically by squamous cell carcinoma) or due to cytokines secreted by osteoclastic metastatic cells (multiple myeloma is a classic example). Cancers at times can cause both types (e.g. breast cancers).
[d]Patients who have high bone turnover rate (e.g., Paget's disease or in children), immobilization can lead to development of significant hypercalcemia (Hypercalcemia of Immobilization).
Abbreviation: PTH, parathyroid hormone

Hypocalcemic disorders

Ca^{2+}	PO_4^-	PTH	Vitamin D	Diagnosis
Low	↑	**Low**	N	**Primary hypoparathyroidism** (Etiology: DiGeorge syndrome, thyroidectomy complication, parathyroidectomy, polyglandular autoimmune syndrome, etc.)
Low	↑	↑ [e]	Low	Chronic renal failure[a]
Low	↑	↑ [e]	N	???[b]
Low	Low	↑ [e]	Low	Vitamin D deficiency (osteomalacia in adults and rickets[c] in children)
Low	Low	↑ [e]	**N or ↑**	Vitamin D resistant rickets[d]

[a]In renal failure, there are two primary mechanisms: (1) retention of PO_4^{2-} (which chelates calcium), (2) decrease in vitamin D production.
[b]Looks like it is a PTH-related disorder with calcium and phosphorus in opposite direction. Calcium is low even though PTH is high. So, PTH must not be working at all. Dx is **pseudohypoparathyroidism,** where there is a defect in PTH receptor, so even if PTH is present, it does not exert its effect.
[c]For rickets, look for frontal bossing, bowed legs, and enlargement of costochondral junction.
[d]Primary pathology is defect in vitamin D receptors, so even though vitamin D level is normal or high there is lack of effect.
[e] ↑ = secondary hyperparathyroidism (Elevated alkaline phosphatase is present in all cases except in pseudohypoparathyroidism.)

Clinical Case Scenarios

	Ca²⁺	PO₄⁻	PTH	Vitamin D	Diagnosis
A pediatric patient presents with frontal bossing, bowed legs, and enlargement of costochondral junction.	N	Low	N/↑	**N**	Hereditary **hypophosphatemic** rickets[a]
An old patient's x-ray shows diffuse thinning of bone.	N	**N**	N	**N**	Osteoporosis

[a]Heritable disorder in which the primary problem is significant phoshaturia (phosphate wasting).

In a nutshell

Miscellaneous info on calcium-related disorders:

- Hydrochlorothiazide can cause mild serum hypercalcemia by increasing urinary calcium reabsorption.
  This hypocalciuric effect is helpful in prevention of stone formation in hypercalciuric recurrent calcium phosphate stones.

- Differences in clinical features of hyper-/hypocalcemia

Hypercalcemia	Hypocalcemia
• Decreases neuromuscular conduction and signaling pathways	• Increases neuromuscular conduction
• Constipation, fatigue, lethargy, muscle weakness, cardiac arrhythmias, etc.	• Muscle cramps, paresthesia, tetany, cardiac arrhythmias, etc.
• Blunts ADH signaling pathway which may lead to nephrogenic diabetes insipidus (polyuria, polydipsia)	

Abbreviation: PTH, parathyroid hormone.

Hypercalcemia
Clinical features

- **Gastrointestinal:** constipation, abdominal pain, pancreatitis, etc.
- **Renal:** polyuria/polydipsia.
- **Neurological symptoms** depending upon severity: difficulty concentration → fatigue, weakness → altered mental status → seizures, coma.
- **Cardiac:** arrhythmias can also occur.

Normal serum calcium is ≤ 10.2 mg/dL

Management

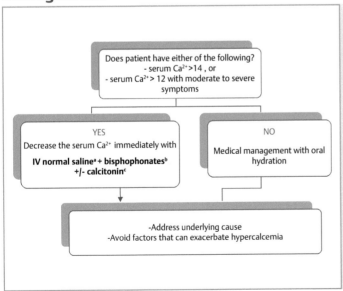

[a]Furosemide (Lasix) is not routinely indicated in management of hypercalcemia. If patients develop volume overload with IV normal saline, it can be judiciously used.

[b]**Bisphosphonates** decrease osteoclastic activity. As opposed to calcitonin, it takes at least few days for the hypocalcemic effect to kick in, but it is more sustained. It is contraindicated in severe renal failure.

Bisphosphonates are also indicated in patients with symptoms related to bone resorption, for example, patient with acute back pain due to metastatic osteolytic lesion. Denosumab is an alternative treatment of persistent hypercalcemia of malignancy refractory to bisphosphonates.

[c]IV calcitonin is mostly recommended in patients with serum Ca²⁺ > 14. It decreases calcium levels faster than bisphosphonates do, but its efficacy is reduced after 48 hours.

In severely hypercalcemic patients, hemodialysis can be done as a treatment of last resort.

[15]If PTH is low or low-normal, NSIDx- check PTHrP, vit D levels (1,25 and 25-OH forms).

[16]If 24-hour urinary calcium is low, the dx is **Familial hypocalciuric hypercalcemia:** High calcium, via calcium-sensing receptors should generally decrease PTH secretion from parathyroid glands and increase calcium excretion from kidneys.
In this rare disorder, calcium-sensing receptors in the parathyroid gland and kidneys are defective. These patients have high normal or high PTH level and low 24-hour urinary calcium excretion, despite high serum calcium. Genetic testing is confirmatory.

The MCC (most common cause) of hypercalcemia in nonhospital outpatient setting is primary hyperparathyroidism.
The MCC of hypercalcemia in hospital setting is malignancy. "

Primary Hyperparathyroidism

Etiology: MCC is parathyroid adenoma. Other causes include parathyroid hyperplasia/malignancy.

Presentation: hypercalcemia.

Workup: After detecting elevated calcium levels, NSIDx is to check serum PTH level.[15] If elevated or upper side of normal range, NSIDx is 24-hour urinary calcium measurement. If 24-hour urinary calcium is elevated the dx is primary hyperparathyroidism.[16]

Management of Primary Hyperparathyroidism

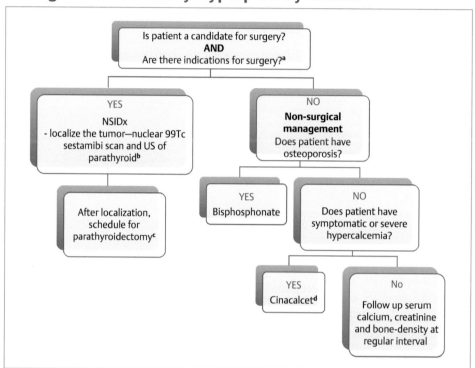

[a] Symptomatic hypercalcemia is an obvious indication. In **asy**mptomatic patients, the following are indications for surgery:
- Young patients < 50 years of age with no comorbidities, who have low risk for surgery
- Pregnant patients
- Calcium phosphate renal stones, nephrocalcinosis or 24-hour urinary calcium > 400 mg/day
- Serum calcium level of 1 mg/dL or more above the upper limit of normal
- Osteoporosis
- Reduced renal function (eGFR < 60 mL/minute)

[b]Other options are CT or MRI scan of parathyroid gland. Localization of tumor is not necessary in patients undergoing nonsurgical management.

[c]A potential complication of removal of parathyroid adenoma is **hungry bone syndrome.** (7 to 10 days after surgery with precipitous decline in PTH levels, bones can go into a rapid remineralization phase with increased uptake of calcium and phosphates, resulting in serum hypocalcemia and hypophosphatemia. This is usually self-remitting and transient.)

[d]Cinacalcet decreases PTH secretion by activating calcium-sensing receptors in parathyroid glands (it acts by "mimicking" calcium).

Hypocalcemia

Additional etiologies of hypocalcemia

Etiology	Underlying mechanism
Multiple units of blood transfusion	Citrate (a negatively charged ion), which is used as an anticoagulant in blood bags, binds with free Ca^{2+} causing hypocalcemia
Acute hypoxemia (e.g., pulmonary embolus) or panic disorder with increased respiratory rate	**Respiratory alkalosis**: in alkalosis, there is depletion of positively charged ions (e.g., H^+ ion) and abundance of negatively charged ions (e.g., HCO_3^-). Hence, Serum albumin becomes more negatively charged, and more free Ca^{2+} binds with albumin, decreasing the free calcium level
Patient is an alcoholic or is malnourished	**Hypomagnesemia** inhibits PTH secretion
Nephrotic syndrome	This is due to loss of cholecalciferol (vitamin D)-binding protein in urine

Presentation: Acute hypocalcemia leads to generalized neuromuscular and cardiac hyperexcitability.

Sensory nerve excitation	⇒	Tingling sensation in perioral area, hands, and feet
Motor nerve excitation	⇒	In milder cases, spasms are only inducible, e.g., measuring blood pressure in arm can induce carpopedal spasm and facial nerve tapping can induce facial muscle spasms In severe cases, it can progress on to generalized tetanus–like condition and seizures
Cardiac	⇒	Increased cardiac contractility and heart failure. Electrocardiography classically reveals prolonged QT interval

Management: Treatment of acute hypocalcemia is with IV calcium gluconate or calcium chloride. Maintenance is with oral calcium.

 MRS

Potassium-calcium-magnesium and QT interval always go in opposite directions. If potassium, magnesium or calcium is low, QT interval is prolonged.

2.4 Thyroid Hormone

Thyroid hormone controls the basal metabolic rate and Na^+–K^+–ATPase pump in all our cells.

In hyperthyroidism, everything is fast	In hypothyroidism, everything is slow
Weight loss despite increased appetite (due to increased basal metabolic rate)	Weight gain despite decreased appetite (due to decreased basal metabolic rate)
Heat intolerance due to increased basal metabolic rate and increased intrinsic heat production (even minimal external heat makes patients uncomfortable)	Cold intolerance
Tachyarrhythmias	Bradyarrhythmias
Diarrhea due to increased GI motility	Constipation
Increased deep tendon reflexes	Slow deep tendon reflexes, slow speech and movement
Excessive production and expression of β_1 adrenergic receptors leads to increased β_1 adrenergic activity = sweating, tachycardia, anxiety, and tremors The drug of choice to control these symptoms is β blockers	Additional features: sparse hair, croaky voice, puffy looking face, and myxedema
Note: Both hypo- and hyperthyroidism can cause proximal muscle myopathy.	

Terminology
Toxic = hyperthyroid
Goiter = enlargement of thyroid gland

2.4.1 Thyrotoxicosis and Primary Hyperthyroidism

Etiology of primary hyperthyroidism

Condition	Pathophysiology	Morphological changes in thyroid gland	Radioactive iodine uptake (RAIU)
Graves' disease (diffuse toxic goiter[a])	Autoimmune disease with production of **TSH** receptor **antibody** (**TRab**), which can continuously stimulate thyroid cells leading to gland enlargement (goiter) and increased thyroid hormone production	Diffuse goiter	Diffuse uptake Source: Three modes of image production. In: Gunderman R. Essential radiology. Clinical presentation, pathophysiology, imaging. 3rd ed. Thieme; 2014.
Toxic adenoma	Single autonomously functioning thyroid nodule[b]	Single nodule in thyroid	This scan shows a focus of increased uptake ("hot nodule") and mild suppression of remaining gland. Source: Yürekli Y, Cengiz A, Güney E. Graves disease induced by radioiodine therapy for toxic nodular goiter: a case report. Mol Imaging Radionucl Ther. 2015.
Toxic multinodular goiter[c] (Plummer's disease)	Multiple autonomously functioning nodules in thyroid[b]	Multiple nodules in thyroid	Increased focal uptake in multiple areas

[a]Features unique to Graves' disease are exophthalmia (proptosis due to retro-orbital tissue deposition) and dermopathy (pretibial myxedema).

[b]These nodules may have somatic "gain-of-function mutation" of TSH receptor, which leads to autonomous hyperactivity.

[c]Nontoxic nodular goiter can transform into toxic nodular goiter.

Clinical features

- Young patients usually present with symptoms of nervous system such as tremors, anxiety, heat intolerance, etc.
- In old patients, cardiovascular and myopathic symptoms predominate. They can present with arrhythmias or muscle weakness.[17]
- Cardiovascular effects include increased cardiac output, systolic HTN, and increased pulse pressure.
- Bone loss—thyroid hormones activate the osteoclasts, resulting in osteoporosis, hypercalcemia and secondary hypoparathyroidism.

[17]Old patients with Graves' disease typically do not have dermopathy, ophthalmopathy, or symptoms of nervous system. This is called the **"apathetic Graves."**

Sequential workup of hyperthyroidism[18]:

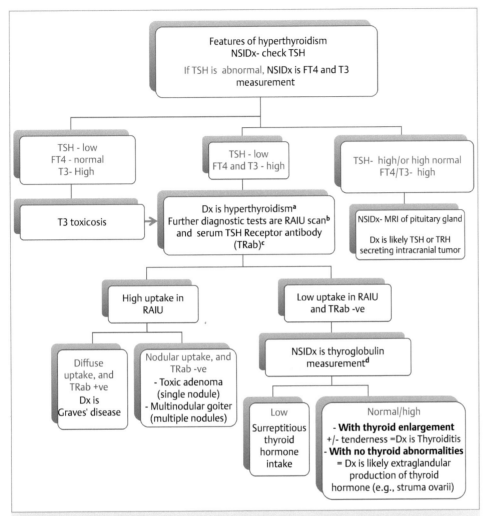

[18] The best initial and most sensitive test to assess thyroid function is TSH (thyroid stimulating hormone). If TSH is normal, then patient is euthyroid.

[a] After hyperthyroidism is confirmed, NSIM is to alleviate patient's symptoms by prescribing β **blockers** prior to scheduling any further diagnostic tests.

[b] Radioactive iodine uptake (RAIU) scan; aka radionuclide thyroid scan is contraindicated in pregnancy. In pregnant patients, perform ultrasound to assess thyroid blood flow.

[c] TSH receptor antibody (TRab) is found in Graves' disease. Various tests are available to detect TRab such as thyroid-stimulating immunoglobulin assay, thyrotropin-binding inhibiting immunoglobulin, etc.

[d] What C-peptide is to insulin, thyroglobulin is to thyroid hormone.

Abbreviations: NSIM, next step in management; NSIDx, next step in diagnosis; FT4, free thyroxine; T3, tri-iodothyronine; RAIU, radioactive iodine uptake scan, aka radionuclide thyroid scan; TRH, thyrotropin (TSH)-releasing hormone

Management of primary hyperthyroidism (Graves', toxic adenoma and toxic multinodular goiter)

- First SIM is β blockers (atenolol/metoprolol/propranolol, etc.)
- With significant symptoms, or in older patients with heart disease, NSIM is to decrease thyroid hormone production as soon as possible. Initiate antithyroid medications (known as thionamides) such as methimazole, carbimazole, or propylthiouracil. Methimazole is generally preferred over propylthiouracil because of its beneficial pharmacology (except in 1st trimester of pregnancy when propylthiouracil is preferred)
- Follow serum TSH, free T4 and T3.
- After euthyroid state is achieved, NSIM is radioiodine ablation (definitive treatment). In patients **without** significant symptoms, radioiodine treatment can be done without pretreatment with antithyroid drugs.
- Antithyroid therapy (without thyroid ablation) can be offered in patients with mild disease, small goiter, and Graves' in children and adolescents, in hopes of achieving spontaneous remission. They might not end up needing radioiodine ablation or surgery.

Radioiodine Treatment

[19]In Graves' disease, as the whole gland is hyperactive, radioactive treatment often results in hypothyroidism, because it destroys most of the thyroid cells.

- Hyperactive thyroid gland rapidly uptakes the radioactive iodine, resulting in radiation-induced death of the hyperactive thyroid cells. Antithyroid drugs need to be stopped few days before the procedure because they block the uptake of radioactive iodine thus decreasing its efficacy.
- After radioiodine treatment, follow TSH levels. If patient develops hypothyroidism (elevated TSH), then thyroid hormone should be replaced with **levothyroxine**.[19]
- Ophthalmopathy in Graves' disease gets worse after treatment with radioactive iodine. In patients with significant ophthalmopathy, treatment of ophthalmopathy with steroids or surgery/radiation might be necessary **before** radioiodine treatment.

Contraindications: pregnancy[20], severe ophthalmopathy, and children < 5 years of age.

Thyroid Surgery

[20]Pregnant patients are usually continued on antithyroid drugs. If pregnant patients cannot tolerate antithyroid medications, then only surgery is done.

Indication: Recommended in patients with severe hyperthyroidism and a large goiter, and in patients with contraindication to thionamides or radiation (children, severe ophthalmopathy, etc.).

Clinical Case Scenarios

A 65-year-old male with no significant prior medical hx presents with transient acute atrial fibrillation with rapid ventricular response. He develops congestive heart failure. Exam reveals no proptosis or edema. TSH is found to be low.

4. What is the NSIDx in regard to low TSH?

5. If FT4 and T3 comes back elevated, which medication should be started now?

6. What is the NSIDx?

7. TRab is positive and RAIU scan reveals goiter with diffuse uptake. What is the likely dx?

8. When do we schedule for definitive treatment?

9. The patient was started on methimazole, and few weeks later he develops sore throat and fever. Complete blood count shows neutropenia. What is the first SIM?

10. If the initial test had revealed low uptake in RAIU and TRab was negative, what would be your NSIDx?

11. If serum thyroglobulin was found to be low, what will be your likely dx?

Thyroid Storm

Background: It occurs in untreated hyperthyroid patients and is frequently precipitated by stressful conditions such as surgery, trauma, burns, etc.

Pathophysiology: Thyroid storm is an emergency condition in which the thyroid gland suddenly releases large amounts of thyroid hormone in a short period of time. This can be fatal if not treated.

Clinical features: Look for exaggerated symptoms of hyperthyroidism—hyperthermia, altered mental status, and cardiovascular dysfunction (e.g., hypotension, congestive heart failure).

Management

- First step: IV fluids and supportive treatment (oxygen, cooling blankets).
- Second step: Antithyroid drugs (propylthiouracil is preferred over other drugs as it also reduces T4 to T3 conversion), β blocker and steroids (e.g., hydrocortisone). All these three drugs reduce T4 to T3 conversion. β blockers also block effects of thyroid hormone.
- Third step: Iodine (inhibits thyroid hormone biosynthesis). When the thyroid gland is actively taking up the iodine, it is not making the thyroid hormone. Give iodine only after antithyroid drugs (thionamides block the iodine to become a substrate for new thyroid hormone production). Iodine also reduces T4 to T3 conversion.

 MRS

I Am Blocking Sinister Iodine that makes thyroid hormone.

2.4.2 Hypothyroidism

Etiology: MCC of hypothyroidism (with or without goiter) is Hashimoto's thyroiditis. Another common cause is iatrogenic (result of hyperthyroidism treatment such as surgery or radioiodine ablation). Goitrous hypothyroidism can also be due to amiodarone and dietary iodine deficiency.

Clinical features

Amenorrhea or hypomenorrhea.

Bradyarrhythmia.

Constipation, carpal tunnel syndrome, cold intolerance, CK increase (myopathy with normal erythrocyte sedimentation rate [ESR]).

Depression, dementia, deep croaky voice, delayed deep tendon reflexes, diffuse thinning of hair, dyslipidemia (elevated low-density lipoproteins and triglycerides).

Edema (nonpitting) = myxedema, elevated diastolic blood pressure.

MRS

ABCDE

Newborn with hypothyroidism (due to heritable biosynthetic defects) present differently[21]:
- Umbilical hernia.
- Down facies (facial features that look like Down's syndrome).
- Jaundice.

Management:
- "NSIDx is TSH. If TSH high, NSIDx is FT4 and repeating TSH again. If FT4 is low and TSH is still high, dx is confirmed.

Hypothyroidism can easily be treated with thyroxine (T4) replacement therapy, which can reverse most of the ABCDE features.

[21] All newborn should be screened for hypothyroidism. If not treated promptly, it can lead to permanent impairment of mental/ physical development. This is called cretinism.

Common Drug Interactions of Oral Levothyroxine

Decreases effect of levothyroxine	Increases effect of levothyroxine
Proestrogenic agents (e.g., estrogen, tamoxifen, raloxifene) and pregnancy can increase thyroid-binding globulin synthesis and reduce free active levothyroxine levels	Anabolic steroids (androgens) and glucocorticoids can decrease thyroid-binding globulin levels
Bile acid binders, proton pump inhibitors, and sucralfate can decrease absorption of oral thyroxine	
Cytochrome inducers (e.g., antiepileptics, rifampin) can increase metabolism of thyroid hormone	
Note: You will likely need to increase or decrease levothyroxine dosage when patients are started on the above medication	

> **Clinical Case Scenarios**

12. A 34-year-old male presents with features of ABCDE. Interestingly, thyroid function test reveals high normal TSH and elevated T4/T3. What is the likely dx?

2.4.3 Myxedema Coma

Background: It is the severest form of hypothyroidism that may occur in uncontrolled hypothyroid patients. It is precipitated by stress such as burns or trauma.

Presentation: Hypothermia, bradycardia, altered mental status, and hypotension.

Workup: NSIDx is free T4 level and TSH. Also check cortisol (before and after ACTH administration) to look for coexistent hypocortisolemia.

Management: If myxedema coma is strongly suspected, initiate empiric treatment with T4 and T3 along with empiric corticosteroids (until coexistent adrenal insufficiency has been excluded), before biochemical confirmation.

2.4.4 Thyroiditis

- Hashimoto's thyroiditis (aka chronic lymphocytic thyroiditis).
- Subacute thyroiditis.
- Subacute lymphocytic thyroiditis.
- Riedel's thyroiditis.
- Acute thyroiditis (bacterial/fungal infection) +/– abscess.

2.4.5 Hashimoto's Thyroiditis

Hashimoto's thyroiditis is the MCC of hypothyroidism in developed countries.

Pathophysiology: Chronic autoimmune lymphocytic thyroiditis leads to gradual thyroid failure (with or without goiter formation). This can be associated with other female predominant autoimmune disorders (e.g., primary biliary cirrhosis, rheumatoid arthritis, Sjögren's syndrome, scleroderma, autoimmune hypophysitis, autoimmune adrenalitis, vitiligo, pernicious anemia).

Workup: In patients with no apparent cause of hypothyroidism[22], antithyroid peroxidase antibody (aka antimicrosomal antibody) and antithyroglobulin antibody can be checked; however, it is not routinely necessary.

[22] History of radioactive iodine treatment, thyroid surgery or use of lithium/ amiodarone

Management: supplement with levothyroxine, if hypothyroid.

Complication: increased risk of Hodgkin's lymphoma.

 In a nutshell

Both Graves' disease and Hashimoto's thyroiditis have the following factors in common:

- They are of autoimmune pathophysiology and both are associated with other autoimmune syndromes.
- Both can have antithyroglobulin, antithyroid peroxidase, and anti-TRab antibodies.
- Both can present with diffuse goiter and pretibial myxedema.

Note: Presence of hyperthyroidism and proptosis points to Graves' disease.

MRS

PASs "General IQ test" = Pass GQ = PAinful, Subacute, Granulomatous, De Quervain

2.4.6 Subacute Thyroiditis (aka Subacute Granulomatous, Giant cell and De Quervain Thyroiditis)

Pathophysiology: Subacute process of granulomatous inflammation, possibly induced by viral infection.

Presentation: Painful, tender, enlarged thyroid gland. Patients may have features of transient acute hyper- and/or hypothyroidism. Patients can have a preceding hx of upper respiratory tract infection or viral prodrome (myalgia, fatigue, etc.).

Management Steps

- First SIDx is to look for inflammatory indicators (e.g., elevated sedimentation rate or C-reactive protein).
- Pain relief with aspirin/NSAIDs and if refractory, use steroids.
- If patient has signs of hyperthyroidism, then β blocker is indicated. If symptomatic hypothyroidism develops, short course of levothyroxine is given.

2.4.7 Subacute Lymphocytic Thyroiditis (aka Painless or Silent Thyroiditis)

Pathophysiology: Process is similar to Hashimoto's disease with diffuse lymphocytic infiltrates. There is association with other autoimmune diseases and presence of antithyroid antibodies. If it occurs in pregnant women or within one year of delivery or abortion, it is called postpartum thyroiditis.

Presentation: The clinical course is similar to subacute thyroiditis with transient hyper- then hypo- and then euthyroid state. However, this form of thyroiditis is painless and there is no viral prodrome and ESR is normal. Recurrent attacks of thyroiditis can occur, but are fortunately rare.

Treatment: Similar to subacute thyroiditis, use β blocker and thyroid hormone supplementation as needed.

2.4.8 Riedel's Thyroiditis

It is a rare disorder characterized by intense fibrosis of thyroid gland and surrounding structures. It may be a component of a systemic multifocal fibrosclerosis disease, which can involve other areas such as retroperitoneal or mediastinal fibrosis. Exam will reveal hard enlargement of thyroid gland.

Rx: Thyroid hormone replacement if hypothyroid. Long-term steroids can be used to reduce fibrosis. Surgery may be needed if fibrosis extension compression of esophagus or trachea.

 In a nutshell

How to differentiate different forms of thyroiditis?

Type of thyroiditis	Pain/elevated ESR	Autoimmune antibody	Transient thyrotoxicosis/ hypothyroidism	May result in **chronic** hypothyroidism
Hashimoto's	no	Yes	No	Yes[c]
Subacute lymphocytic	no	Yes	Yes[b]	no
Subacute[a]	Yes	no	Yes[b]	no

[a]Loss of mark: Subacute thyroiditis (aka granulomatous) is a nonantibody-mediated disease different from subacute lymphocytic thyroiditis which is antibody mediated.

[b]Both of these subacute forms can have phase of spillover of thyroid hormones into the blood, causing transient hyperthyroidism (with decreased RAIU). This can later progress to transient hypothyroidism (due to decreased function of thyroid follicle cells from inflammation/necrosis). Hypo- /hyperthyroidism will subside in most of the cases.

[c]In Hashimoto's thyroiditis, hypothyroidism can be permanent as it is a chronic autoimmune process.

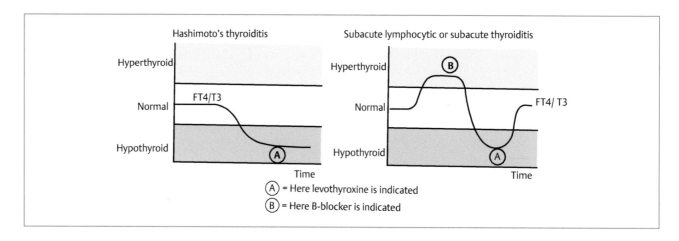

A = Here levothyroxine is indicated

B = Here B-blocker is indicated

Practice Table

TSH	Free T4 and T3	RAIU	Diagnosis
Low	↑	↑ (diffuse uptake)	**Graves' disease**
Low	↑	↑ (focal uptake)	**Toxic functioning adenoma**
Low	↑	Low	**Transient thyrotoxic phase of thyroiditis** (spillover of thyroid hormone): Look for normal or high thyroglobulin **Extrathyroid thyroid hormone production** (e.g., struma ovarii—a dermoid cysts variant): look for normal or high thyroglobulin **Surreptitious thyroxine ingestion** (e.g., patient trying to lose weight by taking thyroid supplements): look for low thyroglobulin
↑	↑	↑	**Pituitary adenoma secreting TSH**
↑	Low	Low	**Primary hypothyroidism** The thyroid gland is not functioning because it is destroyed by: - Inflammation (e.g., Hashimoto's thyroiditis) - Radioactive iodine treatment of Graves' disease - Thyroidectomy
↑	Normal	–	Subclinical hypothyroidism[a]

[a]Indications for thyroid hormone replacement in subclinical hypothyroidism are as follows:

- Clinical symptoms of hypothyroidism
- TSH of > two times the upper limit of normal (this is associated with increased risk of coronary heart disease)
- Patients who are or planning to become pregnant
- Patients with anovulation or infertility
- High levels of antithyroid peroxidase antibody levels (this is more likely to progress onto clinical hypothyroidism)

👥 Clinical Case Scenarios

In an ICU patient, thyroid function test reveals the following: TSH is normal or low, T3 and free T4 are low.

13. What is the likely dx?

14. What is the NSIM?

Management of incidental solitary thyroid nodule

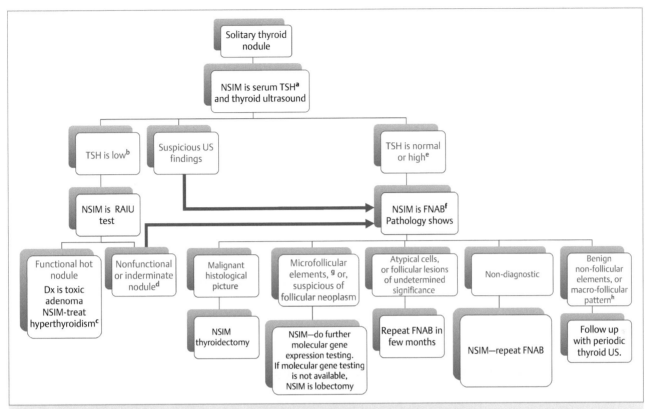

[a]When a thyroid nodule is functioning (i.e., making hormones) it is usually not cancer, because thyroid cancers are typically nonfunctional, so first SIDx is TSH level.

[b]Now if TSH is low, it can be due to following two different scenarios:

- The solitary nodule is a hyperactive nodule (i.e., toxic adenoma).
- The nodule itself might be nonfunctional and the remaining gland is hyperactive.

[c]If the nodule is functional, it will uptake a lot of radioactive iodine (hot nodule) and is typically nonmalignant.

[d]An example scenario would be presence of a nonfunctioning nodule in patient with Graves' disease. (Nonfunctional nodules are more likely to be malignant.)

[e]If TSH is normal or high, the nodule is likely to be nonfunctional. Therefore, in this case there is a possibility that it could be malignant.

[f]FNAB is usually done with ultrasound (US) guidance.

FNAB can be deferred in patients with **nodule size < 1 cm** with no risk for thyroid malignancy and no suspicious US findings. In this case, periodic US follow-up is done. The size of the nodule and/or speed of enlargement are good predictors of the presence of malignancy.

[g]**Micro**follicular pattern needs further exploration, as malignant follicular carcinoma can also have a benign **micro**follicular histologic appearance in aspirate exam. To differentiate, molecular gene testing or lobectomy/thyroidectomy is usually required. For dx of follicular cancer, pathology report of invasion of tumor capsule and blood capillaries is required.

[h]**Macro**follicular pattern is mostly benign.

Abbreviations: NSIDx, next step in diagnosis; NSIM, next step in management; FNAB, fine needle aspiration biopsy.

Patient with hx of Hashimoto's thyroiditis on levothyroxine therapy now presents with sudden enlargement of thyroid gland.

15. What is the NSIM?

16. US reveals 3 cm thyroid nodule and TSH is normal. What is the NSIM?

If biopsy reveals the following, what is the NSIM in each scenario?

17. Macrofollicular pattern?

18. Microfollicular pattern?

19. Nondiagnostic?

20. Atypical cells, or follicular lesions of undetermined significance?

2.5 Thyroid Cancers

MCC of thyroid nodule is **colloid nodule or cysts**. MC type of thyroid malignancy is papillary carcinoma.

Type	Additional info	
Papillary type	Presence of psammoma bodies and Orphan Annie-eye nuclei in histological picture **Risk factors:** hx of head and neck radiation	 Psammoma bodies are of papillary (nipple-like) histomorphology Source: Central nervous system tumors. In: Borsody M. Comprehensive board review in neurology. 2nd ed. Thieme; 2009.
Follicular cancer	A unique characteristic of this carcinoma is that it preferentially metastasizes through hematogenous pathway	
Anaplastic cancer	Malignant cells are highly undifferentiated. This cancer has a very poor prognosis	

General principles of management of thyroid cancer

[23]Medullary cancer of thyroid is managed and followed up differently, as it does not arise from the functioning thyroid cells(discussed on next page).

- Most of the thyroid cancers are treated by total thyroidectomy.
- Postsurgical radioiodine ablation is done to destroy remaining cancerous cells.
- Postsurgery patients will require levothyroxine. (Levothyroxine also suppresses TSH, which theoretically prevents TSH-mediated tumor growth.).
- Serum thyroglobulin concentration and thyroid US is commonly used for follow-up.[23]

2.5.1 Medullary Cancer of Thyroid

Background: It is neuroendocrine cell cancer arising from the parafollicular cells of thyroid gland. This tumor can secrete calcitonin and carcinoembryonic antigen (CEA). It is associated with multiple endocrine neoplasia (MEN) IIa/MEN IIb syndrome *(discussed below)*

Managements steps

- After dx of medullary cancer is made by biopsy, NSIDx is to measure serum calcitonin and CEA (both are used for follow-up).
- Do genetic screening for RET proto-oncogene mutation (to screen for MEN IIa/MEN IIb which have autosomal dominant inheritance). Also measure plasma fractionated metanephrines to screen for pheochromocytoma and serum calcium to screen for parathyroid hyperplasia/adenoma.
- The only effective treatment is thyroidectomy.

Multiple Endocrine Neoplasia Syndromes

They are a group of genetic disorders that typically run in families. They present with development of multiple endocrine tumors that cause over secretion of specific hormones. Genetic testing is usually done. There are three distinct entities.

Types of MEN syndrome	Endocrine tumors associated with the specific types		
MEN I	Parathyroid adenoma	Pancreatic or para-pancreatic* neuro-endocrine tumors E.g., Gastrinoma, insulinoma, vipoma, glucagonoma (see GI chapter for further discussion)	Pituitary tumor
MEN IIa	Parathyroid adenoma	Pheochromocytoma	Medullary carcinoma
MEN IIb	Other • Mucosal or intestinal neuromas • Marfanoid body habitus	Pheochromocytoma	Medullary carcinoma

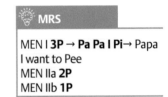

MRS

MEN I **3P** → **Pa Pa I Pi** → Papa I want to Pee
MEN IIa **2P**
MEN IIb **1P**

For patients with suspected MEN I syndrome:

- DNA testing for MEN1 gene mutation is done to help with dx.
- Do regular screening prolactin and serum calcium +/- PTH. Keep vigilance for symptoms of pancreatic tumor +/- imaging.

For patients with suspected MEN IIa/MEN IIb syndrome:

- Do genetic screening for RET proto-oncogene mutation
- Offer prophylactic thyroidectomy
- Screen for pheochromocytoma (check plasma fractionated metanephrine)
- In MEN IIa, screen for parathyroid hyperplasia/adenoma with serum calcium

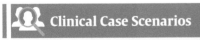 **Clinical Case Scenarios**

21. A patient with history of Hodgkin's lymphoma treated with radiation therapy, now develops hard, fixed thyroid nodule. What is the likely dx?

2.6 Hormonal Disorders Related to Adrenal Gland

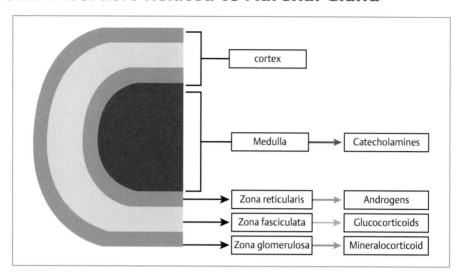

2.6.1 Cushing's Syndrome (Hypercortisolism)

Background: This is a condition resulting from chronic exposure to excess glucocorticoids.

Etiology	CRH[1]	ACTH	Cortisol level
Tertiary hypercortisolism due to CRH[a]-secreting tumor (very rare condition)	↑	↑	↑
• Secondary hypercortisolism due to ACTH-secreting corticotroph pituitary adenoma aka Cushing's disease • Ectopic ACTH production (commonly from small cell cancer of lung or carcinoid tumor)	Low	↑	↑
• Primary hypercortisolism due to adrenal adenoma, hyperplasia, or cancer • Exogenous administration of cortisol (e.g., patient is on oral prednisone for severe persistent asthma). MCC of Cushing's syndrome	Low	Low	↑
[a]Corticotrophin-releasing hormone (CRH) secreted from hypothalamus gland stimulates ACTH secretion from anterior pituitary gland, which in turn stimulates adrenal gland to increase cortisol secretion.			

Clinical effects of hypercortisolemia	Clinical pathophysiology
Severity may range from mild hyperglycemia, prediabetes to overt diabetes	Cortisol hormone promotes gluconeogenesis with help of glucagon
Muscular atrophy	Cortisol hormone promotes protein breakdown in muscle, which provides amino acid substrate for gluconeogenesis
Osteoporosis	Cortisol can stimulate bone resorption
	CCS—patient on chronic steroid treatment presents with acute back pain after minimal trauma. X-ray reveals vertebral compression fracture with diffuse thinning of bone
Fatty tissue redistribution	This can lead to fat deposition, particularly in face (moon facies) and back (buffalo hump)
Apparent mineralocorticoid excess syndromes	Cortisol can act as its close cousin aldosterone, resulting in HTN and hypokalemia
Androgenetic effects	Can act as its close cousin androgen and lead to hair overgrowth and acne
Easy bruising, abdominal striae, and poor wound healing	Cortisol increases collagen breakdown
Leukocytosis	Decreases neutrophil marginalization

Diagnostic work up of Cushing's syndrome, in patients with no apparent cause (e.g., no history of chronic steroid treatment)

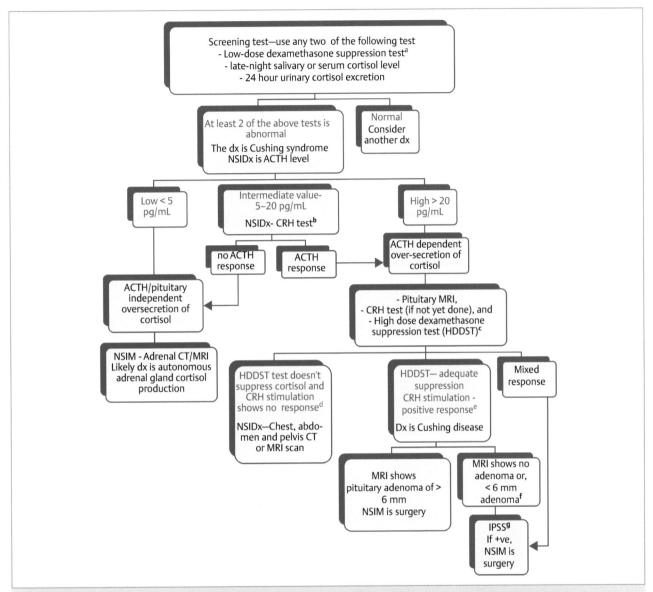

[a]Dexamethasone is preferred over other glucocorticoids, as it does not interfere with laboratory assays of cortisol levels. Dexamethasone given at night should suppress secretion of ACTH by **normal** pituitary gland and decrease intrinsic cortisol production. If AM cortisol (in next morning) is still high, screening test is positive.

[b]**Corticotrophin-releasing hormone (CRH) test:** Only pituitary cells have receptors for CRH. In nonpituitary sources of Cushing's syndrome, the pituitary gland is already suppressed and CRH will not stimulate the pituitary gland. Abnormal pituitary adenomatous cells will respond to CRH test by increasing ACTH secretion, resulting in increased cortisol.

[c]As opposed to low dose dexamethasone, which does not suppress ACTH secretion by pituitary adenomas, high dose can suppress ACTH production from adenomatous pituitary cells. On the other hand, extrapituitary source of ACTH (e.g., small cell cancer) do not have receptors for steroids (dexamethasone), so autonomous ACTH production from these will not be suppressed.

[d]Dx is extrapituitary source of autonomous production of ACTH (e.g., small cell cancer of the lung).

[e]*Both CRH and high dose dexamethasone tests are positive only in pituitary corticotroph adenoma (Cushing's disease).*

[f]In this case, pituitary adenoma is too small. It may not be the culprit tumor causing hypercortisolemia, so confirmation should be done before definitive treatment.

[g]Inferior petrosal venous sinus sampling by catheterization is the most direct way to demonstrate excess ACTH production by pituitary cells. It involves measuring ACTH level directly in the veins draining the pituitary area and comparing it with peripheral venous ACTH level.

Management: Surgical removal of ACTH or cortisol-producing tumor is the treatment of choice. For unresectable tumors, ketoconazole and metapyrone are given to decrease synthesis of cortisol.

2.6.2 Conn's Syndrome (Primary Hyperaldosteronism)

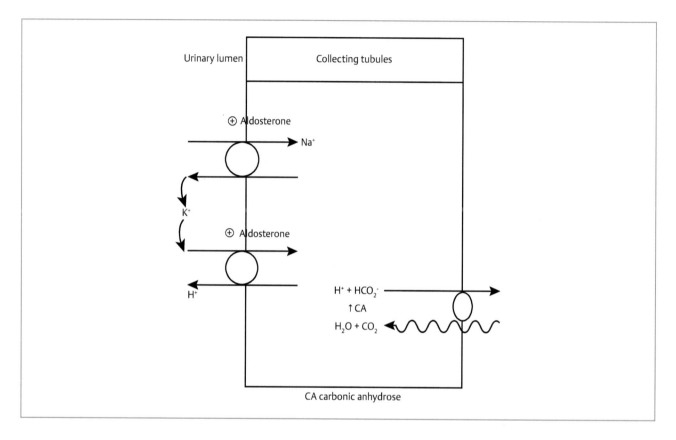

CA carbonic anhydrose

Etiology: Autonomous secretion of aldosterone by adrenal adenoma, primary adrenal hyperplasia, or adrenal cancer.

Pathophysiology: Aldosterone signals kidneys to increase reabsorption of Na^+/water and in exchange, increases excretion of K^+/H^+ in urine.

Presentation: HTN, hypokalemia (muscle weakness), elevated bicarbonate (metabolic alkalosis) +/− mild hypernatremia.

Workup: NSIDx is to measure plasma aldosterone concentration and plasma renin activity (best initial test).

Primary hyperaldosteronism and its differential diagnosis—how to differentiate in between them?

Plasma renin activity	Plasma aldosterone concentration	Dx (all the following can present with HTN, hypokalemia, and metabolic alkalosis)
↑	↑	Secondary hyperaldosteronism due to elevated renin. This can be due to renal disease (autosomal dominant polycystic kidney disease, renal artery stenosism, etc.), or renin-secreting tumor (reninoma)
Low	↑	If aldosterone/renin ratio is ≥ 20, NSIDx is aldosterone suppression test. This is the confirmatory test, which can be done in the following ways: • Oral sodium load and then measure urinary aldosterone secretion • Intravenous sodium loading and measure plasma aldosterone concentration If aldosterone is not suppressed, then autonomous oversecretion of aldosterone is confirmed. • **Dx is primary hyperaldosteronism (aka Conn's syndrome)**

(Continued)

Plasma renin activity	Plasma aldosterone concentration	Dx (all the following can present with HTN, hypokalemia, and metabolic alkalosis)
Low	Low	The following conditions have increased aldosterone pathway activity • Liddle's syndrome (genetic defect causing overactivity of aldosterone pathway) • 11-β-hydroxylase deficiency (congenital adrenal hyperplasia) • Syndrome of apparent mineralocorticoid excess (It is an autosomal recessive genetic disorder with deficiency of kidney isoform of 11-β-hydroxylase enzyme) • Overingestion of licorice (indirectly increases aldosterone receptor activity) • Deoxycorticosterone secreting tumor[a] • Cushing's syndrome[a]

[a]When in excess, deoxycorticosterone and cortisol can also act like aldosterone.

Management of primary hyperaldosteronism

- After biochemical confirmation of Conn's syndrome, NSIDx is adrenal CT or MRI scan.
- If patient does not want surgery or is a poor surgical candidate, medical therapy is indicated with aldosterone antagonists. Eplerenone is the drug of choice (DOC) and is preferred over spironolactone; spironolactone has antiandrogenic side effects (painful gynecomastia and decreased libido) and eplerenone doesn't.
- If patient is a good candidate for surgery, look at the following algorithm:

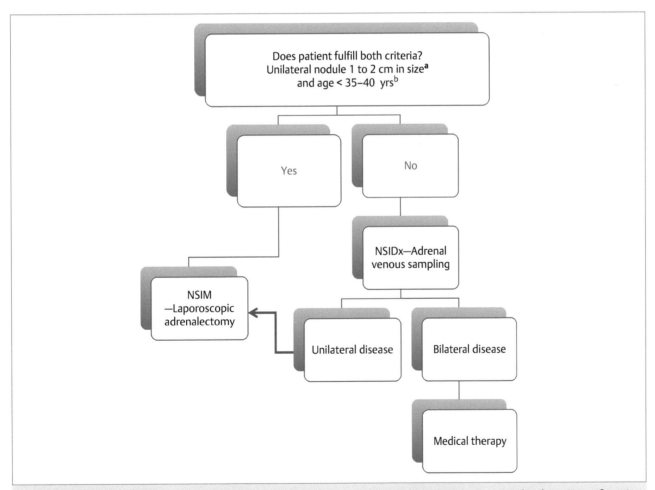

[a]Most adrenal aldosteronomas are sized **1–2 cm**. Adenomas less than 1 cm or larger than 2 cm size are atypical and require confirmation with adrenal venous sampling.

[b]In patients aged >35–40 years, there is a greater likelihood of bilateral adrenal hyperplasia, even if imaging suggests a unilateral disease, hence confirmatory testing is needed.

2.6.3 Pheochromocytoma

Background: Tumor arising from the chromaffin cells of the sympathetic nervous system, which can autonomously secrete norepinephrine, epinephrine, and/or dopamine. Pheochromocytoma is is most commonly found in the adrenal gland (this classically secretes epinephrine). It can also be found in sympathetic ganglia outside of adrenal gland, which classically secretes norepinephrine.[24]

Presentation: Symptoms are typically paroxysmal and related to episodic hypersecretion of catecholamines.

- Patients can present with hx of episodic headache, palpitation (tachycardia), and sweating. They may have no abnormal findings during physician's evaluation, as some have blood pressure elevation only during the attack (*# Physicians can even misdiagnose such patients with panic attacks*).
- Other patients may have stable HTN.

[24]**Familial forms of pheochromocytoma occur in the following conditions:** familial pheochromocytoma, MEN IIa/IIb, neurofibromatosis I and von-Hippel–Lindau syndrome.

Workup and management steps

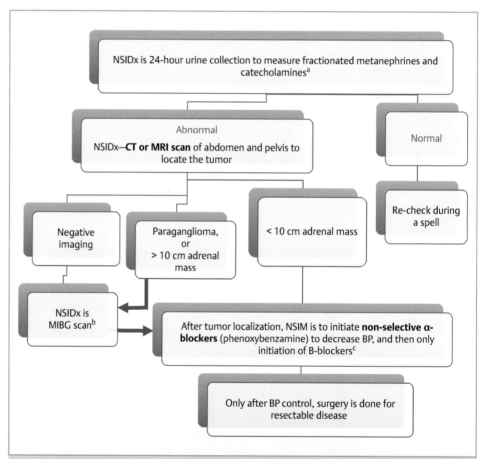

[a]For high-risk patients (e.g., suspected familial forms) use plasma-fractionated metanephrines instead of 24-hour urine collection. In non-high-risk patients, plasma testing has high false positive rates. In high-risk patients, the pretest probability is high enough to use this test.

[b]*MIBG = meta-iodobenzylguanidine scan.* This test is more sensitive. Also, it is useful for detecting metastasis and spread of small tumor cells (more commonly seen in paragangliomas). If adrenal mass is > 10 cm, it is more likely to have metastasized.

[c]β **blockers** should not be initiated until adequate α blockade is achieved. If initiated without adequate α blockade, unopposed α-1 vasoconstriction can occur, leading to malignant HTN. Nonselective α blockers like IV phentolamine can be used for hypertensive crisis.

In a nutshell

Incidental adrenal adenoma

Definition: adrenal mass lesion > 1 cm.

Management:

For an incidentally detected adrenal adenoma, NSIM is to check whether it is functioning or not. Do the following test:

- Twenty-four-hour urinary fractionated metanephrines and catecholamines.
- Low dose dexamethasone suppression test.
- Check plasma aldosterone and plasma renin activity (only if patient has HTN).

For nonfunctioning adrenal adenoma, look at the size to determine management

- If > 4 cm, surgery is considered.
- If < 4 cm with smooth contours and homogenous density, it is usually benign. Follow-up with repeat imaging after 6 to 12 months.

Clinical Case Scenarios

A 35-year-old man presents with long-standing severe HTN. Multiple prior serum electrolyte panels have revealed hypokalemia and elevated bicarbonate.

22. What is the NSIDx?

23. Patient's plasma renin activity/plasma aldosterone concentration ratio was found to be 20. What is the NSIDx?

24. CT scan revealed 3 cm left adrenal mass. What is the NSIM?

25. Adrenal venous sampling shows bilateral increase in aldosterone secretion from both adrenal glands. What is the best SIM?

26. A 25-year-old male was diagnosed with primary hyperaldosteronism. He was found to have 1.5-cm adenoma in the left adrenal gland. What is the NSIM?

2.6.4 Adrenal Insufficiency

Type	Etiology	Which adrenal hormones are affected
Primary adrenal insufficiency (aka Addison's disease)	Destruction of adrenal gland by infection, autoimmune inflammation, tumor, hemorrhage, or infarction • Infection: CMV, HIV, MAC, CMV, *Cryptococcus*, Kaposi's sarcoma, TB, etc. • Autoimmune adrenalitis • Hemorrhagic necrosis in *Neisseria meningitidis* infection (aka Waterhouse–Friedrichsen syndrome) • Metastatic bilateral invasion of adrenal gland (most commonly from lung cancer)	All hormones secreted by adrenal cortex are affected = low aldosterone, low cortisol[a] and low testosterone
Secondary adrenal insufficiency	ACTH deficiency due to any cause of hypopituitarism (e.g., pituitary macroadenoma, Sheehan's syndrome)	Low ACTH → low cortisol. Aldosterone and testosterone are not affected[b]
Tertiary adrenal insufficiency	• Deficiency of CRH due to hypothalamic pathology (e.g., brain tumor) • Abrupt cessation of steroid use[c]	Low CRH → low ACTH → low cortisol. Aldosterone and testosterone are not affected

[a]Electrolyte abnormalities and hypotension is more likely to be present in Addison's disease (due to double whammy of aldosterone and cortisol deficiency) as opposed to secondary to tertiary adrenal insufficiency.

[b]As name giveth all; adrenal-CORTI-co-trophic hormone (ACTH) only controls secretion of CORTIsol; not aldosterone or testosterone.

[c]MCC of adrenal insufficiency is abrupt cessation of chronic steroid use. Steroid use depresses the CRH–ACTH–adrenal axis.[25]

[25]FYI this suppression can last weeks to months.

Presentation

The MC electrolyte abnormality in adrenal insufficiency is hyponatremia.

- Nonspecific anorexia, fatigue, weight loss, and chronic malaise.
- Hyponatremia is due to concurrent increase in ADH.
- Specific features due to low cortisol are hypoglycemia, eosinophilia, and increased risk of hypotension (cortisol increases sensitivity of blood vessels to intrinsic vasoconstrictors).

Features unique to Addison's disease (primary adrenal insufficiency)

[26]Hypotension is less problematic in secondary and tertiary type.

- Due to deficiency of aldosterone: hypotension,[26] hyperkalemia (weakness, paraesthesias, cramping, etc.), and metabolic acidosis.
- GI symptoms are more common: nausea, vomiting, abdominal pain, and diarrhea alternating with constipation (possibly due to electrolyte disturbances).
- Hyperpigmentation ("sun-tanned skin"): the byproduct of increased ACTH production is increased melanocyte-stimulating hormone production.

Workup: NSIDx is ACTH, morning cortisol level, and cosyntropin stimulation test.

ACTH	Baseline cortisol	Cortisol level after cosyntropin administration	Dx	Additional test	
Low	Low	Cortisol may or may not rise depending upon chronicity[a]	Secondary or tertiary adrenal insufficiency	NSIDx is CRH[b] stimulation test	**Positive ACTH response:** pituitary is intact = CRH deficiency = tertiary adrenal insufficiency **Etiology:** hypothalamic pathology (brain tumor) or abrupt cessation of steroid use
					Negative ACTH response: pituitary is damaged = secondary adrenal insufficiency due to hypopituitarism **Etiology:** pituitary macroadenoma, Sheehan's syndrome, etc.
↑	Low	No rise in cortisol	Primary adrenal insufficiency (aka Addison's disease)	NSIDx is to asses for presence of mineralocorticoid deficiency: check plasma renin activity, and serum aldosterone concentration	

[a]In later stages of untreated secondary/tertiary hypoadrenalism, adrenal atrophy will develop, which will manifest as no rise in cortisol hormone after cosyntropin is given.

[b]CRH = corticotropin releasing hormone (secreted by hypothalamus). Think of CRH as ACTH releasing hormone (Corticotropin is ACTH).

Treatment: Glucocorticoid replacement (hydrocortisone or prednisone is commonly used). In Addison's disease, fludrocortisone (a mineralocorticoid) should also be added.

Stress dosing of steroids: If patients with hypoadrenalism have concurrent acute illness or if patients are undergoing surgery, increase steroid dosage to prevent adrenal crisis. This is called stress dosing of steroids.

2.6.5 Adrenal Crisis

Background: This can occur in patients with-
- Abrupt withdrawal of chronic steroids
- Chronic adrenal insufficiency and ongoing stress (e.g., infection/surgery)
- Bilateral adrenal infarction/hemorrhage
- Sudden catastrophic pituitary pathology (pituitary apoplexy) due to surgery, hypotension, direct trauma (e.g., motor vehicle accident)

Pathophysiology: Acute mineralocorticoid deficiency is the main issue, so adrenal crisis is seen mainly in primary adrenal insufficiency. However, it can also occur in secondary adrenal insufficiency when loss of pituitary function is sudden and severe, such as in pituitary apoplexy.

Presentation: Shock, altered mental status, and GI disturbances (nausea, vomiting, and abdominal pain). Due to aldosterone deficiency, there is hyperkalemia.

It is not stress that kills Addison, it is the absence of reaction to it

Management

- NSIDx is to obtain **baseline cortisol and ACTH level (!)**
- NSIM is volume (IV fluids) and electrolyte replacement.
- After obtaining blood sample for ACTH and cortisol level, start on IV hydrocortisone. Hydrocortisone is preferred over other steroids as it has good mineralocorticoid activity.
- Fludrocortisone is started after stabilization. (Note that its effect will take some days, hence not needed emergently.)

> ⚠ **Caution**
>
> (!) Do not choose cosyntropin stimulation test as answer.

Differential diagnosis

	Adrenal crisis	Myxedema coma	Thyroid storm
Hypotension		Present in all	
Altered mental status			
Tachycardia	+/–	No (bradycardic)	Present
Fever	May be present[a]	No (hypothermic)	Present
Hypoglycemic	Present	Present	No

[a]If inciting cause of adrenal crisis is infection.

👥 Clinical Case Scenarios

A patient with history suggestive of bitemporal hemianopsia presents with sudden onset of severe headache, nausea, vomiting, and meningeal signs (stiff neck, Kernig's and Brudzinski's signs) (!).

27. What is the likely dx?

28. If patient develops hypotension, what is the NSIDx and NSIM?

Patient presents with 6 months hx of dry cough, fatigue, and GI complaints. Exam reveals hyperpigmented skin. CT abdomen reveals bilateral adrenal mass.

29. What is the NSIDx to find out the underlying cause?

> ⚠ **Caution**
>
> (!) This is similar in presentation to subarachnoid hemorrhage. Features that points toward pituitary apoplexy are rapidly worsening visual field deficits and prior history suggestive of pituitary adenoma.

🌐 In a nutshell

	Aldosterone excess	Aldosterone deficiency
Blood pressure	HTN	Hypotension
K+ and H+	Low potassium (hypokalemia) Low H+ = metabolic alkalosis	hyperkalemia + metabolic acidosis
Causes	• Primary hyperaldosteronism • Apparent mineralocorticoid excess syndromes	Addison's disease and crisis

2.7 Hyperkalemia/Hypokalemia

Etiology of Hyperkalemia/hypokalemia

Underlying pathophysiology	Hyperkalemia	Hypokalemia
Shift of K^+ in between intracellular and extracellular fluid compartment	In acidosis, excess H^+ ion goes inside the cell in exchange for potassium, which comes out to the extracellular compartment	In alkalosis, potassium goes inside the cell in exchange for H^+ ion, which subsequently buffers the excess base in extracellular fluid
	Low insulin	• **Insulin** promotes potassium and glucose entry into cells • β_2 **agonist** promotes potassium entry into the cells
	K^+ is released from dying cells (hyperkalemia can occur when cell death occurs in large numbers such as in rhabdomyolysis or tumor lysis syndrome)	Potassium uptake occurs when cells are being made. Hypokalemia can occur in treatment with: • Granulocyte colony-stimulating factor (in patients with neutropenia) • While initiating treatment of vitamin B12 deficiency with IM vitamin B12 (increased K^+ uptake by cells for granulopoiesis / erythropoiesis)
Urinary potassium excretion	**Decreased urinary excretion** due to • Hypoaldosteronism (Addison's disease, salt-wasting type of congenital adrenal hyperplasia, etc.) • Renal failure • Drugs that block K^+ excretion: ACE inhibitors and K^+-sparing diuretics (amiloride, triamterene, spironolactone, and eplerenone) • Other drugs: cyclosporine, heparin, digoxin, NSAIDs, nonselective β blockers, succinylcholine, and Bactrim (trimethoprim component)	**Increased urinary excretion** • Hyperaldosteronism/hypercortisolism • All diuretics, except the K^+-sparing ones • Osmotic diuresis: in DKA or HONK • Hypomagnesemia[a] (These stimulate distal convoluted tubules of kidney to increase Na^+ reabsorption and K^+/H^+ excretion)
Miscellaneous	Increased intake of K^+ containing foods, particularly in patients with renal failure	**Increased GI losses:** vomiting, nasogastric tube aspiration, diarrhea, etc.

[a]Hypomagnesemia also causes decrease in parathyroid hormone secretion and PTH receptor responsiveness, leading to hypocalcemia. A cumulative effect is refractory hypokalemia and hypocalcemia.

Abbreviations: ACE, angiotensin-converting enzyme; DKA, diabetic ketoacidosis; HONK, hyperosmolar nonketotic coma.

Presentation of hypo/hyperkalemia

	Hyperkalemia	Hypokalemia
Clinical features	• Muscular weakness (if severe, ascending paralysis can occur) • Abnormal cardiac conduction (e.g., ventricular fibrillation)	• Ascending muscle weakness and paralysis • Cardiac arrhythmias • Polyuria and polydipsia (development of nephrogenic diabetes insipidus) • If severe, can result in rhabdomyolysis
EKG changes	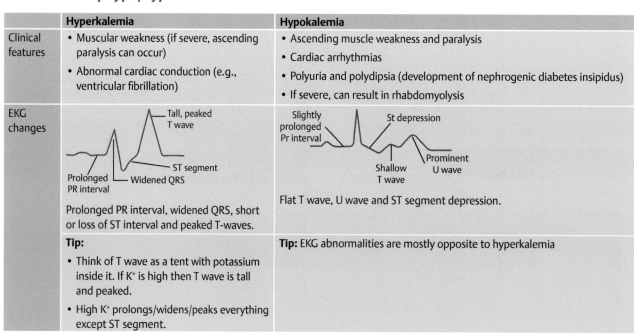 Prolonged PR interval, widened QRS, short or loss of ST interval and peaked T-waves.	Flat T wave, U wave and ST segment depression.
	Tip: • Think of T wave as a tent with potassium inside it. If K^+ is high then T wave is tall and peaked. • High K^+ prolongs/widens/peaks everything except ST segment.	**Tip:** EKG abnormalities are mostly opposite to hyperkalemia

Treatment of hyperkalemia

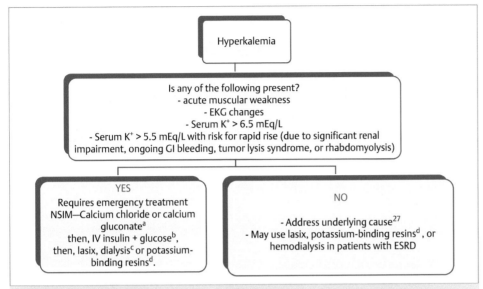

aFirst step is to protect the heart: calcium stabilizes cardiac cell membranes and prevents arrhythmias.

bSecond step is to push the excess potassium inside the cells: **insulin + glucose** is preferred. Inhaled β_2 agonist can be given as adjunctive therapy for severe manifestations.

cThird step is to remove extra K+ from the body with either **furosemide** or hemodialysis in patients with nonfunctioning kidneys.

dPotassium-binding resins, such as patiromer, ZS-9, or kayexalate, can be used. Potential serious adverse effect with kayexalate is intestinal necrosis (avoid this in patients with active bowel disease or in postoperative patients).

Treatment of hypokalemia

- For severe hypokalemia, use IV potassium replacement. IV K+ infusion rate should not exceed > 40 mEq per hour, because rapid infusion can result in arrhythmias.
- For mild cases, use oral replacement.

2.7.1 Polyglandular Autoimmune Syndrome (aka Autoimmune Polyendocrine Syndrome)—Low Yield

Definition: Autoimmune destruction of two or more endocrine glands is known as polyglandular autoimmune syndrome (PGA). There are two main types:

PGA type I aka **APECED** (**A**utoimmune **p**olyendocrinopathy-**c**andidiasis-**e**ctodermal **d**ystrophy)	• Affected endocrine glands are parathyroid gland (hypocalcemia) and adrenal gland (Addison's disease) • Nonendocrine disorder = recurrent mucocutaneous candidiasis
PGA type II	• Autoimmune destruction of β cells of pancreas → diabetes mellitus type I • Autoimmune adrenalitis → adrenal insufficiency • Autoimmune thyroiditis → hypothyroidism

[27]Clinical pearl: Always review medication list in a patient with -hypokalemia.

2.8 Glucose Hemostasis

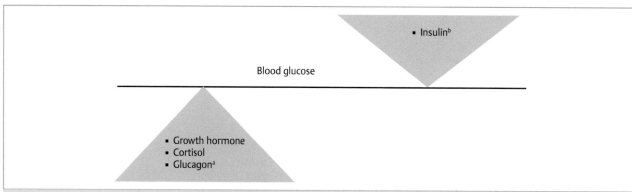

[a]Excess in GH (acromegaly), cortisol (Cushing's syndrome), or glucagon (glucagonoma), depending upon underlying severity, can cause hyperglycemia, impaired fasting glucose/impaired glucose tolerance, or overt diabetes mellitus (DM). Treatment depends upon underlying disorder.

[b]Insulin deficiency or resistance is a more common etiology of hyperglycemia and DM.

2.9 Diabetes Mellitus

Type I DM	Loss of β cells of pancreas (either due to autoimmune destruction or other causes) can lead to absolute deficiency of insulin. Typically, autoimmune antibodies to β cells and/or its components are present (e.g., anti-islet cell antibodies, anti-insulin antibodies)	Usual presentation is a young patient with acute onset of **p**olyuria, **p**olydipsia, and weight loss despite **p**olyphagia (**3Ps** of DM). This presentation can be precipitated by stress, infection, pregnancy, etc.
Type II DM	Primary pathology is decreasing sensitivity to insulin (i.e., increased insulin resistance). Compensatory increase in insulin secretion occurs, but as β cells must work a lot, it leads to increased amyloid deposition in pancreas, culminating in decreased β cell mass. At later stages, absolute insulin deficiency develops.	This type of diabetes occurs typically in the older age group and is associated with metabolic syndrome[a]

[a]Metabolic syndrome (aka insulin resistance syndrome or syndrome X) occurs in patients who are obese, sedentary, who do not exercise, and who frequently eat processed meat, red meat, overcooked or deep fried, high-glycemic-index foods etc., Metabolic syndrome has the following features:

• Central abdominal obesity with increased waist-to-hip ratio.

• Increased insulin resistance and development of overt type II DM.

• Dyslipidemia.

• HTN.

Abbreviation: DM, diabetes mellitus

Clinical effects of chronic hyperglycemia

● Increased nonenzymatic glycosylation of proteins leads to protein dysfunction in various organs. These glycated proteins play an important role in pathogenesis of diabetic vasculopathy, neuropathy, retinopathy, nephropathy, etc.

● HbA_{1c} is one example of glycated protein (in hemoglobin).

● Osmotic damage of cells that contain aldose reductase (e.g., lens of eye, nerve cells): aldose reductase changes glucose into sorbitol, which becomes trapped inside the cells. This leads to osmotic swelling and damage leading to development of cataract and neuropathy.

● Also, Insulin is an anabolic hormone and its absolute deficiency can lead to weight loss despite increase in appetite.

● Uncontrolled serum glucose can cause osmotic diuresis in kidney leading to polyuria and polydipsia.

How diagnosis of DM is made

	Normal	Diagnostic of diabetes	Intermediate values
Fasting plasma glucose	< 100 mg/dL	≥ 126 mg/dL	100–125 mg/dL Dx is impaired fasting glucose (IFG)
Random plasma glucose or 2-hr postprandial glucose (used mostly for screening of gestational DM)	<146 mg/dL	≥ 200 mg/dL	146–199 mg/dL Dx is impaired glucose tolerance (IGT)
HbA1c	< 5.7%	≥ 6.5%	5.7–6.5% = prediabetes

- In symptomatic patients, a single random blood glucose of ≥ 200 mg/dL is diagnostic of DM.
- In asymptomatic patients with abnormal value, recheck fasting plasma glucose or HbA1c to confirm the diagnosis.
- For prediabetes (IFG and IGT), NSIM is life style modifications and metformin.

General Management

- Patient education: stress the benefits of tight glucose control.
- Lifestyle modification:
  - Exercising at least three times a week for at least 30 minutes each session.
  - Eating diet low in dietary AGE[28], red meat, processed meat, and refined carbohydrates.
  - Losing weight if the patient is obese.

Management Strategy of Insulin-Dependent Diabetes Mellitus

- All patients with type I DM need to be on Insulin regimen.
- Insulin formulations are available in various forms with different timing of onset and duration of action.

Insulin formulation	Timing/duration of action	Usage
The following are premeal insulin used for postmeal sugar control		
Lispro or Aspart	Shortest and fastest acting formulation of insulin	Premeal
Regular insulin	Short-acting insulin	• Subcutaneous regular insulin is given premeal • Intravenous regular insulin is used for acute life-threatening conditions such as DKA/HONK and for treatment of severe hyperkalemia
Isophane, glargine, and detemir are used for basal requirement		
Isophane (NPH) insulin	Intermediate-acting insulin Lasts around 8–12 hr	Usually dosed twice daily
Insulin determine, glargine, or degludec	Long-acting insulin for basal insulin needs	Once a day regimen

The following are the commonly use combinations of basal and pre-meal insulin:

- NPH (Isophane) insulin + regular insulin twice a day (Typically 2/3rd of total insulin is given in AM and 1/3rd, given in PM)
- Glargine or detemir (once a day) for basal requirement in combination with lispro/Aspart (before meals) for premeal requirements
- NPH twice a day for basal requirement with lispro/Aspart (before meals)

FYI only- Not needed for boards:
General recommendation on starting-dose-of-insulin
For type I DM, typical range includes 0.2 to 0.6 unit per kg per day of total insulin (basal + pre-meals combined).
For type II DM, 10 units or 0.1 to 0.2 units/kg once daily.

[28] *Dietary AGE = dietary Advanced Glycation End Products.*
Where does dietary AGE come from? Why should we care about it?
Dietary AGE is a new concept of unhealthy food. More dietary AGE is formed, when food containing protein, sugar and/or fat is :-
-cooked for too long period of time,
-at very high temperature, and/or
-at dry conditions
(e.g., grilling, broiling, roasting, searing, and frying). E.g., There is more dietary AGE in fried red meat (higher fat content), chicken curry, General Tso's chicken than in poached chicken.
Increased intake of dietary AGE leads to increased total AGE in body (similar to hyperglycemic glycation of proteins in diabetes), and interacts with cellular Receptors for AGE (RAGE receptors) and increases rates of cellular dysfunction.

All insulin formulations that we are talking about here is subcutaneous. The only time insulin is given in IV drip form is DKA or HONK.

All insulin formulations are excreted renally; if patient has been on stable insulin regimen for a while and develops renal failure, watch out for hypoglycemia

Patients on insulin are asked to monitor blood glucose before meals and before bedtime (AC and HS). Insulin dosage is changed according to the blood glucose levels.

Adjusting NPH and premeal insulin dose in various situations

As a rule:
- If sugars are high throughout the day (including pre-breakfast), increase dose of glargine, detemir, or both AM-PM dose of NPH.
- If only prelunch or predinner sugar is elevated, then increase the dose of previous meal's rapid acting insulin.

Blood sugar	Problem	Solution
Pre-breakfast (aka morning/fasting sugar) (6–7 a.m.)[a]	High	See below in Dawn/Somogyi effect section
	Low	Decrease basal insulin dose (decrease glargine/detemir dose or decrease predinner NPH dose)[b]
Prelunch (11 a.m.–12 p.m.)	High	• If predinner sugar is also high, increase AM NPH • If only this is high, increase prebreakfast short-acting insulin[c]
	Low	• If predinner sugar is also low, decrease AM NPH • If only this is low, decrease prebreakfast short-acting insulin[c]
Predinner (5–6 p.m.)[a]	High	• If prelunch sugar is also high, increase AM NPH • If only this high, increase prelunch short-acting insulin[c]
	Low	• If prelunch sugar is also low, decrease AM NPH • If only this is low, decrease pre-lunch short-acting insulin[b]
Bedtime (9–10 p.m.)	High	• If prebreakfast sugar is also high, increase PM NPH • If only this is high, increase predinner short-acting insulin[b]
	Low	• If prebreakfast sugar is also low, decrease PM NPH • If only this is low, decrease predinner short-acting insulin[b]

[a]NPH BID dosing is usually given during this time. AM NPH affects prelunch and pre-dinner blood sugar. PM NPH (given predinner) affects bedtime and next AM blood sugar (pre-breakfast).

[b]Do the same for nighttime hypoglycemia.

[c]Short-acting insulin are the premeal insulins (lispro, Aspart, or regular insulin).

Clinical Case Scenarios

Patient uses premixed combination of NPH/regular insulin morning and evening. His blood glucose (mg/dL) trend is as follows:

(Note: Goal blood sugar is < 140 mg/dL)

Case	Blood sugar	NSIM
1	6 a.m.: 108 11 a.m.: 180 6 p.m.: 110 9 p.m.: 187	Increase 6 a.m. and 6 p.m. regular insulin. In this case, we do not need to increase AM NPH
2	6 a.m.: 108 11 a.m.: 180 6 p.m.: 160 9 p.m.: 123	Increase AM NPH

Clinical Case Scenarios

Patient is on glargine, degludec or detemir (once a day) for basal requirement, in combination with lispro/Aspart (before meals) for premeal requirements. His blood glucose (mg/dL) trend for 3 days is as follows:

Case	Blood sugar	NSIM
3	6 a.m.: 95, 90, 100 11 a.m.: 182, 190, 184 6 p.m.: 184, 190, 192 9 p.m.: 190, 180, 192	Increase pre-meal lispro or Aspart. Also note that patient might have poor dietary compliance. As morning sugars are good, no need for increasing long-acting insulin. If you increase long-acting insulin, this might result in AM hypoglycemia. FYI- Typically, pre-meal insulins are given either in sliding scale format (higher the sugar, higher the pre-meal dose to be given), or fixed amount before meals.
4	6 a.m.: 180 11 a.m.: 182 6 p.m.: 184 9 p.m.: 190	NSIM: increase long-acting insulin dosage.

Early morning hyperglycemia in diabetic patients on insulin can be secondary to the following two eff ects

MRS

Somogyi is a funny name and hyperglycemia is due to a funny paradoxical mechanism.

Dawn phenomenon	Somogyi effect
This is early morning hyperglycemia due to inadequate insulin dosage	Higher than required dose of basal insulin may lead to nocturnal hypoglycemia. This can lead to compensatory rise in glucogenic hormones (growth hormone, cortisol, glucagon) that can increase blood glucose with subsequent rebound hyperglycemia in morning

= Gluconeogenic hormones likes growth hormones cortisol an glucagon are secreted

How to differentiate between the two?

This can be done by:

- Checking blood glucose at 3 a.m. (during nighttime)
- We can do a trial of **decreasing** the dose of basal insulin dose (glargine or predinner isophane). If early morning blood sugar normalizes then the dx is Somogyi effect. If it does not then dx is Dawn phenomenon

| For Dawn phenomenon, NSIM is to **increase** basal insulin dose (glargine or evening isophane) | For Somogyi effect, NSIM is to **decrease** the dose of basal insulin dose (glargine or evening isophane) |

Pharmacotherapy of type II diabetes mellitus

	Mechanism of action	Additional points
Metformin	Increases sensitivity to insulin	• **Side effects:** GI upset (diarrhea), and life-threatening lactic acidosis[a] • Low risk for hypoglycemia • Does not promote weight gain • Associated with vitamin B12 deficiency
Sulfonylurea (e.g. glipizide, glyburide)	Stimulates insulin secretion	**Side effects:** weight gain, hypoglycemia
Meglitinides (repaglinide)	Increases glucose-dependent insulin release (closely resembles sulfonylureas)	
Thiazolidinedione (e.g., pioglitazone, rosiglitazone)	Increases insulin sensitivity by activating peroxisome proliferator-activated receptors (PPARs)	**Side effects:** edema, CHF, weight gain. Possible increased risk of bladder cancer with pioglitazone and heart attack with rosiglitazone
DPP-IV inhibitors (e.g., sitagliptin, saxagliptin, linagliptin)	Increases endogenous incretins that promote insulin synthesis and release lowers glucagon secretion	Low risk of hypoglycemia and does not promote weight gain
GLP-1 receptor agonist (e.g., sitagliptin, saxagliptin, linagliptin)	Incretin mimetics	• Can cause weight loss • They have lower hypoglycemia risk • Possible risk of pancreatitis and renal failure
Acarbose	Inhibits alpha glucosidase (a brush border enzyme for carbohydrate digestion). This decreases absorption of carbohydrates, so is particularly useful in decreasing postprandial glucose level	Side effects are related to malabsorption (i.e., flatulence and diarrhea) Not commonly used nowadays

[a]Due to increased risk of lactic acidosis, metformin is contraindicated advanced chronic kidney disease" and add annotated side box or if there are risk factors for metabolic acidosis (e.g., severe heart failure, liver failure).

To prevent metformin induced lactic acidosis, it should be held in the following situations:

• 1 to 2 days before surgery, because there is high incidence of lactic acidosis with surgery.
• Before IV contrast for radiological procedures.

Abbreviations: CHF, congestive heart failure; DPP IV, dipeptidyl peptidase IV; GLP-1, Glucagon-like peptide-1.

TIP:
Creatine clearance (CrCl) < 45 mL/min: Donot start metformin. It is ok to continue metformin, that was started prior to the fall in CrCl, but consider reducing the dose. Creatine clearance < 30 mL/min: Donot give any metformin.

FYI- Suggested starting dose of once daily basal insulin is either 10 units or 0.1 to 0.2 units/kg.

[a]Consider insulin as a first-line therapy for patients with type II DM, who have:
• HbA1c > 9.5 %.
• Fasting plasma glucose > 250 mg/dL.
• Random glucose consistently > 300 mg/dL.
• Presence of ketonuria.
[b]In patients with renal dysfunction, use repaglinide, glipizide, or glimepiride.
[c]If HbA1c < 7% (well-controlled diabetes), NSIM is to continue current treatment and follow-up HbA1c at regular intervals.

Step-wise management strategy for type II diabetes mellitus

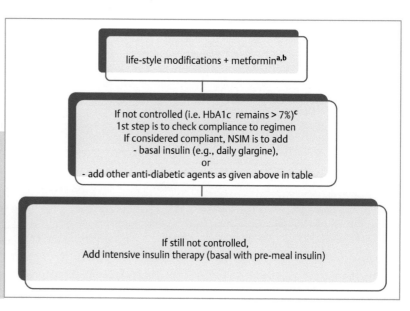

2.9.1 Complications of Diabetes Mellitus

- Diabetic vasculopathy
- Diabetic nephropathy
- Diabetic neuropathy
- Diabetic retinopathy
- Immunosuppression

Diabetic vasculopathy

Macrovasculopathy	Involves major arteries and its braches	It is the major risk factor for atherosclerotic cardiovascular disease (ASCVD) • Coronary artery disease • Peripheral vascular disease • Cerebrovascular disease • Carotid artery disease
Microvasculopathy	Involves small arterioles	Uncontrolled DM is a major predisposing factor of hyaline arteriosclerosis in small arterioles. It leads to diabetic nephropathy, retinopathy, neuropathy, lacunar infarcts in brain, small vessel disease in extremities, etc.

DM is the (most common) MC underlying disorder in coronary artery disease.

Diabetic nephropathy

Pathophysiology: Combination of hyaline arteriosclerosis of afferent/efferent arterioles of glomeruli and angiotensin II-mediated preferential efferent arteriole constriction leads to intraglomerular hypertension, increase in glomerular filtration pressure, and hyperfiltration injury to kidney. It is also characterized by development of diffuse and/or nodular glomerulosclerosis and other histopathologic changes.

Screening: Nephropathy screening in type 2 DM should start at the time of diagnosis and 5 years after diagnosis in type 1 DM. Preferred screening test is spot urine albumin/creatinine ratio and serum creatinine. Urine dipstick is not sensitive enough and cannot be used to monitor effectiveness of treatment.

Management: DOC for preventing or slowing diabetic nephropathy is ACE inhibitor or angiotensin II receptor blocker (ARB), which preferentially dilate the **efferent arterioles.**

DM is the MCC (most common cause) of chronic kidney disease.

Diabetic neuropathy

Neuropathy in DM develops due to two pathologies: microvasculopathy and osmotic damage. Diabetes can have different types of neuropathy which are as follows:

- **Symmetrical distal polyneuropathy:** It is the MC type of neuropathy in DM with features of sensory loss and tingling-pins-needle sensation. It typically affects distal extremities first (glove-stocking distribution). Sometimes symptoms of neuropathy can be very painful and disturbing. Monofilament testing is a sensitive screening test (see picture). **For pain and discomfort,** use gabapentin, pregabalin, or tricyclic antidepressants. Neuropathy increases risk of trauma, diabetic foot ulcers, and neuropathic joint (Charcot joint; see Chapter 11, Rheumatology for further details).
- **Mononeuropathy:** MC singular nerve involvement is cranial nerve III (oculomotor nerve palsy). Patients may also present with foot drop, radial nerve palsy, etc. NSIM is supportive management and tight glycemic control. They usually resolve spontaneously over few months.
- **Autonomic neuropathy:** It can involve autonomic nerves in various organ systems such as:

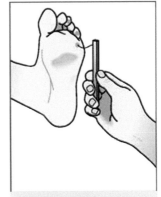

Inability to feel the monofilament suggests sensory neuropathy.

Stomach (gastroparesis)	Stomach fails to empty normally (delayed gastric emptying time)
	Presentation: Postmeal bloating, flatulence, early satiety, and postmeal hypoglycemia. Acute exacerbation can present with acute epigastric pain, nausea, and vomiting
	Diagnosis: It is important to rule out other causes that can obstruct pyloric antrum (e.g., tumor), so NSIDx is endoscopy. Best test is gastric emptying time study.
	Rx: First step is life style modification (including consuming small frequent meals) and tight glycemic control. For continuing chronic symptoms, use metoclopramide. Other agents include erythromycin and domperidone. For acute exacerbation of gastroparesis, use IV erythromycin
Small intestine	Decreased motility predisposes to small bowel bacterial overgrowth that may lead to malabsorptive diarrhea. Treatment is with trial of broad-spectrum antibiotics (e.g., amoxicillin-clavulanic acid)
Large intestine	Decrease in GI motility leads to constipation
Pelvic nerves	Overflow incontinence (DOC is bethanechol)
Heart	Silent angina/MI (always be vigilant in patients with diabetes)
Vascular	Orthostatic hypotension (hx of syncopal attacks)

Diabetic retinopathy

Screening: Start screening with dilated fundoscopy 3 to 5 years after dx of type I DM and immediately in patients with type II DM.

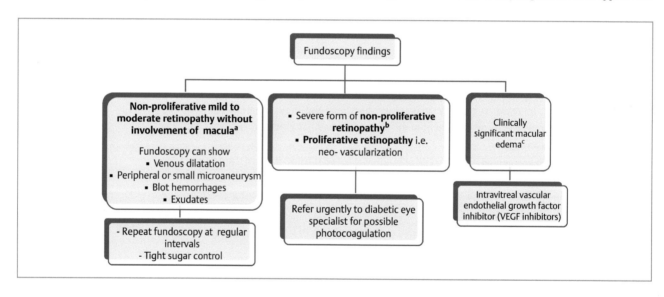

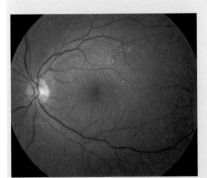

[a]Microaneurysms, fine hard exudates, and dot hemorrhages in mild, nonproliferative diabetic retinopathy

Source: Diabetic retinopathy. In: Tabandeh H, Goldberg M. The retina in systemic disease: a color manual of ophthalmoscopy. 1st ed. Thieme; 2009.

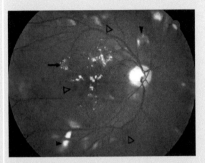

[b]Microaneurysms, intraretinal hemorrhage (open arrowheads), hard exudates representing lipid deposits in the retina (*arrow*), and cotton-wool spots representing nerve fiber infarction (also called soft exudates) (*black arrowheads*)

Source: Diabetic retinopathy. In: Lang G. Ophthalmology. A pocket textbook atlas. 3rd ed. Thieme; 2015.

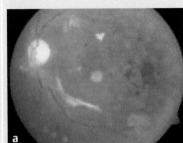
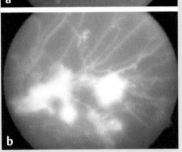

[c](a) Clinically significant macular edema. (b) Picture shows fluorescein angiography of same patient showing neovascularization and macular edema

Various presentation scenarios of visual symptoms in patients with DM

Acute visual loss in DM can be due to intravitreal hemorrhage or retinal detachment. This occurs due to proliferative retinopathy.

Chronic slowly progressive visual loss is likely due to slowly progressive form of diabetic retinopathy or cataract

Uncontrolled sugars can result in osmotic lens swelling and abrupt changes in focal length. Sometimes patients may report that they no longer need glasses or they need higher power glasses to correct their vision

Diabetic foot

Pathophysiology

- Most important **predisposing factor** for a new foot ulcer development is peripheral neuropathy (due to loss of sensory modalities such as position sense, touch, and pain).
- The most important determinant of the fate of **ulcer (healing or extension)** is underlying vasculopathy.
- Systemic immunosuppression and underlying vasculopathy increases risk of infection, contributing to delayed wound healing and wound extension.

Management: All ulcers with necrotic tissue should be debrided. All patients with diabetic foot ulcer should be referred to diabetic foot specialist. Please see cellulitis section in ID chapter for management of infection.

Diabetic foot is the MCC—most common cause of nontraumatic amputation.

In a nutshell

Summary of preventative management in diabetes

	Screening test	Management
Glucose control and compliance	HbA1c at regular interval	If HbA1c > 7%, screen for noncompliance. If considered compliant, step up or increase dosage of therapy
Dyslipidemia	Fasting lipid profile in regular intervals	See Chapter 1, Preventive medicine for further details
Microalbuminuria	- Yearly spot urine albumin/creatinine ratio and serum creatinine - Begin screening for nephropathy at the time of diagnosis in type 2 DM and 5 years after diagnosis in type 1 DM	If +ve, give ACE inhibitor Use ARB, if ACE inhibitor intolerant or allergy
Pneumococcal infection	–	PPSV23 at diagnosis and PCV13 and 2nd dose of PPSV23 at the age of 65 or after 5 years (whichever is later)
Diabetic retinopathy	Start screening with dilated fundoscopy 3–5 years after dx of type I DM and immediately in patients with type II DM	As above
ASCVD of > 10	–	Consider aspirin for primary prevention of ASCVD
Diabetic neuropathy	Monofilament test at regular interval	Tighter control of sugar • May need referral to podiatry if foot ulcer or deformities are present

2.9.2 Acute Metabolic Complications of Diabetes Mellitus

DKA and HONK are the acute metabolic complications.

Diabetic ketoacidosis (DKA)

Background: DKA occurs primarily in type I DM, as absolute deficiency of insulin is a potent stimulator for lipolysis and ketogenesis. In type 2 DM, especially in the earlier course of disease, there is enough insulin to prevent significant ketogenesis. DKA is commonly precipitated by acute stress such as infection, trauma, alcohol ingestion, and insufficient or interrupted insulin.

Pathophysiology

- **Anion gap acidosis:** Absolute deficiency of insulin leads to increased catabolic state, increased lipolysis, and fatty acids production which are converted into ketoacids (acetoacetic acid and beta-hydroxybutyrate). This anion gap metabolic acidosis is partially compensated by respiratory alkalosis.
- **Dehydration and electrolyte imbalance:** Increased blood glucose leads to osmotic diuresis and consequent loss of fluid and electrolytes (particularly potassium) from the urine. Hence there is volume depletion and decreased total body potassium. But note that in DKA, serum potassium might be high or normal, even though the body's potassium stores are depleted. This is because, in acidosis, the excess H$^+$ ions in extracellular fluid enter the cells to be buffered by intracellular proteins, in exchange for K$^+$, which moves out of the cells (transcellular shift). (*Boards love this fact and this is commonly tested*).

Presentation

In a young adult or adolescent patient, suspect DKA when he presents with **abdominal pain, nausea and vomiting,** and has a hx of polyuria and polydipsia.[29]
Exam typically reveals a patient with rapid/deep breathing (Kussmaul sign) +/− confusion.

Management steps

It's an emergency case and as in every emergency never forget the ABCs. Both acidosis and electrolyte imbalance can lead to fatal arrhythmias in severe DKA patients.
NSIDx: Finger stick blood glucose (very easy to do and results are available instantaneously) and check serum/urine ketones, electrolytes, and blood
Diagnostic criteria: Blood pH < 7.3, blood glucose > 250 mg/dL, serum bicarbonate < 20, and positive plasma ketones.

Treatment

- 1st step is to correct volume depletion (give generous IV normal saline)
- If potassium is low, do not give any insulin. Normalize potassium 1st, then only start IV regular Insulin infusion, otherwise dangerous hypokalemia might ensue.
- If potassium levels are within normal limits, give potassium with IV normal saline to replenish body's potassium stores (this will prevent hypokalemia).
- To assess adequacy of treatment, monitor bedside capillary beta-hydroxybutyrate butyrate level, serum anion gap/bicarbonate level, and/or venous pH(!)
- Transition IV insulin infusion to subcutaneous insulin when serum anion gap has closed.

Hyperosmolar Nonketotic Coma (HONK)

Background: HONK is more commonly seen in elderly type II DM patients, as they have enough baseline insulin to prevent fatty acid breakdown and ketogenesis but not enough to prevent hyperglycemia.
Pathophysiology: Hyperglycemia leads to osmotic diuresis resulting in dehydration and electrolyte imbalance.
Presentation: Hyperglycemia (> 600 mg/dL) + polyuria + dehydration + altered mental status without ketones in urine/blood and without acidosis (serum pH is > 7.3).
Management: Similar to DKA, replenish volume (IV normal saline) and control blood glucose (IV insulin drip).

2.10 Hypoglycemia

Etiology: MCC of hypoglycemia is antidiabetic medications and insulin. If patient without hx of DM presents with hypoglycemia, look for the following causes:
- **Ex**ogenous administration of insulin or oral hypoglycemic agents, especially in patients who have access to this drug. For example, nurse, pharmacist, or patient with a relative who has hx of diabetes (think of factitious or malingering disorder).
- **P**ancreatitis (**acute/chronic**): patient will have hx of epigastric pain and tenderness.
- **L**iver failure causes fasting hypoglycemia: patient will have features suggestive of liver disease. *Note: gluconeogenesis occurs in liver.*
- **A**drenal insufficiency (**ACTH** deficiency/**A**ddison's disease).
- **A**lcohol can cause fasting hypoglycemia.
- **I**nsulinoma which is a **n**euroendocrine tumor.
- **N**onpancreatic neoplasm (e.g., retroperitoneal fibrosarcomas).

[29] Board question may not give hx of DM, because, as in real life, this might be first presentation of DM.

MRS

7.3; **DKA** = **3** letters

Caution

(!) Do not choose serum glucose level or blood ketone levels to monitor the response to treatment.

In DKA/HONK remember that elevated serum glucose can lead to pseudohyponatremia. Always calculate corrected sodium level in this case.

MRS

How can we **ExPLAIN** hypoglycemia in a non-diabetic?

Presentation

Low blood sugar supply to the **brain** (neurogenic symptoms)	Dizziness, headache, blurry vision and if severe, may lead to altered mental status and seizures
Low blood sugar stimulates secretion of **adrenergic hormones**	Sweating, tachycardia, anxiety etc. Adrenergic stimulation increases blood sugar

Treatment: If mild, use oral glucose or sugary drinks. If severe, use IV dextrose or glucagon.

Know how to differentiate between common causes of hypoglycemia in a nondiabetic patient

	Exogenous insulin	Insulinoma	Sulfonylurea/ meglitinide
Plasma insulin	↑	↑	↑
C-peptide	low	↑	↑
serum sulfonylurea/ meglitinide level	Absent	Absent	Present

Clinical case scenario of an elderly patient presenting with acute change in mental status is very common. Some of the important dyselectrolytemia causes are the following:
• Hypo- or hypernatremia.
• Hypo- or hypercalcemia.
• Hypo- or hyperglycemia.
Note that all these can also induce seizures.

Clinical Case Scenarios

A young patient presents to clinic with polyuria, polydipsia, and weight loss despite polyphagia.

30. What is the best SIDx to confirm diabetes?

31. If single **random** blood glucose is ≥ 200 mg/dL, is the dx confirmed?

32. An asymptomatic patient with family hx of DM is being screened for diabetes with fasting plasma glucose (Note: HbA1c is an acceptable alternative for screening for DM). Fasting plasma glucose is found to be 126 mg/dL. What is the NSIM?

A 34-year-old female who is a pharmacist comes in with hypoglycemia. She has no other associated clinical features. She found to have elevated insulin and C-peptide level.

33. What is the NSIDx?

34. If serum sulfonylurea is negative, what is the NSIDx?

Answers

1. Large pituitary lactotroph adenoma with secondary hypothyroidism.

2. Primary hypothyroidism and secondary pituitary hyperplasia.

   Explanation

   Hypothyroidism results in compensatory increase in secretion of thyrotropin-releasing hormone, which can lead to pituitary hyperplasia and hyperfunctioning pituitary gland hence increased prolactin secretion. This can also lead to increased secretion of other pituitary hormones.

3. Hypertonic saline

4. FT4 and T3 measurement.

5. β blocker + methimazole (as patient has significant symptoms, initiate thionamides).

6. Check serum TRab and RAIU scan.

7. Apathetic Graves'. Notice that patient does not have the classical proptosis or dermopathy.

8. Follow serum TSH, free T4 and T3. Only after euthyroid state is achieved, schedule for radioiodine ablation (definitive treatment).

9. Stop the medication. All thionamides can cause agranulocytosis or neutropenia.

10. Serum thyroglobulin measurement.

11. Surreptitious thyroid hormone intake.

12. Dx is inherited thyroid hormone resistance or impaired sensitivity to thyroid hormone. This can present later in life too. TSH may be elevated because there is impaired direct negative feedback by T4/T3.

13. **Sick euthyroid syndrome aka low T3 syndrome;** Nonthyroidal significant illness can lead to transient thyroid dysfunction. TSH and T4 may be low, normal or minimally elevated. T3 is usually low.

14. NSIDx: recheck thyroid function within 1-2 weeks. Treatment is considered only if TSH is very low or very high and T4/T3 levels are congruent with TSH abnormality.

15. Thyroid US and TSH.

16. FNAB. Note: patients with Hashimoto's thyroiditis have an increased risk for non-Hodgkin's lymphoma arising from the thyroid gland.

17. Follow-up with periodic thyroid US.

18. Molecular gene expression testing.

19. Repeat FNAB.

20. Repeat FNAB in few months.

21. Papillary carcinoma of thyroid.

22. Check plasma renin activity and plasma aldosterone concentration.

23. Aldosterone suppression test with sodium loading.

24. Adrenal venous sampling.

25. Eplerenone.

26. Left adrenalectomy. The only indication of surgery without the need for adrenal venous sampling is typical 1 to 2-cm size adrenal adenoma in a young patient (< 35–40 years), with classical primary hyperaldosteronism.

27. Pituitary apoplexy

28. NSIDx is to check baseline cortisol and ACTH level. NSIM is volume/electrolyte repletion and IV hydrocortisone.

29. NSIDx is CT scan of chest with IV contrast. This could be due primary lung cancer which commonly metastasizes to adrenal gland.

30. For symptomatic DM, best SIDx is random blood glucose.

31. Yes; no need for further testing.

32. Repeat fasting plasma glucose level or check HbA1C. Diagnosis of DM is not confirmed yet in this asymptomatic patient.

33. Serum sulfonylurea/meglitinide screen.

34. CT abdomen to search for insulinoma.

3. Pulmonology

"The act of breathing is living"

3.1 Acute Respiratory Failure

Acute onset of shortness of breath (SOB) or acute respiratory decompensation is a common emergency condition. This can occur due to multiple etiologies, as following:

- Exacerbation of asthma or chronic obstructive pulmonary disease (COPD).
- Respiratory infection (viral/bacterial).
- Lung injury.
- Foreign body aspiration.
- Heart failure and pulmonary edema.
- Respiratory depressants such as opiate poisoning or barbiturates.
- Tiring diaphgramatic muscles which can occur in all causes of severe persistent hypoxemia, e.g., in later stages of asthma exacerbation or pulmonary embolism.
- Acute neuro-muscular weakness with involvement of diaphgram, that can occur in conditions like myasthenic crisis or Guillain–Barre syndrome.

Lung auscultation is a very powerful diagnostic tool

Lung auscultation findings	In what area?	Causes
Decreased breath sounds	In all lung zones	• Hypoventilation • Complete obstruction of central airway • Severe COPD or asthma
	In specific zones	• Atelectasis • Pleural effusion (additional finding is dullness to percussion) • Pneumothorax (additional finding is tympanic sound on percussion) • Misplaced endotracheal tube
Increased breath sounds (inspiration and expiration equally heard = bronchial breath sounds)	In specific zones	**Consolidation of lung segments** due to lobar pneumonia Additional findings include: • Increased vocal and tactile fremitus[a] • Dullness to percussion
Wheezes or rhonchi	In all lung zones	Bronchospasm, which can be caused by • Asthma • COPD • Parasympathomimetics (e.g., organophosphate poisoning) • β blocker overdose • Bronchiolitis in children • Generalized bronchiectasis
	In specific zones	Localized bronchiectasis
Crackles or rales	Bilateral basilar crackles	• Fluid accumulation in alveoli due to congestive heart failure • Interstitial lung disease with bibasilar predominance (Velcro-crackles)
	In specific zones	• Pneumonia • Atelectasis • Localized bronchiectasis
	Generalized	• Interstitial lung disease (Velcro crackles) • Generalized bronchiectasis
Stridor = noisy breathing (often so loud that it can be heard without a stethoscope)	–	Due to incomplete upper or middle-respiratory tract obstruction • Foreign body • Infection (e.g., epiglottitis, croup) • Laryngomalacia • Subglottic stenosis

[a]These exam findings are due to increased conduction of vibration by consolidated lung. In the consolidated part of the lung
- with auscultation, patient's spoken words and whispered sounds are heard louder (termed as bronchophony and whispering pectoriloquy, respectively)
- with percussion, more vibration is felt (increased tactile fremitus).

Management steps for acute respiratory failure

- **Pulse oximetry (which measures oxy-hemoglobin saturation), chest X-ray (CXR), and** on occasions arterial blood gas (ABG), are important initial diagnostic tools to evaluate the severity and the cause of respiratory compromise.
- **Step up of supplemental oxygen therapy:** This is used to maintain oxygen saturation (SaO_2) to > 88 to 92% or P_aO_2 > 60 mmHg.

How much supplemental oxygen is needed to maintain adequate oxygenation tells us how sick the patient is; for example, the respiratory status of a patient requiring 100% oxygen delivered through a nonrebreather mask is much worse than a patient on 4 L of oxygen by nasal cannula.

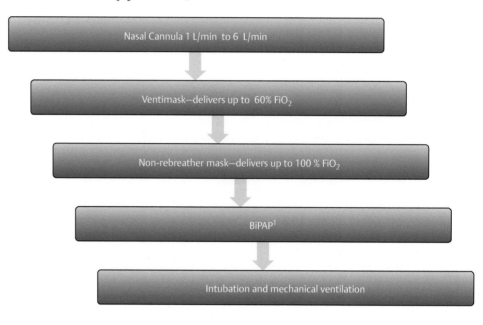

Nasal Cannula 1 L/min to 6 L/min

Ventimask—delivers up to 60% FiO_2

Non-rebreather mask—delivers up to 100 % FiO_2

BiPAP[1]

Intubation and mechanical ventilation

3.1.1 Bilevel Positive Airway Pressure aka Noninvasive Positive Pressure Ventilation

[1] Note that BiPAP cannot be used in following cases:

- **Obtunded** patient who cannot control their airway.
- Patients with **excessive secretions.**
- Agitated or uncooperative patient.
- Hemodynamic instability.

In these cases, NSIM is endotracheal intubation.

Bilevel positive airway pressure (BiPAP) is a noninvasive method of ventilation that can deliver up to 100% oxygen with application of positive airway pressure through a tight-fitting mask. The mask is very easy to put on and take off (since it is a mask), in contrast to invasive intubation. In acute pulmonary edema, BiPAP has the added benefit of decreasing preload. BiPAP increases intrathoracic pressure and decreases venous return to right heart.

3.1.2 Mechanical Ventilation

Indications

- Severe hypoxemia, hypercarbia, or respiratory acidosis unresponsive to general noninvasive measures.
- Patients who have hemodynamic instability (such as hypotension).
- Patients who have altered mental status and cannot protect their airways.

An endotracheal tube is inserted in the patient's airway and connected to a ventilation machine.

In most ventilator settings, the following parameters are looked at

Tidal volume (TV)	It is the volume of air delivered through ventilation machine in each breath. Recommended tidal volume is 6–8 cc/kg of predicted body weight.[2]	
	Too high TV can cause: • Barotrauma • Can increase intrathoracic pressure resulting in decreased venous return to heart, thereby. decreasing cardiac output • Hyperventilation (respiratory alkalosis)	Too low TV can cause atelectasis, and hypoventilation (respiratory acidosis)
Respiratory rate (RR)	It is generally set at **8–14/min**	
	Too high RR can result in: • Incremental air trapping in each successive breath causing auto-PEEP[a] • Hyperventilation (respiratory alkalosis)	Too low RR can cause hypoventilation (respiratory acidosis)
FiO₂ (fraction of inspired oxygen)	Generally preferred at < 60% to decrease risk of oxygen toxicity	
Positive end expiratory pressure (PEEP)	Minimal PEEP of 5 cm H_2O is used in all patients on mechanical ventilation to prevent end expiratory alveolar collapse. As PEEP is increased, it helps to recruit collapsed alveoli to improve gas exchange and oxygenation. Higher levels of PEEP (15–20 cm H_2O) may be required to improve oxygenation, with the goal to reduce higher FiO₂ to prevent oxygen toxicity. However, note that higher PEEP can be associated with the following complications: • Increased risk of rupture of alveoli with subsequent development of tension pneumothorax (pulmonary barotrauma) • Hypotension: high intrathoracic pressure impedes venous return into the right heart, which leads to subsequent decrease in preload of the left heart and cardiac output	

[a]**Auto-PEEP** can occur when the respiratory rate is set too high and/or if there is increased airway resistance (due to COPD, asthma,[3] or narrow endotracheal tube).

In this case, the lungs do not have enough time to expire the inhaled air, and hence, more and more air gets trapped in each consecutive respiratory cycle, incrementally increasing the intrathoracic pressure. This can result in barotrauma and hypotension, similar in pathophysiology to high PEEP.

[2]**Note:** in ARDS the recommend TV is not more than 6 cc/kg of predicted body weight.

[3]To prevent auto-PEEP in COPD/asthma, it is recommended to use lower TV and RR, even at the expense of mild hypoventilation and respiratory acidosis, as long as pH is > 7.2. This strategy is known as permissive hypercapnia.

 In a nutshell

• Tidal volume (TV) and respiratory rate (RR) are used to control ventilation (getting rid of CO_2).

• FiO₂ and positive end expiratory pressure (PEEP) are used to control oxygenation.

• Minute ventilation = RR × TV.

1. An intubated patient is found to be hypoxic and hypotensive. Exam reveals severe wheezing. It appears that ventilator settings needs to be adjusted. What is the likely cause of hypoxia and hypotension in this patient?

2. An intubated patient is found to be hypoxic and hypotensive. Exam reveals no breath sounds on one side of the lung. What is the likely cause of hypoxia and hypotension in this setting?

    Intubated patient has hypoxia and absent breath sounds in one side of the lung.

3. What are the differential dx?

4. How would you differentiate in between them?

---

[4] Do not choose **synchronized-intermittent mandatory ventilation** as a weaning mode for ventilation as this method is not used anymore.

3.1.3 Modes of Ventilation

Assisted-control mode of ventilation (ACMV): This mode is commonly used for starting patient on mechanical ventilation and when patient is ready for weaning[4] (prior to initiation of low-pressure support ventilation). The clinician determines preset TV and RR. Patients may initiate breathing, but preset TV is delivered. Patient can also breathe over the vent.

For example, ACMV mode is set at TV of 500 cc and RR of 12.

● If patient's **own** breathing rate is 10, then patient will get additional 2 breaths delivered with TV of 500 cc each. In this case minute ventilation = 0.5 L × 12/min = 6 L/min.

● If **patient's** own breathing rate is 15, then the extra 3 breaths that patient initiates, he/she will get 500 cc of preset TV in each breath (minute ventilation = 0.5 × 15). In this case, patient is said to be breathing over the vent.

Pressure control ventilation (PCV): The ventilator delivers preset pressure support in each breath. Tidal volume is not specified.

Stepwise management of ventilation

[a] Try to keep the ratio of 60% FiO$_2$ to 10 of PEEP, and 40% FiO$_2$ to 5 of PEEP. Most of the time exam CCS will involve a question with 60 FiO$_2$ with 10 of PEEP scenario.

[b] Reducing FiO$_2$ is the first step to reduce risk of oxygen toxicity. But note that if PEEP was mistakenly set at 20 and FiO$_2$ is set at 60%, and if oxygenation is adequate then NSIM is to decrease PEEP in this case; but this is an extreme example only.

[c] Recommended tidal volume is 6 to 8 cc/kg of predicted body weight. FYI an average adult's normal tidal volume is 500 mL.

[d] Remember permissive hypercapnia in ARDS, COPD, and asthma.

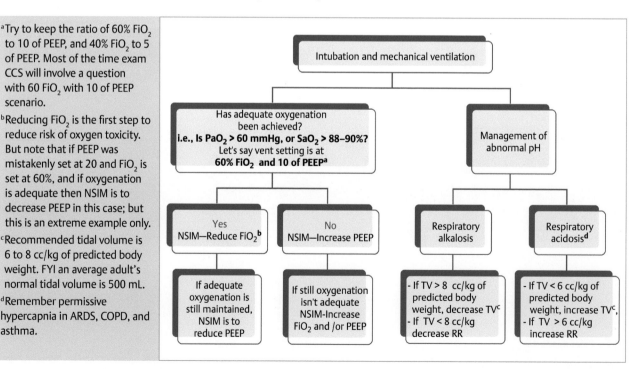

🔍 Clinical Case Scenarios

5. Patient is intubated for ARDS. His vent settings are PEEP of 10, FiO_2 of 80% and RR of 12. ABG reveals PaO_2 of 90. What is the NSIM?

6. A 65-year-old female with asthma exacerbation is currently intubated. RR of 20. ACMV mode is set at RR of 13 per minute and TV of 500 cc. ABG shows pH of 7.26, $PaCO_2$ of 60 mmHg, PaO_2 70 mm Hg. What is the NSIM?

Ventilator Weaning

Consider weaning when the patient

- Can maintain oxygenation with FiO_2 < 40 to 50%, PEEP of ≤ 5 cm H_2O.
- Does not have excessive secretions.
- Is awake enough to control airway.
- Is hemodynamically stable (no or minimal vasopressor support).

To determine whether patient is ready for extubation, a spontaneous breathing trial is used with ventilation mode changed to **low-pressure support ventilation**. It is very similar to BiPAP, with positive pressure given during inspiration and expiration and TV/RR is completely dependent on the patient's own respiratory effort.

During the first few hours of low-pressure support ventilation, **rapid shallow breathing index** (RSBI) ratio is calculated.RSBI = RR/TV (in liters). It is a ratio that is used to assess readiness of a patient to get extubated.

RSBI > 105	Patient is breathing rapidly (high RR) and has shallow breathing (low TV). Patients with RSBI of > 105 are likely to fail extubation[5]
RSBI ≤ 105	Patient is ready for weaning. NSIM is consider extubation

[5]If ventilator weaning fails for more than 7 to 10 days, consider tracheostomy.

Other complications of mechanical ventilation

- **Stress-induced peptic ulcers:** all patients on mechanical ventilation are recommended to get prophylaxis with proton pump inhibitor or H_2 receptor antagonist (e.g., famotidine).
- **Ventilator-acquired pneumonia:** placing patient on semirecumbent position has been shown to decrease incidence.
- **Pneumomediastinum, pneumoperitoneum, and subcutaneous emphysema** are milder forms of barotrauma and generally require supportive care only.

🔍 Clinical Case Scenarios

A 65-year-old male patient is on 5 PEEP and 40% FiO_2 on ACMV mode. ABG done showed PaO_2 of > 60 mmHg. Prior to morning intensive care unit (ICU) rounds the ventilator setting is changed to low-pressure support ventilation. During rounds he is found to have RR of 30 per minute and TV of 200 cc.

7. What is his RSBI?

8. What would you do next?

   Next morning his RSBI is < 105 on low-pressure support. Extubation is attempted after rounds.

   Intubated ARDS patient develops swelling of face and neck and eyelids. Exam reveals crepitus over the neck and face.

9. What is the NSIDx (next step in diagnosis)?

10. If CXR is negative, what is the most likely dx?

VQ mismatch

Ventilation(V) in a lung zone should be matched with perfusion (Q) in that zone. The following are the types of VQ mismatch:

Dead space	Shunt
When perfusion is decreased to a well-ventilated area of the lung, then that part of the lung is defined as a dead space, where the ventilated volume of air will not participate in gas exchange. Think of this as dead air (space), which is useless. Classical example is pulmonary embolus	**Anatomic or vascular shunts**: blood passes from right side of heart to the left side bypassing the lungs/alveoli. This is known as right to left shunt Examples: pulmonary AV malformation, Eisenmenger's syndrome, cyanotic congenital heart disease, etc. **Physiological shunt**: An area with no ventilation, but with continuing perfusion creates intrapulmonary physiologic **shunt**[a]; blood is being passed through an area of lung with no gas exchange. This occurs when the alveoli are: • Collapsed (in atelectasis) • Filled with infiltrates (in lobar pneumonia or ARDS) • Filled with fluid (in pulmonary edema) To counteract this mismatch, reactive hypoxic pulmonary vasoconstriction does occur, but remember that compensation is never complete etc.[1]
Dead space = high V/Q ratio as denominator (perfusion) is low	Shunt= low V/Q ratio as **ventilation is low**.

[a]Hypoxemia due to anatomic/vascular shunts canot be corrected by supplemental oxygen. Physiologic shunting, on the other hand, is usually not a pure shunt. Supplemental oxygen will help in these cases.

How to find out the cause of acute respiratory failure by looking at ABG?

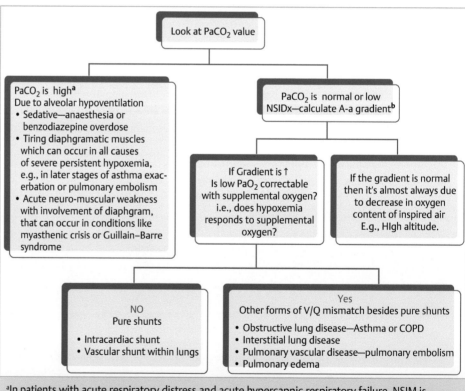

[a]In patients with acute respiratory distress and acute hypercapnic respiratory failure, NSIM is usually BIPAP or intubation. Patients at this stage are usually lethargic or comatose.[6]

[b]A–a gradient = Alveolar (P_AO_2) – arterial (P_aO_2) gradient. As alveolar (P_AO_2) is not easily obtainable, clinically the following formula is used to calculate A-a gradient = **(150 − 1.25 × P_aCO_2) − P_aO_2** (the normal value is < 15 mmHg). Increased gradient (in between the oxygen content of the alveoli and the oxygen content of the systemic arteries) means that there is intrinsic lung pathology. A–a gradient is not increased in hypoventilation or high altitude.

[6]On the other hand, chronic hypercapnia +/− hypoxemia can occur in COPD, obesity hypoventilation syndrome and extrinsic lung disease (e.g., severe kyphoscoliosis). It is usually well compensated by chronic metabolic alkalosis.

3.1.4 Acute Respiratory Distress Syndrome

Background: Any severe local lung injury (e.g. drowning) or severe extrapulmonary pathology (e.g. severe sepsis) can cause oversecretion of inflammatory mediators into the blood stream that can activate neutrophils, which in turn release proteases and free radicals, damaging the endo-thelial and epithelial layers of alveoli. This leads to high protein vascular fluid leakage into the alveoli which eventually fills most of the intra-alveolar space, thereby causing significant areas of shunting. This condition is called ARDS. Histopathological picture is of diffuse alveolar damage.[7]

[7]Possible long-term sequela of ARDS is pulmonary fibrosis.

Etiology

- **Systemic:** severe sepsis, trauma, burns, acute pancreatitis, drug overdose, toxins, transfusion related acute lung injury (TRALI), etc.
- **Pulmonary:** drowning, large volume aspiration, severe pneumonia, etc.

Diagnostic criteria

- Acute onset: within **1** week of initial insult.
- PaO_2/FiO_2 ratio of $\leq$ **200**.
- Bilateral infiltrates present on CXR.
- No clinical evidence of elevated left atrial pressure, or pulmonary capillary wedge pressure (PCWP) is $\leq$ 18 mmHg.

In patients with similar presentation, but PaO_2/FiO_2 ratio is > 200 (and < 300), the dx is acute lung injury (ALI).

Work-up: Transthoracic echocardiogram (TTE), and serum Brain natriuretic peptide (BNP) are good initial tests, as the major differential dx for ARDS is cardiogenic pulmonary edema. TTE is generally adequate to assess for evidence of heart failure. If large body habitus makes it hard to get a good quality TTE images and if assessment of volume status is needed, a Swan-Ganz catheter can help in direct measurement of cardiac pressures.

Rx: Always treat the underlying etiology. Mechanical ventilation is usually necessary. Recommended TV is 6 mL/kg of predicted body weight and plateau pressure (end inspiratory) of $\leq$ 30 cm H_2O, even if it results in mild hypercapnia and respiratory acidosis (permissive hypercapnia is tolerated until pH is < 7.2).[8]

MRS

123 for ARDS/ALI

[8]Lower TV strategy has been shown to have better outcome.

In ARDS of newborns (aka hyaline membrane disease [HMD] of the prematurity), the primary pathology is generalized collapse of alveoli due to deficient surfactant. So CXR picture in HMD of newborn will show ground-glass appearance of the lung as opposed to ARDS of adults that will show bilateral opacities.

Clinical Case Scenarios

A 41-year-old male admitted to ICU for severe pancreatitis now develops acute onset of respiratory symptoms with increasing SOB. ABG in 100% non-rebreather mask reveals PaO_2 of 40 mmHg. CXR shows diffuse bilateral infiltrates (see picture).

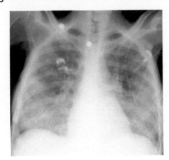

Source: Heart. In: Gunderman R. Essential radiology.
Clinical presentation, pathophysiology, imaging. 2nd ed.
Thieme; 2000.

11. What is the NSIDx?

12. What is the likely dx?

3.2 Pulmonary Function Tests

Indications

- Unexplained pulmonary symptoms.
- Monitoring known pulmonary disease.
- Preoperative assessment prior to lung resection.
- Differentiating between obstructive and restrictive lung disease.[9]

[9]If a patient presents with vague respiratory complaints and has hx of smoking as well as high-risk occupation (such as working in mining industry), test of choice is **spirometry**. It can differentiate between obstructive (COPD) and restrictive (asbestosis associated interstitial lung) disease.

Pulmonary function test includes

- Spirometry.
- Flow volume loop.
- Lung volumes.[10]
- Diffusion-lung capacity for carbon monoxide (DLCO).

[10]Spirometry cannot measure residual volume (RV) and any parameter that requires this value (e.g., function residual capacity or total lung capacity). This requires special techniques.

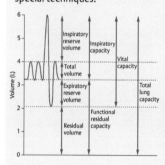

Pulmonary function test values in obstructive and restrictive lung disease

	Obstructive	**Restrictive**
General principle	It is characterized by decrease in **expiratory** flow rates in PFT. Narrowing of airway disproportionately affects expiratory phase, as airway is normally narrower in expiration	One of the classic examples of **restrictive lung diseases** is interstitial lung fibrosis. Imagine the lung as a **thick, stiff, small balloon** which is very hard to inflate (to inhale) and easy to deflate (exhale), as the recoil pressure of the stiff-fibrosed lung is very high
FEV	**Decreased**	**Decreased**
FVC	**Normal (or decreased)**	**Decreased**
FEV1/FVC[a] ratio	**Decreased**	N or ↑
TLC	↑	Decreased
RV	↑	Decreased
Functional residual capacity	↑	Decreased
DLCO[b]	Decreased	Emphysema, bronchiolitis obliterans[c] and bronchiectasis	Decreased	Primary pulmonary restrictive disorder, e.g., diffuse parenchymal lung disease (aka interstitial lung disease)
	Normal	Asthma[d] and chronic bronchitis	Normal	Extraparenchymal lung disorders[e]

[a]FEV_1/FVC = **F**orced **e**xpiratory **v**olume of air in **1** sec/**f**orced **v**ital **c**apacity (most important parameter we need to look at)

[b]DLCO is a measurement of alveolar diffusion capacity. This diffusion capacity is affected by decrease in surface area (e.g., emphysema) or decreased permeability (e.g., interstitial lung disease).[11]

[c]**Bronchiolitis obliterans (aka obliterative bronchiolitis)** is inflammatory condition of smallest airways. It can be either sudden in onset or slowly progressive. It presents with dry cough, SOB, and wheezing. Etiologies include lung, or bone-marrow transplantation, infection, connective tissue disorders, toxic fume inhalation, etc. Treatment is supportive as disease is irreversible and patients may go on to require lung transplantation.

[d]NSIDx after **PFTs suggest obstructive airway disease** is to do bronchodilator challenge (e.g., albuterol). If FEV_1 increases by ≥ 12% and/or increases by 200 mL from baseline, it indicates reversible airway obstruction suggestive of asthma.

[e]Examples

[11]High DLCO occurs in polycythemia and left to right shunt.
Decreased DLCO and normal PFTs can be seen in severe anemia, or primary pulmonary vascular disorder with no parenchymal involvement (e.g., pulmonary hypertension).

 MRS

ABC of the obstructive airway disease:
Asthma
Bronchiectasis, **b**ronchiolitis obliterans
COPD (chronic bronchitis and emphysema)

→ Chest wall disorder	⇒	Kyphoscoliosis
→ Extrinsic compression and restriction of lung movements	⇒	Massive ascites, obesity hypoventilation syndrome
→ Neuromuscular disorders	⇒	Myasthenia gravis or Guillain–Barre syndrome affecting the diaphragm

Note: These values (FEV$_1$, FVC, etc.) obtained from PFT are used for diagnosis, prognosis, evaluating progression of disease, and treatment response. So, PFT is "the" diagnostic test of choice for most of the chronic respiratory disorders.

Abbreviations: DLCO, diffusion capacity of lung for carbon mono oxide; RV, residual volume; TLC, total lung capacity Residual volume.

Let's practice some values

- First trick is to look only at percentage of predicted value. The normal value is usually 80 to 120% (100 +/− 20). Low is <80%. The only exception is forced expiratory volume$_1$/forced vital capacity (FEV$_1$/FVC) ratio, where the cut off for low value is < 70%.
- Second trick is to first look at FEV$_1$/FVC to categorize it as obstructive or restrictive and then look at DLCO to find out the subtype.

MRS

LOAD ratio (LOw FEV$_1$/FVC **ratio** is **o**bstructive **a**irway **d**isease.
If it helps, another way to look at this MRS is to see **70 in LO**; L looks like 7. So, the cut-off value for this ratio is 70, whereas for everything else, it is 80.

FEV$_1$ (%)	FEV$_1$/FVC (%)	DLCO (%)	Diagnosis
75	69	75	FEV$_1$/FVC is low = obstructive airway disease. DLCO low = emphysema, bronchiolitis obliterans, or extensive bronchiectasis disease
75	75	65	FEV$_1$/FVC is normal = restrictive lung disease. DLCO low = diffuse parenchymal lung disease
60	65	80	Asthma or chronic bronchitis. NSIDx is bronchodilator challenge test
70	90	90	Chest wall disorder, neuromuscular issue, massive ascites or obesity hypoventilation syndrome. Note that FEV$_1$ is low (abnormal)
85	90	75	Normal FEV$_1$ with low DLCO = anemia or primary pulmonary vascular disorder

3.2.1 Flow Volume Loop

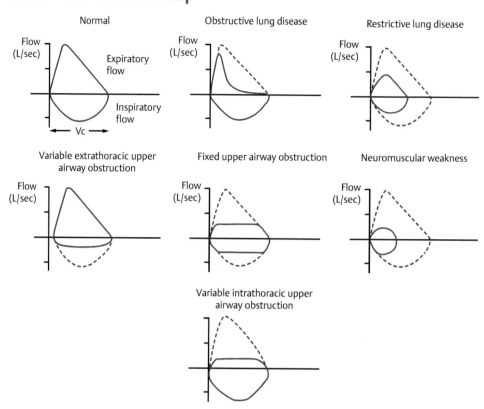

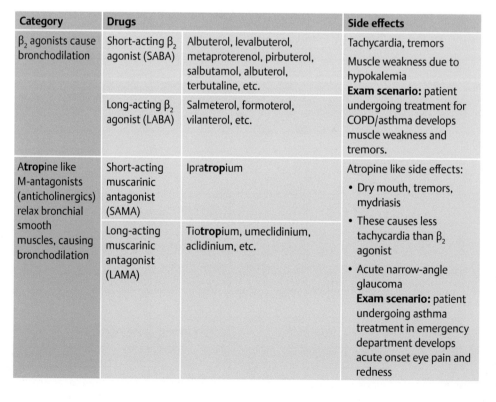

Commonly used medications for obstructive airway disease

ABC of the obstructive airway disease:
Asthma
Bronchiectasis, **b**ronchiolitis obliterans
COPD (chronic bronchitis and emphysema)

 MRS

For β2 agonists, look for suffix +terol

Category	Drugs		Side effects
β₂ agonists cause bronchodilation	Short-acting β₂ agonist (SABA)	Albuterol, levalbuterol, metaproterenol, pirbuterol, salbutamol, albuterol, terbutaline, etc.	Tachycardia, tremors Muscle weakness due to hypokalemia **Exam scenario:** patient undergoing treatment for COPD/asthma develops muscle weakness and tremors.
	Long-acting β₂ agonist (LABA)	Salmeterol, formoterol, vilanterol, etc.	
Atropine like M-antagonists (anticholinergics) relax bronchial smooth muscles, causing bronchodilation	Short-acting muscarinic antagonist (SAMA)	Ipratropium	Atropine like side effects: • Dry mouth, tremors, mydriasis • These causes less tachycardia than β₂ agonist • Acute narrow-angle glaucoma **Exam scenario:** patient undergoing asthma treatment in emergency department develops acute onset eye pain and redness
	Long-acting muscarinic antagonist (LAMA)	Tiotropium, umeclidinium, aclidinium, etc.	

Corticosteroids decrease airway inflammation	Inhaled corticosteroids	Fluticasone, beclomethasone, mometasone, budesonide, flunisolide, ciclesonide	• Low to mid dose-inhaled steroids usually only have local side effects such as dysphonia (changes in voice) and oral candidiasis • High dose can cause systemic side effects similar to oral steroids
	Oral corticosteroids	Prednisone, prednisolone	Frequent use (e.g., in patients with multiple exacerbation) may lead to development of drug-induced Cushing's syndrome
	Intravenous corticosteroids	Methylprednisolone or hydrocortisone	

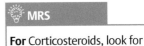

MRS

For Corticosteroids, look for suffix +sone or +ide

3.3 Asthma

Pathophysiology: A disorder of hyperactive airways due to inflammatory response to generally innocuous stimuli (such as allergens, cold, exercise, etc.), which lead to the following changes:

- **B**ronchospasm
- **A**irway edema
- **M**ucosal hypersecretion

Depending upon the stimuli, asthma can be divided into the following categories:

MRS

BAM

Atopic (aka extrinsic or allergic) asthma	• Attacks are precipitated by allergens (e.g., molds, dust mites, pollen, animal dander, feather, dust, food, cockroaches, etc.). MC trigger is **house dust mites.** • Patients may have history of other type I hypersensitivity reactions, such as allergic rhinitis, urticaria, or atopic dermatitis • Complete blood count may show **eosinophilia** • Allergy skin prick testing is recommended to find specific triggers and to avoid them. If not available, blood radioallergosorbent test, (which measures specific IgE levels to common allergens), can be done • Generally, this kind of asthma has better prognosis than late-onset nonatopic asthma
Intrinsic (aka idiosyncratic or nonatopic) asthma	• Attacks are precipitated by nonimmunologic stimuli such as infections, cold air, exercise, emotional upset, etc.
Occupational asthma	• Reaction to chemicals, irritants, or allergen exposure at work • Work-related symptom history should be obtained in all asthma patients • If this dx is suspected, NSIDx is PFTs before and after work or during vacation.
Reactive airway dysfunction syndrome	This can result from a single, accidental inhalation of large amounts of respiratory irritants like gas, smoke, fume, or vapor (chlorine gas, bleach, ammonia, etc.) • Dx is based upon history of exposure, and subsequent development of asthma syndrome in a patient with no prior history of pulmonary disease

Classic presentation: Acute sudden onset of wheezing and shortness of breath[12] that comes and goes. In earlier stages, patients are mostly asymptomatic in between the attacks. If asthma is not properly controlled, it can progress to fixed airway obstruction and at this stage patients can have persistent SOB or wheezing.

[12] Asthma can also present with hx of paroxysms of acute cough episodes (cough-variant asthma).

Diagnosis

- PFT is most helpful in confirming the dx of asthma
- **If FEV$_1$ or FEV$_1$/FVC is reduced (in moderate to severe asthma)**, NSIM is bronchodilator challenge (e.g., albuterol). If repeat PFT shows ≥ 12% increase in FEV$_1$ and/or increase in 200 mL from baseline, this indicates reversibility of airway obstruction, suggestive of asthma.
- **If FEV$_1$ and FEV$_1$/FVC is normal, then NSIDx is either**
  - Bronchoprovocation test by using inhaled methacholine, mannitol or exercise testing.
    or
  - Serial measurement of FEV$_1$ or peak expiratory flow (PEF) at home or in office. A variability of ≥ 20%, corresponding with symptoms is suggestive of asthma.

3.3.1 Principles of Asthma Management

- Prevent exposure to stimuli and treat other associated comorbidities that can worsen asthma (e.g., gastroesophageal reflux disease [GERD], morbid obesity, sinusitis, etc.).
- Prevent asthma attacks (long-term management).
- Treat acute asthma exacerbation.
- Diagnose and manage complications.

Long-term management of asthma

Intensity of therapy depends on frequency and timing of attacks, as shown in the table below.

Frequency of symptoms during daytime	Frequency of symptoms during nighttime	Baseline FEV$_1$	Asthma severity	Treatment
2 or less days/week	2 or less nights/month	Normal	**Intermittent asthma**	No daily medication; just SABA (e.g., albuterol) as needed
> 2 days/week	More than 2 nights/month	Normal	**Persistent asthma (mild)**	Low-dose inhaled steroids (**LDIS**) should be given
Daily occurrence of symptom (acute SOB and wheezing occurring at least once every day)	2 or more nights/week	Low (< 80)	**Persistent asthma (moderate)**	LDIS + LABA[a] If not yet well controlled, NSIM is medium dose inhaled steroids (MDIS) + LABA
Continuous symptoms (SOB and/or wheezing throughout the day)	Frequent (nightly awakening)	< 60	**Persistent asthma (severe)**	High dose inhaled steroids (HDIS) + LABA[b] If not yet well controlled, NSIM is oral steroids[c]

[a]In asthma, LABA is not used alone and is always given in combination with inhaled steroids. Using LABA alone has been shown to increase risk of asthma-related complications. In contrast, LABA can be given alone in COPD.[13]

[b]When patients are on HDIS evaluate for appropriateness of omalizumab (monoclonal IgG antibody to IgE). Omalizumab is indicated in patients who have evidence of allergy in skin testing and IgE levels between 30 and 700 IU/mL. If IgE levels are too low, giving antibody to IgE is useless. If IgE levels are too high, antibodies to IgE are overwhelmed by the amount of IgE .

[c]Some patients with severe asthma might require chronic use of systemic steroids. In these patients an FDA approved procedure, called bronchial thermoplasty can be considered, which consists of bronchoscopy-mediated application of heat to reduce smooth muscle hypertrophy and obstruction.

Abbreviations: LABA, long-acting β$_2$ agonist; SABA, shortong-acting β$_2$ agonist; SOB, shortness of breath.

[13]In asthma, inhaled steroids have been shown to have the maximal benefit on the patient's long-term quality of life. They work by reducing the airway reactivity, edema, and inflammation.

Few notes on long-term management of asthma

- Use of short-acting β_2 agonist (SABA) > two times/week for acute symptoms indicates poor asthma control and signals the need for step-up of therapy.
- If asthma is well controlled, always attempt to reduct dosage or discontinue inhaled steroids. This strategy will reduce incidence of side-effects (step-down management)
- Consider subcutaneous allergen desensitization therapy in patients with persistent atopic asthma.
- In patients with persistent asthma, alternative therapies such as mast cell stabilizers (cromolyn or nedocromil), theophylline, and leukotriene receptor antagonist (zafi rlukast and montelukast) can also be considered.

Clinical Case Scenarios

13. Patient has hx of asthma and is on low-dose inhaled steroids (LDIS). He complains of wheezing and SOB every day for the last one week. What is the severity of asthma? What is the NSIM?

14. Patient has hx of asthma and is on LDIS+ long-acting β_2 agonist (LABA). Currently patient reports that for the last few months, he has had to use his rescue inhaler (albuterol) only two times per week. What is the NSIM?

15. Patient has hx of asthma and is on LDIS. Patient has FEV_1 of 50 in office. She reports that this is her baseline and feels SOB throughout the day. What is the severity of asthma? What is the NSIM?

16. Patient has hx of moderate persistent asthma and is on LDIS +LABA. Patient reports waking up at least two times per week with SOB. What is the NSIM?

3.3.2 Acute Asthma Attack

Example CCS: Patient with hx of asthma comes to emergency department (ED) with acute onset of shortness of breath(sob). Exam reveals diffuse wheezing. Peak expiratory flow rate (PEFR) at beside is 220 L/minute. Patient's predicted PEFR value is 350. Patient's PEFR is 62% of predicted (as 220/350 = 0.62).

Algorithm for guidelines on acute asthma exacerbation management

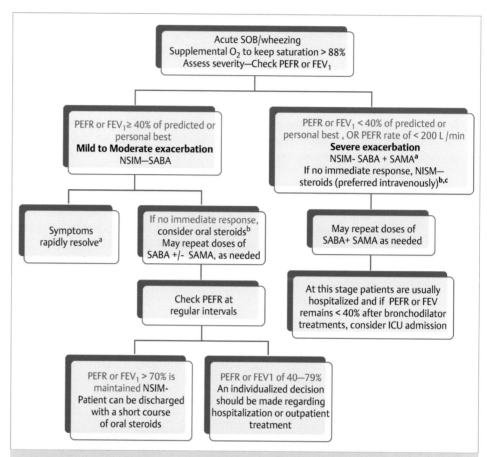

Legend: NSIM, next step in management; SABA, short-acting B$_2$ agonist (albuterol); SAMA, short-acting muscarinic antagonist (e.g., ipratropium); PEFR, peak expiratory flow rate.

[a]If patient improves after the first bronchodilator treatment with **PEFR of > 70%** of predicted or personal best, patient can be discharged without systemic steroids.

[b]After first round of SABA +/− SAMA, if patient still has persistent wheezing and no improvement, NSIM is to give steroids (oral or intravenous). Time to order CXR.[14]

[c]If any of the following signs/symptoms are present, even after adequate bronchodilator therapy, NSIM is to **consider intubation and IV magnesium sulfate.**

- Patient has difficulty talking and cannot complete sentences due to respiratory distress.
- Altered mental status.
- Cyanosis.
- Pulsus paradoxus.[15]
- Inaudible or decreased breath sounds on lung exam: in this scenario, the airway obstruction is so severe that there is no air movement (clinically called **silent chest).**
- PaCO$_2$ is N or ↑ : PaCO$_2$ is low in acute asthmatic attack, due to tachypnea and hyperventilation, but if PaCO$_2$ is **N** or ↑ then it is either due to severe obstruction or patient's respiratory muscles are tiring.[16]

[14]In asthma exacerbation, CXR is usually normal or may just show hyperinflated lungs.

[15]There is so much lung hyperinflation that it is increasing the intrathoracic pressure, leading to greater than expected drop in systolic pulse pressure (> 20 mmHg) on inspiration. (The pathophysiology is similar to auto-PEEP.)

[16]Decision to intubate should not be made based on ABG alone. If ABG shows PaO$_2$ of > 60 mmHg and high PaCO$_2$, but patient is speaking in full sentences and clinically appears better, then intubation is likely not necessary. In this case, patient is likely improving from severe asthma attack and is responding to treatment.

Acute asthma management—additional points

- Prior to discharge remember the indications for vaccination which include flu and pneumococcal vaccination (same schedule as in COPD). Also, assess underlying severity of asthma (to prescribe LDIS or MDIS or LABA, if needed).
- Antibiotics are only indicated if there is hx suggestive of bacterial bronchitis or pneumonia.
- Do not give mast cell stabilizers (nedocromil and cromolyn sodium) for acute episode.

3.3.3 Other Forms of Asthma

Exercise-induced asthma	SOB and wheezing occurring only during or after exercise. It happens because of mast cell degranulation and histamine-mediated airway reactivity induced by exercise **Rx:** SABA or mast cell stabilizers prior to exercise
Nocturnal asthma	Cough and/or SOB only at night **Rx:** General asthma management principles apply here too
Pseudoallergic reaction to aspirin/NSAIDs	**Pathophysiology:** Aspirin/NSAIDs inhibit COX enzyme (cyclooxygenase pathway), but not the LOX (lipoxygenase) pathway. Their use may lead to overactivation of lipoxygenase pathway, with resultant overproduction of leukotrienes, which are proinflammatory to airways. This inflammation can also involve nasal passages leading to development of rhinosinusitis and inflammatory nasal polyps **Presentation scenario:** new-onset episodic SOB and wheezing, and/or nasal congestion and snoring (due to rhinosinusitis/polyp). It can occur in children or adults **Diagnosis:** it is made clinically; look for history of chronic aspirin/NSAIDs use (exam scenario may say some OTC pain medication) **Management:** DOC is leukotriene receptor antagonist (zafirlukast and montelukast). Avoid aspirin or NSAIDs. If underlying condition requires treatment with NSAIDs or aspirin, NSIM is desensitization

Abbreviations: COX, cyclooxygenase; DOC, drug of choice; NSAID, nonsteroidal anti-inflammatory drug; OTC, over the counter; SABA, short-acting β_2 agonist; SOB, shortness of breath.

Conditions presenting with asthma-like symptoms (*low yield*)

Patients with the following conditions can present with **difficult to control asthma** or worsening asthma symptoms in a previously well-controlled patient:

Syndrome	Eosinophilic granulomatosis with polyangiitis (formerly known as Churg–Strauss syndrome)	Chronic eosinophilic pneumonia	Allergic bronchopulmonary aspergillosis (ABPA)
Common to all		Asthma-like presentation + eosinophilia	
Specific organ involvement	Lungs + other organ involvement, such as • **Colon:** colitis • **Nerves:** sensory loss • **Upper airway:** e.g., recurrent otitis media, allergic rhinitis, sinusitis, etc. • **Skin:** palpable purpura	**Only** lungs are involved	**Only** lungs are involved
Additional clues that point toward the diagnosis	Use of leukotriene antagonist therapy leads to worsening of disease	Flu like syndrome (e.g. low-grade fever, malaise), weight loss, night sweats, etc.	Increasing severity of asthma or COPD, with thick-brownish phlegm production
CXR/CT scan picture	Migratory or transient interstitial infiltrates	Infiltrates with peripheral or pleural-based distribution (it is photographic opposite of pulmonary edema which as infiltrates predominant in perihilar region)	• Upper zone opacities • Findings of bronchiectasis • Atelectasis due to mucoid impaction
Workup	• Serum ANCA • Elevated IgE • Biopsy of affected area confirms the dx (e.g., skin or peripheral nerve)	NSIDx is bronchoalveolar lavage which will show ≥ 25% eosinophils	• **1st Screening test:** skin prick test with aspergillus antigen, or check serum anti-aspergillus IgE antibody. • **NSIDx:** check total IgE levels (elevated), peripheral eosinophilia count, and aspergillus-specific IgG antibody • CT scan of chest is also done
Management	Systemic corticosteroids	Systemic corticosteroids	• Systemic corticosteroids • Itraconazole or voriconazole is indicated for patients who cannot be tapered off steroids, or who have acute ABPA exacerbation

Abbreviations: ANCA, antineutrophil cytoplasmic antibodies; COPD, chronic obstructive pulmonary disease.

[17] Of all chronic smokers, 10 to 15% develop COPD. Ninety percent of COPD patients have smoking history.

3.4 Chronic Obstructive Pulmonary Disease

Pathophysiology: Long-term exposure to irritants, such as tobacco smoking, air pollution, exposure to poorly ventilated cooking and heating fires (particularly in developing world), and genetic factors can lead to an inflammatory response in the lungs, causing COPD.[17] It presents with chronic SOB and exercise intolerance. It typically worsens over time.

COPD comprises of emphysema and chronic bronchitis.[18]

[18] Patients with COPD may not have a clear-cut emphysema or chronic bronchitis. These frequently coexist and the management is similar.

	Emphysema	**Chronic bronchitis**
Pathology	Destruction of alveolar walls and respiratory bronchioles with subsequent loss in diffusion surface area	Chronic airway inflammation with mucosal hypersecretion (chronic productive cough) and hypertrophy (obstruction)
Clinical features	Patients have normal oxygenation (pink) but as the lungs are hard to deflate (due to poor lung recoil and diaphragmatic flattening), patients typically must puff out the air (puffers). Hence known as "Pink puffers"	**Early stage:** chronic sputum production (*look for this to make a clinical dx of chronic bronchitis*) **Late stage:** chronic hypoxemia (blue cyanotic) → reactive chronic pulmonary vasoconstriction → pulmonary HTN → right heart failure → edema (bloating) Hence known as blue bloaters.
CXR findings	• Decreased pulmonary vascular markings • Hyperinflation with diaphragmatic flattening (diaphragmatic flattening increases the work of breathing)	Increased pulmonary vascular markings
Main differentiating feature in PFT[a]	DLCO is decreased	DLCO is normal

[a]**The diagnosis of COPD is made with PFT:** FEV_1/FVC ratio remains < 70% after bronchodilator challenge (signifying irreversible obstruction).

Abbreviations: DLCO, diffusion lung capacity for carbon monoxide; HTN, hypertension; PFT, pulmonary function test.

3.4.1 General Principles of COPD Management

- Smoking cessation (**most important** intervention that increases long-term survival rate).
- Symptomatic control to improve quality of life.
- Pulmonary rehabilitation program is recommended in patients with FEV_1 < 50% of predicted. This has been shown to improve SOB and quality of life.
- Pharmacological measures (see section below).
- Treatment of acute exacerbation of COPD.
- Long-term home oxygen therapy (increases long-term survival rate) in select patients.
- **Vaccination:** flu vaccine is given every year. For pneumococcal vaccine give PPSV23 alone at diagnosis. After 5 years or at the age of 65 (whichever comes late) give PCV13 followed by PPSV23 (booster dose).[19]

[19] All chronic lung diseases have this same schedule (e.g., asthma, bronchiectasis, interstitial lung disease, etc.)

Pharmacological measures to improve symptoms in COPD

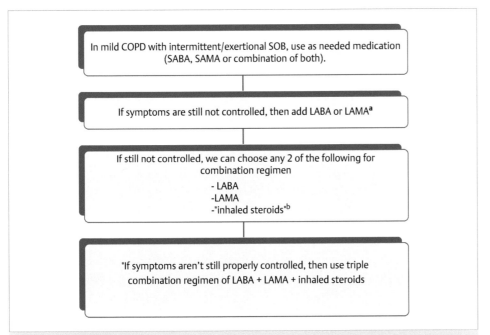

In mild COPD with intermittent/exertional SOB, use as needed medication (SABA, SAMA or combination of both).

If symptoms are still not controlled, then add LABA or LAMA[a]

If still not controlled, we can choose any 2 of the following for combination regimen
- LABA
- LAMA
- "inhaled steroids"[b]

"If symptoms aren't still properly controlled, then use triple combination regimen of LABA + LAMA + inhaled steroids

[a]LAMA is generally preferred because it is associated with reduced rate of exacerbation and it is also a once daily medication. Unlike asthma, in COPD inhaled steroids isn't the 1st line therapy. In COPD, inhaled steroids have not been shown to alter long-term decline in FEV1; in-fact in old patients with advanced disease, inhaled steroids may actually increase the risk of pneumonia.[20]

[b]In patients with evidence of reversibility of airway obstruction (asthmatic component), a combination regimen with LAMA or LABA + inhaled steroids might be preferred.

Abbreviations: NSIM, next step in management; SA BA/LABA, short-acting/long-acting B[2] agonist; SAMA/LAMA, short-acting/long-acting muscarinic antagonist.

[20] In COPD, inhaled steroids should not be used alone: use only in conjunction with either LABA or LAMA. In asthma, LABA should not be used alone: use only in conjunction with inhaled steroids.

Other treatment modalities for refractory disease

Theophylline: It can be considered in patients with poor exercise tolerance despite triple therapy.

• Coadministration of drugs that inhibit cytochrome enzyme pathway (e.g., erythromycin, H[2] blockers, macrolides, quinolones, etc.) may result in high drug levels and increased toxicity. • Symptoms of toxicity are related to stimulation of various systems, as aminophylline is a stimulant drug. Symptoms are as follows: - **Central nervous system stimulation:** headache, insomnia, and seizures - **Cardiovascular stimulation:** arrhythmias - **Gastrointestinal stimulation:** nausea, vomiting, and diarrhea	Coadministration of cytochrome enzyme pathways inducers (e.g., phenobarbitals, rifampin) will result in low therapeutic levels

Roflumilast (oral phosphodiesterase inhibitor)	• It is indicated in patients with severe COPD with chronic bronchitis and frequent exacerbations, despite triple therapy. It has been shown to reduce the frequency of exacerbations. exacerbations it is not used for patients with primary emphysema • It is contraindicated in patients with moderate to severe liver cirrhosis and depression
Chronic low-dose azithromycin therapy	Azithromycin also has anti-inflammatory effect. This can be considered, in-lieu of roflumilast in patients with frequent COPD exacerbations. Avoid this in patients with prolonged QT-interval.
Lung volume reduction surgery	In some carefully chosen patients with **severe emphysematous disease** who are good surgical candidates, this has been shown to improve quality of life and exercise capacity. Other alternative is placement of endobronchial valves.
Lung transplantation	Appropriate in patients with advanced COPD who are good surgical candidates, i.e., young patients with no major comorbidities. Active substance abuse is absolute contraindication.

Quick note:
Think of bronchiolitis obliterans when patients with hx of lung transplantation present with progressive SOB, several years after lung transplant. This is a result of chronic allograft rejection.

[21] Acute pulmonary infection can lead to acute inflammation and development of generalized acute bronchospasm.

[22] Patients with acute SOB should always have an EKG done (to rule out angina equivalent).
In patients with acute COPD exacerbation, EKG may reveal atrial arrhythmias like multiple atrial tachycardia (narrow-complex tachycardia with different P waves), or atrial flutter/fibrillation.

[23] These are the same organisms that commonly cause sinusitis, bronchitis, and otitis media, hence same antibiotics are given.

[24] Unlike in asthma, patients with COPD might have chronic hypercapnia, hence normal or elevated P_aCO_2 itself is not an indicator of severe COPD.

Quick note:
In patients with recurring COPD exacerbations or recent multiple hospitalizations, consider causes such as ongoing significant tobacco abuse, infection with hard to treat or resistant organisms (e.g. pseudomonas, stenotrophomonas), Mycobacterium avium complex (MAC) infection, Allergic bronchopulmonary aspergillosis (ABPA), aspiration, etc.

3.4.2 Acute Exacerbation of COPD

Definition: It is characterized by acute worsening of respiratory status more than patient's baseline.

Etiology: Pulmonary infection (MCC of exacerbation[21]), continuing tobacco abuse, heart failure, pulmonary embolism, sinusitis, etc.

Presentation: Typically presents with increased SOB, and auscultatory finding of **bilateral wheezing** or, absent/decreased breath sounds. Look for symptoms of underlying cause (e.g., increased yellow phlegm production in patients with acute infection).

Management steps

- Immediate step in management (SIM) is supplemental oxygen.
- NSIDx is pulse oximetry, CXR, and electrocardiography (EKG)[22] +/− ABG.
- **Bronchodilators:** The most effective immediate treatment is combination of inhaled short-acting muscarinic antagonist (SAMA; ipratropium bromide) + SABA (albuterol).
- **Corticosteroid therapy** (IV or oral): It decreases the intensity of symptoms and reduces the duration of hospital stay. Usually short course is recommended (5–7 days).
- **Empiric antibiotic therapy:** it is indicated in patients with history of increased sputum volume or purulence. Use any of the following: azithromycin, third-generation cephalosporins (cefpodoxime, cefdinir), respiratory fluoroquinolones (e.g., levofloxacin), trimethoprim-sulfamethoxazole, or doxycycline. These cover *Streptococcus pneumoniae*, *Haemophilus Influenzae*, and *Moraxella catarrhalis*.[23]

After general treatment measures (mentioned above), if patient continues to have moderate to severe dyspnea with use of accessory muscles, paradoxical abdominal wall motion, severe respiratory acidosis (pH < 7.35[24]) **and/or** RR of > 25/minute, look at the following management algorithm:

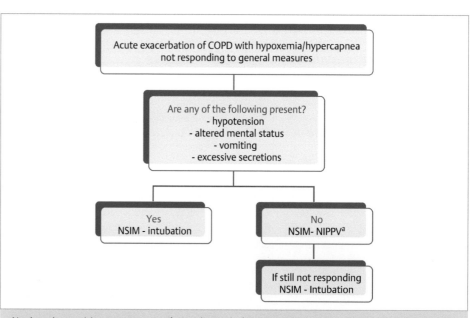

[a] Noninvasive positive pressure ventilation (NIPPV) aka BiPAP is given through a tight-fitting mask. Intubation carries its own risks and needs to be avoided when possible.

Predictors of poor prognosis in COPD

- FEV_1 after bronchodilator inhalation is the best predictor of survival; the lower FEV_1, worse the prognosis.
- **Rapid rate of FEV_1 decline:** all patients should have regular follow up spirometry. If there is a rapid decline, then assess for compliance and most importantly, make sure patient is not continuing to **smoke.**
- Presence of comorbidities, emphysema in CT scan and poor exercise tolerance also predict poor outcome.

Indications for long-term oxygen therapy in chronic lung disease

	Use either or PaO_2 or SaO_2	
	Resting PaO_2	Resting SaO_2
General indications	≤ 55 mmHg	≤ 88%
In patients who have any of the following complications of lung disease, use lower cut-off values: Pulmonary HTN, cor pulmonale (P-pulmonale on EKG), or hematocrit > 55% (polycythemia)	≤ 59 mmHg	≤ 89%

Patients who desaturate (SaO_2 ≤ 88%) with ambulation and feel SOB may benefit from supplemental oxygen.

3.4.3 Alpha-1 Antitrypsin Deficiency

Pathophysiology: Genetic deficiency of this protease inhibitor protein leads to excessive destruction of lung and/or liver tissue by proteolytic enzymes such as elastase.

Presentation and clinical features

- Onset is at 45 years of age or earlier.
- Positive family hx of lung and/or liver disease.
- No occupational risk factor or significant smoking history.
- Presence of panlobular emphysema[25] with bibasilar predominance (see MRS box).
- Coexisting unexplained liver disease (e.g., neonatal hepatitis, cirrhosis).[26]

Work-up: Measure serum alpha-1 antitrypsin levels. If low, NSIDx is genetic testing.

Management: Intravenous human alpha-1 antitrypsin is indicated for select patients. Smoking cessation is important.

 MRS

Smoking is an inhalation related injury; smoke levitates up and predominantly cause upper lung injury. In alpha-1 antitrypsin deficiency, there is predominantly bibasilar emphysema (as shown below)

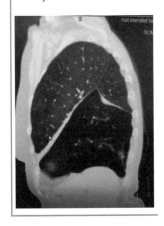

[25] Emphysema due to smoking is centrilobular.
[26] Absence of liver disease does not exclude alpha-1 antitrypsin deficiency.

Pulmonology

Clinical Case Scenarios

17. Patient with hx of asthma comes to your office with SOB and wheezing. After administration of one dose of albuterol, patient's SOB resolves with no residual symptoms. What is the NSIM?

    A. Oral steroids.

    B. Administer inhaled albuterol + ipratropium combination.

    C. Assess underlying severity of asthma.

    D. Repeat inhaled albuterol.

18. Patient with hx of asthma comes to ED with SOB. PEFR is 220 L/minute. (predicted PEFR value is 350 L/minute). 220/350 = 0.62. Patient's PEFR is 62% of predicted. What is the immediate NSIM?

    A. Oral steroids.

    B. Administer inhaled albuterol + ipratropium combination.

    C. Administer inhaled albuterol.

19. Patient with hx of asthma comes to ED with acute onset severe SOB. Patient appears cyanotic. Lung exam reveals poor air movement and no wheezing. What is the immediate NSIM?

    A. Intubation.

    B. Administer inhaled albuterol + ipratropium combination.

    C. Administer inhaled albuterol.

    D. IV steroids.

20. A 75-year-old male with hx of COPD comes in for regular follow-up. In office, his oxygen saturation on room air is 88%. Patient reports that this is how he generally feels at baseline. What is the NSIM?

21. A 65-year-old male with COPD exacerbation is brought in by emergency medical service on 100% non-rebreather oxygen mask. Patient is obtunded. His pulse oximetry reveals 100% oxygen saturation. What is the likely diagnosis?

    A. Acute hypercapnic respiratory failure due to severe COPD exacerbation.

    B. Acute hyperoxic hypercapnic respiratory failure.

22. A 65-year-old female patient is in the hospital receiving treatment for acute asthma/COPD exacerbation. 2 to 3 days later complete blood count (CBC) reveals elevated WBCs and neutrophilia. Patient reports that she has had no fever and is feeling better day by day. What is the likely cause of leukocytosis?

23. Patient, currently hospitalized for severe exacerbation of COPD/asthma, develops palpitations, muscle weakness, and tremors. What is the most likely cause of this side effect?

    A. Steroids.

    B. Albuterol.

    C. Ipratropium.

24. A 75-year-old male with hx of COPD comes in for regular follow-up. Exam reveals bilateral clubbing. What is the NSIM?

25. A patient with COPD presents with symptoms of urinary tract infection. He receives ciprofloxacin. Few days later he presents with nausea, vomiting, and an episode of seizure. What is the likely diagnosis?

3.5 Bronchiectasis

Background: Chronic destruction of bronchial walls leading to permanent dilatation of small and medium sized bronchi.

27

Involvement	Etiology
Localized bronchiectasis	As a sequela of lung infection that was severe, recurrent or chronic (e.g., tuberculosis, fungal infection, lung abscess, recurrent postobstructive pneumonia, foreign body aspiration)
Generalized bronchiectasis	Most often develops in patients with genetic and/or immunologic defects that affect the airways • Cystic fibrosis (discussed on next page) • Kartagener's syndrome (immotile cilia syndrome) • Alpha-1 antitrypsin deficiency (can cause both COPD and bronchiectasis) • Immunodeficiency syndromes: IgA deficiency, IgG deficiency (common-variable immune-deficiency syndrome), selective IgG deficiency, etc. If hx is suspicious for these disorders, check immunoglobulin levels and IgG subclass level . Subclass levels will help to diagnose selective IgG deficiency, as total IgG leves can be normal in this case.

Normal bronchi

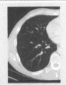

There should not be large bronchi like bronchioles in the periphery
Source: Lung. In: Gunderman R. Essential radiology. Clinical presentation, pathophysiology, imaging. 3rd ed. Thieme; 2014.

Advanced bronchiectasis in the lower lobe

Some airways are partially filled with secretions
Source: Dyspnea. In: Siegenthaler W. Siegenthaler's differential diagnosis in internal medicine: from symptom to diagnosis. 1st ed. Thieme; 2007.

Presentation: Patients typically have hx of daily mucopurulent sputum production over months to years. They may also present with complications such as acute hemoptysis or recurrent pulmonary infection.

Work-up

- CXR will classically reveal increased pulmonary vascular markings, ring shadows, peribronchial thickening and/or linear atelectasis.
- **Best step in Dx** is high-resolution CT scan (HRCT).[27]
- Sputum gram stain and culture should be sent for bacteria, mycobacteria, and fungi along with acid fast bacilli stain times three.[28]
- In case of localized bronchiectasis of unclear cause, NSIM/NSIDx is flexible bronchoscopy.

Management of acute exacerbation of bronchiectasis

[28]Primary infection with nontuberculous mycobacteria (e.g., mycobacterium avium complex) can cause bronchiectasis.

Mild pulmonary infection	Patients present with increased cough and mucus production only. In this case use different antibiotic with each episode. This is called rotatory antibiotic regimen, which diminishes emergence of bacterial resistance. Use amoxicillin–clavulanic acid, trimethoprim–sulfamethoxazole, doxycycline, azithromycin, or third-generation cephalosporins[MRS-I]
Hospitalized patient with pulmonary infection	• Presents with fever, increased purulent sputum production, and prominent changes in CXR. In this case, use an antibiotic that covers pseudomonas • In very sick patients, double antipseudomonal regimen can be considered. Possible combinations include: - Piperacillin/tazobactam +/– aminoglycosides or ciprofloxacin - Cefepime +/– aminoglycosides or ciprofloxacin

MRS

[MRS-I]These are the same antibiotics given in otitis media, sinusitis, bronchitis and in COPD patients.

Treatment strategy in all bronchiectasis patients

- Bronchodilators and chest physiotherapy to facilitate drainage of bronchial secretions.
- Surgical therapy may be considered for localized bronchiectasis.
- In patients with more than two exacerbations per year, preventive macrolide therapy is indicated.
- Vaccination: flu and pneumococcal vaccine (same schedule as in COPD).
- Long-term oxygen therapy for hypoxic patients.

Complications

- Chronic hypoxemia that can lead to cor pulmonale or secondary polycythemia.
- Massive hemoptysis (it may be acute and life threatening).
- Secondary amyloidosis.

3.6 Cystic Fibrosis

Background: An autosomal recessive genetic disorder caused by mutation of **c**ystic **f**ibrosis **t**ransmembrane-conductance **r**egulator (CFTR) gene in chromosome 7. This leads to combination of defective chloride secretion and increased sodium reabsorption across epithelial cells in exocrine glands of lung, pancreas, liver, intestinal epithelium, etc. Increased Na⁺ reabsorption results in increased water reabsorption. This leads to formation of thick, viscous mucus that is hard to clear out, causing plugging (inspissation) and predisposes to recurrent inflammation/infection.

Various presentation scenarios

Clinical Tip: Patients can present with symptoms of cystic fibrosis for the first time as an adult.

- Meconium ileus, intussusception, and small bowel obstruction (in infants and children).
- Recurrent respiratory infections: recurrent sinusitis, inflammatory nasal polyps, otitis media, recurrent pneumonia leading to bronchiectasis, and chronic infection with *Staphylococcus aureus*, *Pseudomonas*, and *Burkholderia*.
- Acute pancreatitis → chronic pancreatitis → pancreatic insufficiency → malabsorption, steatorrhea, weight loss, and diabetes mellitus.
- Chronic bile duct inflammation due to bile inspissation may lead to biliary cirrhosis. Patients may end up needing transplantation.
- Infertility: It is due to defective sperm transport and/or incompletely developed or absent vas deferens, in men. In women, it is due to thick cervical mucus and cachexia leading to menstrual abnormalities.

[29] Cystic fibrosis can be caused by various mutations; thus, DNA studies are not that reliable.

Work-up: NSIDx is **sweat chloride test** (Cl⁻ ≥ 60 mEq/L is diagnostic). In this test, topical pilocarpine is used to induce sweating.[29]

Management of lung disease

- For persistent airway secretions, NSIM is treatment with aerosolized human recombinant DNase. This is useful to break up inspissated mucus. Hypertonic saline along with SABA and chest physiotherapy are also recommended.
- In patients with bronchiectasis, manage as given in bronchiectasis section.
- Consider lung transplantation if disease progresses despite conservative management.

3.7 Hemoptysis

Etiology of massive hemoptysis (large amount and/or rapid rate of hemoptysis)

- Bronchiectasis (MCC), tuberculosis, bronchogenic carcinoma—*these are the three most common cause of massive hemoptysis.*
- Lung abscess, fungal infection (histoplasmosis or blastomycosis), and aspergilloma.
- Severe bronchitis with underlying coagulopathy.
- Pulmonary emboli causing pulmonary infarction, in those who are on anticoagulation.
- Granulomatous polyangiitis, microscopic polyangiitis, Goodpasture syndrome.
- Pulmonary arteriovenous malformation (AVM) (e.g., in patients with hereditary hemorrhagic telangiectasia).
- Septic pulmonary emboli.
- Severe pulmonary HTN (e.g., in mitral stenosis).

Algorithm: management of hemoptysis

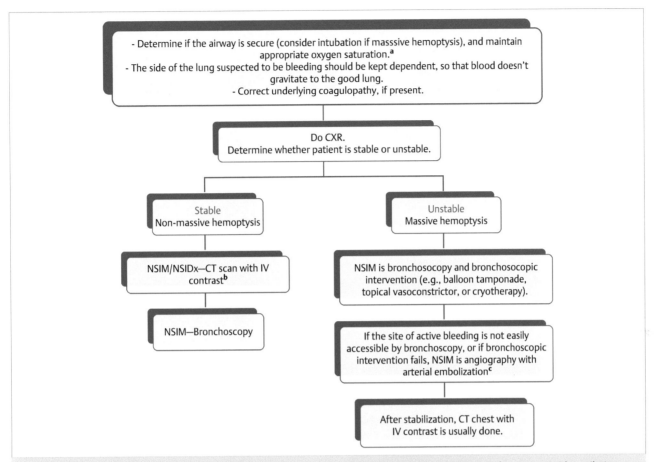

- Determine if the airway is secure (consider intubation if masssive hemoptysis), and maintain appropriate oxygen saturation.[a]
- The side of the lung suspected to be bleeding should be kept dependent, so that blood doesn't gravitate to the good lung.
- Correct underlying coagulopathy, if present.

Do CXR.
Determine whether patient is stable or unstable.

Stable
Non-massive hemoptysis

Unstable
Massive hemoptysis

NSIM/NSIDx—CT scan with IV contrast[b]

NSIM is bronchosocopy and bronchosocopic intervention (e.g., balloon tamponade, topical vasoconstrictor, or cryotherapy).

NSIM—Bronchoscopy

If the site of active bleeding is not easily accessible by bronchoscopy, or if bronchoscopic intervention fails, NSIM is angiography with arterial embolization[c]

After stabilization, CT chest with IV contrast is usually done.

[a] In most patients with massive hemoptysis, death occurs not due to bleeding, but airway obstruction and compromised ventilation.

[b] This provides road map for bronchoscopy. In a stable patient, we have time to get CT chest.

[c] Most common (MC) origin of massive hemoptysis is usually bronchial artery. This belongs to the systemic arterial circulation which has high pressures, as opposed to low pressure vascular system of pulmonary veins and pulmonary arteries.

 In a nutshell

[30] Look for coexistent superficial telangiectasias.

Pulmonary arteriovenous malformation

Background: abnormal vascular connections between the pulmonary arteries and veins which bypass the pulmonary capillary system and thus bypass gas exchange (these are pure shunts).

Etiology: idiopathic or due to hereditary hemorrhagic telangiectasia, hepatic cirrhosis, etc.

Presentation scenarios[30]:

- Hemoptysis.

- Asymptomatic incidental pulmonary nodule.

- Clinical features of pulmonary shunt: clubbing, cyanosis, polycythemia, and paradoxical emboli (in which venous thromboembolism, such as deep venous thrombosis, can lead to arterial emboli, causing transient ischemic attack, stroke or ischemic colitis).

- Platypnea (dyspnea upon standing up, which improves with lying down; this is opposite of orthopnea).

Management: Large AVM can be treated with embolization or surgery.

A GAP in my life due to dry cough.

3.8 Chronic Dry Cough

Differential dx of chronic cough with sputum production is different from chronic nonproductive cough. Common causes of chronic dry cough include the following:

ACE inhibitor	**Pathophysiology:** inhibition of degradation of bradykinins results in elevated bradykinin levels, causing cough. Similar pathophysiology can result in angioedema in susceptible individuals.
	Rx: discontinue ACE inhibitors. Do not choose CXR as an option (it is not needed at this stage). If cough persists even after discontinuation of ACE inhibitor, then only do CXR
GERD	Coughing paroxysms that occurs especially at night[a]
Asthma	Paroxysms of dry cough might be the presenting complaint in cough-variant asthma
Postnasal drip	Look for hx of chronic nasal congestion

[a]Differential dx here is nocturnal cough in variant asthma. Look for coexistent morning sore throat and horse voice that points toward GERD.

Abbreviations: ACE, angiotensin-converting enzyme; GERD, gastroesophageal reflux disease.

Quick note: Diseases that look similar on exam question

- **Cystic fibrosis and Kartagener's syndrome:** both have recurrent respiratory tract infection and infertility. Kartagener's syndrome is associated with situs inversus and there is no pancreatic involvement.
- **Cystic fibrosis and IgA deficiency:** both can present with recurrent respiratory tract infections. Presence of recurrent gastrointestinal or genitourinary infections and absence of other features related to cystic fibrosis point towards IgA deficiency.
- **COPD and bronchiectasis**

	COPD	Bronchiectasis
• Sputum production (both can have chronic cough with sputum production)	• Mostly nonpurulent sputum production • Purulent sputum production may occur in acute exacerbation	• Patients can have mucopurulent and voluminous sputum production at baseline
Hemoptysis	Small amount of hemoptysis might be present	Mild to massive hemoptysis
Physical exam finding	Diffuse wheezing	In diffuse bronchiectasis, diffuse wheezing and diffuse crackles might be present
Clubbing	Absent	Present

Clinical Case Scenarios

26. Patient presents with chronic dry cough. Patient has hx of rheumatic heart disease with **mitral stenosis**. EKG reveals left atrial dilatation. What is the likely cause of the cough?

27. A 7-year-old female with cystic fibrosis is brought in by her mother for a fever of 104°F. She has recent onset cough with copious sputum production. This is the second time in the last 3 months that she had similar symptoms. Upon exam, she is thin appearing with wheezing heard throughout the lung fields. What is the likely organism causing her respiratory infection?

    a) *S. aureus.*

    b) *H. Influenzae.*

    c) *Pseudomonas aeruginosa.*

    d) *S. pneumoniae.*

3.9 Atelectasis

Definition: Collapse of alveoli, lung segments, or a whole lobe. This results in loss of diffusion surface area.

Clinical features: It depends on the extent of involvement, speed of development of atelectasis, and underlying cardiopulmonary reserve. For example, in patients can present with acute respiratory distress in acute massive atelectasis or patients may be asymptomatic especially in slowly progressive small-size atelectasis.

Exam may reveal tracheal deviation (if massive)[31] and dullness to percussion, with decreased breath sounds on the affected side.

[31] Tracheal deviation to the affected side of homogenous opacification is an important clue. This is massive atelectasis.

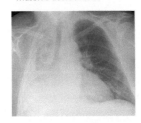

Atelectasis due to	Clinical situations and management
Poor inspiratory effort	**In immediate postop period (due to anesthesia and lack of coughing):** In all postop patients, recommend preventive incentive spirometry and encourage ambulation
	Rib fracture (especially in the elderly): Prevention with adequate analgesic therapy and incentive spirometry is recommended
	Massive ascites: NSIM is paracentesis in this case
Obstruction	**Mucus plug,** for example, in asthma patients: CCS- Patient presents with severe asthma attack with severe respiratory failure. CXR reveals atelectasis of major portion of left lung
	Intrabronchial or extrabronchial lung tumors or extrinsic compression of airway by enlarged lymph node, for example, in lymphoma
	Foreign body aspiration: typically occurs in pediatric population

For acute case of massive atelectasis, NSIM is usually rigid bronchoscopy (remove the mucus plug/foreign body causing the atelectasis)

3.10 Pulmonary Nodule, Mass and Lung Cancer

Solitary pulmonary nodule (SPN) versus mass

	Solitary pulmonary nodule	Mass
Size	≤ 3 cm, NOT associated with lymphadenopathy or other lung opacities	> 3 cm
NSIM	Seek older CXR/CT scan	Generally needs to be biopsied

MCC of SPN are infectious granuloma or hamartoma.

3.10.1 Solitary Pulmonary Nodule

Radiological features	Benign solitary pulmonary nodule	Malignant solitary pulmonary nodule
Border	Smooth	Spiculated (spikes on the surface) or irregular Source: Opacities in the lung. In: Eastman G, et al. Getting started in clinical radiology. From image to diagnosis. 1st ed. Thieme; 2005.
Consistency	Dense, solid, homogenous	Ground glass opacity, heterogeneous, or mixed (subsolid+ solid components)
Calcification	Bulls eye (central) or concentric/lamellar/laminated calcifications are more likely due to granulomatous reaction to prior infection (known as infectious granulomas).[a] Central Laminated	**Eccentric or speckle**d calcification, or absence of calcification Speckled calcification Eccentric calcification
	Popcorn calcification or diffuse amorphous calcification are more likely hamartomas[b] Popcorn	
	Diffuse calcification Diffuse	
Doubling time	Less than 1 month (likely infectious/inflammatory nodule), or > 1 year (benign nodule)	1 month to 1 year

[a]**Infectious granulomas** are likely to be asymptomatic. Common infections that often result in granulomas or healed scars include:

- Fungal (histoplasmosis or coccidioidomycosis) in endemic areas.
- Tuberculosis (in endemic areas or immigrants).

[b]**Hamartoma** is the most common **benign lung tumor**. It is composed of cartilage surrounded by connective tissue and fat. CXR/CT scan typically show **lobulated** solitary pulmonary nodule +/- "popcorn" calcification.

3.10.2 Management of SPN (Solitary Pulmonary Nodule)

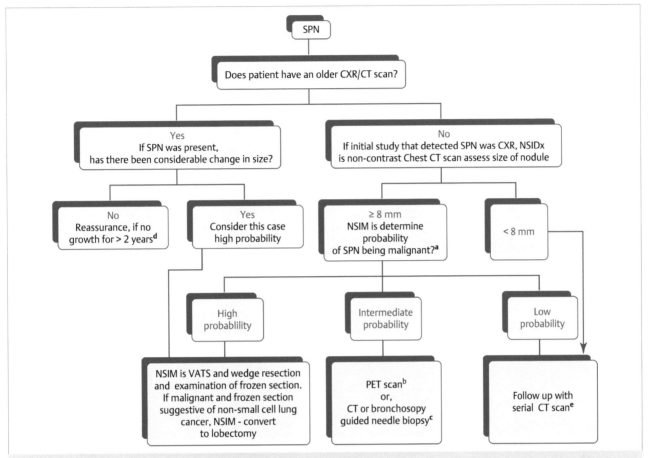

[a]Presence of the following increase the probability of the SPN being malignant:

Clinical characteristics	Radiological characteristics
Age > 60 years	SPN size is ≥ 2 cm
Significant smoking history	Spiculated or other radiological features suggestive of malignancy
Hx of extrathoracic malignancy	Upper lobe location (likely to be malignant)

In addition, always consider the presence of following factors:

• Unexplained weight loss or other symptoms suggestive of malignancy.

• Significant family history of lung cancer.

• Exposure to asbestos or radon.

[b]Positron emission tomography (PET) scan is not used when lesion is < 1 cm as it can be negative.

[c]If **nodule** is centrally located, use bronchoscopy-guided biopsy: endobronchial ultrasound-guided (EBUS) transbronchial biopsy is preferred over conventional bronchoscopy.
If peripherally located, use CT-guided biopsy.

[d]Exception is ground glass nodular opacity or partly solid nodule which can be low-grade **slowly growing** adenocarcinoma or other forms of indolent carcinoma and requires at least 5 years of follow-up.

[e]Use Fleischner society recommendations for follow-up of SPN.

Abbreviations: NSIM, next step in management; NSIDx, next step in dx; SPN, solitary pulmonary nodule; VATS, video-assisted thoracoscopic surgery.

Nodule size (mm)	< 6	6–8	> 8
Solid nodule	Usually no follow-up needed • For certain high-risk patients consider repeating CT scan after 1 year	Repeat CT scan after 6–12 months and, consider repeating CT scan at 18–24 months in higher risk cases If no change, no further follow-up needed	Repeat CT scan in 3 months, then 9 months, and at 24 months.
Partly solid or subsolid nodule	No follow-up needed	Repeat CT scan in 3–6 months; If nodule is unchanged, but if solid portion is persistently > 8 mm, consider biopsy or resection Otherwise, repeat CT scan annually for 5 years	
Ground glass nodule	Usually no follow-up needed • For certain high-risk patients consider repeating CT scan after 2 and 4 years	Repeat CT scan after 6–12 months and then every 2 years for total of 5 years	

Clinical Case Scenarios

This is a very simplified approach to a complicated topic of SPN management. Let's try to practice some CCS that should help you to understand these concepts.

A 57-year-old male who has never smoked, found to have a 2-cm smooth central hilar nodule on CXR.

28. What is the best initial step?

29. If old CXR is not available, what is the NSIDx?

30. Is it with contrast or noncontrast?

31. What is the best SIM?

32. A 4-mm SPN detected in CT scan in a nonsmoker patient with no other risk factors for malignancy. What is the NSIM?

33. A 65-year-old male with 45 pack-year smoking history who is still smoking, is found to have a 2.4 cm spiculated noncalcified nodule. What is the best SIM?

34. A 45-year-old female nonsmoker with a solid smooth 1.1 cm SPN. What is the NSIM? What if the size of the nodule was 6 mm?

35. A 63-year-old patient, with 60 pack-year smoking hx, has a CXR showing spiculated 3.5 cm lung nodule. What is the best SIDx?

36. For the previous question, what is NSIDx?

3.10.3 Lung Cancers

Type of lung cancer	Histological feature	Other characteristics
Small cell lung cancer (aka oat cell cancer)	Round cells with granular cytoplasm	• Central and perihilar location
Squamous cell lung cancer	Can vary from well-differentiated squamous cell neoplasm with keratin formation and intercellular bridges to poorly differentiated forms	• Central and perihilar location • MC lung cancer in patients with hx of smoking
Adenocarcinoma	Cancerous cells with glandular architecture and mucin production	• Peripheral location • This is more likely to involve pleura and to cause pleural effusion • MC lung cancer in patients with no hx of smoking
Adenocarcinoma with lepidic growth (used to be classified under bronchioalveolar carcinoma)	Lepidic predominant growth pattern carcinoma that are minimally invasive (hence have better prognosis)	• Peripheral location • They fill alveolar spaces, can have air bronchograms, and can be misdiagnosed as pneumonia
Large cell carcinoma	Poorly differentiated sheets or nests of **large polygonal or giant multinuclear cells** • One histological subtype is large cell neuroendocrine carcinoma	• Peripheral location

• Lung cancer is the MCC of **mortality due to malignancy** in the United States.
• Smoking cessation is the most effective way to reduce the risk of lung cancer.

Presentation: Cough, SOB, hemoptysis, significant weight loss, etc.

Workup: If lung cancer is suspected, NSIM/NSIDx is CT scan with intravenous (IV) contrast. Tissue biopsy is very important in evaluating suspected cancer.

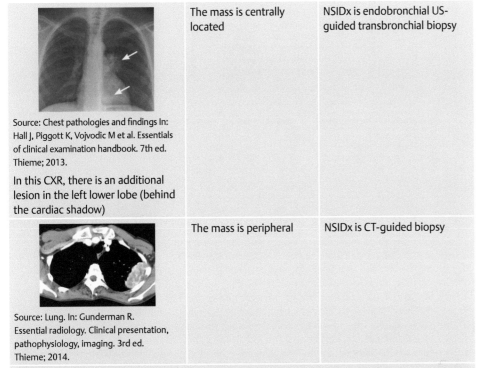

	The mass is centrally located	NSIDx is endobronchial US-guided transbronchial biopsy
Source: Chest pathologies and findings In: Hall J, Piggott K, Vojvodic M et al. Essentials of clinical examination handbook. 7th ed. Thieme; 2013. In this CXR, there is an additional lesion in the left lower lobe (behind the cardiac shadow)		
Source: Lung. In: Gunderman R. Essential radiology. Clinical presentation, pathophysiology, imaging. 3rd ed. Thieme; 2014.	The mass is peripheral	NSIDx is CT-guided biopsy

If the procedures above do not give a definitive tissue diagnosis, then more invasive procedures like VATS or mediastinoscopy can be done.

After-tissue diagnosis of lung cancer, look at the following algorithm for management

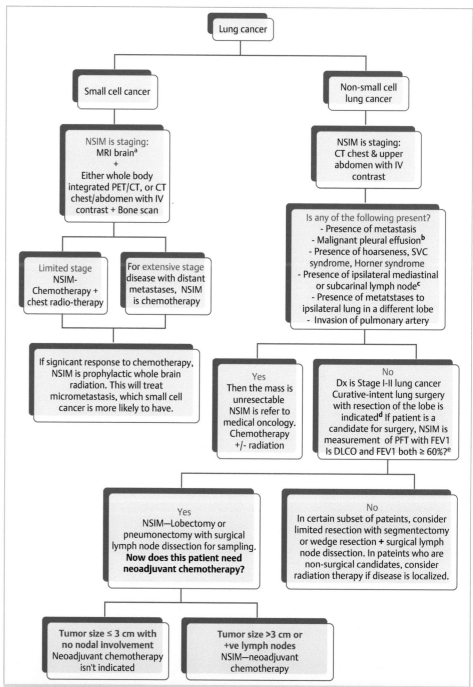

Lung cancer

Small cell cancer

Non-small cell lung cancer

NSIM is staging:
MRI brain[a]
+
Either whole body integrated PET/CT, or CT chest/abdomen with IV contrast + Bone scan

NSIM is staging:
CT chest & upper abdomen with IV contrast

Is any of the following present?
- Presence of metastasis
- Malignant pleural effusion[b]
- Presence of hoarseness, SVC syndrome, Horner syndrome
- Presence of ipsilateral mediastinal or subcarinal lymph node[c]
- Presence of metatstases to ipsilateral lung in a different lobe
- Invasion of pulmonary artery

Limited stage
NSIM-Chemotherapy + chest radio-therapy

For extensive stage disease with distant metastases, NSIM is chemotherapy

Yes
Then the mass is unresectable NSIM is refer to medical oncology. Chemotherapy +/- radiation

No
Dx is Stage I-II lung cancer Curative-intent lung surgery with resection of the lobe is indicated[d] If patient is a candidate for surgery, NSIM is measurement of PFT with FEV1 Is DLCO and FEV1 both ≥ 60%?[e]

If signicant response to chemotherapy, NSIM is prophylactic whole brain radiation. This will treat micrometastasis, which small cell cancer is more likely to have.

Yes
NSIM—Lobectomy or pneumonectomy with surgical lymph node dissection for sampling.
Now does this patient need neoadjuvant chemotherapy?

No
In certain subset of pateints, consider limited resection with segmentectomy or wedge resection **+** surgical lymph node dissection. In pateints who are non-surgical candidates, consider radiation therapy if disease is localized.

Tumor size ≤ 3 cm with no nodal involvement Neoadjuvant chemotherapy isn't indicated

Tumor size >3 cm or +ve lymph nodes NSIM—neoadjuvant chemotherapy

[32] Invasion of chest-wall or diaphragm is still stage II NSCLC.

Nowadays, patients with NSLC are tested for genetic mutations, such as lung cancer anaplastic lymphoma kinase (ALK) and epidermal growth factor receptor (EGFR), because it can predict response to targeted gene therapies. Targeted therapies include tyrosine kinase inhibitors, such as crizotinib, afatinib, gefitinib, erlotinib, etc.

[a] In small cell lung cancer, do routine brain MRI for screening of brain metastases. In contrast, in non-small cell lung cancer (NSLC), routine MRI brain might only be indicated in patients with advanced disease or with symptoms.

[b] In patients with apparently localized disease and coexistent pleural effusion, thoracentesis and cytology to evaluate for malignant pleural involvement is done.

[c] Metastasis to ipsilateral hilar or intrapulmonary/bronchopulmonary nodes is still stage II NSLC.[32] Metastasis to ipsilateral **subcarinal or mediastinal** nodes is stage III. If PET scan shows increased uptake in **mediastinal or subcarinal lymph nodes** in a patient with otherwise apparently localized disease, NSIM is to find out if cancer had actually spread into these lymph nodes, as it makes a difference in staging and treatment. Endoscopic bronchial US-guided needle biopsy of lymph nodes can be done.

[d] PET scan, or whole-body integrated PET/CT, can be considered in patients with large primary tumor or poor surgical candidates to rule out metastases and confirm staging.

[e] New American Thoracic Society guidelines suggest this cut-off value.

Paraneoplastic syndromes associated with lung cancer

CCS: Lung mass + ... ↓	Dx	Pathophysiology	Most common in
Ptosis, proximal muscle weakness, and decreased or absent reflex	**Eaton–Lambert syndrome**	Antibody against **presynaptic** voltage-gated calcium channels	Small cell cancer
Proximal muscle weakness and **normal reflex**	**Polymyositis or dermatomyositis**	Autoimmune myositis	Various
Encephalomyelitis (e.g., ataxia, transverse myelitis)	**Autoimmune encephalitis or myelitis (but first, rule out metastatic disease with MRI of brain and spinal cord)**	Autoimmune mechanisms against CNS cells	Small cell cancer
Hyponatremia	**SIADH**	Overproduction of ADH from malignant cells	Small cell cancer
Presentation: abdominal pain, bone pain, psychosis, etc. **Lab** reveals hypercalcemia, low or normal phosphate, low or normal vitamin D and low PTH	**Pseudohyperparathyroidism**	Production of PTH-related peptide which acts like PTH	Squamous cell cancer
Bilateral painful and tender wrist joint, thickening of distal fingers and clubbing	**Hypertrophic osteoarthropathy**	–	Various
Breast enlargement +/– pain	**Gynecomastia**	Ectopic b-HCG and prolactin production	Large cell carcinoma
Buffalo hump, moon facies, osteoporosis, hyperglycemia, etc.	**Cushing's syndrome**	Ectopic ACTH production	Small cell cancer

Abbreviations: ACTH, adrenocorticotropic hormone; ADH, antidiuretic hormone; b-HCG, beta human chorionic gonadotropin; CNS, central nervous system; PTH, parathyroid hormone; SIADH, syndrome of inappropriate antidiuretic hormone secretion.

Non-paraneoplastic conditions associated with lung cancer

CCS: Lung mass + ... ↓	Dx	Pathophysiology	Most common in
• Lid lag + miosis = Horner's syndrome, and/or • Pain in the region of ulnar nerve in the upper extremity (brachial plexus involvement), and/or • Hoarse voice (recurrent laryngeal nerve involvement)	**Superior sulcus tumor (pancoast tumor)** Source: Clinical aspects. In: Galanski M, Dettmer S, Keberle M, et al. Direct diagnosis in radiology. thoracic imaging. 1st ed. Thieme; 2010.	Direct compression of sympathetic nerve chain (Horner's syndrome), lower thoracic nerve, and/or recurrent laryngeal nerve by the mass	Squamous cell cancer or adenocarcinoma
Plethora/swelling in face and neck + large venous collaterals	**Superior vena cava obstruction syndrome**	Direct compression of superior vena cava (this same syndrome can occur in lymphomas too)	Small cell cancer

3.10.4 Metastatic Disease to the Lungs

- Lung is a common site for metastasis.
- **Presentation:** hemoptysis and cough.
- Metastasis is suspected when imaging (CXR or chest CT scan) reveals multiple nodules or masses (canon ball metastasis).

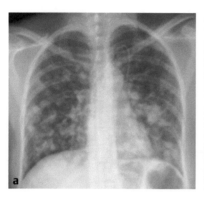 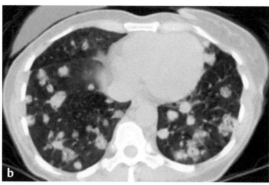

Source: Lung. In: Gunderman R. Essential radiology. Clinical presentation, pathophysiology, imaging. 3rd ed. Thieme; 2014.

- After suspecting a diagnosis, look for the primary source of cancer. *Head/neck, thyroid, breast, kidney, colon, uterus, testis, and skin (melanoma) cancers can metastasize to lung.*
- Treatment usually depends on the type of primary cancer. Solitary lung metastasis from sarcomas, renal cell carcinoma, breast cancer, and colon cancer can be treated with surgical resection and has been shown to improve survival.

 In a nutshell

Lymphangitic carcinomatosis: Primary lung cancer or metastatic disease to lung can invade and spread through the pulmonary lymphatic system. This is lymphangitic intrapulmonary spread of cancer. Patients can present with progressive SOB and dry cough. It has a unique radiological pattern. CXR will reveal reticular or reticulonodular opacification, often with associated septal lines (Kerley A and B lines) and lymphadenopathy.

Clinical Case Scenarios

37. A 29-year-old female with hx of elective termination of pregnancy 9 months ago presents with SOB and hemoptysis. CXR shows multiple various sized nodules. What is the most likely dx?

38. In the previous question, what is the NSIDx?

39. A 20-year-old male patient presents with massive hemoptysis. Exam reveals cryptorchidism. What is the likely dx?

3.11 Mediastinal Tumors

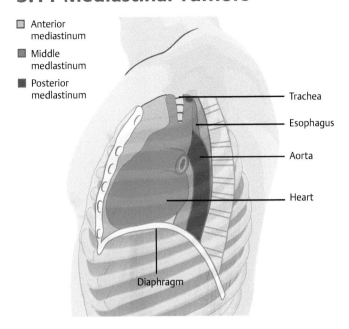

☐ Anterior mediastinum

◩ Middle mediastinum

■ Posterior mediastinum

- Trachea
- Esophagus
- Aorta
- Heart
- Diaphragm

Location	Tumor
Anterior mediastinum	Thyroid or parathyroid tumor
	Thymoma (benign or malignant) Treatment of choice is resection. Thymomas are associated with myasthenia gravis and pure red cell aplasia
	Teratoma (germ cell tumor) Radiology may reveal teeth-like material present inside the mass
Middle mediastinum	**L**ymph node tumors or enlargement: lymphoma, metastatic lymphadenopathy, lymphadenopathy associated with granulomatous disease (tuberculosis, sarcoidosis, silicosis, etc.)
	Cysts (bronchogenic or pericardial cyst)
Posterior mediastinum	Tumors arising from esophagus and neural tissue
	• **E**sophagus: cancer or benign tumors can arise from the following components of esophagus:
	- Epithelial cells: esophageal carcinoma
	- Muscle: leiomyomas (benign smooth muscle tumor) or leiomyosarcoma (malignant muscle tumor)
	- Connective tissue: fibromas
	• **N**eural tissue: neuroblastoma, neurofibromas, schwannoma (neural sheath tumors)

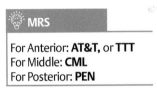

MRS

For Anterior: **AT&T,** or **TTT**
For Middle: **CML**
For Posterior: **PEN**

👥 Clinical Case Scenarios

40. A 45-year-old male is found to have anterior mediastinal mass. CBC reveals anemia with normal platelet and WBC count. Reticulocyte count is very low. What is the likely dx?

3.12 Pleural Disorders

3.12.1 Pleural Effusion

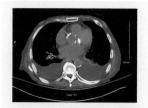

[33] Bilateral pleural effusion on chest CT.

Definition: Presence of fluid in the pleural space.

Presentation: Depending on the size of pleural effusion and associated cardiopulmonary co-morbidities, patients can be asymptomatic or have severe respiratory compromise (dyspnea and tachypnea). Exam will reveal an area of decreased breath sounds, dullness to percussion, and decreased tactile fremitus.

Work-up: NSIDx is CXR (always look at the right and the left cardiodiaphragmatic angle on any CXR. If the acute angle is obliterated and there is fluid layering, then it is likely a pleural effusion).

Bilateral pleural effusion[33]: This is most commonly due to systemic conditions, such as heart failure, advanced chronic kidney disease, hypoalbuminemia.In these cases, NSIM is treatment of the underlying cause.

Unilateral pleural effusion: Usually requires diagnostic thoracentesis (see algorithm below).

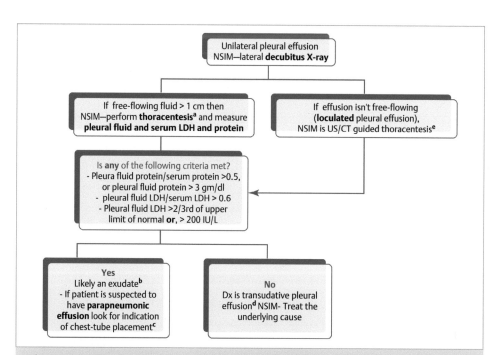

[a]Whenever possible US-guided thoracentesis is always preferred over blind thoracentesis. For free-flowing pleural effusion blind thoracentesis can be done if US is not available; but for loculated pleural effusion one should not attempt blind thoracentesis.

[b]Causes of exudative pleural effusion are: infection, malignancy, connective tissue disorders, pulmonary infarction, and hemothorax. These develop as a result of increased capillary permeability or decreased lymphatic drainage due to obstruction.

[c]For suspected **parapneumonic effusions**, look for the following indications of chest tube insertion:

- Loculated pleural effusion (if multiloculated VATS might be necessary).
- pH < 7.2.
- Gross pus present in the pleural aspirate.
- Glucose < 60 mg/dL.
- Gram stain or pleural-fluid culture is positive for bacteria.

[d]Due to increased hydrostatic pressure or decreased oncotic pressure (see above in section of bilateral pleural effusion).

[e]For multiloculated pleural effusion chest tube is usually indicated.

MRS

LDH, Di-Hundred = 200

MRS

LPG[3] Liquid Petroleum Gas. If present, it means pneumonia infection has reached the pleural space; we need to drain this infected fluid very well by inserting a chest tube.

Additional points on analysis of pleural fluid

Low pleural fluid glucose (< 60 mg/dL) and low pH (< 7.2)	In addition to parapneumonic effusion, also seen in rheumatoid arthritis, malignancy, tuberculosis, and esophageal rupture[a,b]
Lymphocytes predominant pleural fluid	Think about chronic inflammation due to malignancy, tuberculosis, sarcoidosis, rheumatoid pleurisy, and chylothorax Do cytology. If tuberculosis is suspected, do AFB stain & culture, adenosine deaminase enzyme assay, and *M. tuberculosis* polymerase chain reaction from pleural fluid[c]
Pleural fluid Hct > 50%	Indicates hemothorax. NSIM is chest tube placement
Elevated pleural fluid amylase	Occurs in pleural effusion of gastrointestinal source. For example, acute pancreatitis, esophageal perforation, or pancreaticopleural fistula
Pleural fluid triglyceride of > 110 mg/dL	It is suggestive of chylothorax. This can be seen in lymphangioleiomyomatosis

[a]In these cases, low glucose and low pH are not an indication for chest tube placement. "The LPG[3]" applies only to suspected parapneumonic effusion.

[b]*The metabolic activity of abundant inflammatory cells, bacteria, and/or cells result in active anaerobic glucose utilization, leading to low pleural fluid glucose and pH of < 7.2 (due to lactic acidosis).*

[c]Pleural biopsy is the most sensitive test for pleural tuberculosis, but is invasive and is not usually done unless necessary.

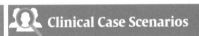 **Clinical Case Scenarios**

41. Patient with hx of stage IV lung cancer has rapidly reaccumulating and/or recurrent pleural effusion. What is the NSIM?

3.12.2 Empyema

Definition: pus in the pleural space.

Etiology: bacterial pneumonia, rupture of lung abscess, bronchopleural fistula, hepatic subphrenic abscess, or due to secondary infection of hemothorax. The most common involved microbes are *S. pneumoniae*, *S. Aureus*, and anaerobes.

Presentation: fever, SOB, pleuritic chest pain, etc. Look for history pointing toward the etiology (e.g., motor vehicle accident few weeks ago).

Management steps

- Best initial diagnostic test is CXR, which will typically show multiloculated pleural effusion.

Cover for MRSA and pseudomonas if there are risk factors, e.g., hospital-acquired pneumonia, post-procedural empyema, etc.

- NSIDx is CT scan of chest with IV contrast, which will better define extent of involvement, loculations, and whether the cavities are thick or thin rimmed.
- NSIM is broad-spectrum antibiotics that cover anaerobes (e.g., piperacillin/tazobactam) + one of the following interventions:

Clinical situation	Preferred intervention
Uncomplicated empyema	• Chest tube insertion for pus drainage If no clinical or radiological improvement in 24 hours, NSIM is intrapleural thrombolytics (tPA or streptokinase + deoxyribonuclease)[a]
CT scan shows multiloculated and thick pleural peel empyema, or patient who is being managed with chest tube is not getting better, and drainage through the chest tube is not adequate	VATS: with VATS the loculations in the pleural space can be disrupted with a thoracoscope and the pleural space can be drained
• Presence of extensive adhesions or • Thick pleural peel entrapping the lung and not allowing it to expand	Thoracotomy and decortication

[a]Fibrinolytics may be contraindicated in patients with a recent hx of major trauma. These patients can have empyema that developed as a complication of hemothorax.

Abbreviation: VATS, video-assisted thoracoscopic surgery.

3.12.3 Spontaneous Pneumothorax

Background: Spontaneous rupture of alveoli can result in air being trapped within the visceral pleura, forming subpleural or pleural blebs. These blebs, with thin walls, can then spontaneously rupture and cause pneumothorax.

Notice the absence of lung markings in this patient with pneumothorax.

Source: Chest pathologies and findings. In: Shi Y, Sohani Z, Tang B, et al. Essentials of clinical examination handbook. 8th ed. Thieme; 2018

Definition

Primary pneumothorax	Pneumothorax that occurs in patients with no preexisting lung disease. Smoking is the MC risk factor. Other causes are Marfan's syndrome, cocaine use, etc. Classical patient is a tall, thin young patient who is a smoker.
Secondary pneumothorax	Pneumothorax that occurs in patients with preexisting lung disease. MC underlying disorder is COPD. Others include cystic fibrosis, *Pneumocystis jirovecii* infection in HIV patients, lymphangioleiomyomatosis, etc. Compared to primary pneumothorax, this has a higher risk of expansion and hemodynamic instability, as well as higher risk of recurrence.

Presentation: Acute sudden-onset sharp pleuritic chest pain. Chest exam will reveal diminished breath sounds, tympanitic percussion, and decreased tactile fremitus in the affected area.

Management steps

All patients with pneumothorax who have dyspnea should receive supplemental oxygen prior to any evaluation.

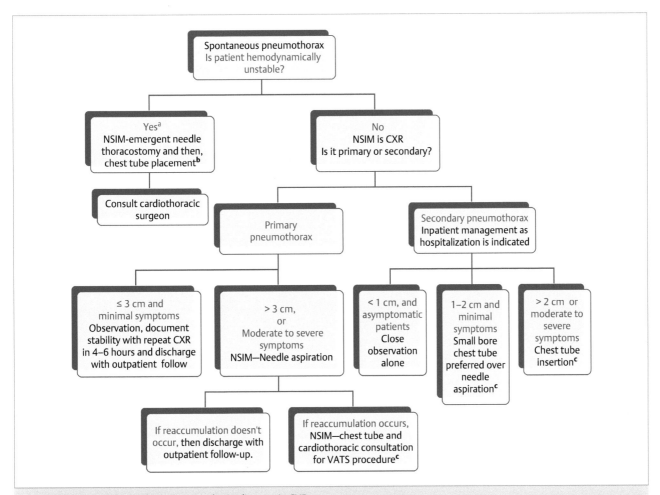

[a]If unstable, you might not have time to obtain diagnostic CXR.

[b]Hemodynamic instability is due to development of tension pneumothorax. This typically presents with hypotension, increasing oxygen requirements, tracheal deviation, and absent breath sounds on one side. If unrecognized or if severe, it can progress to pulseless electrical activity.

[c]**Intervention to prevent recurrence** Includes VATS with "stapling of blebs or bleb removal" and procedure to induce pleurodesis (surgical abrasion or chemical pleurodesis). It is indicated in first episode of secondary pneumothorax and primary pneumothorax with reaccumulation or recurrence. Chemical pleurodesis via the chest tube is an alternative in poor surgical candidates.

3.13 Venous Thromboembolism (DVT and PE)

Background: Venous thromboembolism (VTE) is an umbrella term for development of clot in the venous system (deep venous thrombosis [DVT]), which can embolize to the pulmonary arteries leading to pulmonary embolism (PE). VTE also accounts for disorders such as Budd–Chiari syndrome, mesenteric vein thrombosis, etc.

Risk factors: Remember Virchow's triad of coagulation which promotes clotting.

In this chapter VTE will refer mostly to PE/DVT.

VTE can cause arterial embolism in patients with right to left shunt or pulmonary arterio-venous malformations.

Stasis	Stasis occur in the following situations: • Prolonged immobilization: surgery or long-haul travel (e.g., international flights) • Venous incompetence: varices in legs
Vessel wall damage	Central venous catheters, major surgery, trauma, etc.
Hypercoagulability[a]	• Hereditary thrombophilia (see box below) • Acquired hypercoagulable states: cancer, nephrotic syndrome, pregnancy, heparin-induced thrombocytopenia, oral contraceptive pills, etc.

[a]Although most of these disorders increase risk of venous thromboembolism, some conditions have been associated with both arterial and venous thrombosis. These include antiphospholipid antibody syndrome, hyperhomocystienemia, heparin-induced thrombocytopenia, paroxysmal nocturnal hemoglobinuria, and malignancy.

 In a nutshell

Hereditary thrombophilia

These disorders increase risk of venous thrombosis.

 MRS

CLAPS

C =protein C deficiency	Protein C is an anticoagulant
L =factor V Leiden	Factor V Leiden is the MC hereditary thrombophilia. It is caused by mutation of the gene encoding factor V, which makes it resistant to anticoagulant effect of protein C
A = antiphospholipid antibody syndrome (APAS)	See hematology chapter—page for further information
P = prothrombin gene mutation	This mutation results in increased prothrombin levels
S = protein S deficiency	Protein S is an anticoagulant

3.13.1 Deep Venous Thrombosis

[34]Absolute contraindications to anticoagulation are active bleeding (excluding menses), platelet count of <25,000/µl, recent hemorrhagic stroke, recent high-risk surgery/ invasive procedure or major trauma, and severe bleeding disorder.
Note: in patients with remote hx of intracranial bleeding, anticoagulation may be given.

Background: The MC sites of DVT are distal leg veins (**below-knee-veins**); but the MC site of thrombus that leads to pulmonary embolism is proximal leg veins (**above knee veins**), i.e., iliofemoral veins.

Presentation: Commonly presents with asymmetric pitting edema of an extremity +/− erythema and/or pain. DVT of calf vein can present with tender, swollen, and red calf. Dorsiflexing the foot may elicit calf pain (Homan's sign).

Work-up: NSIDx is compression US of leg vein.

Rx:

● If anticoagulation is contraindicated,[34] then NSIM is Inferior vena cava (IVC) filter to prevent the clot from traveling to pulmonary circulation.

- If there are no contraindications, NSIM is anticoagulation. Use any of the following:
  - **Warfarin + parenteral agent** (e.g., low-molecular-weight heparin (LMWH),[35] fondaparinux, or heparin) for bridging therapy, as it takes few days to reach therapeutic international normalized ratio (INR). INR should be in therapeutic range for 2 consecutive days prior to discontinuation of the bridging therapy.
    OR
  - **Edoxaban and dabigatran**: these require parenteral anticoagulation (e.g., LMWH) for at least 5 days prior to its initiation.
    OR
  - **Apixaban and rivaroxaban**: these do not require parenteral anticoagulation prior to initiation.
- In patients with massive DVT with risk for venous gangrene and limb loss, catheter-directed thrombolysis might be considered.

[35]In patients with VTE and active malignancy, LMWH was traditionally preferred over other agents, however recent studies have shown that DOACs (direct oral acting anticoagulants) such as apixaban, rivaroxaban, edoxaban are also acceptable alternatives (except in patients with gastrointestinal malignancy, in which there is increased risk of bleeding with DOACs). LMWH is also preferred in pregnant patients.

3.13.2 Prophylaxis of VTE

Indication	Therapeutic agents
In most hospitalized patients (including surgical and internal medicine patients), benefits of DVT prophylaxis outweigh the risk of bleeding. If contraindications to anticoagulation is present, consider pneumatic sequential compression devices	Heparin, low-molecular-weight heparin (LMWH), fondaparinux, etc.
In patients who had knee/hip surgery, major trauma or spinal cord surgery, VTE prophylaxis is indicated for 3–4 weeks after surgery	Warfarin, LMWH, heparin, fondaparinux, or novel oral anticoagulants

3.13.3 Pulmonary Embolism

Presentation scenarios

- Patient presents with sudden onset pleuritic chest pain (MC symptom), tachypnea (MC sign), and SOB. Exam reveals tachycardia. Hemoptysis might also be present.
- 7th-day postop patient suddenly collapses while getting up from bed. Note: Sudden collapse in a bed-ridden patient after trying to get up from bed is a classical CCS of massive PE. PE can present with sudden syncope or pulseless electrical activity arrest.

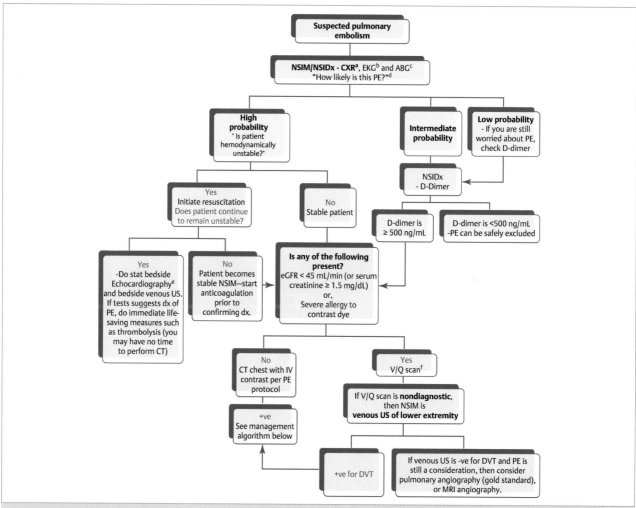

[a]In most of the cases of PE, CXR will be normal. CXR can also help to rule out other differential diagnosis for acute onset SOB (e.g., ARDS and pulmonary edema). Pleural effusion, if present in PE, can be unilateral and is usually associated with pleuritic chest pain. In subset of patients with PE who have pulmonary infarction, CXR may show a wedge-shaped opacity in the periphery which is known eponymously as the Hampton hump.

[b]MC EKG finding in PE is sinus tachycardia with nonspecific ST-T changes. Note, that patients may present with new-onset atrial arrhythmias, such as multifocal atrial tachycardia, aflutter, or a-fib.

In large PE, EKG can reveal signs of increased strain on right ventricle, as evidenced by

- Right ventricular strain pattern (T wave inversion in V_1-V_3).
- Right bundle branch block ("M"-shaped QRS wave in right oriented leads like V_1 and V_2).
- Right axis deviation.
- $S_1Q_3T_3$ syndrome = deep S wave in lead V_1, presence of Q wave and T wave inversion in V_3.

[c]The most consistent finding of PE in ABG is hypoxemia (P_aO_2 ↓) with hypocarbia (P_aCO_2 ↓). The hypocarbia is due to tachypnea and hyperventilation.

[d]To risk-stratify the probability of PE, various scoring systems such as "Well's criteria" are available but memorizing them is not needed for exam purposes. To simplify this, we can use the following strategy:

Probability of PE	Scenario
High probability	Presenting clinical scenario is classical and laboratory data (CXR, EKG, ABG) is compatible with dx of PE
Intermediate probability	Presenting clinical symptoms is compatible with dx of PE, but laboratory data suggest other diagnosis; or vice-versa (laboratory data suggest PE, but clinical scenario is not classical)
Low probability	Presentation is not compatible with dx of PE and there is an alternative explanation for respiratory deterioration, such as pneumonia or pneumothorax

[e]TTE may reveal findings suggestive of increased right ventricular (RV) pressure and strain: RV dilatation, functional TR, septal deviation to left ventricle, etc. Sometimes you can actually see a clot in transit in right side of the heart. RV failure can decrease cardiac output and lead to cardiogenic shock or pulseless electrical activity.

[f]In V/Q scan, perfusion defect with no associated ventilation defect suggests PE.

Finding associated with poor prognosis in PE are elevated BNP, troponin, and evidence of acute RV strain.

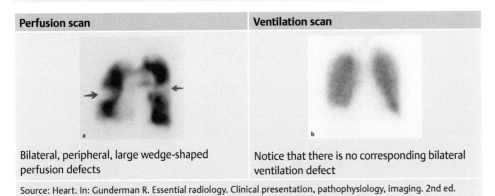

Perfusion scan	Ventilation scan
Bilateral, peripheral, large wedge-shaped perfusion defects	Notice that there is no corresponding bilateral ventilation defect

Source: Heart. In: Gunderman R. Essential radiology. Clinical presentation, pathophysiology, imaging. 2nd ed. Thieme; 2000.

How to workup PE in pregnant patients?

In pregnant patients, radiation is not desired, so the first SIDx is venous US of lower extremities.
- If US is negative and CXR is clear, NSIDx is VQ scan.
- If US is negative and CXR is significantly abnormal, NSIDx is CT scan with IV contrast per PE protocol. (If CXR is abnormal, VQ scan has poor accuracy for dx of PE).

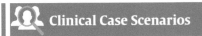 **Clinical Case Scenarios**

42. Hx of motor vehicle accident and multiple long-bone fractures less than 3 days ago. Patient now has a new onset SOB. CBC reveals thrombocytopenia. VQ scan is positive for perfusion defect without ventilation defect. What is the likely Dx?

Treatment of Pulmonary Embolism

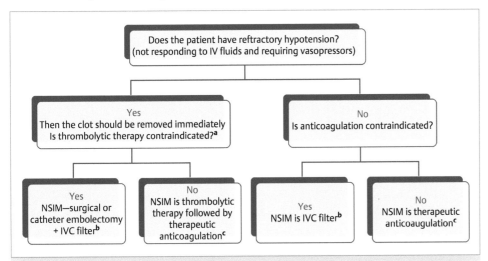

Does the patient have reftractory hypotension? (not responding to IV fluids and requiring vasopressors)

Yes — Then the clot should be removed immediately. Is thrombolytic therapy contraindicated?[a]

No — Is anticoagulation contraindicated?

Yes — NSIM—surgical or catheter embolectomy + IVC filter[b]

No — NSIM is thrombolytic therapy followed by therapeutic anticoagulation[c]

Yes — NSIM is IVC filter[b]

No — NSIM is therapeutic anticoaugulation[c]

Remember, PE can occur in immobilized patients after debilitating hemorrhagic stroke or major surgery within 3 weeks. Thrombolysis and anticoagulation in these situations are contraindicated.

[a]Try to remember and write down the list of contraindications for thrombolysis, and compare your list to information given in stroke section of neurology chapter.

[b]Other indication for IVC filter is recurrent PE despite adequate anticoagulation. Also, it may be considered in patients in whom another episode of PE would likely be fatal (e.g., massive PE with a large lower extremity DVT).

[c]See above in DVT section for choices of anticoagulation.

Duration of anticoagulation for VTE (DVT/PE)

Scenario	Duration of anticoagulation
First episode of VTE, with reversible risk factors (transient immobilization, surgery, trauma, pregnancy, use of hormones, etc.)	Continue for 3–6 months or as long as risk factor is present (whichever is later)
First episode of idiopathic or unprovoked VTE	Treatment is generally lifelong, unless the risk of bleeding outweighs the benefit of anticoagulation
More than 1 episode of VTE or VTE with underlying hypercoagulable disorder	

3.13.4 Chronic Thromboembolic Pulmonary Hypertension

Presentation: chronic SOB and features of pulmonary HTN/cor pulmonale.

Diagnostic evaluation: Best initial test is VQ scan, which has higher sensitivity than CT chest with IV contrast in cases of chronic thromboembolisc pulmonary hypertension. Direct pulmonary angiography or right heart catheterization can also be done.

Rx: lifelong anticoagulation. All patients should be referred to specialty centers for possibility of surgical thromboendarterectomy (definite treatment).

> ### Clinical Case Scenarios
>
> A 66-year-old male presents with acute PE and severe right heart strain. Two days later he develops acute right leg pain. Exam reveals diminished right leg arterial pulses. Angiogram shows an arterial thrombus in the right lower extremity.
>
> 43. What is the NSIDx to determine the likely cause of this presenation?
>
> 44. What is the likely Dx?

3.14 Diffuse Parenchymal Lung Disease aka Interstitial Lung Disease

Background: Diffuse parenchymal lung disease (DPLD) is a group of various conditions that affect almost all tissues in the lung (e.g., alveolar epithelium, basement membrane, interstitium, capillary endothelium, pulmonary parenchyma, pleura, perivascular, and perilymphatic tissues). They are all noninfectious and have varying severity and acuity.

DPLD can be broadly categorized into the following groups *(do not memorize the following table. This is just for your understanding and is a low-yield for USMLE):*

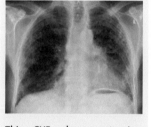

This CXR shows extensive, primarily reticular, and honeycomb interstitial changes. Source: Clinical aspects. In: Galanski M, Dettmer S, Keberle M, et al. Direct diagnosis in radiology. Thoracic imaging. 1st ed. Thieme; 2010.

Associated with specific disease or exposure	• Associated with connective tissue disorder (e.g., systemic lupus erythematosus, rheumatoid arthritis, scleroderma, etc.) • Drug toxicity: amiodarone, methotrexate, nitrofurantoin, bleomycin, etc. • High-risk occupations (pneumoconiosis) • Radiation-induced • Hypersensitivity pneumonitis • Acute eosinophilic pneumonia
Idiopathic DPLD	• **Chronic and fibrosing forms** are idiopathic pulmonary fibrosis (MC form of idiopathic DPLD) and idiopathic nonspecific interstitial pneumonia • **Acute/subacute forms** are bronchiolitis obliterans organizing pneumonia (BOOP)/cryptogenic organizing pneumonia (COP), and acute interstitial pneumonia • **Smoking-related forms** are respiratory bronchiolitis interstitial lung disease, desquamative interstitial pneumonia, pulmonary Langerhan's cell histiocytosis
Granulomatous DPLD	An example is sarcoidosis.
Other forms	Lymphangioleiomyomatosis, histiocytosis X, etc.

Clinical classification of DPLD

Acute forms	Chronic forms
DPLDs that present **acutely** are: acute interstitial pneumonia, acute eosinophilic pneumonia, acute hypersensitivity pneumonitis, bronchiolitis obliterans organizing pneumonia (BOOP)/cryptogenic organizing pneumonia (COP), and vasculitis	Other forms of DPLD usually present with progressively worsening dyspnea and cough over a course of several months

Common features

All of the DPLD can have the following features in common:
- Symptoms of exertional dyspnea and dry cough.
- Exam may reveal coarse/fine crackles and (+/−) clubbing.
- In chronic forms, pulmonary HTN or right heart failure can develop.
- **Lab findings:**
  - CXR: fine, diffuse, nodular infiltrate or reticulonodular opacities.
  - ABG: increased A–a gradient.
  - PFTs: usually restrictive pattern (FEV_1/FVC ratio > 70%), with decreased DLCO.
- **Workup:**
  - High-resolution CT scan.
  - Bronchoscopy with bronchoalveolar lavage or VATS with biopsy can be done to make a definitive diagnosis.

3.14.1 Hypersensitivity Pneumonitis aka Extrinsic Allergic Alveolitis

Pathophysiology: Cell-mediated type IV hypersensitivity reaction to inhaled organic dusts (antigen).

Sub-types are classified depending upon the inciting agent[36]	Additional info
Farmer's lung	Due to **inhalation of** dust that contain spores of **thermophilic actinomycetes**
Bird breeder's lung	Exposure to pigeons, cockatoos, parakeets, etc.
Lab worker's lung	Allergy to aerosolized mice feces
Hot tub pneumonitis	Inhalation of water aerosols containing non-tuberculous mycobacteria (particularly Mycobacterium avium complex)
Byssinosis	Exposure to cotton dust
Other subtypes include machine operator's lung, cheese washer's lung, potato worker's lung, veterinary lung, grain worker's lung, construction worker's lung, etc.	

[36]Hx of exposure is very important for diagnosis, and it is usually given in exam question.

Presentation

Fever, dry cough, SOB and headache.
- Acute presentation occurs after 4 to 8 hours of high-level exposure to dust.
- Subacute/chronic forms are due to low level chronic exposure; may additionally have weight loss and malaise.

Diagnostic evaluation

- **CXR:** interstitial markings with fine, diffuse, and nodular infiltrates.
- **HRCT:** diffuse reticulonodular and ground glass opacity. Chronic forms can have fibrosis and severe forms can have honeycomb changes.
- Patients with unclear etiology and significant disease may need transbronchial biopsy. Histological picture is loosely formed granulomas centered around the airways and mononuclear infiltrate.

Management: Best SIM is to avoid allergens. Steroids are indicated in severe cases.

Clinical Case Scenarios

A 55-year-old male presents with several days hx of low-grade fever, SOB, and dry cough. Patient just started breeding pigeons in his house which is poorly ventilated. Physical exam reveals bilateral diffuse crackles. CXR shows diffuse ill-defined patchy infiltrates. His serologic testing for *Chlamydia psittaci* is negative.

45. What is the likely diagnosis?

46. What is the best SIM?

Miscellaneous types of diffuse parenchymal lung disease—low yield

Forms of DPLD	Clinical situation	Unique imaging and histological features	Management
Pulmonary Langerhans cell histiocytosis	• Young male with recurrent pneumothorax • Occurs in smokers	• **CT:** thin-walled pulmonary cystic nodules with accompanying satellite nodules • **Electron microscopy findings:** Langerhan's cells with pentalaminar infolding of cell membrane, Birbeck's granules, and highly convoluted nuclear membrane	
Desquamative interstitial pneumonia	Occurs in smokers	• **HRCT** diffuse ground glass appearance with scant fibrosis • **Biopsy** shows airspaces filled with macrophages containing lipid, periodic acid-Schiff (PAS)-positive granules, and lamellar bodies (surfactant)-smokers' macrophages. There is an accompanying interstitial pneumonitis, and desquamation of epithelial cells into alveoli	Smoking cessation. Oral steroids can be tried for progression of symptoms despite smoking cessation
Respiratory bronchiolitis-associated interstitial lung disease	• Occurs in smokers • Milder disease	• **CT scan:** centrilobular micronodules, and diffuse or patchy ground glass opacities • **Biopsy** will reveal presence of pigmented macrophages within the lumen of respiratory bronchioles	
Pulmonary alveolar proteinosis • It is characterized by accumulation of PAS positive lipoprotein material in the distal airspaces probably due to impaired clearance • This is associated with presence of antibodies to granulocyte-macrophage colony stimulating factor	• Patients may have hx of occupational exposure, e.g., to silica dust	Bronchoalveolar lavage (bronchoscopy sample) will reveal opaque or milky fluid with PAS positive material	For severe cases, lung lavage is done

(Continued)

Forms of DPLD	Clinical situation	Unique imaging and histological features	Management
bronchiolitis obliterans and organizing pneumonia (BOOP) • BOOP histology might be associated with connective tissue disorder or infection • BOOP of idiopathic type is known as cryptogenic organizing pneumonia (COP)	Patient present with **recurrent episodes** of **pneumonia** that do not respond to antibiotics	• **CT/CXR:** Waxing and waning pulmonary alveolar infiltrates • **Biopsy** will show patchy organizing exudates filling the alveolar lumen	It is mostly responsive to corticosteroids or immunosuppressive
Acute interstitial pneumonia or idiopathic diffuse alveolar damage Rare and fulminant form of DPLD that presents with rapidly progressive severe respiratory failure over days to weeks; most cases result in death[a]		• **Biopsy** reveals diffuse alveolar damage (interstitial edema, acute and chronic inflammation, and hyaline membrane formation)	Supportive treatment similar to ARDS; if intubation is required, use low tidal volume.
Nonspecific interstitial pneumonia (NSIP) Often associated with underlying connective tissue disorder (e.g., scleroderma, SLE, rheumatoid arthritis), HIV, drugs (e.g., amiodarone, nitrofurantoin), or can be idiopathic. • This has better prognosis than usual interstitial pneumonia	Weeks to months of progressive dyspnea and cough	• **CT:** bilateral ground glass infiltrate • **Lung biopsy:** diffuse and uniform interstitial and chronic inflammation, with or without fibrosis	Responsive to corticosteroids +/- immunosuppressive therapy (e.g., cyclophosphamide)
Usual interstitial pneumonia (UIP)[MRS-II] • Causes: SLE, rheumatoid arthritis, drugs (e.g., amiodarone, nitrofurantoin), systemic sclerosis, asbestosis, or idiopathic. • ! UIP of unknown cause is called idiopathic pulmonary fibrosis	Slowly progressive dyspnea and cough	• **CT scan** subpleural cyst formation with honeycombing pattern and traction bronchiectasis with bibasilar predominance. Ground glass opacities might be present in patients with acute exacerbation. • **Biopsy** will reveal areas of mild chronic inflammation, **fibrosis,** +/- honeycombing	See idiopathic pulmonary fibrosis section below

[a]*Presentation is similar to acute respiratory distress syndrome (ARDS) and both have the same pathology of diffuse alveolar damage. Think of it like this—ARDS of unknown etiology is acute interstitial pneumonia.*

3.14.2 Idiopathic Pulmonary Fibrosis

Background: Idiopathic chronic inflammatory lung disease, which leads to pulmonary fibrosis.
Presentation scenario: 68-year-old female presents with progressively worsening SOB for the last 8 months. She now feels SOB just walking around the room. She also notes dry cough and weight loss. Exam reveals clubbing and bilateral crackles at lung bases. CXR shows bilateral diffuse reticulonodular densities (This is a classical presentation of interstitial lung disease).

Diagnostic evaluation

- NSIDx is HRCT scan of chest. Characteristic CT findings are honeycombing in subpleural location with peripheral and basal predominance, traction bronchiectasis, and reticular opacities (see image).
- Idiopathic pulmonary fibrosis is a diagnosis of exclusion, which includes ruling out disorders that can cause usual interstitial pneumonia. Look for high-risk occupation, and hx suggestive of connective tissue disorders, sarcoidosis, etc.

MRS

[MRS-II]Name giveth all

Usual = most common form of interstitial lung disease

Pneumonia = radiological lung abnormalities (fibrosis and ground glass opacities)

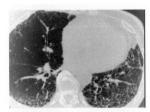

Red arrows show traction bronchiectasis
Source: Imaging. In: Gunderman R. Essential radiology. Clinical presentation, pathophysiology, imaging. 2nd ed. Thieme; 2000.

- If a patient has characteristic clinical and radiologic findings with exclusion of other disorders, lung biopsy can be deferred.
- If diagnosis is still in question, NSIDx is VATS to perform **lung biopsy**, which will show changes typical of usual interstitial pneumonia.

Management

- Supportive care: supplemental oxygen, vaccination, and pulmonary rehab therapy.
- Nintedanib and pirfenidone can slow down reduction in lung function. They are indicated in patients with mild to moderate lung function loss. They are not recommended in advanced disease due to high cost and questionable benefit in this group.
  - Nintedanib is a tyrosine kinase receptor blocker which decreases expression of fibrogenic growth factor.
  - Pirfenidone inhibits transforming growth factor beta (TGF-b)-stimulated collagen synthesis.
- Only intervention to improve survival is lung transplantation.
- Antacid therapy for acid reflux may be beneficial.
- In patients with acute exacerbation, consider high dose steroids.

3.14.3 Lymphangioleiomyomatosis

Background: It is a low-grade pulmonary neoplasm of smooth muscle cells throughout the lungs and its' vessels, lymphatics, pleurae, etc. It can be associated with tuberous sclerosis
Presentation: Women of childbearing age with spontaneous pneumothorax, chylothorax, and/or hemoptysis.
Diagnostic evaluation: HRCT will reveal diffuse thin walled small cysts.
Management: There is no specific therapy. Lung transplantation is done in select patients.

3.14.4 Occupational Lung Diseases (aka Pneumoconiosis)

Definition: A group of DPLD related to chronic **inorganic dust** exposure.

> **MRS**
>
> - Silly TB: Silly = Silicosis
> - Berries are circular and round = granulomas

Asbestosis	• Can be seen in patients who had worked in plumbing, shipyard, insulation or mining. It can take 10–15 years for symptoms to develop
	• Look for pleural or peritoneal plaques. Biopsy, if done, will show ferruginous bodies
	• All patients should be advised to stop smoking, as there is a synergistic risk for development of cancer with smoking[a]
Silicosis	• Hx of exposure to silicon particles in mining, tunneling, sandblasting, quarrying (stone workers), glass and pottery making
	• CXR will typically show nodules prominent in upper lobes (similar to tuberculosis)
	• All patients with silicosis should be screened yearly for tuberculosis with Interferon-gamma release assay.
	• Silicosis is also associated with increased risk of autoimmune disorders
Coal worker's pneumoconiosis	• Features of restrictive lung disease in a patient with a hx of work-related exposure to coal
Berylliosis	• It is a major differential diagnosis of sarcoidosis, because biopsy will typically reveal noncaseating granulomas. Presence of high-risk occupation, like work in aerospace industry, nuclear reactor, semiconductor, or light bulb factories will help to distinguish between the two
	• May respond to steroid treatment

[a]MC cancer associated with asbestosis is squamous cell cancer (not mesothelioma); however, mesothelioma (pleural and peritoneal) is seen almost exclusively with asbestosis.

Mesothelioma

Background: Carcinoma arising from mesothelial cells (either from pleura or peritoneum). It is almost always associated with significant asbestos exposure.

Presentation: MC symptom is chest pain due to early parietal-pleural involvement. Other common symptoms include SOB and weight loss. CXR/chest CT scan may show large pleural effusion with diffuse pleural thickening and multiple pleural plaques. The tumor can be seen encasing the lung (inset picture).

Diagnostic steps

- If significant pleural effusion is present, NSIDx is thoracentesis +/− pleural biopsy.

- If biopsy from above procedure is negative or if there is no significant pleural effusion, VATS and biopsy might be needed.[37]

Management: Chemotherapy and, in select cases, pneumonectomy.

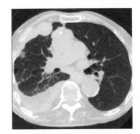

Source: Clinical aspects. In: Galanski M, Dettmer S, Keberle M, et al. Direct diagnosis in radiology. Thoracic imaging. 1st ed. Thieme; 2010.

[37] Pathology will reveal epitheloid or sarcomatous elements with spindle cell morphology.

3.14.5 Sarcoidosis

Definition: Sarcoidosis is an idiopathic inflammatory disorder characterized by development of noncaseating granulomatous inflammation in various organs (lymph nodes, eyes, skin, lungs, etc.).

Presentation: Depends upon the location, extent, and severity of underlying granulomatous inflammation. Nonspecific inflammatory symptoms (fever, night sweats, and weight loss) are commonly present.

Organ involved	Clinical features
Pulmonary (MC organ involved)[a]	Dry cough, SOB etc.
Lymph nodes and reticuloendothelial system	• Bilateral hilar lymphadenopathy[a] • Hepatosplenomegaly
Skin	Erythema nodosum and lupus pernio
Eye	Iritis, uveitis (eye pain, photosensitivity) ! Slit lamp examination should be done in all patients with suspected sarcoidosis
Musculoskeletal	Acute and/or chronic arthritis or myositis
Peripheral neuropathy	Example: facial nerve palsy, foot drop, etc.
Central nervous system	Aseptic meningitis, seizures, and focal neurological deficits
Heart	Restrictive cardiomyopathy and heart block
Bone marrow	Pancytopenia
Biochemical effect of increased number of granulomas	Granulomas contain enzyme that metabolize vitamin D to its active form, leading to hypercalcemia and hypercalciuria. They can also produce angiotensin-converting enzyme (ACE), which may lead to high ACE levels[b]

[a] **CXR** is the best initial test for suspected cases. Classical finding is bilateral hilar lymphadenopathy. Patients may also have reticulonodular opacities (suggestive of DPLD), consolidation, cavitation, etc.

[b] However, note that the absence of hypercalcemia, hypercalciuria, and elevated ACE does not exclude sarcoidosis.

Establishing diagnosis: Biopsy of the most accessible site is done: skin lesions (except for erythema nodosum), palpable lymph nodes, parotid gland, lacrimal gland, etc. If there are no peripheral lesions, bronchoscopy (+/− endobronchial ultrasound) with biopsy or mediastinoscopy with lymph node biopsy might be necessary.

Since granulomatous inflammation can be seen in multiple other conditions, sarcoidosis is a dx of exclusion. The diagnosis of sarcoidosis is made on basis of compatible clinical and radiologic findings, supported by histologic evidence of noncaseating granulomas in the absence of organisms or particles; therefore, all biopsy tissue should be sent for bacterial, mycobacterial, and fungal stain and culture. Tuberculosis screening should also be performed.

Management

- Most patients with sarcoidosis do not require any specific treatment as high proportion of patients have asymptomatic, or non-progressive disease or experience a spontaneous remission. However, the need for treatment may arise, if the disease acuity or severity is high. Look for the following indications for steroids:
  - Optic neuritis, severe uveitis.
  - Central nervous system involvement.
  - Cardiac involvement.
  - Chronic moderate to severe hypercalcemia.
  - Progressive or symptomatic pulmonary sarcoidosis.
  - Other forms of sarcoidosis with moderate to severe symptoms.
- In patients who do not respond to or are intolerant of steroids due to side effects, other immune-modulating agents such as methotrexate, azathioprine, mycophenolate can be used.
- Topical steroids can be used in skin lesions and anterior uveitis.
- Refer to ophthalmology for eye involvement in sarcoidosis.

 In a nutshell

There are two distinct forms of **acute sarcoidosis**:

Lofgren syndrome	⇒	CCS: Patient presents with recent onset fever with bilateral **ankle pain.** He has recent hx of left wrist pain and swelling. Physical exam reveals tender **red nodules in lower extremities.** CXR reveals bilateral **hilar lymphadenopathy**
Heerfordt–Waldenström syndrome	⇒	CCS: Patient presents with recent onset fever with eye pain, photophobia (**anterior uveitis**), **parotid gland enlargement** + **facial nerve palsy** (due to compression by enlarged parotid gland) +/− joint pain

These classical presentations have such a good diagnostic accuracy that biopsy may not be required.

3.14.6 Granulomas

Pathologically, granulomas are divided into the following two groups:

Noncaseating granulomas	Caseating granulomas (mostly infectious)[38]
Crohn's disease	Tuberculosis
Berylliosis	Syphilis
Sarcoidosis	Histoplasmosis
Hypersensitivity pneumonitis	Brucellosis
Lymphomas (HL or NHL)[a]	Cryptococcus

(Continued)

Noncaseating granulomas	Caseating granulomas (mostly infectious)[38]
	Blastomyces

[a]Lymphomas can have a presentation very similar to sarcoidosis with fever, weight loss, bilateral hilar lymphadenopathy, and high ACE/vitamin D levels.[39] Presence of skin, eye, and pulmonary parenchymal involvement will point toward sarcoidosis. Look for high LDH in lymphoma.

[39] All conditions with granulomatous inflammation may have elevated vitamin D (hypercalcemia or hypercalciuria) and ACE levels.

 In a nutshell

Other causes of bilateral hilar lymphadenopathy:

- **Infections:** tuberculosis, fungal infection.

- **Malignancy:** lymphomas, mediastinal tumors.

- **Inorganic dust exposure:** berylliosis or silicosis.

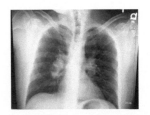

Clinical Case Scenarios

47. A 64-year-old male, who works in mining, presents with increasing SOB for last 4 months and weight loss. Exam reveals bilateral fine crackles. CXR shows multiple bilateral pleural plaques with a perihilar mass. What is the most likely dx?

    a. Squamous cell cancer.

    b. Pleural mesothelioma.

48. CXR reveals upper lobe nodules in a patient with history of high-risk occupation. Patient is being screened for yearly tuberculosis. What is the like dx?

    a. Silicosis.

    b. Berylliosis.

    c. Asbestosis.

    d. Coal worker's pneumoconiosis.

49. Biopsy of a patient with bilateral hilar lymphadenopathy reveals noncaseating granulomas. Which of the following pneumoconiosis is the like dx?

    a. Silicosis.

    b. Berylliosis.

    c. Asbestosis.

    d. Coal worker's pneumoconiosis.

50. A 40-year-old female patient presents with dry cough, dyspnea, fever, night sweats for 2 months. CBC reveals mild pancytopenia, with low reticulocyte count. What is the best initial test?

    a. CT scan of chest.

    b. CXR.

    c. Bone marrow biopsy.

3.15 Sleep Apnea

Obstructive sleep apnea (OSA)

Etiology: In obese patients, this is caused by airway blockage from excess fatty tissues in the neck. Look for increased neck circumference.

Other causes are **anatomic airway obstruction** (look for this particularly in patients with low or normal BMI):

- Nasal obstruction that may result from many causes including allergies, polyps, deviated septum, enlarged adenoids, and enlarged nasal turbinates
- Obstruction can also be in the area of the soft palate, tonsils, and uvula

Airway blockage is more likely to occur when patient is supine and sleeping

Central sleep apnea (CSA)

Pathophysiology: Impaired response of respiratory center to changes in blood $PaO_2/PaCO_2$ levels, which commonly occurs while sleeping.

- MC form is Cheyne–Stokes respiration characterized by initial phase of progressively increasing tidal volume followed by a phase of gradual decrease in tidal volume and termination of the cycle with a temporary stop in breathing (apnea). This is due to increased sensitivity to $PaCO_2$ and subsequent hyperventilation, which drives down the $PaCO_2$ level so low that it effectively ceases respiratory effort

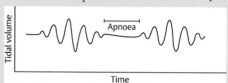

Risk factors: Conditions like a-fib, heart failure, advanced CKD, stroke, brainstem lesions, and use of sedatives predispose to this condition

Presentation

- Daytime somnolence—due to poor sleep quality
- HTN
- Pulmonary HTN with cor pulmonale (in severe sleep apnea, nocturnal oxygen desaturation causes reactive pulmonary vasoconstriction, resulting in chronic arteriopathy)
- Congestive heart failure
- Erythrocytosis
- Partner may witness periods of apnea or frequent/loud snoring

Management steps

- First step in management is to advice patients to avoid sedatives and alcohol before sleep. Sedatives (alcohol, benzodiazepines, valproic acid, etc.) can cause both OSA (due to poor muscle tone in upper airway) and central apnea (due to respiratory depression)
- NSIDx and best SIDx is nocturnal polysomnography (overnight sleep testing)

Findings in polysomnography: Repetitive periods of apnea (absence of airflow), or hypopnea (decreased airflow) despite adequate respiratory effort and/or respiratory-effort related multiple arousals is diagnostic of OSA

Findings in polysomnography: Absence of respiratory effort at least for 10 seconds is diagnostic of CSA

Management

- Next step in evaluation is to look for correctable conditions, particularly in patients who are nonobese. Example includes anatomic lesions which can be surgically corrected (significant deviated nasal septum can be corrected with septoplasty; enlarged tonsils or adenoids with tonsillectomy or adenoidectomy)
- In patients with allergic symptoms, treatment with nasal steroids may be helpful
- In obese patient, the best SIM is weight reduction
- Avoid supine posture while sleeping[a]
- If adequate weight loss cannot be achieved, positive airway pressure, either in the form of CPAP or BiPAP[b] (which keep the airway open while sleeping), is the most effective therapy for OSA.
- Uvulopalatopharyngoplasty (surgical enlargement of upper airway) might be considered in patients who have failed CPAP/BiPAP

Management

- NSIM: treat underlying condition (e.g., if patient has underlying decompensated heart failure, NSIM is Lasix)
- If it persists despite treatment of underlying cause, use CPAP, BiPAP, or adaptive seroventilation +/− nocturnal oxygen. Note that BiPAP or adaptive seroventilation is contraindicated in patients with heart failure with reduced ejection fraction
- For patients who do not tolerate positive airway pressure, respiratory stimulants like acetazolamide can be used with caution

[a]In someone who is actively snoring, NSIM is to change his position from supine to lateral decubitus or prone.

[b]BiPAP might be needed if CPAP fails to adequately maintain airflow, or in patients cannot tolerate CPAP. Some patients are more comfortable with BiPAP which provides different pressures during inspiration and expiration as opposed to a constant pressure given by CPAP.

Abbreviations: BiPAP, bilevel positive airway pressure; BMI, body mass index; CKD, chronic kidney disease; CPAP, continuous positive airway pressure; HTN, hypertension.

3.16 Obesity Hypoventilation Syndrome aka Pickwickian Syndrome

Pathophysiology: Obesity hypoventilation (OHS) occurs in patients with **body mass index (BMI) > 30**. Increased abdominal girth/contents lead to increased abdominal resistance causing increased diaphragmatic workload and restriction of lung movements.

Diagnosis: Look for baseline serum bicarbonate > 27 mEq/L in an obese patient. If present, NSIDx is baseline ABG. Baseline daytime $PaCO_2$ > 45 mmHg is suggestive of OHS. It is a diagnosis of exclusion and look for other causes of chronic hypoventilation that could explain hypercapnia; obtain PFTs (OHS will show restrictive pattern in PFT with normal DLCO), TSH, CXR, etc.

Management: CPAP or BiPAP is indicated in all patients. Weight loss is the best SIM.

Complications: It is similar in complications to obstructive sleep apnea (OSA; e.g., polycythemia, pulmonary HTN, right-sided heart failure).

3.17 Cor Pulmonale

Definition: Right ventricular failure due to increased pulmonary pressures, commonly as a result of chronic pulmonary hypoxemia.

Etiology: Any disorder that causes chronic hypoxia can lead to cor pulmonale. COPD is the MCC. Other causes include, chronic forms of DPLD, severe diffuse bronchiectasis, OSA, Pickwickian syndrome, severe kyphoscoliosis, etc.

Pathophysiology: Chronic pulmonary hypoxemia → chronic vasoconstriction → arterial smooth muscle hypertrophy → chronic pulmonary HTN. This leads to RV strain → RV hypertrophy → RV failure.[40]

Management: Supplemental oxygen is the first SIM. Treat the underlying disease.

[40] Right-sided heart failure due to left-sided heart disease or congenital heart disease is NOT considered cor-pulmonale.

🔍 Clinical Case Scenarios

A morbidly obese patient with BMI of > 40 comes in with bilateral lower leg edema and scrotal swelling. He also complains of excessive snoring and daytime somnolence. TTE shows RV dilatation.

51. What is the cause of edematous state?

52. What are the two likely underlying cause?

53. What is NSIDx to find out the underlying cause?

3.18 Pulmonary Hypertension

Definition: Resting mean pulmonary artery pressure of ≥ 25 mmHg.

Classification by etiology

- Primary pulmonary arterial HTN[41]
    - HIV.
    - Connective tissue disorder.
    - Portal HTN.
    - Drugs (fenfluramine, methamphetamine, cocaine).
    - Congenital heart disease.
    - Idiopathic.
- Pulmonary HTN (pHTN) due to left heart pathology (pulmonary venous HTN leads eventually to pulmonary arterial HTN).
- pHTN owing to primary lung disease and/or hypoxia (cor pulmonale).

[41] Pathophysiology of pulmonary arterial HTN: intimal fibrosis in the walls of small pulmonary arteries and plexiform arteriopathy.

- pHTN due to chronic thromboembolic pulmonary HTN.
- pHTN associated with other disorders: metabolic (e.g., heritable enzyme disorder), systemic (e.g., sarcoidosis), hematologic (e.g., myeloproliferative disorder, chronic hemolytic anemias), etc.

Presentation

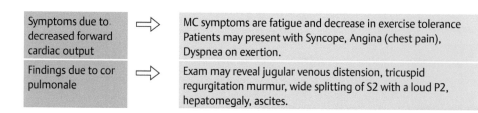

Symptoms due to decreased forward cardiac output	⇒	MC symptoms are fatigue and decrease in exercise tolerance. Patients may present with Syncope, Angina (chest pain), Dyspnea on exertion.
Findings due to cor pulmonale	⇒	Exam may reveal jugular venous distension, tricuspid regurgitation murmur, wide splitting of S2 with a loud P2, hepatomegaly, ascites.

MRS

pHTN presents like aortic stenosis (SAD on exertion) and sounds like ASD (wide-split S2)

Labs may reveal secondary erythrocytosis (chronic hypoxemia stimulates erythropoiesis).

Diagnostic evaluation

Initial workup consists of CXR, PFTs,[42] ABG, and EKG. Also check for HIV (antigen/antibody assay), connective tissue disorder (ANA, rheumatoid factor, ANCA), portal HTN (LFTs), etc.

[42] PFT in pulmonary arterial hypertension and chronic thromboembolic pHTN will show **decreased DLCO with normal spirometry.**

- CXR typically shows prominent pulmonary vascular markings and enlarged right heart border.
- TTE can measure pulmonary pressures indirectly and rule out significant left heart pathology. It typically reveals RA/RV dilatation and functional TR.
- VQ scan should be done to rule out chronic thromboembolic pulmonary HTN.
- Nocturnal polysomnography (sleep study) should be done to evaluate for sleep disorders.
- Cardiac catheterization is the gold standard for diagnosis: resting mean pulmonary artery pressure of ≥ 25 mmHg is diagnostic.
- If all of the above tests fail to reveal an underlying disorder that could lead to pHTN, then dx is likely idiopathic or heritable form of pulmonary arterial HTN.

General management principles

[43] Advanced therapy is used in pulmonary arterial HTN. It can be considered on a case-by-case basis in chronic thromboembolic pHTN, and pHTN associated with other disorders.
Do not use advanced therapy in patients with pHTN due to left heart failure or primary lung disease.

- Supportive: diuretics when there is evidence of congestive heart failure and supplemental oxygen for hypoxemia.
- Therapeutic anticoagulation is recommended in in chronic thromboembolic pHTN. Consider anticoagulation in pulmonary arterial hypertension on a case-by-case basis.
- Advance therapy, as shown below in algorithm, is indicated in **pulmonary arterial HTN.**[43]

Management of pulmonary arterial HTN

[a]Inhaled nitric oxide is preferred as it selectively decreases pulmonary artery pressures than other agents.
[b]Drugs with suffix "entan" are **en**dothelin receptor **ant**agonist: ambrisentan, bosentan, and macitentan. Note, endothelin is a powerful vasoconstrictor.
[c]Drugs with suffix "afil" are sildenafil and tadalafil. They are phosphodiesterase inhibitor which increases nitric-oxide-mediated vasodilation.
[d]Epo**prost**enol and treprostinil are **prost**acyclin analogues, which may confer the greatest improvement in survival in New York Heart Association (NYHA) classification IV.
Lung +/– heart transplantation might be needed in patients with end stage pHTN with refractory NYHA grade III or IV.

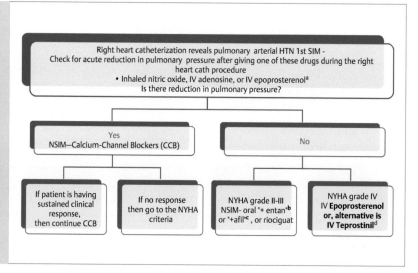

🌐 In a nutshell

Pregnancy and pulmonary arterial HTN

- Females with pulmonary arterial HTN are recommended to avoid pregnancy, as it can worsen underlying condition.

- Entans and riociguat are absolutely contraindicated in pregnancy.

---

1. Auto-PEEP.

2. Tension pneumothorax.

3. Tension pneumothorax, misplacement of endotracheal tube when it is placed too far (into the right, or less commonly in left bronchus[44]), or lung atelectasis.

4. Coexistent hypotension points towards tension.

5. Decrease FiO_2 ($FiO_2 < 60\%$ reduces risk of oxygen toxicity from free radicals).

6. Continue current management. Patient is hypercapnic and has low pH, but it is not < 7.2. Permissive hypercapnia is recommended to prevent auto-PEEP and barotrauma.

7. His calculated RSBI is = 30/0.2 = 150 (remember that in this ratio tidal volume is expressed in liters).

8. The decision is made to continue ventilation for today. His ventilation mode is changed back to ACMV.

9. CXR should be ordered to rule out pneumothorax.

10. Subcutaneous emphysema. NSIM is supportive care.

11. Serum BNP and TTE.

12. ARDS; notice on CXR, there is no evidence of pleural effusions (absence of costophrenic angle blunting in both sides).

13. This is moderate persistent asthma. Add LABA to LDIS.

14. We can discontinue LABA and continue LDIS + short-acting PRN bronchodilators. If asthma is well controlled, step-down treatment to avoid side effects.

15. This is severe persistent asthma. Change regimen to HDIS +LABA. If hx of atopic asthma, time to consider omalizumab.

16. Change LDIS to MDIS (moderate dose inhaled steroids).

17. (c) Assess underlying severity of asthma.

    No indication for short course of steroids here. Prior to discharge remember the indications for vaccination, which includes flu and pneumococcal vaccines and assess severity of underlying asthma to prescribe LDIS or MDIS or LABA, if needed.

18. (c) Administer inhaled albuterol.

    This is mild to moderate asthma exacerbation. SABA (e.g., albuterol) is indicated as the first step. Steroids do not provide immediate relief as it takes some time for it to act.

19. (b) Administer inhaled albuterol + ipratropium combination.

    NSIM is SABA + SAMA administration (bronchodilator therapy can rapidly improve respiratory status). If patient does not improve after this treatment and continues to have danger signs, consider intubation.

20. Long-term home oxygen supplemental therapy. Remember the numbers—55, 59, 88, and 89 for indication of home oxygen therapy.

21. (b) Acute hyperoxic hypercapnic respiratory failure.

    In patients with chronic hypercapnia (e.g., in COPD), use of high-flow supplemental oxygen may lead to excessive CO_2 retention causing respiratory acidosis and decreased mental status. This is known as acute hyperoxic hypercapnic respiratory failure. Several mechanisms have bene implicated; increased V/Q mismatch, decreased ventilator drive, changes in CO_2–Hb dissociation curve, etc. So, in patients with lung disease causing chronic hypercapnia (e.g., COPD), target SaO_2 is 88 to 92%.

[44] This can lead to local barotrauma due to high pressures delivered to only one side of the lung .

If this patient was hypoxemic, the likely dx would have been acute hypercapnic respiratory failure due to severe COPD exacerbation.

22. Dx is steroid induced leukocytosis, which presents as neutrophilia (usually without bandemia). Steroids also can cause lymphopenia/eosinopenia.

23. (b) Albuterol.

   These are side effects related to use of β_2 agonists, e.g., albuterol. It can cause muscle weakness (by inducing hypokalemia) and tremors.

24. Low-dose CT scan of the chest. As opposed to bronchiectasis, COPD usually does not cause clubbing. If clubbing is present in a COPD patient, think about lung cancer.

25. Aminophylline toxicity. NSIDx is check serum aminophylline level. Ciprofloxacin is a cytochrome inhibitor.

26. Enlarged left atrium is pushing up the bronchus, causing persistent cough.

27. (c) Pseudomonas aeruginosa.

   The most common cause of respiratory infection in a child with cystic fibrosis is *S. aureus*. In adults, the MCC is *Pseudomonas* infection.

28. Look for older CXR.

29. Chest CT scan.

30. Noncontrast CT scan. IV contrast is not required to evaluate SPN.

31. PET scan or endobronchial ultrasound and transbronchial biopsy (as the nodule is central). This is an intermediate probability case.

32. No follow-up is required.

33. High probability case. Best SIM is VATS with wedge resection and examination of frozen section.

34. Low-probability case. NSIM: follow-up CT scan in 3 to 6 months. Follow-up CT scan in 6 to 12 months.

35. VATS biopsy.

36. NSIDx is CT chest. Note: Best SIDx is different from NSIDx.

37. Choriocarcinoma with metastasis to the lung.

38. US of uterus.

39. Dx is testicular cancer with metastasis to the lung.

40. Pure red cell aplasia related to thymoma.

41. Consider chemical pleurodesis (obliteration of pleural space) with talc, or pleural catheter placement.

42. Fat emboli. The ways to differentiate PE from fat emboli is that fat emboli typically happen shortly after trauma and are usually associated with petechiae and thrombocytopenia.

43. TTE with bubble study that will likely show PFO with right to left shunt.

44. Dx is paradoxical emboli. PE can cause acute severe pHTN, leading to elevated pressures in the right side of the heart and development of right to left shunt in a patient with preexisting PFO.

45. Extrinsic allergic alveolitis — Bird breeder's lung. LOM with atypical pneumonia caused by *C. psittaci*.

46. Avoid bird exposure.

47. (a) (perihilar mass is likely squamous cell cancer). Pleural plaques are common in patients with asbestosis.

48. (a) (Silicosis).

49. (b) (Berylliosis). Even though silicosis might present with bilateral hilar lymphadenopathy, it will not have noncaseating granulomas.

50. (b) CXR is the best initial test. Think of sarcoidosis.

51. Cor pulmonale.

52. OSA and Pickwickian syndrome. If patient has hx of OSA, assess for compliance to CPAP.

53. Baseline ABG, PFTs, and nocturnal polysomnography.

4. Cardiology

"*All great artists draw from the same resource:* **the human heart, which tells us that we are all more alike than we are unalike.**"- *Maya Angelou*

4.1 Atherosclerosis

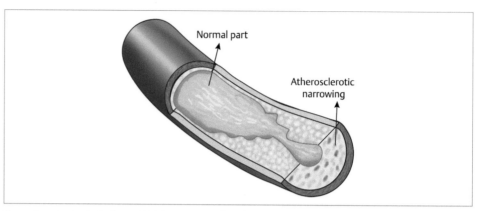

Source: Hypertension. In: Luellmann H, Mohr K, Hein L. Pocket atlas of pharmacology. 4th ed. Thieme; 2010.

Pathophysiology: It is a slow and progressive pathologic process with buildup of lipid-filled plaques, accompanied with interstitial changes in the walls of medium- and large-sized arteries. This is secondary to years of accumulative arterial wall damage and inflammation.

- These plaques can cause chronic narrowing of arteries and limit blood supply, resulting in ischemic complications.
- At times the plaques can rupture or ulcerate, leading to acute formation of **thrombus** which can cause:
  - Acute luminal narrowing resulting in infarction or worsening ischemia.
  - If the plaque dislodges, it can form an **embolus** that blocks blood supply wherever it goes.

Risk factors

- Age > 45 years in males and > 55 years in females.
- Family hx of symptomatic atherosclerotic disease.
- Diabetes.
- Dyslipidemia.
- Smoking.
- Hypertension (HTN).

Diabetes, dyslipidemia, smoking, and HTN are modifiable risk factors. Smoking has the highest impact on the progression of atherosclerosis.

4.1.1 Atherosclerotic Cardiovascular Disease

Background: Atherosclerotic plaques can form virtually anywhere, but usually they form in areas where vascular anatomy predisposes to increased turbulence of blood flow, producing shearing forces that cause continuous microendothelial injury (e.g., in areas of bifurcation of major arteries).

Clinical effects depend on the location of the plaques

Coronary artery disease	Plaques form in coronary arteries, causing signs and symptoms of myocardial ischemia or infarct
Peripheral arterial disease	Plaques form in arteries of lower extremities. This can present with leg pain at rest that may be triggered by exertion (vascular claudication), nonhealing ulcer, or gangrene
Cerebral vascular disease	Presents with transient ischemic attack or stroke

Progression of coronary artery disease

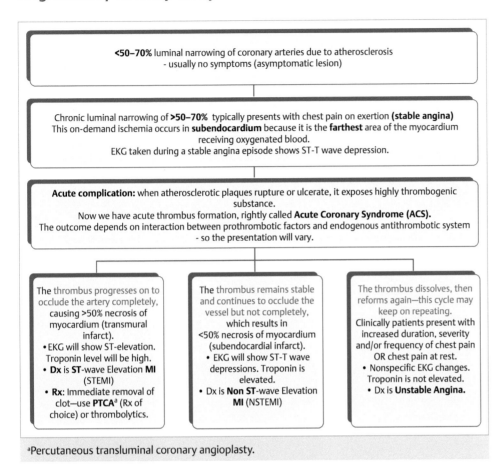

<50–70% luminal narrowing of coronary arteries due to atherosclerosis
- usually no symptoms (asymptomatic lesion)

Chronic luminal narrowing of **>50–70%** typically presents with chest pain on exertion **(stable angina)**
This on-demand ischemia occurs in **subendocardium** because it is the **farthest** area of the myocardium receiving oxygenated blood.
EKG taken during a stable angina episode shows ST-T wave depression.

Acute complication: when atherosclerotic plaques rupture or ulcerate, it exposes highly thrombogenic substance.
Now we have acute thrombus formation, rightly called **Acute Coronary Syndrome (ACS).**
The outcome depends on interaction between prothrombotic factors and endogenous antithrombotic system - so the presentation will vary.

The thrombus progresses on to occlude the artery completely, causing >50% necrosis of myocardium (transmural infarct).
• EKG will show ST-elevation. Troponin level will be high.
• **Dx** is **ST**-wave Elevation **MI** (STEMI)
• **Rx:** Immediate removal of clot—use **PTCA**[a] (Rx of choice) or thrombolytics.

The thrombus remains stable and continues to occlude the vessel but not completely, which results in <50% necrosis of myocardium (subendocardial infarct).
• EKG will show ST-T wave depressions. Troponin is elevated.
• Dx is **Non ST**-wave Elevation **MI** (NSTEMI)

The thrombus dissolves, then reforms again—this cycle may keep on repeating.
Clinically patients present with increased duration, severity and/or frequency of chest pain OR chest pain at rest.
• Nonspecific EKG changes. Troponin is not elevated.
• Dx is **Unstable Angina.**

[a]Percutaneous transluminal coronary angioplasty.

• Coronary artery disease (CAD) is the most common cause (MCC) of death in the United States and worldwide.
• MC underlying condition that predisposes to CAD is diabetes mellitus.
• MC underlying condition that predisposes to stroke is HTN.

4.2 Stable Angina

Pathophysiology: With underlying significant atherosclerotic narrowing of coronary vessel (> 50–70%), cardiac ischemia and chest pain can develop whenever there is increase in oxygen demand. Oxygen demand increases when the heart must work more due to increase in preload, afterload, and/or increase in heart rate.[1]

The following conditions can precipitate chest pain in patients with stable angina by increasing adrenergic activity and cardiac workload:

● Physical exertion.
● Anxiety.
● Cold exposure (epinephrine and norepinephrine are secreted in response to cold to maintain body temperature).
● Large meals.

Factors that lower oxygen content in blood may aggravate underlying ischemia, for example, anemia and carbon monoxide poisoning.

[1]Increase in heart rate not only increases myocardial oxygen demand, but also decreases myocardial blood supply, as heart spends less time in diastole. Note: Most of the myocardial blood supply occurs during **diastole.**

MRS

It **BANS angina.** All stable angina patients should be on BANS therapy, unless contraindicated.

Pharmacotherapy of stable angina

β-blockers	Primarily work by decreasing heart rate, thereby decreasing myocardial O$_2$ demand
Antiplatelet agents (e.g., aspirin, clopidogrel, ticagrelor)	Prevent platelet aggregation in the event of plaque rupture or ulceration **Aspirin** confers maximal mortality benefit in comparison to other treatment strategies
Nitrates (sublingual), as needed for chest pain	These primarily dilate venous capacitance vessels, thereby decreasing the preload. It also dilates large coronary vessels, which improves coronary blood flow Long-acting nitrates are used in patients who continue to have angina despite having adequate control of baseline heart rate (HR)
Statins	Stabilize plaques and reduce low-density lipoproteins levels

Ranolazine: It is indicated only in refractory stable angina (i.e., when symptoms persist despite optimal management). It decreases cardiac oxygen demand by inhibiting Na$^+$ channels and indirectly inhibiting calcium-mediated contraction.

Chest pain

Work-up: Any patient who presents with chest pain needs an electrocardiography (EKG), even if the pain is atypical.[2]

Now, let us say the EKG is normal. When do we investigate further for coronary artery disease (CAD)?

First, we need to answer the following questions:

- Is the chest pain typical?
  - Typical angina chest pain is crushing, heaving, substernal chest pain, radiating to left arm or jaw, exacerbated by exertion/emotion and relieved by rest. It usually does not have any relation with position or breathing.
- Does the patient have any risk factors for atherosclerotic cardiovascular disease (ASCVD)? *See the risk factors listed in the beginning of the chapter.*
- What is the age and sex of the patient?

Let us try some clinical case scenarios:

[2]Remember you cannot miss a diagnosis like angina or myocardial infarction (MI). It is the leading cause of death in developed countries.

CCS	Clinical assessment	NSIM (next step in management)
A 37-year-old male presents with periodic substernal burning chest pain not associated with exertion. He does not have any risk factors for CAD	Atypical chest pain in a patient with low likelihood of CAD	Cardiac stress test is not needed. Search for other causes of chest pain
Male older than 45 years of age (or female older than 55 years of age) presents with atypical chest pain. Patient is a smoker and has HTN (or has other additional risk factors for CAD)	Atypical chest pain in a patient with CAD risk factors	This CCS is medium probability for CAD. Schedule for cardiac stress test. The diagnosis of CAD cannot be missed
Male older than 45 years of age (or female older than 55 years of age) presents with typical chest pain associated with exertion. Patient has hx of multiple risk factors for CAD	Typical chest pain in a patient with CAD risk factors	The probability of stable angina is high. Initiate BANS therapy and schedule cardiac stress test for risk stratification

In a nutshell

Silent angina or myocardial infarction (MI): Patients with diabetes (and underlying autonomic neuropathy), postsurgery patients (on analgesia), and elderly patients can have atypical presentation of CAD. They may not present with classical anginal chest pain. These patients can present with the following symptoms:

- Sudden onset of shortness of breath.

- Profound weakness or diaphoresis.

- Jaw pain or left arm pain/heaviness.

- Epigastric pain.

- Confusion (usually in elderly).

This is known as silent angina or MI. Also, these patients are likely to present directly with complications of MI.

Management algorithm of stable angina

Legend: NSIM, next step in management; NSIDx, Next step in diagnosis

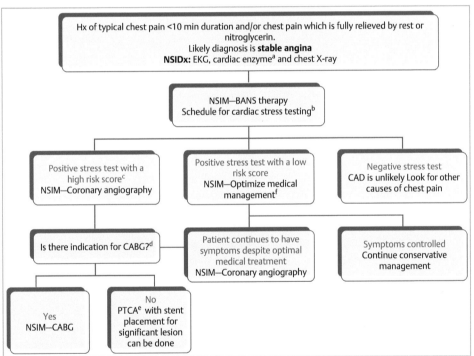

 MRS

For coronary artery bypass grafting (CABG) purpose, internal mammary artery graft is preferred over vein graft as the arterial graft lasts longer.

[a]Patients with stable angina typically present after an episode of chest pain, hence baseline EKG can be normal. Also, cardiac enzymes are normal by definition in angina.

[b]Patients who have high-risk occupations (e.g., pilots, bus drivers, train operators,) and who have presentation suggestive of high probability CAD can proceed directly to coronary catheterization, as missing angina in these cases may be catastrophic. Also, see next section on how to choose the right stress test.

[c]Early onset of chest pain or ST wave changes, large areas of ischemia, or hemodynamic instability during stress testing are considered high-risk features.

[d]Indications for **c**oronary artery bypass **g**rafting (CABG) are:

- Left main coronary artery stenosis of **> 50%.** (As left main artery is considered crucial, the cutoff for significant lesion is lower).

- Left main equivalent (≥ **70%** stenosis of proximal left anterior descending coronary artery [LAD] and proximal left circumflex).

- Three vessel disease (stenosis of **50%** or more in all three major coronary arteries)

- **More than 70%** proximal LAD stenosis + either EF < 50% or demonstrable ischemia on noninvasive testing.

- One- or two-vessel disease, a large area of viable myocardium **and** high-risk criteria in noninvasive testing.

[e]In stable angina, percutaneous transluminal coronary angioplasty (PTCA) has been shown to improve symptoms, but not mortality.

[f]Target resting HR should be around 55–60 beats per minute. Use beta blocker (preferable) and/or cardioselective calcium channel blocker (e.g. verapamil, diltiazem). If angina is still not controlled, use long-acting nitrates, followed by ranolazine on a step-by-step basis.

MRS

BANS CaLoRie Ca = **Cal**cium channel blocker.
Lo = **Lo**ng-acting nitrates.
Rie = **R**anolaz**ie**ne.

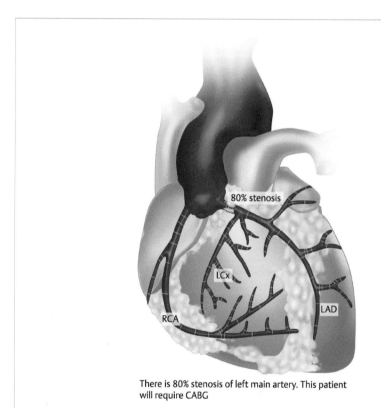

There is 80% stenosis of left main artery. This patient will require CABG

Clinical Case Scenarios (CCS)

1. Patient presents with problematic stable angina symptoms. He is on maximal dose of a beta blocker, full-dose aspirin, sublingual nitroglycerin as needed, and high-intensity statin therapy (BANS therapy). His resting heart rate is 90 beats per minute. What is the NSIM?

2. Above patient comes back to the office and reports that he continues to have problematic stable angina symptoms. His resting heart rate is 60 beats per minute. What is the NSIM?

3. In a patient with angina not controlled with optimal medical management, coronary angiography shows 65% proximal left main coronary artery stenosis. What is the NSIM?

How to choose the right stress test?

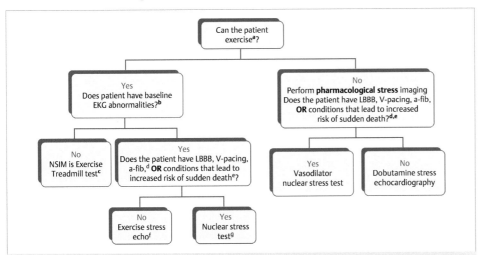

[a]Whenever possible, do exercise testing. It allows assessment of functional capacity of the patient. Some patients cannot exercise due to orthopedic or pulmonary issues.

[b]Conditions mentioned below typically have baseline EKG abnormalities (e.g., ST-T wave depression ≥ **1 mm**) where EKG cannot be interpreted[3]

- Left bundle branch block (LBBB).
- Certain cardiac drugs, such as digitalis, procainamide, can cause ST-T wave depression.
- Left ventricular hypertrophy with significant ST-T wave abnormalities.
- Wolff–Parkinson–White syndrome.
- Ventricular pacing.

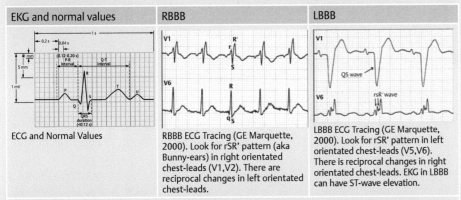

EKG and normal values	RBBB	LBBB
ECG and Normal Values	RBBB ECG Tracing (GE Marquette, 2000). Look for rSR' pattern (aka Bunny-ears) in right orientated chest-leads (V1,V2). There are reciprocal changes in left orientated chest-leads.	LBBB ECG Tracing (GE Marquette, 2000). Look for rSR' pattern in left orientated chest-leads (V5,V6). There is reciprocal changes in right orientated chest-leads. EKG in LBBB can have ST-wave elevation.

Source: The precordial exam. In: Shi Y, Sohani Z, Tang B, et al. Essentials of Clinical Examination Handbook. 8th ed. Thieme; 2018.

[c]Exercise Treadmill Test (ETT) is always preferred over other modalities, as it is low cost, easy to do, and does not involve radiation. But this can only be done in patients who can exercise and who have no significant baseline EKG abnormalities.[4]

[d]V-pacing and LBBB can produce false positive results on **exercise echocardiogram**. In patients with atrial fibrillation, dobutamine can worsen the arrhythmia.

[e]The following conditions can present with chest pain. They also predispose to sudden onset of ventricular fibrillation and have higher risk of sudden death on exertion or stress. Dobutamine or exercise stress test are contraindicated in these cases:

- Hypertrophic obstructive cardiomyopathy (HOCM)[5]
- Hx of sustained ventricular arrhythmia.
- Severe symptomatic aortic stenosis.
- Severe valvular disease.

[f]After exercise, ischemic areas become hypokinetic which is detected by echocardiography. *Note: if patient is known to have has extensive baseline wall motion abnormalities at rest, then echo imaging is not really helpful. In this case nuclear imaging is done.*

[g]Nuclear stress test includes the use of:

- Radionuclide contrast (thallium or technetium-99m) that helps in directly visualizing coronary blood flow; hence it is aka radionuclide myocardial perfusion imaging (rMPI)
+
- Vasodilator (adenosine or dypiridamole[6]) or exercise.

[3]If patients with these conditions and significantly abnormal baseline EKG, present with symptoms of ongoing ischemia, EKG changes can be obscured. Consider bedside echocardiography to look for hypokinesia or akinesia of the ventricular walls.

[4]Stress tests in order of preference are ETT > echocardiographic studies > nuclear imaging
Nuclear stress imaging involves radiation exposure that is approximately 15–20 times more than an average CT scan of head.

[5]CCS of young male athlete with chest pain—think of HOCM.

[6]Contraindications for adenosine or dipyridamole:
- Active bronchospastic airway disease.
- Sick sinus syndrome and high degree AV block (no pacemaker yet).
- Oral dipyridamole use.
Theophylline should be held for 48 hours and no caffeinated drinks for 12 hours before the procedure.

119

[7]Unlike adenosine or dypiridamole, nitrates cause vasodilation primarily in large epicardial vessels, thus there is less likelihood of coronary steal phenomenon.

"Coronary Steal Phenomenon"

Nuclear vasodilator test is based on this phenomenon. Stenosed coronary arteries, affected by atherosclerosis, are maximally dilated to compensate for decreased blood supply. Administration of a coronary vasodilator causes dilation of normal vessels and redirection of flow, "stealing" blood away from ischemic regions of the heart, resulting in decreased perfusion to these areas.[7]

Uniform distribution of radioactive thallium at rest but decreased radioactivity in certain areas after dipyridamole or adenosine injection is diagnostic of CAD.

Clinical situation *Tip: First try to answer if patient is able to exercise or not?*	Presence of other abnormalities	What stress test to order?
No orthopedic or pulmonary issues	RBBB with < 1 mm ST-T wave depression	ETT (Exercise Treadmill Test)
	• Patient has left bundle branch block (LBBB) • Extensive wall motion abnormalities were seen in previous echocardiography	Exercise nuclear stress test *(exercise whenever possible)* - Here we cannot do ETT because of LBBB and cannot do stress echocardiogram because of baseline wall motion abnormalities and LBBB
History of below knee amputation	No LBBB, no V-pacing, no baseline wall motion abnormalities or atrial fibrillation	Dobutamine echocardiography
Chronic pulmonary fibrosis	Has LBBB or V-pacing	Vasodilator nuclear stress test

Exercise treadmill test

Preparing for test: Medications that decrease heart rate (e.g., β-blockers, calcium channel blockers) should be withheld 48 hours prior to scheduled exercise treadmill test (ETT), as this might produce false negative result.

Test description: While patient is running on a treadmill or pedaling a bicycle, we monitor patient's vital signs (e.g., blood pressure, heart rate), and do a realtime EKG to look for signs of ischemia.

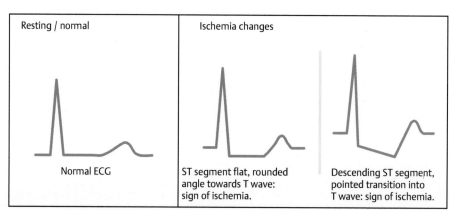

Remember these signs of ischemia:
- Altered mental status (e.g., confusion), or dizziness.
- Shortness **of** breath (SOB) or chest pain with ST-T wave depression ≥ **1 mm**.
- Hypotension.

- ST-T wave elevation in non-Q wave lead.
- Other high-risk features include development of high-grade atrioventricular (AV) block, ventricular arrhythmia, and/or left bundle branch block (LBBB).

If any of the above features develop, NSIM is to stop the test. Dx of stable angina is made.

- ETT is considered adequate if patient's heart rate reaches at least 85% of maximal heart rate.[8]
- If no signs of ischemia develop with target heart rate, then the dx of CAD is unlikely.
- If test fails to achieve at least 85% of the maximal heart rate, the test is considered to be inadequate to rule out CAD.

[8]The maximal heart rate = 220 − patient's age. 85% of maximal heart rate = target heart rate for ETT.

4.3 Acute Coronary Syndrome

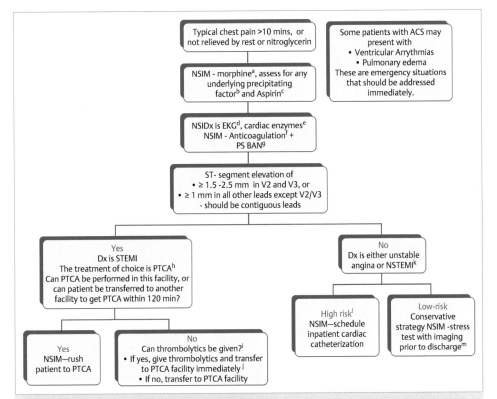

[a]Morphine is given to alleviate chest pain. Alleviating pain decreases accompanying sympathetic activity, which decreases cardiac myocardial oxygen demand. Morphine also acts as a direct venodilator, reducing the preload. If chest pain persists despite morphine and sublingual nitroglycerin, NSIM is intravenous nitroglycerin.

[b]If patient develops chest pain in the setting of acute massive gastrointestinal (GI) bleeding, NSIM is blood transfusion. Do not give aspirin in this setting.

- If patient develops chest pain in the setting of tachyarrhythmia, then controlling heart rate should be the primary goal.

[c]**Aspirin** confers the highest mortality benefit. It should be given in all chest pain patients as soon as possible, after excluding active bleeding, even before any diagnostic work-up. The first aspirin tablet should be chewed.

[d]If EKG can't be interpreted due to some preexisting condition (see optimal cardiac stress test chapter), NSIDx is bedside echocardiogram.[9]

[e]Cardiac enzymes are creatine kinase-muscle/brain (CK-MB) and cardiac troponins T or I. They can be normal in early MI, as it can take up to 4 to 12 hours after the MI event for the levels to be abnormal. Hence, normal cardiac enzyme levels cannot exclude MI in the first few hours after MI.

[f]In patients who are going for coronary catheterization, anticoagulation with unfractionated heparin or bivalirudin is preferred over low-molecular weight heparin (LMWH) due to easy reversibility and shorter duration of action. In low-risk patients for which conservative strategy is planned LMWH is preferred.

[9]Note that LBBB (new or old) is not considered a ST-elevation myocardial infarction (STEMI) equivalent anymore, as new studies suggest that only a small number of patients with new LBBB are ultimately diagnosed with acute MI.

MRS

PS BAN (PleaSe BAN chest pain for me)

[10] Platelet receptor (adenosine diphosphate receptor) blockers are ticagrelor, clopidogrel, and prasugrel.

[11] β-blockers are contraindicated in patients who present with acute congestive heart failure (particularly when patient is β-blocker naïve), hypotension, severe bradycardia, and heart block (other than first degree).

MRS

The recurrent number here is 3.

[g] Platelet receptor blockers,[9] statins, β-blockers,[10] aspirin, and nitrates are mainstay of treatment of acute coronary syndrome (ACS). Most patients with ACS are recommended to get dual antiplatelet therapy with aspirin+ platelet receptor blockers.

[h] Two treatment modalities have been shown to increase survival in STEMI:

- Percutaneous transluminal coronary angioplasty (PTCA) with stent placement (aka percutaneous coronary intervention [PCI]).
- Thrombolytics (administration of tissue plasminogen activator).

PTCA has been shown to have better outcome than thrombolytics, so whenever available, PTCA is the treatment of choice.

[i] Absolute contraindications for thrombolytics are:

- Active internal bleeding (excluding menstrual bleeding).
- Hx of **hemorrhagic** stroke anytime.
- Hx of **ischemic** stroke within the last 3 months.
- Significant closed head/facial trauma within 3 months.
- Suspected aortic dissection.
- Intracranial malignancy or vascular lesion.

Relative contraindications are:

- Poorly controlled HTN (systolic blood pressure > 180 mmHg).
- Ischemic stroke more than 3 months ago.
- Cardiopulmonary resuscitation for >10 minutes, or major surgery within < 3 weeks ago.
- Recent (within 3 weeks) internal bleeding.
- Recent invasive procedure.
- Noncompressible vascular puncture.
- Pregnancy.
- Active peptic ulcer.
- Pericarditis or pericardial fluid.
- Current use of anticoagulants—the higher the international normalized ratio (INR), the higher the risk of bleeding.
- For streptokinase: prior exposure (more than five days previously) or prior allergic reaction to these agents.
- Age > 75 years.
- Diabetic retinopathy.

[j] Studies have shown better outcomes in patients transferred to PCI facility immediately after thrombolysis, as rescue PCI may be needed if thrombolysis is not successful. The indicators of successful reperfusion therapy are resolution of chest pain, normalization of ST-segment, and development of transient benign accelerated idioventricular rhythm (reperfusion arrhythmia).

[k] Difference between unstable angina and non-STEMI is that in unstable angina, cardiac enzymes are not significantly elevated.

[l] Consider preangiography glycoprotein IIb/IIIa inhibitor (eptifibatide or tirofiban) if patient has persistent chest pain and/or persistent EKG changes despite optimal medical treatment.

[m] In selected unstable angina patients, who have no further episodes of chest pain and no troponin elevation, risk stratification with stress test can be done. If stress testing shows high-risk findings or EF of < 40%, coronary angiography is recommended.

ECG Evolution during Acute Q-Wave MI

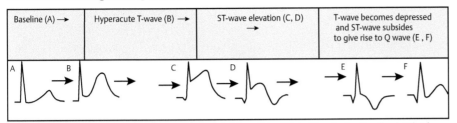

Baseline (A) →	Hyperacute T-wave (B) →	ST-wave elevation (C, D) →	T-wave becomes depressed and ST-wave subsides to give rise to Q wave (E, F)

Source: The precordial exam. In: Shi Y, Sohani Z, Tang B, et al. Essentials of Clinical Examination Handbook. 8th ed. Thieme; 2018.

4.3.1 Additional Notes on ACS Management

- What are the treatment modalities that decrease mortality and increase survival in acute coronary syndrome (ACS) patients?

β-blocker	• IV is preferred in patients with **ongoing** ischemia, chest pain, or EKG changes, particularly when patients have high heart rate or blood pressure. Then, oral maintenance therapy is long term • Cardioselective β-blockers like metoprolol are preferred in patients with COPD/asthma
Drugs that decrease platelet function	• Dual antiplatelet therapy with combination of aspirin and platelet receptor blockers has been shown to have better outcomes[a] • Usually aspirin is given lifelong, whereas duration of platelet receptor blocker is variable, depending on clinical situation
Statins	High-intensity statin therapy
ACE inhibitors or angiotensin II receptor blockers	Have been shown to improve mortality only in patients with EF of ≤ 40% (systolic dysfunction). They reduce ventricular remodeling
PTCA and thrombolytics	These drugs improve mortality only in STEMI patients

[a]Platelet receptor blockers are ticagrelor, clopidogrel, and prasugrel. *Recent recommendations prefer ticagrelor over clopidogrel in most of the clinical situations (except when thrombolytics are given, where clopidogrel is preferred).*

- Patients with CAD may have concomitant vascular impotence (same risk factors) and might be using phosphodiesterase inhibitors, such as sildenafil. **Nitrates** should not be given within **24 hours** of sildenafil use, as it can lead to dangerous hypotension, which can worsen myocardial infarction (MI).
- Postinfarct or post-revascularization chest pain is always considered unstable angina and treated as such. Measuring CK-MB level is very helpful for diagnosing reinfarction because it has short half-life and levels return to normal within 3 days.

 MRS

TropoNin return to baseline in TEN days.

Complications of coronary angiography or peripheral arterial catheterization

Clinical case	Dx	Additional info
Acute kidney injury few days after coronary catheterization	Can be due to contrast-induced nephropathy or renal atheroemboli (aka cholesterol emboli syndrome)	Renal atheroemboli occurs when dislodged atherematous plaque (commonly from abdominal aorta) leads to occlusion of renal vasculature. This can be spontaneous or due to arterial manipulation (as in angiography procedures). Look for additional features of atheroemboli, such as digital ischemia (blue-toes) or livedo reticularis (purple-brown, mottled skin rash). Eosinophilia might be present. Rx: usually supportive
Patient presents with acute low back pain after coronary angiography. Exam reveals pain on hip flexion	Retroperitoneal hematoma	NSIDx: CT scan of abdomen Rx: conservative management with avoidance of anticoagulation
Patient develops pulsatile mass in groin area, where catheterization was done a day earlier. Exam reveals systolic bruit over the swelling	Femoral artery pseudoaneurysm	NSIDx: ultrasound doppler Rx: usually managed conservatively, unless expanding rapidly or becomes very large, then surgical repair is recommended

Clinical Case Scenarios

4   A 59-year-old male presents with chest pain. After receiving nitroglycerin patient develops hemodynamic instability with hypotension. What medication is the patient likely taking at home?

4.3.2 Myocardial Infarction, Arterial Territories, and Complications

Mechanical complications of MI were commonly seen prior to the era of interventional cardiology, but fortunately, they are not that common anymore.

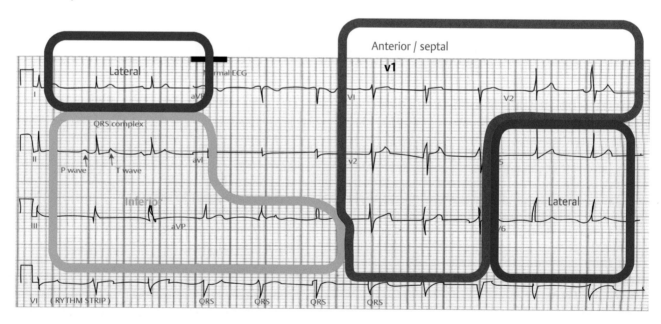

Artery	Areas supplied	EKG changes	Complications		Additional points
Right coronary artery (RCA)	• SA and AV node • Right ventricle (RV) • Inferior wall of left ventricle • Posterior portion of interventricular septum	**II, III, AVF** = inferior wall involvement **V1 and V2** = RV involvement[a]	Complete heart block and possible development of asystole due to AV node infarction		Hypotension, bradycardia **Rx:** Pacemaker
			Acute RV failure • RV infarction → decrease in compliance of RV (as RV fails to relax) → decrease in RV output → decrease in blood return to left ventricle → then total decrease in cardiac output → hypotension		Hypotension, tachycardia, and JVD with Kussmaul sign[b] Clear lungs on exam and clear CXR **Rx:** IV fluids and dobutamine
			Within few days/week after acute MI, patient develops acute heart failure and/or cardiogenic shock. This can be due to following factors →	Rupture/dysfunction of posterior **papillary muscle** of mitral valve with development of acute mitral regurgitation	Pansystolic murmur heart best at mitral area radiating to axilla
				Acute VSD due to rupture of interventricular septum	Pansystolic murmur heard best at left sternal border with palpable systolic thrill
Left circumflex artery	Lateral wall infarction	AV**L**, **I**, V5, V6	Nonspecific		
Left anterior descending (LAD) artery	• Anterior wall of left ventricle • Anterior portion of interventricular septum	V1 to V6	The anterior wall constitutes the major contractile portion of left ventricle; hence infarction may lead to following →	Acute heart failure and/or cardiogenic shock presenting on the first day of MI	Presents with acute pulmonary edema or hypotension (cardiogenic shock), without any characteristic murmur
				Low ejection fraction that leads to increased stasis and increased risk of intracardiac thrombus formation[c]	Development of acute stroke, intestinal ischemia, or acute leg pain in a patient with recent hx of anterior wall MI. (This is a late complication)
			Within few days to 2 weeks after acute MI, patient develops acute heart failure and/or cardiogenic shock →	Free wall rupture resulting in hemopericardium and cardiac tamponade	Hypotension, JVD, pulsus paradoxus,[d] muffled heart sounds CXR and chest exam are unremarkable NSIM is emergent pericardiocentesis
				Acute VSD due to rupture of interventricular septum[e]	Pansystolic murmur heard best at left sternal border with palpable systolic thrill
			Left ventricular aneurysm In large anterior wall MI, the ventricular wall can become weak and develop outpouching		Can present with progressive heart failure, systemic cardiac embolism, and/or sustained ventricular tachycardia Look for double apical impulse in physical exam and **sustained ST-wave elevation** in EKG[f] NSIDx: TTE

Posterior descending artery	Posterior wall	Horizontal ST-wave depression in V1-V3 might suggest posterior wall STEMI	Nonspecific It is usually associated with complications related to either RCA or left circumflex territory as posterior descending artery can be a branch of either one of these arteries

[a]If ST-T wave elevation in V1 taller than V2, suspect right ventricular infarction. NSIDx is to place EKG leads in right side of the chest. Most specific finding for RV infarction is ST-T wave elevation in right-sided leads.

[b]Kussmaul sign = paradoxical increase in jugular venous pressure (JVP) on inspiration.

[c]Warfarin or newer generation anticoagulants is recommended in patients with EF of < 30% and severe anteroapical wall motion abnormality (high risk of thrombus formation). Anticoagulation is also reasonable in patients with EF of ≤ 40% and severe wall motion abnormalities, particularly if patient has low risk for bleeding.

[d]Pulsus paradoxus= more than expected fall in systolic blood pressure (≥10 mm Hg) during inspiration.

[e]Most specific diagnostic finding for VSD is the presence of left-to-right shunt on right heart catheterization.

[f]This aneurysm may enlarge and mature over time; a mature true left ventricular aneurysm rarely ruptures because of the dense fibrosis in its wall.

Management: Medical treatment with afterload reduction for small- to moderate-sized aneurysm. Consider aneurysmectomy + coronary artery bypass grafting (CABG) for patients with persistent heart failure or intractable ventricular arrhythmias, who failed medical management or percutaneous interventions. In patients with severe left ventricular (LV) dysfunction or presence of a clot, anticoagulation is recommended.

Abbreviations: AVF, augmented Vector Foot; CXR, chest X-ray; EKG, electrocardiogram; JVD, jugular venous distension; MI, myocardial infarction; VSD, ventricular septal defect.

Differentiating different causes of acute heart failure and/or cardiogenic shock in acute MI

Diagnosis	High-grade heart block	Right ventricular infarction	Free ventricular wall rupture → hemopericardium → cardiac tamponade	Acute ventricular septal defect	Acute mitral regurgitation	Anterior wall MI
Arterial territory	RCA (or LAD[a])	RCA	LAD	LAD (or RCA)	RCA or LAD	LAD
Pointers to diagnosis	EKG shows high-grade heart block (heart rate < 60/min)	• Clear lungs on exam and clear CXR[b] • JVD • Heart rate >60/min (they usually develop tachycardia) • Positive Kussmaul sign, Pulsus paradoxus[c]		Biventricular failure occurs; hence lungs might be clear. They mostly present with hypotension (cardiogenic shock)	Acute pulmonary edema, S3, JVD, and bibasilar crackles	
Characteristic cardiac auscultation	NA	Might have functional murmur of TR due to tricuspid annular dilatation	Muffled heart sounds	Loud holosystolic/ pansystolic murmur heart best at left sternal border. (Sometimes it is best heard at mitral area and can be hard to differentiate from MR)	Loud holosystolic/ pansystolic murmur heart best at mitral area, radiating to axilla	Might have functional murmur of MR due to annular dilatation
Management (including supportive care)	Pacemaker	IV fluids +/- inotropes (dobutamine)	Rapid bedside TTE and pericardiocentesis. If pericardiocentesis is bloody, immediate surgery is indicated	NSIDx: emergent TTE. NSIM: afterload reduction, IABP, and emergent surgery	Pressure support and IABP, if needed	

[a]Complete heart block can also occur in extensive anterior wall MI, which has a poorer prognosis.

[b]In acute pericardial tamponade due to myocardial rupture, the classic sign of big globular heart in CXR might not be evident, as adequate time hasn't passed by for pericardial stretching to occur.

[c]Pulsus paradoxus and Kussmaul sign have very similar causes (e.g. constrictive pericarditis, restrictive cardiomyopathy, pericardial tamponade)

Abbreviations: CXR, chest X-ray; IABP, intra-aortic balloon pump; JVD, jugular venous distension; LAD, left anterior descending artery; MI, myocardial infarction; MR, mitral regurgitation; RCA, right coronary artery; TR, tricuspid regurgitation, TTE, transthoracic echocardiography; VSD, ventricular septal defect.

> ⚠ **Caution**
>
> Know how to differentiate them. Think about the ones that cause pulmonary edema (crackles in exam and CXR with bilateral infiltrates) versus the ones that do not.

4.3.3 Other Complications of Acute Coronary Syndrome

Ventricular Fibrillation (VF)

It is the most common cause (MCC) of death in CAD and MI is VF. Arrhythmias usually occur within first 24 hours of MI. Mechanism of arrhythmia is reentrant circuit formation (ischemic/infarct area have different conduction properties than viable/normal myocardium).

- β-blockers decrease risk of ventricular arrhythmias.
- Lidocaine should **NOT** be given prophylactically as it can increase risk for asystole.
- Automated implantable cardioverter-defibrillator (AICD) placement is indicated in VF and sustained ventricular tachycardia (VT) that occur after 48 hours of index-MI.

[12] By similar mechanism, intracardiac thrombus can form in:
- Atrial fibrillation (stasis of blood in the left atrium).
- Dilated cardiomyopathy (all of the heart chambers are dilated and hypokinetic).
- LV aneurysm.

Cardioembolic phenomenon

With loss of major contractile portion of the heart that occurs particularly in anterior wall MI, resultant stasis increases risk of thrombus formation in the left ventricle.[12] Development of thrombus can lead to the following complications:

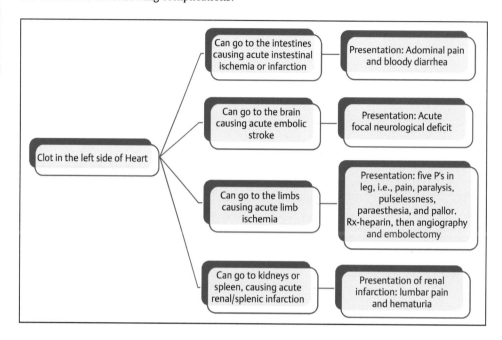

Post-MI pericarditis: Section 4.6.5, Pericarditis

Clinical Case Scenarios

Patient had an anterior wall MI 3 weeks ago. She now presents with sudden onset left-sided weakness and aphasia. EKG reveals sustained ST-wave elevation.

5. What is the NSIDx to look for the underlying cause?

6. What is the likely underlying cause?

Other causes of chest pain

Clinical case	Clues	Dx and additional info	Management
Young patient presents with chest pain along with features of sympathetic hyperactivity (sweating, pupil dilation, agitation, psychosis, etc.) *"Usually after a party"*	**Exam** may reveal multiple track marks in the arms, nasal bleeding, and/or septum perforation. Troponin is elevated	**Cocaine-induced vasospasm** resulting in acute MI Patients *can deny illicit drug use (favorite red-herring in exam question)* Cocaine can also cause seizures, hemorrhagic stroke, and arryhthmias	**D**iazepam (decreases the stimulatory effects of cocaine), **a**spirin, and **n**itrates β-blocker is contraindicated because it can cause unopposed α-1 vasoconstriction leading to severe HTN and worsening ischemia When suspected, urine drug screen should be done

(Continued)

Clinical case	Clues	Dx and additional info	Management
Young patient with no risk factors for atherosclerotic disease presents with chest pain **mostly at night**	When EKG is taken during an episode of chest pain, it can reveal **transmural ischemia** in the form of ST elevation in the respective arterial territory in which vasospasm is occurring. Most common artery involved is **RCA**	**Variant angina aka Prinzmetal's angina** The vasospasm commonly remits on its own, but sometimes it can progress to MI or arrhythmias. It occurs due to abnormal vasomotor reactivity, and can be associated with other vasospastic conditions such as Raynaud's syndrome or migraine	NSIM is calcium channel blockers (drug of choice) or nitrates. **Avoid** aspirin or β-blockers as they might aggravate vasospasm To confirm the dx, do **coronary angiography** with provocative testing (acetylcholine or ergonovine induce vasospasm in these patients). Hyperventilation can also induce chest pain
Patient presents with chest pain after a severe physical or emotional stress/trauma	EKG may show ST-T wave elevation. Typically, there is significant troponin elevation. TTE: decreased left ventricular systolic function with apical hypokinesis and ballooning. Angiography reveals normal coronary arteries	**Stress-induced cardiomyopathy (aka Takotsubo syndrome)** Pathophysiology: Surging stress hormones (e.g., epinephrine) can essentially "stun" the heart triggering changes in myocardial contractility and/or coronary blood vessel	If EF < 40%, start β-blocker and ACE inhibitor Repeat TTE in few weeks. Generally the hypokinesis resolves with time
Old person with chest pain on exertion	Physical exam reveals ejection systolic murmur	**Aortic stenosis**	NSIDx is TTE Schedule for coronary angiography and aortic valve surgery, as chest pain due to aortic stenosis is an indication for surgery
Perimenopausal female patient presents with chest pain (at rest and/or exertion)	Tread mill test induces ST depression. Coronary angiography is unremarkable	**Cardiac syndrome X**	β-blocker and reassurance
Patient presents with atypical chest pain	Exam reveals a click followed by a systolic murmur	**Mitral valve prolapse**	Usually reassurance and lifestyle modification (avoidance of alcohol, stress, and caffeine). β-blockers have not shown to be effective in this case
Patient presents with chest pain that gets worse when taking deep breaths	Exam reveals costochondral tenderness. EKG is unremarkable	**Costochondritis**	NSAIDs

Note: Other causes of chest pain are aortic dissection (discussed later in this chapter), esophagitis/esophageal syndrome (see Chapter 9), spontaneous pneumothorax and pulmonary embolism (see Chapter 3).
Abbreviations: ACE, angiotensin-converting enzyme; EKG, electrocardiogram; HTN, hypertension; NSAIDs, nonsteroidal anti-inflammatory drugs; RCA, right coronary artery; ETT; TTE, transthoracic echocardiography.

4.4 Heart Failure

Definition: Primary life-sustaining work of our heart is to receive blood (diastole) and then to pump it (systole). Heart failure can occur when heart fails to relax adequately to receive enough blood (diastolic failure/dysfunction) or to pump enough blood (systolic heart failure/dysfunction). It might also fail to do both.

Clinical features of heart failure

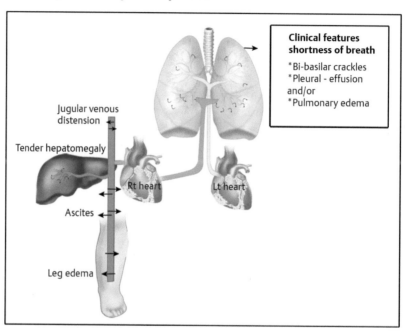

Clinical features
shortness of breath

*Bi-basilar crackles
*Pleural - effusion
and/or
*Pulmonary edema

Jugular venous distension

Tender hepatomegaly

Rt heart   Lt heart

Ascites

Leg edema

Clinical pathophysiology

[13] The predominant symptom of the left heart failure is SOB.

[14] Lying flat increases venous return, thereby increasing preload pressure and putting strain on a weak heart.

MCC of right heart failure is left heart failure, as left heart pathology is more common. Increased left-sided pressure due to left heart failure eventually increases right-sided heart pressure.

- **Increase in backward pressure from left heart failure:** Increased pressure in pulmonary vascular system results in fluid leakage into the alveoli, causing gas exchange problem and SOB (shortness of breath).[13]
  Depending upon severity of heart failure, SOB can initially be present only on exertion, later progress to paroxysmal nocturnal dyspnea (SOB 1–2 hours after lying down) → orthopnea (SOB immediately after lying flat)[14] → SOB at rest.
  Severe left heart failure can cause acute respiratory failure and acute pulmonary edema. Exam may reveal bibasilar crackles and S3. (S3 is one of the most specific finding in heart failure.)
- **Increase in backward pressure from right heart failure:** This results in increased pressure in the systemic veins and presents with jugular venous distension, hepatomegaly, ascites, and bilateral pitting edema.
- **Decrease in forward cardiac output:** All patients with heart failure have symptoms related to decrease in cardiac output. This presents with SOB and limitation of physical activity.

New York Heart Association functional classification of heart failure

NYHA grade	Description
I	No limitation of physical activity (i.e., no symptoms with ordinary exertion)
II	Slight limitation of physical activities (i.e., ordinary activity causes SOB)
III	Marked limitation of physical activity (i.e., less than ordinary activity causes SOB)
IV	SOB at rest

Work-up: For any patient who presents with abovementioned clinical features, the NSIDx is transthoracic echocardiography (TTE).

Heart failure (HF) classification by ejection fraction[15]

Classification	EF ≤ 40% = systolic heart failure (aka heart failure with reduced EF)	EF > 40 %= diastolic heart failure (aka heart failure with preserved EF)
Major causes	• Dilated cardiomyopathy • Ischemic heart disease Note: Almost all causes of diastolic HF, if untreated can lead to systolic HF	Hypertension, valvular heart disease, hypertrophic obstructive cardiomyopathy, restrictive cardiomyopathy, right ventricular infarction[a]
Extra heart sound heard[b]	S3	S4
Echocardiography findings	**Akinetic** or **hypokinetic** myocardium	Impaired relaxation of cardiac wall with thickened myocardium
Medical therapy	• **ACE inhibitors** (DOC) or ARB. (They decrease afterload, so that the ventricles can contract easily.) • **β-blockers** (discussed further on next page)	• Spironolactone has been shown to be beneficial • Other medications such as β-blockers, ACE inhibitors, and ARBs lack proven benefit, but can be used to treat underlying cause such as HTN

[a]In right ventricular (RV) infarction, the primary pathologic mechanism is the failure of the right heart to relax. The systolic function of RV is not that important, as RV is not required to generate a lot of force to pump blood through low-pressure pulmonary system.

[b]*Practice listening to the S3/S4 heart sounds as it is high yield. They are available in Google videos/ YouTube.*

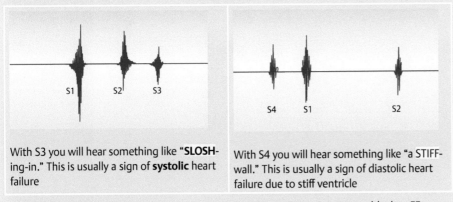

With S3 you will hear something like "**SLOSH**-ing-in." This is usually a sign of **systolic** heart failure

With S4 you will hear something like "a STIFF-wall." This is usually a sign of diastolic heart failure due to stiff ventricle

Abbreviations: ACE, angiotensin-converting enzyme; ARB, angiotensin receptor blocker; EF, ejection fraction; HTN, hypertension.

[15]MUGA scan (a nuclear medicine scan) is the most accurate test for assessment of EF. However, it is rarely done, as TTE is a pretty good test.

MRS

Triple load: Triple = 3 = S3, which is due to volume overload and systolic CHF. For compliance reasons. For = four= S4 is due to compliance issue of ventricles.
The loudest heart sound is always the S1 which corresponds with "SLOSH" and "STIFF"

4.4.1 Systolic Heart Failure Management

Legend: NSIM, next step in management: ACE-I, angiotensin-converting enzyme inhibitor: ARB, angiotensin receptor blocker

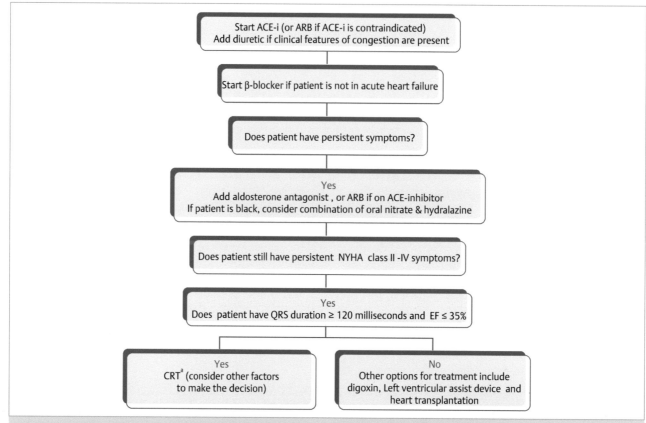

Start ACE-i (or ARB if ACE-i is contraindicated)
Add diuretic if clinical features of congestion are present

Start β-blocker if patient is not in acute heart failure

Does patient have persistent symptoms?

Yes
Add aldosterone antagonist , or ARB if on ACE-inhibitor
If patient is black, consider combination of oral nitrate & hydralazine

Does patient still have persistent NYHA class II -IV symptoms?

Yes
Does patient have QRS duration ≥ 120 milliseconds and EF ≤ 35%

Yes
CRT[a] (consider other factors
to make the decision)

No
Other options for treatment include
digoxin, Left ventricular assist device and
heart transplantation

[a]Cardiac resynchronization therapy (CRT): Strongest consideration is given for patients with LBBB morphology and QRS duration of ≥ 150 milliseconds.

How does CRT work? Prolonged QRS interval on EKG signals that left and right ventricles are not working in synchrony. CRT (biventricular pacing) consists of placing pacer leads in both ventricles in order to make them contract simultaneously. Synchronous contractions are more effective, resulting in increased cardiac output.

Automated implantable cardioverter-defibrillator (AICD)

Failing heart is prone to life-threatening ventricular arrhythmias, and AICDs improve survival by cardioverting life-threatening ventricular arrhythmias.

	Indications
Primary prophylaxis	• NYHA grade II and III and EF of ≤ 35%[1] • NYHA III and IV with indication for CRT (EF of ≤ 35% and QRS duration of duration ≥ 120 milliseconds)[a] • Ischemic cardiomyopathy, EF of ≤ 30–35% and NYHA I. If recent hx of MI, reevaluate EF at least 40 days post MI
Secondary prophylaxis	• Resuscitated cardiac arrest thought to be due to ventricular arrhythmias. • Hemodynamically unstable ventricular arrhythmias in whom a completely reversible cause is not identified • Spontaneous sustained ventricular tachycardia in presence of structural heart disease (e.g., cardiomyopathies) or channelopathies

[a]In patients with NYHA class IV heart failure and no indication for CRT, AICD alone is not recommended due to poor prognosis.

Abbreviations: CRT, cardiac resynchronization therapy; EF, ejection fraction; MI, myocardial infarction; NYHA, New York Heart Association; VT/VF, ventricular tachycardia/ventricular fibrillation.

Medications that have been shown to decrease mortality in patients with systolic heart failure

ACE inhibitors and angiotensin-II receptor blockers	They halt progression of LV dysfunction and prevent cardiac remodeling by blocking negative effects of renin-angiotensin-aldosterone system
β-blockers	Carvedilol, long-acting metoprolol, and bisoprolol were studied in patients with systolic heart failure, hence they are preferred
Aldosterone antagonists (in patients with NYHA II–IV)	• Spironolactone can have antiandrogen side effects • Eplerenone can be used if patient develops gynecomastia
Isosorbide dinitrate + hydralazine combination	Indications: • In black patients with NYHA class III or IV, or • In all patients with systolic heart failure, who cannot tolerate ACE inhibitor, ARB, or aldosterone antagonist due to advanced CKD or hyperkalemia
Combination of ARB + neprilysin inhibitor (valsartan + sacubitril)	A new study reported that this combination was superior to ACE inhibitor in reducing mortality in patients with systolic heart failure. Guidelines regarding this medication is evolving

Note: CRT and AICD are cardiac devices that also have been shown to improve mortality in a subset of patients with systolic heart failure.

Abbreviations: ACE, angiotensin-converting enzyme; AICD, automated implantable cardioverter-defibrillator; ARB, angiotensin receptor blocker; CKD, chronic kidney disease; NYHA, New York Heart Association

⚠ **Caution**

Diuretics and digoxin provide symptomatic benefit and reduce hospitalization rates; however, these medications have not been shown to improve survival.

All patients with EF <40% should be on β-blockers (one of the 3 mentioned) + ACEi or ARB.

🔍 Clinical Case Scenarios

A 65-year-old male black patient has chronic systolic heart failure with NYHA class II functional status. He was started on an angiotensin-converting enzyme (ACE) inhibitor. In **8 weeks, his creatinine has increased by more than 30%** above baseline.

7. What is the NSIM regarding ACE-i?

8. What should be started next?

A 65-year-old male with hx of systolic heart failure, on lisinopril for the last few months, comes in to the clinic with lip swelling for 1 day.

9. What is the likely diagnosis?

10. What medication will you start after stopping ACE-i?

4.4.2 Acute Decompensated Heart Failure

Presentation: Hallmark of presentation is worsening SOB (more than baseline). When severe, it can progress to pulmonary edema and acute respiratory failure.[16]

Causes of acute decompensation of heart failure

- Inadequate diuretic dosage or noncompliance.
- Excessive dietary salt intake: The first SIM of heart failure patient is to decrease salt intake.
- Brady- or tachyarrhythmias.
- Myocardial ischemia or infarction.
- Thyrotoxicosis (check thyroid-stimulating hormone [TSH] when suspected).

[16]*CCS: 75-year-old male presents with acute respiratory failure requiring 4 L of oxygen via nasal cannula. Physical exam reveals elevated jugular venous pressure, S3 heart sound and extensive crackles are heard throughout lung. Patient is also bringing up pink frothy sputum at bedside.*

- Infection.
- Anemia.
- Uncontrolled HTN.
- Medications such as nonsteroidal anti-inflammatory drugs (NSAIDs), thiazolidinediones, etc.

Management

[17]Brain natriuretic peptide (BNP) is secreted by the ventricles in response to volume overload and stretching of the cardiomyocytes.
- BNP level of <100 often excludes decompensated heart failure as the etiology for SOB.
- BNP of >400 has high positive predictive value for heart failure as the etiology of SOB.
Note: BNP cannot be used to differentiate in between systolic and diastolic heart failure. Also in morbidly obese patients BNP might be falsely low.

For acute presentation with significant worsening of symptoms, NSIDx is EKG, chest X-ray (CXR), and serum brain natriuretic peptide (BNP).[17] TTE should also be done later.
- Address underlying factor (e.g., correction of atrial fibrillation with rapid ventricular rate).
- For severe cases follow the following management plan:
  - **L**oop diuretics (intravenous): Lasix (furosemide), bumetanide, etc. (Furosemide is not only a loop diuretic, but also causes venodilation, thereby decreasing preload, even before the onset of its diuretic action.)
  - **M**orphine: Consider this in patients who appear very short of breath (distress) It decreases accompanying sympathetic activity and acts as a direct venodilator.
  - **N**itroglycerin paste, IV nitroglycerin, or nitroprusside drip, can be used to decrease preload, particularly in patients acute severe heart failure and in presence of comorbidities such as severe HTN, acute mitral regurgitation, etc.
  - **O**xygen (high flow) → BIPAP → intubation (depending upon severity).
  - **P**osition patient to keep the head of bed elevated: A simple technique of increasing the angle of the patient's bed to > 45 degrees decreases venous return and improves symptom.

MRS

LMNOP

Further management

- In hospitalized patients with severe acute heart failure who are not responding to aggressive high-dose diuretics, consider hemodialysis with ultrafiltration to remove extra fluid.
- The following modalities can be considered in patients with progressive severe heart failure, especially in patients with signs of end-organ dysfunction in the setting of a low cardiac output, as a bridging therapy for heart transplantation:-
  - Inotropes such as, sympathomimetic drugs (dobutamine or dopamine), or phosphodiesterase inhibitors (amrinone or milrinone)
  - biventricular pacing, or
  - left ventricular assist device (LVAD)

Electrolyte abnormalities in patients with heart failure

MRS

Potassium-sparing diuretics are **s**pironolactone, **a**miloride, and **t**riamterene.
SAT with potassium

This is common because of concurrent use of diuretics and associated comorbidities.

Hyperkalemia[a]	Can be caused by ACE-i, ARB, and/or potassium-sparing diuretics
Hypokalemia[a]	Can be caused by all diuretics except the potassium sparing ones.
Hyponatremia	Neurohormonal activation leads to increase in ADH and renin-aldosterone activity, which results in excess water retention and hyponatremia. It is often associated with severe heart failure and poor prognosis.

[a]Abnormal potassium level can precipitate arrhythmias and worsen heart failure.

Abbreviations: ACE-i, angiotensin-converting enzyme inhibitor; ADH, antidiuretic hormone; ARB, angiotensin receptor blocker.

4.5 Arrhythmias

Presentation: Depending on the severity of underlying arrhythmia, brady/tachyarrhythmias can present with missed heartbeat, palpitations, chest pain, SOB, exercise intolerance, presyncope (dizziness), and syncope. Very severe arrhythmias can present with sudden onset clinical deterioration and hemodynamic instability.

Work-up: NSIDx for suspected arrhythmia is EKG. If EKG is unremarkable, NSIDx is Holter or event loop monitoring.

4.5.1 Acute Tachyarrhythmias

Main mechanisms are:

- **Reentrant arrhythmic circuit:**[18] Difference in electrical conduction can occur between normal and abnormal myocardium (e.g., due to ischemia, fibrosis, accessory pathway). This can, at times, create an electrical positive feedback loop that can cause persistent action potential propagation and development of arrhythmia.

- **Increased automaticity: This** can occur with excessive adrenergic stimulation, muscarinic blockade, etc.

[18] This is the most common mechanism of arrhythmia.

Algorithm: Approach to Management of Acute Tachyarrhythmias

Legend: NSIM, next step in management; DOC, drug of choice

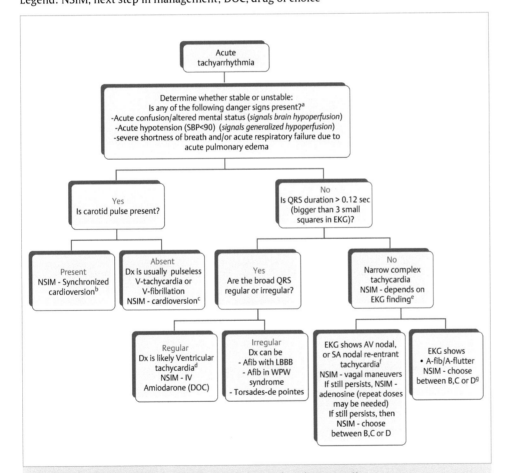

[a] In presence of "danger" signs, NSIM is always electrical cardioversion.[19]

[b] When pulse is present, NSIM is to do synchronized cardioversion, which delivers shock during systole. When cardioversion is not properly synchronized to systole, it can trigger dangerous ventricular tachycardia.

[c] If pulse is absent, there is nothing to synchronize cardioversion with; hence no need for synchronization.

[19] Note, hemodynamically unstable tachyarrhythmias are usually >150 beats per min.

[d]Wide-complex tachycardia with AV dissociation (atria and ventricles beat independently of each other in their own rhythm and rate) is pathognomonic for ventricular tachycardia. **Amiodarone** is the drug of choice (DOC). Other choices are lidocaine, procainamide, and sotalol.

[e]For narrow complex tachycardia look at the EKG to determine next plan of action:

Rhythm	R-R interval	P waves	EKG
Sinus tachycardia and SA nodal reentrant tachycardia	Regular	Present	
AV-nodal reentrant tachycardia (AVNRT)	Regular	No P waves	Source: Abnormalities of cardiac excitation. In: Michael J, Sircar S. Fundamentals of medical physiology. 1st ed. Thieme; 2010.
Atrial flutter	Can be Regular (*inset picture*), or irregular (with variable AV block)	Saw-tooth flutter waves (usually prominent in lead II and V1)	Source: Abnormalities of cardiac excitation. In: Michael J, Sircar S. Fundamentals of medical physiology. 1st ed. Thieme; 2010.
Atrial fib	Always irregular	No P-waves	Source: Tachyarrhythmias. In: Siegenthaler W. Siegenthaler's differential diagnosis in internal medicine: from symptom to diagnosis. 1st ed. Thieme; 2007.

[f]In SA or AV nodal reentrant tachycardia (SANRT or AVNRT), primary micro-reentrant circuit occurs inside the SA node or the AV node. If we block the SA or AV node (even for short period of time), you can terminate the arrhythmia.[20]

- NSIM is vagal stimulation by doing carotid sinus massage (*but wait!! auscultate the carotids before doing that. If carotid bruit is present, avoid doing massage*). Other methods of vagal stimulation include Valsalva maneuver or drinking ice cold water.

- If the tachycardia still persists after vagal maneuvers, NSIM is **a**denosine (a drug that specifically blocks the nodes). This drug has a very short half-life, so repeat dose can be give within few minutes, if still tachycardic.

- If still not controlled, then any of the following can be given:
  - **β**-blocker (do **not** give in patients with obstructive airway disease like compulsive obstructive pulmonary disorder [COPD] and asthma).
  - **C**alcium channel blockers (diltiazem is commonly used).
  - **D**igoxin: this is a third line drug preferred only in patients with associated **systolic** heart failure or relative hypotension.

[g]For atrial fibrillation or atrial flutter,[21] NSIM is to choose between **B, C, (or D)**. These drugs primarily block the AV node conduction, which helps to control the ventricular rate.

4.5.2 Types of Tachyarrhythmias

Multifocal Atrial Tachycardia

EKG description: Three or more P waves of different shapes, with irregularly irregular R-R interval.

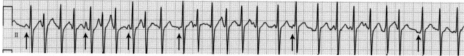

Source: Modified from Jer5150, CC BY-SA 3.0, via Wikimedia Commons.

Side notes:

[20]Sinus tachycardia and SA nodal re-entrant tachycardia may be virtually indistinguishable by looking at EKG; pointers to the latter are abrupt initiation and termination of rhythm and its responsiveness to vagal stimulation or adenosine.

MRS

ABCD

[21]In a-fib/flutter, the extra-nodal circuits are not terminated by transient nodal blockers like vagal stimulation or adenosine.

Premature atrial complexes (PACs) or Premature ventricular complexes (PVCs)
- Most of the time benign.
- Check electrolytes if patient has risk factors for electrolyte abnormalities (e.g., patients on diuretics)
- Reassurance alone is usually enough.

Etiology: Usually related to pulmonary issues (COPD, pulmonary HTN), or electrolyte abnormalities.

Management: Correct hypoxemia, if present and check for electrolyte abnormalities. If tachycardic, use calcium channel blocker. (β-blockers can worsen underlying bronchospastic airway disease.)

Atrial Fibrillation/Atrial Flutter[22]

Etiology of AF

- MCC is HTN.
- Hyperthyroidism: check TSH in all patients presenting with AF. If hyperthyroid, DOC are β-blockers (propranolol or metoprolol).
- Atrial dilatation due to valvular heart disease, dilated cardiomyopathy, etc.
- Pulmonary disorders such as COPD, pulmonary embolism.
- Sick sinus syndrome.
- Wolff–Parkinson–White (WPW) syndrome.

[22] Legend: For this section AF denotes both atrial fibrillation and atrial flutter.

Physical exam may reveal

- Irregularly irregular pulse (atrial fibrillation or atrial flutter with variable AV block).
- Regular (atrial flutter with fixed heart block).

EKG: absent P waves (atrial fibrillation) or saw-tooth P waves (atrial flutter).

Most common structural abnormality which predisposes to atrial flutter is left atrial dilation.

Management of AF includes the following scenarios

- New onset hemodynamically stable AF.
- Chronic AF.
- Anticoagulation in AF.

Approach to management of new onset hemodynamically stable AF

Hemodynamically stable new onset A-fib/A-flutter
Consider cardioversion[a]

Onset <48 hrs
NSIM- Cardioversion ASAP

Onset >48 hrs or unknown
Then we can follow either of the following strategies

CHADVAS[c]
score of 0 or 1
- May not require anticoagulation

CHADSVASc
score of ≥ 2
NSIM -initiate anticogulation

At least 3 weeks of anticoagulation, followed by electrical or pharmacological cardioversion

TEE[b] to rule out intracardiac thrombus, followed by electrical cardioversion

Continue anticoagulation for at least 4 weeks after cardioversion

CHADSVASC of 0, or 1
NSIM- may discontinue anticoagulation

CHADSVASc score of ≥ 2
NSIM- continue anticoagulation

[a]A trial of cardioversion is recommended in most patients aged < 80 years (especially if patient is deemed to have lower risk of recurrence, as evidenced by identification of reversible cause such as hyperthyroidism, pulmonary embolism, or absence of atrial dilatation or absence of major heart pathology).

[b]Transesophageal echocardiography (TEE). Note that noninvasive TTE is not sensitive enough to exclude presence of intracardiac thrombus.

[c]CHADSVASc scoring is discussed on next page.

Management of Chronic AF

- **Rate control** is the preferred approach. Aim is to control heart rate to target of <110 beats/minute, with the use of AV nodal blocking agents (**BCD).**
- **Rhythm control** is a strategy to give antiarrhythmics to maintain sinus rhythm and prevent further AF episodes. It is considered only in patients who continue to have symptoms (dizziness, palpitations, etc.) despite rate control approach. Different antiarrhythmic drugs can be used for this purpose (e.g., amiodarone, sotalol, and dronedarone).
- If patient continues to have symptoms despite medical treatment, a procedure called radiofrequency ablation can be offered. Pathological structure or tissue is changed into a scar tissue.
  - Atrial fibrillation frequently originates from **tissues around the pulmonary veins.** This is where ablation is commonly performed. If ablation fails, then ablation of the His bundle with ventricular pacemaker insertion may be done (essentially creating a complete heart block to stop atrial impulses from reaching ventricles, and using the pacemaker to maintain ventricular rate).
  - In atrial flutter, the usual target area for ablation is the **tricuspid annulus**—a body of fibrous tissue in the lower atrium between the inferior vena cava and the tricuspid valve.[22]
- In some patients with infrequent, asymptomatic episodes of AF, observation alone can suffice.

[23]*Atrial flutter ablation is usually more successful compared to atrial fibrillation ablation. However, heart rate in atrial flutter is harder to control with medications than in atrial fibrillation.*

Management of anticoagulation in AF

Patients with AF have increased risk of mural thrombus formation. It is very important to understand when to use anticoagulation to prevent devastating cardioembolic complications, such as stroke. A clinical prediction rule called CHA_2DS_2VASc score is used to identify patients who will benefit from anticoagulation in patients with **nonvalvular AF.**

 MRS

The numbers to remember are 0, 1, 2

	Comorbid condition	Points
C	Congestive heart failure (or left ventricular systolic dysfunction)	1
H	HTN	1
A	Age ≥ 75 years	**2**
D	Diabetes mellitus	1
S	prior stroke, TIA, or systemic arterial thromboembolism	**2**
V	Vascular disease (e.g., peripheral artery disease, myocardial infarction, and aortic plaque)	1
A	Age 65–74 years	1
Sc	Sex category (female)	1

CHA_2DS_2VASc score	Management
≥ 2	Chronic anticoagulation is recommended
1	Determined on a case-by-case basis
0	No anticoagulation is recommended

Choices of oral anticoagulation

Nonvalvular AF	⇨	Warfarin or Newer-generation oral anticoagulation like dabigatran, rivaroxaban, apixaban, etc.
Prosthetic heart valve, rheumatic mitral valve disease, mitral stenosis of any cause and decompensated valvular disease	⇨	Only warfarin is recommended[a]

[a]New generation anticoagulants (e.g. dabigatran, rivaroxaban, apixaban) are not recommended for thromboprophylaxis in a-fib in these situations.[24]

[24]*In a study of patients with mechanical heart valves, dabigatran showed an excess of bleeding and thromboembolic events as compared to warfarin.*

11. A 75-year-old male was diagnosed with chronic atrial fibrillation. He has no other medical history. What is the NSiM?

12. A 66-year-old male is diagnosed with an episode of transient atrial fibrillation. He has no other medical history. What is the NSiM?

Ventricular Tachycardia (VT) and Ventricular Fibrillation (VF)

Definition of VT

For this section, VT refers to monomorphic VT. For polymorphic ventricular tachycardia see Torsades de pointes section on next page.

Definition

VT	⇒	≥ three consecutive PVCs with rate of more than 100 beats/min
Nonsustained VT	⇒	VT that lasts < ½ min
Sustained VT	⇒	VT that lasts > ½ min. This has higher risk of progression into VF.

Abbreviations: VF, ventricular fibrillation; VT, ventricular tachycardia

> **MRS**
>
> Single and couplet PVCs aren't considered VT.

Common causes of ventricular tachycardia/ventricular fibrillation (VT/VF)

- CAD, with ischemia or infarction.
- Left ventricular dilatation (e.g., dilated cardiomyopathy).
- Aortic stenosis.
- Hypertrophic obstructive cardiomyopathy (HOCM).[25]
- Mitral valve prolapse (MVP).[25]

[25] In patients < 50 years of age presenting with VT/VF, or sudden cardiac death, think HOCM or MVP.

EKG findings

	EKG description	
VT	Wide-complex tachycardia with AV dissociation, which is pathognomonic for ventricular tachycardia AV dissociation is when atria and ventricles are beating in its own rhythm and rate, independent of each other. On EKG, the following features are suggestive of it: • **Fusion beats:** occur when a supraventricular impulse and a ventricular impulse coincide to produce a hybrid complex (*red arrows*). • **Capture beats:** occur when the atrial impulse by chance depolarizes the ventricles to produce a QRS complex of normal duration (*black arrow*).	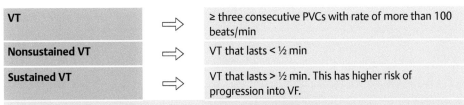 Source: Modified from W.G. de Voogt, MD, PhD, SLAZ, The Netherlands, CC BY-SA 3.0, via Wikimedia Commons.
VF	Erratic electrical activity with no P- QRS-T complexes	Source: Abnormalities of cardiac excitation. In: Michael J, Sircar S. Fundamentals of medical physiology. 1st ed. Thieme; 2010.

Abbreviations: AV, atrioventricular; EKG, electrocardiography; VF, ventricular fibrillation; VT, ventricular tachycardia.

Management of VT and VF

- For hemodynamically unstable patients (VT/VF), NSIM is **electrical cardioversion**. After that arrange for AICD placement.
- For hemodynamically stable patients (VT):

Sustained VT	Non-sustained VT
First step is to convert rhythm by giving antiarrhythmics (ALPS)[a] and start β-blockers[b] In patients with structural heart disease, in whom clearly identified reversible cause is not found, schedule for AICD placement (it has been shown to improve mortality). For recurrent symptomatic episodes or AICD firings, give antiarrhythmics (APS)[c] or do catheter ablation	If symptomatic, give β-blockers.[b] If no effect, use CCBs (diltiazem or verapamil). If still having symptoms, can give antiarrhythmics (APS)[c] or perform catheter ablation

[a] Antiarrhythmics agents for VT/VF are **a**miodarone (DOC), **l**idocaine, **p**rocainamide, or **s**otalol.

[b] β-blockers are indicated in all patients with VT/VF, as they reduce the rate of recurrence.

[c] APS (Amiodarone, procainamide and sotalol) is commonly used for prevention of VT. Lidocaine (IV infusion) is used only for acute treatment of persistent VT.

MRS

ALPS of VT/VF

Clinical Case Scenarios

13. A 28-year-old woman presents with hx of palpitations and dizziness during exercise. Exercise stress test reveals transient VT with LBBB morphology. TTE shows **no** evidence of structural heart disease. What is the likely dx?

Torsade de pointes (aka Polymorphic Ventricular Tachycardia)

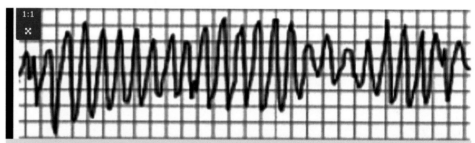

EKG shows arrhythmia with varying QRS morphology, which appears to twist around the baseline
Source: The precordial exam. In: Shi Y, Sohani Z, Tang B, et al. Essentials of clinical examination handbook. 8th ed. Thieme; 2018.

Background: This arrhythmia occurs in patients with prolonged QT interval, which can be caused by the following factors:
- Drugs that prolong QT interval: class Ia (quinidine, procainamide, and disopyramide) or III antiarrhythmics (amiodarone, sotalol, ibutilide, and dofetilide), antipsychotics, tricyclic antidepressants, lithium, antibiotics (e.g., azithromycin, quinolones), etc.
- Severe electrolyte abnormality.
- Inherited long QT syndrome (discussed later).

Presentation: It can be self-terminating or can progress to frank v-fib, causing syncope or sudden death.

Management

- As with all tachyarrhythmias, in hemodynamically unstable patients NSIM is **electrical cardioversion**.
- If hemodynamically stable, then follow the steps below:
  - Stop all medications that can prolong QTc interval.
  - IV magnesium sulfate (even if serum magnesium was within normal range).
  - Check serum electrolytes.
  - If persistent, NSIM is temporary transvenous overdrive pacing (pace at around 100/min), or **isoproterenol drip (both** shorten QT interval).
  - Class Ib antiarrhythmics like lidocaine or phenytoin can also be used. They shorten QT interval.

Wolff–Parkinson–White (WPW) Syndrome aka Preexcitation Syndrome

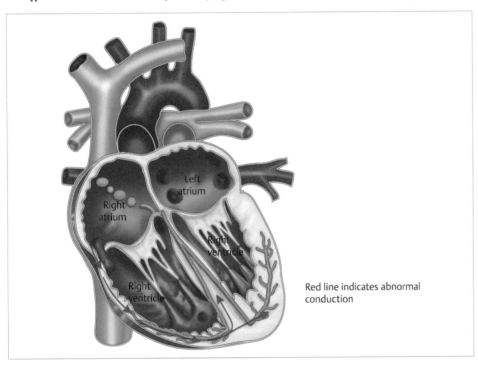

Red line indicates abnormal conduction

Pathophysiology: Normally AV node blocks the atrial impulse for some time and then only conducts it to the ventricles. This safety mechanism makes sure that the atria and the ventricles do not contract at the same time. In WPW syndrome the atrial impulses bypass AV node and reach ventricles, without the delay, through an abnormal accessory conduction pathway between atria and ventricles. The accessory pathway is usually located along the mitral or tricuspid annulus. As the AV node and the accessory pathway can have different refractory periods, reentrant circuit arrhythmias can develop.

Baseline-EKG finding: Absence of PR interval, which is seen as a Delta wave.

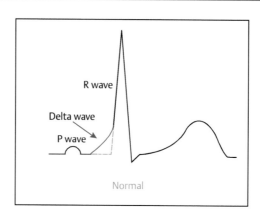

Various presentation scenarios

- Atrial fibrillation with very rapid ventricular response.
- Hx of intermittent palpitations and/or syncope.
- Sudden cardiac death can occur in patients with WPW syndrome due to ventricular fibrillation. It can occur after an episode of atrial fibrillation with very rapid ventricular response, which degenerates into VT or VF.

Management

- For acute tachyarrhythmias:
  - If hemodynamically unstable, NSIM is cardioversion.
  - If hemodynamically stable, NSIM is procainamide, amiodarone, or ibutilide.[26]
- Most patients will require catheter ablation of the accessory pathway.

Hereditary Arrhythmia Syndromes

If a young patient presents with palpitations, presyncope/syncope, or sudden cardiac arrest and there is a family history of sudden cardiac death, think of the following diagnosis.

[26] In WPW syndrome with atrial fibrillation/flutter, AV node blockers (e.g., BCD = β-blocker, CCB, and digoxin) can increase conduction of atrial impulses through abnormal pathway, leading to increased ventricular rate, hemodynamic instability, sometimes converting rhythm to VT or VF.

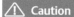 **Caution**

Presentation is similar to HOCM.

Diagnosis	Clues to diagnosis	Treatment *(low yield for exam)*
Congenital long QT interval syndrome • Various types, as there are different forms of inherited ion channel disorders. Some forms can be associated with hearing loss	Hx of episodes precipitated by sudden noise, sleep, or exercise. EKG reveals baseline prolonged QTc interval (> 460 msec). May show polymorphic VT in acute cases	Rx of choice is β-blocker + avoidance of competitive sports and strenuous activities. Dual chamber pacemaker is also commonly placed Indications for AICD placement: • **If patient has cardiogenic syncope or polymorphic VT while on β-blocker therapy** • Hx of sudden cardiac arrest • Strong family hx of sudden cardiac death
Brugada syndrome (autosomal dominant inheritance)	EKG reveals ≥ 2 mm ST-segment elevation in V1-V3. Acute cases can present with VT/VF.	All patients with hx of **cardiac syncope thought to be due to ventricular arrhythmia,** or sudden cardiac arrest will require AICD placement. In low risk patients, electrophysiology study can be done to stratify risk

(Continued)

Diagnosis	Clues to diagnosis	Treatment *(low yield for exam)*
Arrhythmogenic right ventricular cardiomyopathy/ dysplasia (It is caused by fibro-fatty infiltration of right ventricle)	Cardiac MRI or TTE shows abnormal RV size	Indications for AICD placement **• If patients have hx of cardiogenic syncope, thought to be due to ventricular arrhythmia or sudden VT** • Hx of sudden cardiac arrest • Strong family hx of sudden-cardiac death

Abbreviations: AICD, automated implantable cardioverter-defibrillator; MRI, magnetic resonance imaging; TTE, transthoracic echocardiography; VF, ventricular fibrillation; VT, ventricular tachycardia

 MRS

Remember the common indications for AICD in most of these disorders.
• Hx of sudden cardiac arrest.
• Strong family hx of sudden cardiac death.
• Other indications specific to the condition are given above in bold text.

Medications Used in Tachyarrhythmias

Digoxin

Mechanism of action: It inhibits Na^+/K^+–ATPase, thereby increasing intracellular Ca^{2+} and cardiac contractility. It also reduces AV nodal conduction.

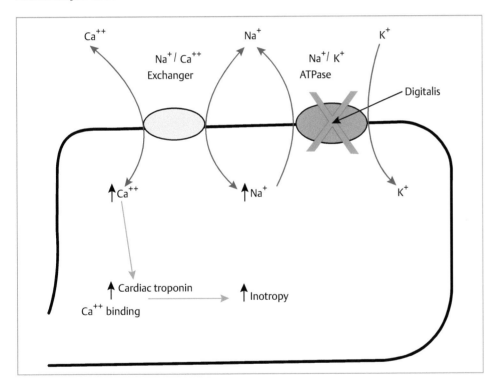

- Diuretics are more likely to cause hypokalemia/hypomagnesemia: **di**uretics **d**ouble **d**igoxin effect.
- **C**alcium works with **d**igoxin; potassium and magnesium work against digoxin.

Digoxin interaction

	Digoxin effect	Mechanism
Hypokalemia and hypomagnesemia	↑	Increases sensitivity of myocardium to digoxin
Hypercalcemia	↑	
Quinidine, verapamil, diltiazem, and spironolactone	↑	Decreases clearance of digoxin
Cholestyramine, colestipol	↓	Binds digoxin in gastrointestinal tract preventing absorption of digoxin
Increased creatinine (decreased renal function)	↑	Decreased renal clearance **Clinical pearl:** when patients on digoxin have acute renal failure, it is very important to check digoxin level and/or reduce digoxin dose

Digoxin toxicity

Presentation

[27] Most common arrhythmia associated with digoxin toxicity is frequent premature ventricular beats.
- Most **specific EKG** finding in digoxin toxicity is atrial tachycardia with AV block

- Gastrointestinal disturbances (anorexia, nausea, vomiting, and abdominal pain): MC presentation of digoxin toxicity.
- Visual symptoms are alterations in color vision, development of scotomas, or even blindness.
- Mental status changes.
- Arrhythmias: *almost any form of arrhythmia can occur (sinus bradycardia, sinus block/arrest, ectopic atrial tachycardia with AV block, atrial fibrillation/flutter, junctional tachycardia, ventricular beats, bidirectional VT, VF, etc.).*[27]

Management steps

- NSIDx is EKG, serum electrolytes, and serum digoxin level.
- Supportive treatment with correction of electrolytes, if needed.
- Indications for Digibind (monoclonal antibody to digoxin):
  - All symptomatic bradycardias or life-threatening arrhythmias (VT, VF, Mobitz II block, complete heart block).
  - Hyperkalemia (> 5–5.5 mEq/L) (!).
  - Evidence of end organ dysfunction (altered mental status, renal failure).

⚠ Caution

(!) Do not give calcium gluconate as calcium increases digoxin effect.

Amiodarone

It is a very powerful wide-spectrum antiarrhythmic drug, which can be used for treatment of different arrhythmias, such as ventricular arrhythmias, atrial flutter or fibrillation, etc.

Side effects: This is high yield for "Boards." Amiodarone can cause the following:

[28] Amiodarone should be avoided in patients with preexisting chronic lung disease.

- **Pulmonary toxicity:** It can range from pneumonitis to pulmonary fibrosis. If biopsy is done, it may reveal foamy macrophages, which have amiodarone/phospholipid intracellular complexes. This is known as lipoid pneumonitis.[28]
- Hypo- or hyperthyroidism (TSH levels should be regularly checked in patients taking amiodarone).
- **Corneal deposits:** In this case, discontinuation is **not** required, as vision is not usually affected.

Notable Side Effects of Other Antiarrhythmic Medications

Procainamide	Agranulocytosis and drug-induced lupus
Lidocaine	Altered mental status and seizures
Quinidine	Cinchonism (blurred vision, nausea, vomiting diarrhea, and tinnitus). *Clinical symptoms are similar to digoxin toxicity.*

4.5.3 Acute Bradyarrhythmia

Legend: *NSIM, next step in management*

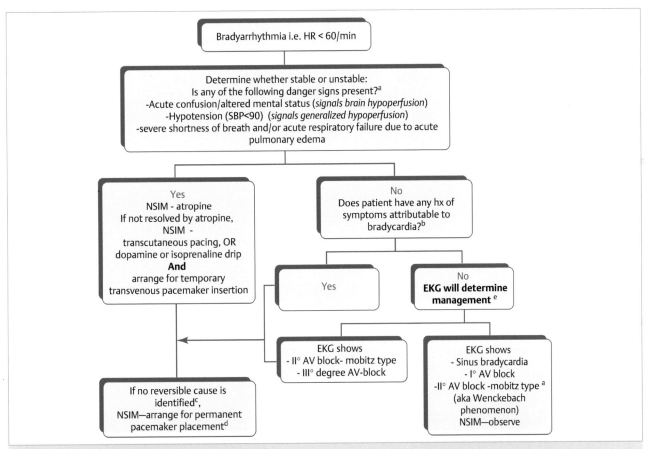

Explanation of the algorithm:

[a]Note that the indications for immediate early management of bradyarrhythmias are the same as for tachyarrhythmias.

[b]Dizziness, lightheadedness, syncope, fatigue, poor exercise tolerance that can be attributed to bradyarrhythmia.

[c]Reversible causes are Lyme's disease, drugs (β-blocker, CCB, or digoxin) toxicity, electrolyte imbalance, hypothyroidism, acute cardiac ischemia/trauma, etc. While these patients may require temporary cardiac pacing for continuing symptoms, permanent pacemaker placement is seldom required.

[d]The decision to implant a pacemaker should be done only after few days of observation to determine if the pathology is transient or permanent.

[e]In **asymptomatic** bradycardias, EKG will determine the need for pacemaker (as outlined in the following table):

Type of bradycardia	EKG	Management
Sinus bradycardia	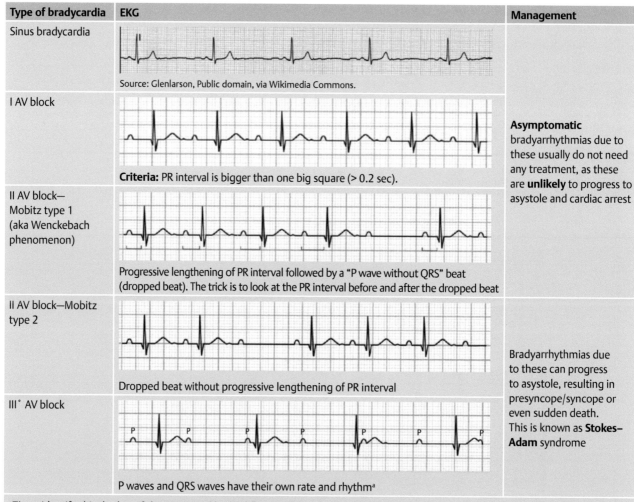 Source: Glenlarson, Public domain, via Wikimedia Commons.	**Asymptomatic** bradyarrhythmias due to these usually do not need any treatment, as these are **unlikely** to progress to asystole and cardiac arrest
I AV block	**Criteria:** PR interval is bigger than one big square (> 0.2 sec).	
II AV block— Mobitz type 1 (aka Wenckebach phenomenon)	Progressive lengthening of PR interval followed by a "P wave without QRS" beat (dropped beat). The trick is to look at the PR interval before and after the dropped beat	
II AV block—Mobitz type 2	Dropped beat without progressive lengthening of PR interval	Bradyarrhythmias due to these can progress to asystole, resulting in presyncope/syncope or even sudden death. This is known as **Stokes–Adam** syndrome
III° AV block	P waves and QRS waves have their own rate and rhythm[a]	

[a]Tip to identify this rhythm: If the PR interval looks different in each beat, always try to march the P waves and the QRS waves.

Note: practice with different variations of this rhythm in Google image.

Since management of asymptomatic bradycardia depends on EKG, practice with as many EKGs that you can find! Use Google image ☺ and see all the variations.

Source: Abnormalities of cardiac excitation. In: Michael J, Sircar S. Fundamentals of medical physiology. 1st ed. Thieme; 2010.

Clinical Case Scenarios

A 54-year-old man presents with ongoing dizziness and chest pain for the last 30 minutes. His heart rate is 30 beats/minute.

14. What is the immediate NSIM?

15. Patient did not respond to atropine. His heart rate is still 40 beats/minute. He continues to have dizziness and chest pain. What is the immediate NSIM?

16. What is the NSIM, after stabilization?

4.5.4 Sick Sinus Syndrome

Definition: Malfunction of the sinus node that can lead to various brady- or tachyarrhythmias. Common causes are advanced age and ischemia-related degenerative process with replacement of sinus node by fibrous tissue.

Presentation: It can lead to the following arrhythmias:

- Sinus pauses, sinus arrest, sinoatrial exit-block due to sinus node dysfunction.
- Frequent periods of severe bradycardia.
- Alternating bradycardia and atrial tachyarrhythmias ("Tachy-brady syndrome").[29]

Management steps

- NSIDx is EKG.
- If EKG is nondiagnostic, NSIDx is Holter monitoring.
- After dx is confirmed, NSIM is permanent pacemaker placement.

[29] Atrial fibrillation is the MC form of atrial tachycardia, associated with sick sinus syndrome. At times, spontaneous termination of atrial fibrillation is followed by a prolonged sinus pause. This may present as palpitations followed by presyncope or syncope.

4.6 Valve Disorders

Evaluation of incidental finding of murmur

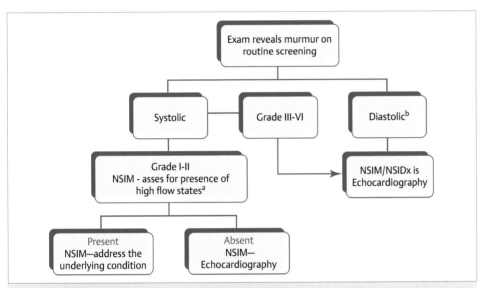

[a] Anemia, hyperthyroidism, pregnancy, and innocent murmur in children. This systolic murmur is heard best in right upper sternal border (aortic area).

[b] Know that diastolic murmurs are always abnormal.

General principles on valvular disorders[30]

- All significant valvular disorders can present with the following:
  - Progressive heart failure with dyspnea, exercise intolerance, and/or bilateral lower extremity edema.
  - Arrhythmias (palpitations, dizziness, syncope, and/or SOB).

Right-sided valvular heart pathology (in TR, TS, PR, PS): clinical features of venous congestion (JVD, ascites, and leg edema) are more predominant	**Left ventricular outflow tract pathology** (HOCM, AR, AS): clinical features of exertional dyspnea and chest pain are more predominant and present earlier during disease course

[30] **Legend**
- TR/TS, tricuspid regurgitation/ stenosis
- PR/PS, pulmonic regurgitation/ stenosis
- MR/MS, mitral regurgitation/ stenosis
- AR/AS, aortic regurgitation/ stenosis
- HOCM, hypertrophic obstructive cardiomyopathy
- MVP, mitral valve prolapse

- Mitral regurgitation (MR) and mitral stenosis (MS) are commonly associated with left atrial dilatation and can present with symptoms of atrial arrhythmias.

Valvular disorders that are associated with **increased afterload** (e.g., AS, HOCM) lead to concentric left ventricular hypertrophy. S4 is more common *! Similar pathophysiological process occurs in coarctation of aorta and HTN*	Valvular disorders (MR/AR) that are associated with **volume overload** lead to eccentric hypertrophy (cavity dilatation and decrease in wall thickness/chamber-dimension ratio). S3 is more common

	Aortic stenosis	Aortic regurgitation	Mitral regurgitation	Mitral stenosis	Mitral valve prolapse
Murmur	Midsystolic diamond-shaped crescendo–decrescendo murmur	• Early diastolic murmur (see *black arrow* in phonogram below) • Mid or late diastolic rumbling murmur can be heard (see *blue arrow*). This is due to the regurgitant blood flow impinging on the inner surface of mitral valve causing functional mitral stenosis (This murmur is similar to murmur of mitral stenosis, and is known as Austin Flint murmur) • High-flow early systolic murmur can also be heard after S1	Pansystolic (holosystolic) murmur	• Opening snap (OS)—Note that interval between the S2 and opening snap is shorter in severe MS. (Atrial pressure builds up early.) • Middiastolic rumble heard after the opening snap	Midsystolic **click** +/− murmur. (Maneuvers that decrease preload increases laxity of mitral valve, so prolapse occurs earlier in systole. This results in earlier initiation of click and longer duration of systolic murmur that follows the click)
	Normal phonogram: note the vibration of S1/S2				
Location of murmur	A, Aortic area = second right intercostal space (right upper sternal border) Murmur radiates to carotid arteries (neck area)	N, Neoaortic area = third left intercostal space Best heard when patient is leaning forward	M, Mitral area = apex aka point of maximal intensity (PMI) Murmur radiates to axilla	Apex (PMI) Heard best in left lateral decubitus position	Apex (PMI)
	T= Tricuspid area P, pulmonic area				
Additional physical exam finding	• Heaving apex beat • S4 • Pulsus parvus et tardus (slowly rising carotid pulse)	• S3 and S4 • Widened pulse pressure[d] • hyperdynamic circulation • Water-hammer pulse, collapsing pulse • Pistol-shot femoral pulse	• Low S1 • S3 can be heard even without clinical heart failure	• Tapping apex beat (the tap is due to loud and palpable S1) • Weak pulse	

	Aortic stenosis	Aortic regurgitation	Mitral regurgitation	Mitral stenosis	Mitral valve prolapse
Echocardiographic findings	• Transvalvular pressure gradient is increased and aortic valve area is <1.5 cm^2 • Concentric LVH	• Diastolic blood flow into the left ventricle from aorta • Concentric and eccentric LVH	• Systolic backflow into left atrium from left ventricle • Mostly eccentric hypertrophy	• Left atrioventricular pressure gradient is increased • Prominent left atrial dilatation[f] • Mitral valve area is decreased, and calcified leaflets are seen	Enlarged floppy mitral valve with prolapse +/− mitral regurgitation
Etiology *Legend: MC, most common; MCC, most common cause*	• **Age < 60 yr:** bicuspid aortic valve • **Age > 60 yr:** age-related calcification of aortic valve (MCC of aortic stenosis) • It is the MC valvular heart disease in developed countries	• In the developing world, MCC is rheumatic heart disease • In developed countries, MCC is aortic root dilation (due to long standing HTN, bicuspid aortic valve, Marfan syndrome etc.) • MC congenital cause is bicuspid aortic valve • Endocarditis	• MCC in United States is mitral valve prolapse • Other causes include CAD, rheumatic heart disease, collagen vascular disease and severe mitral annular calcification • Functional MR[e]	• MCC is rheumatic heart disease	• Myxomatous degeneration of mitral valve (i.e., deposition of glycosaminoglycans in valve leaflets) • MC valvular heart disease in young people in developed countries

Indications for surgery in asymptomatic patients[a]
Legend: LVEF, left ventricular ejection fraction
	• Asymptomatic very severe aortic stenosis (mean transvalvular pressure gradient of ≥ 60 mmHg or aortic V$_{max}$ ≥ 5 m/s) with low surgical risk
	• Asymptomatic severe aortic stenosis (mean transvalvular pressure gradient of ≥ 40 mmHg or aortic V$_{max}$ ≥ 4 m/s. Aortic valve area is typically ≤ 1 cm[b]) + one of the following
	  – LVEF < 50%
	  – Rapidly progressive stenosis
	  – Abnormal exercise treadmill test (development of syncope, angina, dyspnea, significant ST-T wave depressions or hypotension with exercise)
	• Aortic V$_{max}$ ≥ 3 m/s, or mean transvalvular pressure gradient of ≥ 20 mmHg at the time of other cardiac surgery
		• LVEF < 50%
		• LV dilatation (end systolic diameter of > 55 mm or end diastolic of > 75 mm)
			• LVEF < **60%**
			• LV end systolic diameter is >40 mm
			• Pulmonary artery hypertension (systolic PA pressure ≥ 50 mmHg at rest and ≥ 60 mmHg at exercise)
			• New-onset atrial fibrillation with left atrial dilatation
				• Pulmonary artery hypertension (systolic pulmonary artery pressure ≥ 50 mmHg at rest and ≥ 60 mmHg at exercise)	• MVP alone is not an indication for surgery
					• Surgery might be required for coexisting MR (see indications for surgery for MR)

	Aortic stenosis	Aortic regurgitation	Mitral regurgitation	Mitral stenosis	Mitral valve prolapse
Surgery of choice[b]	Aortic valve replacement	Aortic valve replacement	• Do mitral valve repair when anatomy is favorable (i.e., when there is limited calcification, limited stenosis, limited prolapse, and incomplete papillary muscle rupture) • When anatomy is not favorable do mitral valve replacement (e.g., complete papillary muscle rupture)	• Valvular replacement will be needed if patient has coexistent moderate to severe MR, extensive valve calcification, or persistent thrombus despite adequate anticoagulation • If above factors are absent, do mitral valve repair	
Adjunctive treatment[c]	Medications that reduce afterload can be used with **caution** in patients with LV systolic dysfunction, and HTN	Afterload reduction is recommended especially when patients have HTN	Afterload reduction	All patients with atrial fibrillation with MS should get Coumadin with target INR of 2–3, regardless of CHADSVASC score	Usually reassurance and lifestyle modification (avoidance of alcohol, stress, caffeine) should suffice. ! Do not choose β-blocker in patients with chest pain as it has no role. However, β-blocker can be used for documented arrhythmias

[a] In any valvular disorder, surgery is indicated in presence of symptoms. For example, if patient develops acute heart failure in the setting of valvular disorder, NSIM is diuretics, salt restriction, and arrange for surgical intervention, especially if patient is a good surgical candidate. For asymptomatic patients, specific indications are given in the table.[31]

[b] Generally, prior to any open cardiac surgery, coronary angiography is done to screen for CAD, particularly when patient is at risk. We should not miss the opportunity of surgical access to thorax to perform CABG if indicated by coronary anatomy.

[c] In AS, MR, and AR supportive medical treatment is to decrease afterload, which also decreases murmur intensity. Afterload reduction is achieved with arteriolar dilators like ACE inhibitors (preferred), hydralazine or vasoactive CCB like nifedipine or amlodipine. In MR, when peripheral arterial resistance is lowered, relatively greater part of stroke volume is pumped forward through aortic valve, than through the leaky mitral valve. Also, Coumadin is indicated and preferred over newer generation anticoagulation in patients with trial fibrillation/flutter with severe valvular heart disease or any severity of mitral stenosis.

[d] If the difference between systolic blood pressure and diastolic blood pressure is >40 mmHg, it is considered to be widened. Other causes of widened pulse pressure are isolated systolic hypertension, thyrotoxicosis, patent ductus arteriosus, AV fistula, beriberi, and anemia.

[e] Marked dilatation of valvular annulus can lead to incomplete closure of the valve, leading to valvular regurgitation, which is known as functional murmur. For example, dilated cardiomyopathy can cause TR and MR: Systolic right heart failure/dilatation can cause TR.

[f] In patients with long-standing mitral stenosis, significant left atrial enlargement can occur. This can lead to compression of surrounding structures and may present as hoarseness of voice (laryngeal nerve compression), dysphagia (compression of esophagus), and/or elevated left main stem bronchus.

Abbreviations: ACE, angiotensin-converting enzyme; CABG, coronary artery bypass grafting; CAD, coronary artery disease; HTN, hypertension; INR, international normalized ratio; LVH, left ventricular hypertrophy; MR, mitral regurgitation; MS, mitral stenosis; MVP, mitral valve prolapse; TR, tricuspid regurgitation.

[31] As a general rule, surgery is indicated in patients with decreased systolic function or LV dilatation.

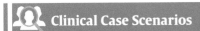 **Clinical Case Scenarios**

17. You hear a midsystolic murmur, early diastolic murmur, and a late middiastolic rumble in a 3-year-old patient. What is the most likely dx?

18. A young patient is found to have characteristic murmur of aortic regurgitation (AR). He recently immigrated to United States from Nepal many years ago. What is the most likely cause?

 MRS

Two arms = **Di ARMS** or another MRS is **ARMS DIE** = **Di**astolic murmurs occur in **a**ortic regurgitation and **m**itral **s**tenosis.
Practice listening to various kind of murmur (Google videos). Some multimedia questions in board-exam need identification of murmur.

Maneuvers that change murmur intensity

This is a heavily tested topic in "board exams," because knowing this implies good understanding of basic cardiac mechanics and pathophysiology.

	Maneuvers	Leg raising, lying down flat, or squatting	Valsalva maneuver or abrupt standing	Phenylephrine, handgrip, or isometric hand exercise	Amyl nitrite
	Effect on preload or afterload	Increases preload	Decreases preload	Increases afterload[c]	Decreases afterload
Effect on murmur intensity	Aortic stenosis[a]	↑	Decreases	Decreases	↑
	MVP/HOCM[a]	Decreases	↑	Decreases	↑
	AR/MR/VSD[b]	↑	Decreases	↑	Decreases

[a]Note that both aortic stenosis and HOCM can have midsystolic murmur and similar presentation, so important ways to differentiate are given.

[b]Both VSD and MR can have pansystolic murmur, and both can occur as a mechanical complication 3–7 days post MI.

[c]Increase in afterload (increased systemic arterial pressure) leads to the following effect:

- Decrease in ventricular output through aorta, results in relatively greater part of stroke volume passing through VSD or MR.
- Increase in retrograde regurgitant diastolic flow from aorta to ventricles results in increased AR murmur intensity.
- Decreased forward output → increase in intraventricular volume → decreased intensity of murmur in HOCM and MVP.

Abbreviations: AR, aortic regurgitation; HOCM, hypertrophic obstructive cardiomyopathy; MR, mitral regurgitation; MVP, mitral valve prolapse; VSD, ventricular septal defect

Most murmurs increase in intensity with preload increase, and vice versa (decrease in intensity when preload decreases), except in MVP and HOCM.

Note that handgrip or amyl nitrite can be used to differentiate systolic murmur of MR versus AS.

4.6.1 Calcific Aortic Stenosis

Pathophysiology: Aortic stenosis (AS) is a result of degenerative atherosclerotic-like changes that occur in aortic valve which develops after years of accumulative microendothelial injury. It has similar pathology with mitral annular calcification and ASCVD.

Presentation scenarios

- **S**yncope/presyncope, **a**ngina, and/or **d**yspnea on exertion.
- Incidental finding of ejection systolic murmur heard best at aortic area (right upper sternal border).

NSIDx: Echocardiography.

MC presenting symptom for HOCM or AS is dyspnea on exertion.

MRS

SAD

MRS

SAD presentation of aortic stenosis requires surgical intervention.
Here the magic no is 1. The A in AS is the 1st letter of alphabet. Severe AS ≤ 1 cm². The average rate of AS progression is 0.1 cm² per 1 yr.

Before all cardiac surgeries, do coronary angiography to assess the need for CABG at the same time.

Management

Indication for surgery are:
● All symptomatic patients with AS.
● Asymptomatic very severe AS (mean transvalvular pressure gradient of ≥60 mmHg or aortic V_{max} ≥ 5 m/second) with low surgical risk.
● Asymptomatic severe AS (mean transvalvular pressure gradient of ≥40 mmHg or aortic V_{max} ≥ 4 m/s. Aortic valve area is typically ≤1 cm²) + one of the following:
  – LVEF < 50%.
  – Rapidly progressive stenosis.
  – Abnormal exercise treadmill test (development of syncope, angina, dyspnea, significant ST-T wave depressions or hypotension with exercise).
● Aortic V_{max} ≥ 3 m/s, or mean transvalvular pressure gradient of ≥ 20 mmHg at the time of other cardiac surgery.

If patient is a poor candidate for cardiac surgery offer transcatheter aortic valve implantation/repair (TAVI/TAVR).

Differential diagnosis: Calcific aortic sclerosis and calcific aortic stenosis both can present with midsystolic murmur radiating to carotids.

	Calcific aortic sclerosis[a]	Calcific aortic stenosis
Symptoms (hx of exertional presyncope/syncope, exertional chest pain, or exertional SOB)	Absent	Present
Left ventricular hypertrophy	Absent	Present
Significant aortic–valvular pressure gradient	Absent	Present

[a]Calcific aortic sclerosis may progress into hemodynamically significant aortic stenosis.
Abbreviation: SOB, shortness of breath.

4.6.2 Bicuspid Aortic Valve

Definition: Aortic valve normally has three cusp (leaflets). In this congenital heart disorder, there are two valve cusps. It is associated with coarctation of aorta, dilatation of aorta, and Turner's syndrome.

Pathophysiology: Two leaflets must do the work of three leaflets resulting in early progressive degenerative changes and AS. It is associated with aortic root dilatation and coexistence of AR.

Presentation: features of AS in a young patient. Exam may reveal coexistent AR murmur.

Management

● Balloon valvotomy can be considered in patients < 30 years of age who have severe AS without significant valvular calcification.
● Patients undergoing surgery for symptomatic or severe AS/AR might require aortic surgery for aortic root dilatation at the same time.

A 62-year-old female with no prior cardiac hx presents with increasing dyspnea on exertion and lower extremity edema. Exam reveals S3, 3/6 holosystolic murmur at the apex occurring after a midsystolic click, soft bibasilar crackles, and jugular venous distension (JVD).

19. What is the NSIDx?

20. What is the immediate NSIM?

TTE reveals severe MR with minimal calcification and mild MVP.

21. What is the best SIM?

   a. Mitral valve surgery.

   b. Mitral valve repair.

   c. Medical management.

Clinical Case Scenarios

22. A 55-year-old male patient is found to have significant three-vessel CAD. During coronary catheterization, he is also incidentally found to have AS with transvalvular mean gradient of 30 mmHg. What is the NSIM?

   a. CABG + aortic valve replacement.

   b. CABG + aortic valve repair.

   c. CABG alone.

   d. Aortic valve replacement alone.

23. A 67-year-old male has chronic AR. His TTE reveals ejection fraction (EF) of 55% and LV end diastolic diameter of 50 mm. What is the NSIM?

24. A 75-year-old male has asymptomatic chronic severe MR. Recent TTE shows EF of 55% and there is limited calcification and prolapse. What is the best NSIM?

   a. Mitral valve surgery.

   b. Mitral valve repair.

   c. Medical management.

25. A 25-year-old male has a systolic murmur. He has widely split-fixed S2, and fixed systolic ejection murmur that does not change with Valsalva, inspiration, or handgrip. What is the likely dx?

Clinical Case Scenarios

A 35-year-old female is found a have a midsystolic click followed by a systolic murmur. The murmur decreases with squatting and increases with Valsalva maneuver.

26. What is the likely dx?

27. What will happen to the click and the murmur with handgrip?

Valve Replacement and Anticoagulation

The choice between mechanical or bioprosthetic valve replacement requires balancing the risk between higher chances of early valve failure with biological valves and increased thrombotic complications associated with mechanical valves.

- Mechanical valve is generally used in younger patients with low bleeding risk, as it requires lifelong anticoagulation.

	Mechanical heart valve replacement	Bioprosthetic heart valve replacement
Aortic valve	Target INR 2–3	2–3
Mitral valve	**2.5–3.5[a]**	2–3
Duration of anticoagulation	Lifelong	All patients receive anticoagulation for initial 3 months after surgery. If additional risk factors are present[b] then warfarin should be continued. If absent, can discontinue anticoagulation
Low dose aspirin	This is recommended in all patients with low-risk of bleeding, regardless of the type of valve replacement	

[a]The only scenario when target INR is 2.5 to 3.5 is with mechanical mitral valve. In all other indications for warfarin target INR is 2 to 3 (including pulmonary embolism and DVT)

[b]Risk factors include atrial fibrillation, prior thromboembolism, EF of <30% and a hypercoagulable state.

MRS

Mechanical mitral valve = MM = double M (mortality) = double trouble, which has higher risk of thrombotic complication, hence higher target of INR.

4.7 Cardiomyopathies (Hypertrophic-Obstructive, Restrictive, and Dilated Cardiomyopathy)

General principles on cardiomyopathies: All cardiomyopathies are due to primary pathology in the myocardium, affecting the contractile portion of the heart. The best initial test to diagnose any of the cardiomyopathies is TTE (Trans-Thoracic Echocardiography). The gold standard for diagnosis is endomyocardial biopsy; however, it is rarely done, since clinical situation, laboratory and other noninvasive testing are often sufficient to establish the diagnosis.

4.7.1 Hypertrophic Obstructive Cardiomyopathy

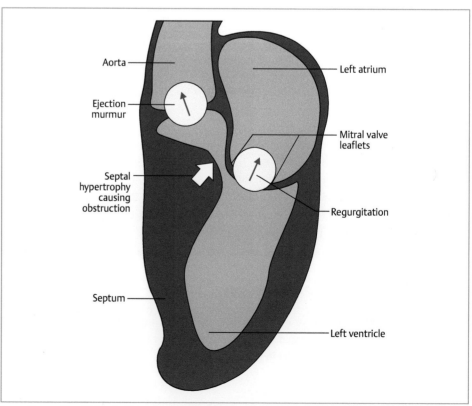

Source: Causes of heart failure. In: Siegenthaler W. Siegenthaler's differetial diagnosis in internal medicine: From symptom to diagnosis. 1st ed. Thieme; 2007.

Pathophysiology: More than 50% cases have autosomal dominant inheritance of gene mutation that codes for β-myosin heavy chain in myocardium. This results in asymmetric thickening of interventricular septum leading to subaortic valve obstruction of LV outflow and increased risk of ventricular arrhythmias.

Various presentation scenarios[32]:

- Sudden cardiac arrest in an active athletic young individual.
- Young patient with syncope, angina, and dyspnea on exertion.
- Screening physical exam reveals a murmur consistent with HOCM (crescendo-decrescendo systolic murmur which decreases in intensity with hand-grip and increases with Valsalva maneuver).

[32] Look for family history of sudden death.

Cardiac imaging: Echocardiography will show asymmetric septal hypertrophy (marked hypertrophy of the interventricular septum). It may have concurrent LV hypertrophy, which is less severe than the septal part. Doppler echocardiography may reveal systolic anterior motion of anterior mitral leaflet which can also contribute to LV outflow obstruction and may cause coexistent mitral regurgitation. Patients with severe HOCM can develop dilated cardiomyopathy.

Management

- Most asymptomatic patients require no specific treatment. They are, however, recommended to avoid competitive sports or strenuous activities.
- In **symptomatic** patients, the treatment of choice is β-**blocker** or cardioselective CCB (e.g., diltiazem)[33]
- If patient continues to have progressive symptoms despite adequate heart rate control, NSIM is septal myomectomy or septal ablation.
- Indications for AICD placement include the following:
  - Previous cardiac arrest.
  - Hx of sustained VT or VF.
  - Strong family hx of sudden cardiac death.
  - Unexplained syncope (!).

[33] Decreasing heart rate increases preload by prolonging diastole, thus giving heart more time to fill up. Increasing preload decreases outflow ract obstruction.

⚠ **Caution**

(!) Exertional chest pain or dyspnea in HOCM are not indicators for AICD placement.

Screening of family members of HOCM patient

In 1st degree family relatives of HOCM patient, begin annual screening after 12-18 years of age with physical exam, EKG, and periodic TTE. If no echocardiographic evidence of HOCM, genetic testing can be done, given that a known gene mutation, associated with HOCM, is identified in the family. Gene testing can identify at risk members.

4.7.2 Restrictive Cardiomyopathy

Pathophysiology: Progressive deposition of substances (e.g., amyloid or iron) in the myocardium, which slowly makes the myocardium stiff and rigid, and unable to relax properly. This leads to reduction in diastolic ventricular volume and increase in intraventricular pressure. Elevated pressure in cardiac chambers results in early biatrial dilatation.

Etiology of restrictive cardiomyopathy	Progressive deposition of the following substances (deposition can also occur in other organs)	Underlying pathology
Amyloidosis	Amyloid protein[a]	**Primary amyloidosis:** primary idiopathic disorder of excess amyloid production and deposition **Secondary amyloidosis:** chronic inflammatory conditions can increase amyloid production and subsequent deposition in organs. Most common conditions associated with secondary amyloidosis are rheumatoid arthritis, chronic osteomyelitis, and multiple myeloma
Sarcoidosis	Granulomas	Idiopathic disorder of granulomatous inflammation
Fibrosis	Fibrous replacement of tissues (including myocardium)	**Carcinoid syndrome:** high levels of circulating serotonin stimulates fibroblast proliferation **Systemic scleroderma:** it is a collagen vascular disorder associated with replacement of body's normal tissues with fibrous tissue **Others:** **Endomyocardial fibrosis** (unknown cause of fibrosis found in poor rural population) **Eosinophilic myocarditis (aka Loeffler endocarditis)** due to hypereosinophilic syndromes: primary (clonal stem-cell/myeloid disorder), or secondary (parasitic infection, lymphoproliferative disorder, drug reaction, etc.)
Hemochromatosis[b]	Iron	**Hereditary hemochromatosis** aka primary hemochromatosis:- genetic disorder with inability to downregulate iron absorption despite excess total iron **Secondary hemochromatosis:** gain of excess iron, commonly due to underlying condition that requires periodic blood transfusion (e.g., β-thalassemia major)

[a]TTE can reveal speckled pattern (unique for amyloidosis).

[b]Restrictive cardiomyopathies tend to have a poor prognosis, except for hemochromatosis, which can be treated with deferoxamine or phlebotomy.

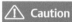 **Caution**

(!) Do not confuse with constrictive pericarditis, which presents similarly but is very different in treatment and prognosis.

Presentation: Patient presents with slowly progressive biventricular failure (bilateral lower extremity edema, SOB). Exam reveals paradoxical increase in jugular venous pressure (JVP) with inspiration (Kussmaul sign) and forceful apical impulse (!). Deposition of substances in conductive pathway can cause heart blocks.

Cardiac imaging

- TTE will show reduced diastolic filling and increased ventricular end diastolic pressure. Presence of biatrial enlargement points toward this diagnosis. Ventricular walls may be symmetrically thickened or might be normal earlier in the course. Echogenic deposits may or may not be seen in the myocardium.
- Cardiac involvement and deposition can be confirmed with cardiac magnetic resonance imaging (MRI).

General treatment principle of restrictive cardiomyopathies: First step is a trial of β-blocker or CCB, which reduces heart rate and improves diastolic filling. But note that in some patients maximal diastolic filling is fixed, so negative chronotropic agents may actually decrease cardiac output and worsen symptoms.

4.7.3 Dilated Cardiomyopathy (DCM)

Pathophysiology: Primary pathology is weakening of the myocardium that eventually leads to dilatation of the heart chambers. Frequently the problem starts with left ventricle, and goes on to involve other chambers of the heart.

Etiology: Any form of heart disease, when severe, can eventually lead to dilated cardiomyopathy in late stages (e.g., hypertensive heart disease, late-stage restrictive/HOCM, HIV, ischemic cardiomyopathy,).

Presentation: Patients present with progressive biventricular failure.

Work-up: NSIDx is echocardiography. Findings include diffuse hypokinesis (all the four chambers of the heart are hypocontractile and hypokinetic). It is primarily a systolic dysfunction, so ejection fraction is reduced.

Management: See systolic heart failure section for general treatment principles.

 MRS

Other specific causes of DCM –ABCD
- **A**—**A**lcohol, **A**uto-immune
- **B**—**C**oxsackie **B**, *Borrelia burgdorferi* infection (check Lyme antibody in endemic areas)
- **C**—**C**hagas, **C**ocaine abuse, **C**hildbirth (peripartum cardiomyopathy), **C**ollagen vascular disorders, **C**oronary artery disease
- **D**—**D**oxorubicin

CCS may give clues to the specific cause

CCS	Additional info
Hx of recent viral upper respiratory tract infection with new onset of heart failure in an otherwise healthy patient. No hx of alcohol or cocaine abuse	One potential complication of viral infection is subclinical myocarditis and acute DCM. MCC is coxsackie virus
Hx of chronic alcohol ingestion	Alcohol is a myocardial poison. NSIM is avoidance of alcohol (stops the progression of DCM)
Peripartum period	If prepartum, best SIM is delivery. Avoid ACE inhibitor or ARB in pregnancy, which are teratogenic
Hx of frequent palpitations or, hx of atrial fibrillation or atrial flutter with uncontrolled heart rate	Tachycardia-induced cardiomyopathy (chronic tachycardia can lead to ventricular systolic dysfunction). If suspected, best SIM is aggressive efforts to achieve heart rate control or restore sinus rhythm. Achieving good heart rate control usually leads to significant improvement in ventricular function
Hx of hypothyroidism or hyperthyroidism	TSH should always be checked in patients with DCM
Young healthy patient with no precedent hx of viral infection presents with acute heart failure. TTE reveals DCM. There is no history of cocaine or alcohol abuse. All lab test, including nuclear stress test is unremarkable	The most common cause of idiopathic DCM is myocarditis. (The initial viral infection might have been subclinical.)

Abbreviations: ACE, angiotensin-converting enzyme; ARB, angiotensin receptor blocker; DCM, dilated cardiomyopathy; TTE, transthoracic echocardiography.

Complications of dilated cardiomyopathy (DCM)

- Arrhythmias: these can lead to atrial flutter or VT/VF.
- Increased risk for mural thrombus formation due to relative stasis.
- Congestive heart failure.

[34]Myocarditis is often associated with pericarditis Patients can present with features that suggest concurrent myocarditis and pericarditis (myopericarditis).

[35]If underlying pathology persists, any of the causes of acute pericarditis can lead to chronic constrictive pericarditis.

4.7.4 Myocarditis

Definition: Infection and/or inflammation of myocardium.

Causes: MCC is coxsackie virus. Other causes include rheumatic fever, Lyme's disease, collagen vascular disease, drugs, fungi infection, parasitic infection, etc.

Clinical features: Fever and chest pain; pain may radiate to jaw or left hand. If underlying pathology is severe, patients can present with acute heart failure, life-threatening arrhythmias and even sudden cardiac death.

Lab findings: EKG may reveal ST wave elevation in nonspecific pattern (similar to pericarditis). There is troponin elevation.[34]

Establishing diagnosis: Often, diagnosis is made with noninvasive measures. Myocardial biopsy is recommended if presentation is severe (e.g., patient has refractory heart failure) and when cause is not identified.

Management: treat symptoms (e.g., heart failure) and address the underlying cause.

4.7.5 Pericarditis

Definition: Infection and/or inflammation of pericardium.

Causes: Uremia, viruses (e.g., coxsackie, cytomegalovirus [CMV], HIV), bacterial (e.g., pneumococcus, TB), inflammatory (e.g., systemic lupus erythematosus [SLE], post MI), malignancy, drugs (e.g., penicillin, hydralazine), recent heart surgery, radiation, etc. Disseminated fungal infection in immune-compromised host can also lead to myopericarditis.[35]

Presentation: Patient can present with chest pain that radiates to jaw or left hand. Note that this pain characteristics is similar to MI, however unlike in MI, the pain here is pleuritic. (It changes in intensity with position and inspiration. It is usually relieved by sitting up and leaning forward and exacerbated by breathing in, coughing, or lying on the back.)

Findings

● Cardiac auscultation may reveal pericardial friction rub (best heard when patient is sitting and leaning forward).

● Typically, EKG will reveal **diffuse** nonspecific upward sloping elevation. PR depression is a specific EKG finding for pericarditis.

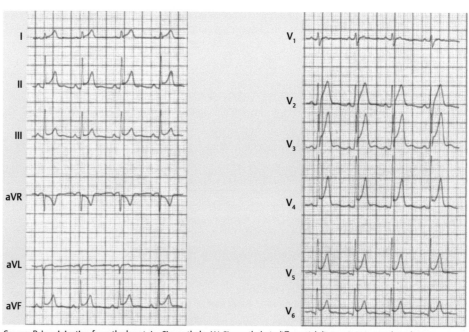

Source: Pain originating from the heart. In: Siegenthaler W. Siegenthaler's differential diagnosis in internal medicine: From symptom to diagnosis. 1st ed. Thieme; 2007.

Establishing diagnosis: EKG and history are the most important tools in diagnosing pericarditis Look for elevated CRP and ESR. Do TTE; presence of even a small pericardial effusion points towards pericarditis.

Management: Identify underlying cause which directs treatment (as shown below).

Features of pericarditis occurring in the following situation	Management
• Hx of viral upper respiratory tract infection (MCC is coxsackie virus infection) • Idiopathic pericarditis	Colchicine[a] + aspirin or NSAIDs[b]
• Significantly increased serum creatinine and BUN – Dx is uremic pericarditis	Dialysis
• In the first week of anterior wall MI – It is due to direct irritation of pericardium by inflamed myocardium	Colchicine + aspirin • NSAIDs/steroids are avoided in peri-MI period
• After 1 week to few months post MI or cardiac surgery/ trauma – Dx is postcardiac injury syndrome. Pathophysiology is development of autoimmune pericarditis (used to be known as Dressler's syndrome- when autoimmune pericarditis occurred after MI). Patients can also have pleuritis.	Colchicine[a] + aspirin or NSAIDs[b] (NSAIDs can be given at this stage)

[a]Colchicine has been shown to prevent recurrence of pericarditis

[b]If symptoms are refractory to ASA/NSAIDs, change to oral steroids.

Abbreviations: BUN, blood urea nitrogen; MI, myocardial infarction; NSAIDS, nonsteroidal anti-inflammatory drugs.

 In a nutshell

Difference between myocarditis and pericarditis

	Pericarditis	Myocarditis
EKG	Both can have diffuse nonspecific ST wave elevation	
Chest pain	Sharp pleuritic	Dull vague
Cardiac enzymes	Normal	Elevated

Pericardial Tamponade (aka Cardiac Tamponade)

Etiology

- Any cause of pericarditis can lead to increased capillary permeability and pericardial effusion. If effusion is large enough, it can cause cardiac tamponade.
- Hemopericardium can develop due to chest trauma, acute MI with ventricular free wall rupture, aortic dissection, etc.
- Malignancy (e.g., lung cancer, breast cancer, lymphoma).

Presentation

Think of cardiac tamponade when the following triad is present:

1. Hypotension.
2. Increased JVP.
3. Muffled heart sounds in auscultation.

Additional features may include:

- Pulsus paradoxus: more than expected fall in systolic blood pressure on inspiration.[36]
- Nonpalpable apex beat.

[36]FYI pulsus paradoxus is a misnomer, as it is not paradoxical; because decrease in systolic blood pressure after inspiration is expected.

- EKG features
  - Electrical alternans: beat-to-beat change in QRS amplitude due to swinging of the heart in the fluid-filled pericardium. This is pathognomonic of pericardial tamponade.
  - Low-voltage QRS complexes.

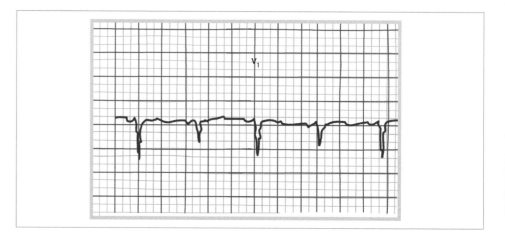

Management steps

- NSIDx is immediate bedside **echocardiography**.
- NSIM is pericardiocentesis (pericardial window).

Constrictive Pericarditis

Pathophysiology: It is a pathologic process that occurs as a result of chronic inflammation of pericardium leading to obliteration of pericardial space with fibrotic tissue. This restraints ventricular diastolic expansion leading to impaired filling.

Etiology: In developed countries, the MCC is idiopathic, or due to postthoracic radiation. In developing countries, the MCC is tuberculosis.

Presentation: They present with chronic progressive biventricular failure. Exam will typically reveal paradoxical increase in JVP during inspiration (aka Kussmaul sign)[37] and early S3 (pericardial knock). CXR will likely show pericardial calcification.

[37] This finding also seen in pericardial tamponade. Also, both pericardial tamponade and constrictive pericarditis have equalization of diastolic pressure in left and right heart.

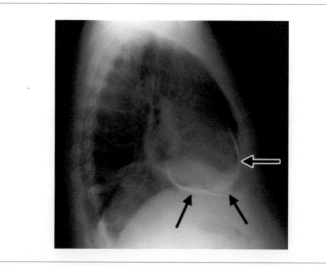

Source: Clinical aspects. In: Claussen C, Miller S, Riessen R, et al. Direct diagnosis in radiology. Cardiac imaging. 1st ed. Thieme; 2007.

Management steps

- NSIDx is TTE, which can reveal to-and-fro motion of interventricular septum during diastole (right and left ventricle are competing for limited space for diastolic expansion).
- Chest CT/MRI scan will show obliteration of pericardial space. Imaging is useful in guiding pericardiectomy.
- Best SIM is surgical decompression (pericardiectomy).

Differential diagnosis: Loss of mark (LOM) with restrictive cardiomyopathy. Both can present with progressive biventricular failure, and have Kussmaul sign and pulsus paradoxus. Absence of atrial dilatation and ventricular hypertrophy points toward constrictive pericarditis. In restrictive cardiomyopathy, biatrial dilatation is usually present +/− left ventricular hypertrophy (LVH). Look for presence of risk factors for constrictive pericarditis, for example, hx of TB (or immigrant to USA) or hx of thoracic radiation (e.g., hx of lymphoma).

4.8 Rheumatic Fever and Rheumatic Heart Disease

4.8.1 Rheumatic Fever

Background: It is an autoimmune inflammatory process, which typically develops as an immunologic sequela to streptococcal infection (most commonly pharyngitis). This preventable condition is more common in more developing countries, due to problems with access of healthcare and subsequent failure to get prompt diagnosis and treatment for strep throat.

The major criteria

- Carditis: endocarditis, myocarditis, pericarditis, or pancarditis. If myocardial biopsy is done, pathology might reveal Aschoff bodies (fibrinoid necrosis). Myocarditis, which results in acute heart failure and predisposes to ventricular arrhythmias, is the MCC of early death in rheumatic fever.
- Arthritis is usually migratory in nature.
- Subcutaneous nodules (aka erythema nodosum) develop due to subcutaneous fat tissue inflammation. Look for tender red nodules or lumps on extensor surfaces of upper or lower extremities.
- Erythema marginatum: red erythematous skin rash.
- Sydenham chorea is a neurological movement disorder, and usually presents late in disease course.

Minor criteria: **P**yrexia (fever), **a**rthralgia, **p**rolonged PR interval in EKG, and **e**levated **ESR** or CRP

Essential criterion: documented infection with *Streptococcus pyogenes*—positive throat culture or elevated serum antistreptolysin O (ASO) or DNase titer.

Diagnosis is made when there is essential criterion

+

two major **OR** one major and two minor manifestations

Major **CASES** of rheumatic fever.

CASES on **PAPEr** of rheumatic fever.

4.8.2 Rheumatic Heart Disease

Background: Recurrent attacks of rheumatic fever can lead to scarring and deformity of valves resulting in development of chronic valvular heart disease. All valves can be affected, with mitral valve involvement being the most common (MR or MS).

How to prevent Rheumatic heart disease or halt it's progression? Give prophylactic monthly intramuscular injections of benzathine penicillin G to patients with rheumatic fever. The following table outlines duration of prophylaxis:

Rheumatic fever	Prophylaxis indicated for
Without carditis	5 years
With mild carditis and no residual heart disease	For 10 years or until 21 years of age (whichever is later)
Residual heart disease	For 10 years or until 41 years of age (whichever is later)

Clinical Case Scenarios

A 13-year-old male who had recent history of lower extremity tender red nodules and migratory joint pain is found dead in his house. His mother reported that he was complaining of dull chest pain and SOB for the last few days.

28. What is the immediate cause of death?

29. What is the likely diagnosis?

4.9 Hypertension

The diagnosis is based upon two or more separate blood pressure readings. MC presentation is asymptomatic elevation of blood pressure found during routine examination.

New updated classification	Systolic (mmHg)		Diastolic (mmHg)	NSIM (next step in management)	
Normal	< 120	and	< 80	No treatment needed. Regular blood pressure screening	
Elevated BP	≥ 120	and	< 80	Lifestyle modifications only and reassess within few months	
Stage I HTN	≥ 130	or	≥ 80	ASCVD 10-year score <10% and no other risk factor (lower risk population)	Lifestyle modifications only and reassess within few months
				Presence of any of the following- ASCVD, DM, CKD, heart failure, age ≥ 65 years, or ASCVD 10-year score ≥ 10% (Higher risk population)	Start one antihypertensive medication and reassess within few months
Stage II HTN	≥ 140	or	≥ 90	Initiate 1 anti-hypertensive medication (in lower-risk) or 2 (in higher-risk patient) as initial treatment + lifestyle modification	

Abbreviations: ASCVD, atherosclerotic cardiovascular disease; CKD, chronic kidney disease; DM, diabetes mellitus.

Work-up: All newly diagnosed cases of hypertension (HTN) should undergo the following baseline testing to detect complications or evidence of end organ damage.

- Urinalysis for presence of proteinuria, hematuria, or glycosuria.
- Complete blood count (CBC).
- Serum electrolytes: Low K^+ points toward hyperaldosteronism. Elevated creatinine points toward end organ damage or chronic kidney disease (CKD) as the cause of HTN.
- EKG for presence of LVH.
- Screen for diabetes mellitus (DM) and dyslipidemia to assess for presence of risk factors for ASCVD.

Always try to identify reversible causes of HTN, e.g., oral contraception, NSAIDs use, alcoholism.

Lifestyle modifications: Given in order of effectiveness in reducing blood pressure.

1. Weight reduction in patients with BMI of more than 30 is the most effective lifestyle modification.
2. DASH diet: consume diet rich in fruits, vegetables, grains, and reduce sodium intake.
3. Exercise.
4. Decrease sodium intake.
5. Moderation of alcohol consumption.

4.9.1 Pharmacological Management of Hypertension

Legend: CKD, chronic kidney disease; DM, diabetes mellitus; ACE-I, ACE inhibitors; ARB, angiotensin receptor blockers

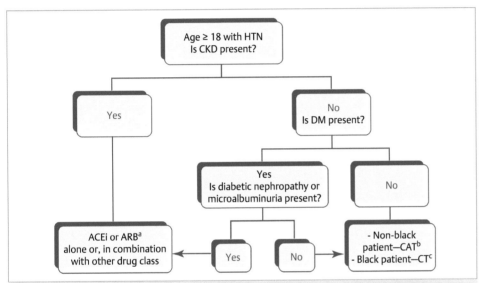

[a]ACE inhibitor or ARB is indicated as first-line therapy in patients with CKD stage 3 or higher without edema,[38] stage 1 or 2 with albuminuria (>300 mg/day), and diabetic nephropathy.

[b]It is very important to know the drugs that have been shown to decrease mortality and hence increase survival in HTN patients.

Calcium channel blockers (CCB)	Dihydropyridines: amlodipine, felodipine, etc. (+ dipine)
	(Note: Nondihydropyridines CCBs, such as verapamil and diltiazem, are more commonly used for heart rate control)
ACE inhibitors or ARBs	ACE-i = suffix "pril" = lisinopril, captopril, benazepril, etc.
	ARB = suffix "artan" = losartan, candesartan, valsartan, etc.
Thiazide-type diuretics	Hydrochlorothiazide, chlorthalidone

[c]CT = CCB or **T**hiazide-type diuretic. CT is preferred over ACE-i or ARB in black patients.[39]

[38] In patients with CKD and edema, use a loop diuretic such as furosemide.

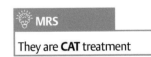

They are **CAT** treatment

[39] A study showed that in black patients' subgroup, CCB and thiazide diuretics were more effective in improving combined cardiovascular outcomes compared to ACE-i.

4.9.2 Individualized Antihypertension Treatment

HTN with the following comorbidities	Drug of choice
CAD, e.g., stable angina or acute coronary syndrome	β-blocker, or ACE-i/ARB
CAD with low ejection fraction (i.e., < 40%)	ACE-i or ARBs and β-blocker
Tremor	noncardioselective β-blocker (e.g., propranolol)
Osteoporosis or, with multiple risk factors for osteoporosis[a]	Thiazide-type diuretic
Claudication (i.e., leg pain on exertion or rest)	Dihydropyridines like amlodipine
Obstructive urinary symptoms due to benign prostatic hyperplasia	Alpha blockers such as doxazosin, prazosin
They relax smooth muscles in prostate, bladder neck, and urethra
Hyperthyroidism	β-blocker
Raynaud's phenomenon	CCB such as nifedipine
Pregnancy	Methyldopa or clonidine. Use IV hydralazine or labetalol for severe HTN. (Note: ACE-i or ARBs are absolutely contraindicated in pregnancy.)
Migraines	CCB or β-blocker

[a]What are the risk factors for osteoporosis? Write it down and compare your list with the one given in preventative medicine chapter.

Abbreviations: ACE, angiotensin-converting enzyme; ARB, angiotensin receptor blocker; CAD, coronary artery disease; CCB, calcium channel blocker.

Common side effects of antihypertensives

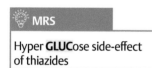

MRS

Hyper **GLUC**ose side-effect of thiazides

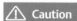

Caution

Avoid hydrochlorothiazide in patients with gout or hyponatremia

| Thiazide type diuretic | Hyper**G**lycemia, high **L**DL, hyper**U**ricemia, hyper**C**alcemia
Hyponatremia |
|---|---|
| CCB (dihydropyridines) | Lower extremity edema |
| β-blockers | - They have negative effects on metabolic profile; increases LDL, decreases HDL, and worsens glucose control. *Exceptions are labetalol, carvedilol, and nebivolol which have a favorable effect on metabolic profile, as they also have α-blocking properties. These might be the preferred β-blockers in diabetes*
- Depression
- May worsen bronchospasm |
| ACE-i | - Chronic dry cough (NSIM is change to ARB).
- Angioedema |

Rebound HTN: Abrupt withdrawal of catecholamine blockers (particularly short-acting ones like clonidine or propranolol) may lead to **rebound** catecholamine surge. This can present with high blood pressure and tachycardia. Risk of rebound HTN with various antihypertensive medications in descending order are: clonidine and propranolol > metoprolol > atenolol (*atenolol is a longer-acting β-blocker*).

Caution: When clonidine and a β-blocker is used together, abrupt discontinuation of clonidine can lead to very severe rebound HTN, as resultant catecholamine surge leads to unopposed alpha-1 activity

Abbreviations: ACE-i, angiotensin-converting enzyme inhibitor; CCB, calcium channel blocker; COPD, compulsive obstructive pulmonary disorder; LDL, low-density lipoproteins; HDL, high-density lipoproteins.

After initiation of antihypertensive medication, patient needs to be reassessed within few weeks

- If average blood pressure reaches the goal value,[40] continue the treatment.
- If goal blood pressure is not achieved:
  - NSIM is to check for **compliance to medical regimen**[41] **and continuing alcohol, NSAIDS, or oral contraceptive** use. (They are the common causes of failure of response to treatment). If patient is obese, obstructive sleep apnea should also be taken into consideration.

If above factors are excluded, NSIM is to either increase the dose of the initial antihypertensive medication (if patient is not on optimal dose), or add another medication (if the patient is on optimal dose of first antihypertensive medication).

4.9.3 Complications of Hypertension

Following complications can develop when HTN is not properly treated in a timely manner:

- **Cerebrovascular complications:** uncontrolled HTN predisposes to transient ischemic attack (TIA), ischemic stroke, lacunar stroke, hemorrhagic stroke, and subarachnoid hemorrhage.[42]
- **Cardiac complications:** uncontrolled HTN → increased afterload → concentric hypertrophy with decrease in luminal size of left ventricle → isolated diastolic dysfunction. This can later progress to dilated cardiomyopathy, if underlying HTN is severe and is left untreated.
- **Renal complication:** hypertensive **nephrosclerosis** is the second MCC of CKD after DM.
- **Aortic root dilatation and dissection:** HTN is the MC predisposing condition.
- **Hypertensive retinopathy:** depending on the severity of underlying retinopathy, patients can have blurred vision, scotomas (visual field defects), and even blindness.

Retinopathy grading by fundoscopy

Grade I	**S**ilver wiring (arteriolar thickening)
Grade II	**A**rteriovenous nicking (now arteriolar thickening is severe thick enough to cause pressure on vein)
Grade III	**C**otton wool exudates (appear as fluffy white patches on the retina): *inset picture-black arrows*
Grade IV	**Pa**pilledema (optic disc swelling with blurring of optic margins)

Source: Hypertensive retinopathy and sclerotic changes. In: Lang G, ed. Ophthalmology. A pocket Ttextbook atlas. 3rd ed. Thieme; 2015.

Clinical Case Scenarios

30. A 40-year-old male is in clinic for regular screening visit. His blood pressure is 140/85 mmHg. He is surprised with elevated blood pressure reading, because when he checks his blood pressure at home and at his local pharmacy it is always <120/80 mmHg. What is the dx and NSIM?

31. A 40-year-old male has noticed multiple blood pressure readings of >140/90 mmHg at home. His blood pressure during the last visit was 120/70 mmHg. Blood pressure measured in office today is 125/75 mmHg. What is the dx and NSIM?

32. A 55-year-old female has multiple blood pressure reading of >135/85 mmHg. Patient is on OCP (alternatively, hx of heavy NSAIDs use). NSIM?

33. A 58-year-old male has HTN and ongoing alcohol abuse. NSIM?

34. A 55-year-old black male presents with multiple readings of >150/90 mmHg. He has no hx of NSAIDs use or alcohol abuse. NSIM?

35. A 67-year-old male with hx of medical noncompliance presents with SOB on exertion and decreased exercise tolerance. His blood pressure is 175/86 mm Hg. CXR is unremarkable. EKG shows LVH and strain pattern. Echocardiography shows normal EF and evidence of concentric LVH. What is the DOC?

[40] *Target BP depends on patient characteristics. This is an evolving field, so unlikely be asked on exam. In a frail elderly patient with increased comorbidities target SBP might be <150, but in a young healthy patient target SBP is lower (<130/80). Also, in patients with significant large cerebral vessel occlusion, be careful in reducing BP too much as higher BP might be needed to perfuse critical brain areas.*

[41] An important cause of noncompliance is development of adverse effects, so always ask patients, as they might not volunteer the information at first.

[42] HTN is the MC underlying cause for stroke

MRS

SAC PAck

4.9.4 Hypertensive Emergency (Old-Term: Malignant HTN) and Hypertensive Urgency

If a patient presents with systolic blood pressure of ≥180 and/or diastolic blood pressure is ≥120 mmHg, NSIM is to screen for end organ damage.

Assess for presence of the following signs and symptoms	Target organ damage	NSIDx
Chest pain or angina equivalent	Acute coronary syndrome Aortic dissection	EKG, cardiac enzymes, and CXR
Blurred vision	Papilledema (this finding is required for the dx of malignant HTN). This can lead to permanent blindness if not treated promptly	Fundoscopy
SOB Exam reveals bibasilar crackles	Congestive heart failure	CXR, BNP, transthoracic echocardiography
Confusion, seizures, or focal neurological deficit	Intracerebral or subarachnoid hemorrhage - hypertensive encephalopathy	CT scan of head
Nonspecific (e.g., lethargy)	Acute renal failure or kidney injury. Malignant nephrosclerosis	BMP (serum creatinine) and urinalysis (can reveal hematuria and proteinuria)

Abbreviations: BMP, basic metabolic panel; BNP, brain natriuretic peptide; CXR, chest X-ray; EKG, electrocardiography; SOB, shortness of breath.

If evidence of one or more end-organ damage, Dx is hypertensive emergency	If no evidence of end organ damage, Dx is hypertensive urgency[a]
Pathology: Blood pressure that is so high that within a short period of time (within few weeks to few months) it is causing end organ damage to various organs **Rx:** NSIM is to hospitalize patient and start intravenous antihypertensive agent (e.g., nitroprusside,[b] nitroglycerin, nicardipine, labetalol, enalapril). Note that blood pressure should not be lowered too rapidly (target reduction of mean arterial pressure is 10-20% in the 1st hour of treatment; target reduction of total 25% in first 24 hours). If lowered too fast it can compromise cerebral or coronary perfusion	NSIM assess for increased risk of cardiovascular events (e.g., hx of aortic or intracranial aneurysms) **If present,** blood pressure reduction should be lowered over a period of few hours (target reduction of 20–30 mmHg). Short- and fast-acting oral antihypertensive medications such as oral furosemide, clonidine or captopril can be used. (Note sublingual nifedipine should not be used its effect can be unpredictable). **If absent,** blood pressure reduction can be done over a period of days. In most patients who are not on any antihypertensive medication, a combination regimen is recommended (e.g., amlodipine + benazepril)

[a]Patients might have mild headache but mostly it is relatively asymptomatic.

[b] **Side effect of nitroprusside:** prolonged infusion can lead to cyanide toxicity (presents with acute confusion and lactic acidosis).

4.10 Secondary Hypertension

Secondary HTN should be suspected in following cases:
- Patients are hypertensive despite taking adequate dose of three or more antihypertensive medications.[43]
- Severe HTN (accelerated or malignant HTN).

[43] Advanced CKD is the MCC of secondary HTN and typically requires multiple antihypertensives to control blood pressure.

- Young (<30 years), nonobese, non-black patient, with no family history of HTN.
- Onset before puberty in any patient.
- Acute worsening of previously stable HTN.
- Presence of features suggestive of secondary HTN (*look at table below*)

In a **very old patient** with poorly controlled HTN, dx can be **calcific arteriosclerosis**. The arteries are so stiff that the blood pressure monitor cuff cannot compress them.

Presentation	Most likely cause of secondary HTN	NSIDx
Obese patient with increased neck circumference. Hx of daytime somnolence and headaches	**Obstructive sleep apnea**	Sleep lab testing (polysomnography)
Hx of heat intolerance, anxiety, and weight-loss despite increased appetite. Blood pressure reveals widened pulse pressure	**Hyperthyroidism due to hyperdynamic circulation**	Serum TSH
Young patient, with hx of epistaxis, headaches, and lower extremity claudication. Exam reveals increased blood pressure in upper extremities and low blood pressure in lower extremities	**Coarctation of aorta**	CXR + transthoracic echocardiography
Exam reveals bruit in paraumbilical or renal area. Lab reveals low K+ and high bicarbonate levels. • In a young female patient, think of fibromuscular dysplasia. • In an old patient with multiple risk factors of ASCVD, think of atherosclerotic narrowing of renal arteries	**Renal artery stenosis with secondary hyperaldosteronism**	Renal duplex USG in nonobese patient or CT/MRI angiography
Hx of muscle weakness, hypokalemia, and metabolic alkalosis (! similar electrolyte profile to secondary hyperaldosteronism)	**Primary hyperaldosteronism, aka Conn's syndrome**	Serum aldosterone/renin levels
Hx of episodic panic attacks, headaches, diaphoresis, and palpitations	**Pheochromocytoma**	Plasma fractionated metanephrine (most sensitive test) or 24-hour urine test for fractionated metanephrines and catecholamines (more specific test)
Exam reveals cutaneous striae, moon face, and buffalo hump	**Cushing's syndrome**	Use any two of the following test: Low-dose dexamethasone suppression test, late-night salivary or serum cortisol level, or 24-hour urinary cortisol excretion
Exam reveals protruded jaw, enlarged hands, and feet	**Acromegaly (growth hormone excess)**	IGF-1 (somatomedin C) levels
Hx of renal stones, psychosis, and abdominal pain. Lab test reveals hypercalcemia and/or hypophosphatemia	**Primary hyperparathyroidism**	Serum PTH level
Hx of renal disease in family. Exam reveals bilateral renal masses. Urinalysis reveals proteinuria and hematuria	**Adult onset autosomal dominant polycystic kidney disease**	Renal US

Abbreviations: ASCVD, atherosclerotic cardiovascular disease; CXR, chest X-ray; IGF-1, insulin-like growth factor 1; PTH, parathyroid hormone; TSH, thyroid-stimulating hormone; USG, ultrasonography.

4.10.1 Renal Artery Stenosis (RAS)

Etiology

Fibromuscular dysplasia	Nonatherosclerotic, noninflammatory condition, with unclear pathogenesis, that causes narrowing (stenosis) and enlargement (aneurysm) of medium-sized arteries. Virtually any artery can be involved; however, most common involvement is renal artery followed by carotid arteries. Extrarenal presentations may include stroke, TIA, or even mesenteric angina. Classic image pattern is "string of beads" appearance of the arteries	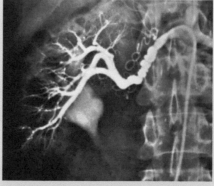 Source: Secondary hypertension. In: Siegenthaler W. Siegenthaler's differential diagnosis in internal medicine: From symptom to diagnosis. 1st ed. Thieme; 2007.
Atherosclerotic renal artery stenosis (*inset picture-red arrow*)	Same pathophysiology as CAD, PVD, and ASCVD	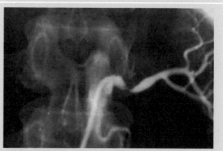 Source: Secondary hypertension. In: Siegenthaler W. Siegenthaler's differential diagnosis in internal medicine: From symptom to diagnosis. 1st ed. Thieme; 2007.

Pathophysiology: Decreased blood supply to the involved kidney → increase in renin secretion → rise in angiotensin and aldosterone to maintain renal blood flow → development of HTN and increased propensity for hypokalemia and metabolic alkalosis.

Presentation scenarios

- CCS: A 32-year-old female was found to have HTN. No hx of oral contraceptive use. ACE-i was initiated. In follow-up visit, blood pressure is still elevated. Her lab work reveals an increase in serum creatinine of greater than 30% above baseline. (In this case, suspect renal artery stenosis due to fibromuscular dysplasia).
- CCS: An elderly patient with previously controlled HTN has been having worsening control over the last few months. He has hx of multiple risk factors for ASCVD.
- Renal artery stenosis (RAS) can also present with recurrent flash pulmonary edema and/or refractory heart failure.
- Exam may reveal continuous murmur in the paraumbilical region.

Management steps

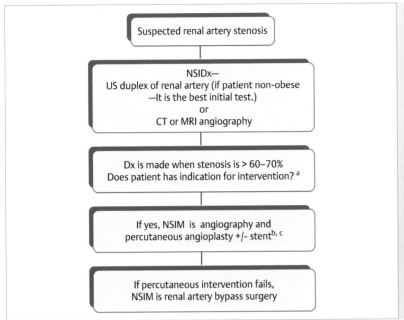

Suspected renal artery stenosis

NSIDx—
US duplex of renal artery (if patient non-obese
—It is the best initial test.)
or
CT or MRI angiography

Dx is made when stenosis is > 60–70%
Does patient has indication for intervention? [a]

If yes, NSIM is angiography and
percutaneous angioplasty +/- stent[b, c]

If percutaneous intervention fails,
NSIM is renal artery bypass surgery

[a]Indication for intervention
- Failure of optimal medical treatment to control blood pressure.
- Intolerance to medical therapy.
- A short duration of blood pressure elevation prior to the dx (this is the strongest clinical predictor of return of blood pressure control after intervention).
- Hx of recurrent flash pulmonary edema and/or refractory heart failure.

[b]In patients with atherosclerotic RAS, angiography with stenting is recommended (angioplasty alone is usually not effective in this patient group). In fibromuscular dysplasia, angioplasty alone can be done +/– stent placement. Angioplasty: a deflated balloon attached to a catheter is passed into the stenotic area and the balloon is then inflated.

[c]If the arterial anatomy is complex, do bypass surgery instead.

Additional points on management of RAS

- Aggressive risk factor management with control of HTN, dyslipidemia, and smoking cessation should be done in all patients with ASCVD-related RAS.
- Medical treatment of HTN with ACE-i and ARB, which blocks renin-angiotensin pathway, are effective in treating this type of secondary HTN. ACEi/ARB can be used even in bilateral RAS; however, serum creatinine needs to be closely monitored after initiation.

4.11 Diseases of the Aorta

4.11.1 Aneurysm

Definition: Aneurysms are localized dilation of artery due to vessel wall weakness.

	Ascending aortic aneurysm	Aneurysm of descending aorta and abdominal aorta
Background	• Occurs in patients with heritable disorders such as Marfan's syndrome, Ehler–Danlos syndrome, bicuspid aortic valve, or coarctation of aorta. • Other cause; aortitis due to syphilis, autoimmune arteritis, etc. • Occurs less commonly due to ASCVD	It occurs mostly in patients with atherosclerotic cardiovascular disease (ASCVD)
	Aortic regurgitation can coexist due to aortic ring dilatation	
	Note: Aortic aneurysm in a young patient with no risk factors can be a result of **blunt trauma**	
	Aneurysms increase risk of dissection	
Work-up	• For asymptomatic thoracic (ascending or descending) aneurysms test of choice is CT or MR angiography. • For abdominal aortic aneurysm, do ultrasound of abdomen	
General management	• Tight control of blood pressure and heart rate • Address underlying cause	• Tight control of blood pressure and heart rate • For ASCVD-related aneurysm, do aggressive risk factors modification[a]

[a]There is no evidence that this can prevent aneurysm expansion, but it may help in decreasing other ASCVD-related complications. Smoking, however, is strongly associated with increased risk of aneurysmal expansion and rupture.

Indications for surgical correction of aortic aneurysm

All aneurysms	• Accelerated growth rate (≥ 1 cm/yr), or growth of ≥ 0.5 cm in 6 months
	• Evidence of dissection
Ascending aortic aneurysm	Size > 5 to 6 cm[a]
	• An ascending aortic aneurysm > 4.5 cm in diameter at the time of aortic valve surgery is also an indication
Descending aortic aneurysm	Size > 6 to 7 cm[a]
Abdominal aortic aneurysm	Size > 5.5 cm[a]

[a]These cutoff sizes represent aneurysms that are more likely to enlarge and rupture. Higher cutoffs are used for patients with higher risk of surgery.

Follow-up: If surgical correction is not indicated, do regular surveillance with US (for abdominal aneurysm), or CT or MR angiography (for thoracic aneurysms).

4.11.2 Thoracic Aortic Dissection

Background: It is an intimal tear in the aortic wall that creates another pathway within which the blood runs, creating a false lumen between the layers of the aortic wall.

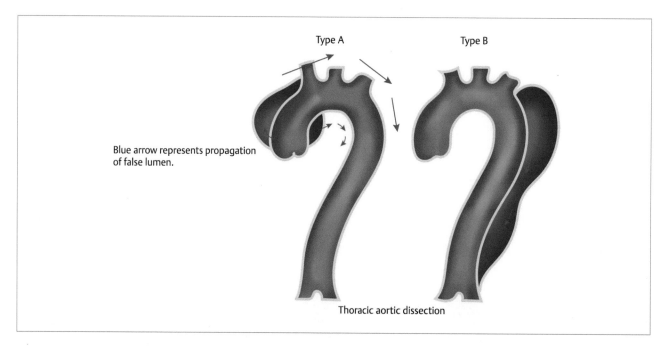

Blue arrow represents propagation of false lumen.

Thoracic aortic dissection

MC predisposing and aggravating condition for aortic dissection is HTN. It can also occur in pregnancy. In young patients with aortic dissection, suspect conditions like Marfan's syndrome, Ehler–Danlos syndrome, or coarctation of aorta.

Presentation: Sudden onset severe/intense tearing or ripping chest pain radiating to the back/interscapular area.

As the dissection progresses with propagation of false lumen, it can obstruct vessels arising from the aorta, which can cause the following complications:

Coronary ostia	RCA territory ischemia/infarction • Look for ST-T wave changes in II, III, AVF	
Can rupture into pericardium	Hemopericardium and pericardial tamponade	More common in type A
Subclavian artery	Exam will reveal decreased blood pressure and pulse pressure in one arm	
Carotid artery	Hypoperfusion to the brain can result in stroke	
Can cause dilatation of aortic ring	Acute aortic regurgitation • Look for diastolic murmur in cardiac exam	
Intercostal arteries which also supply spinal arteries	Paraplegia	
Mesenteric arteries	Intestinal/colonic ischemia	
Renal arteries	Hematuria, lumbar pain	
Iliac arteries	Pain and decreased pulse in lower extremities	

Abbreviations: RCA, right coronary artery; AVF, augmented vector foot.

Management steps

NSIDx is to check blood pressure in both arms. **CXR** will show mediastinal widening.

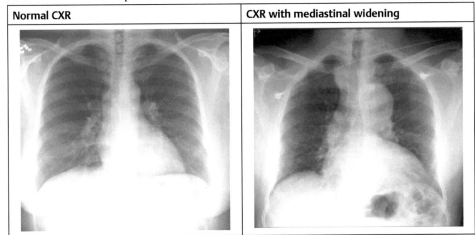

| **Normal CXR** | **CXR with mediastinal widening** |

Source: Aorta. In: Gunderman R. Essential radiology. Clinical presentation, pathophysiology, imaging. 3rd ed. Thieme; 2014.

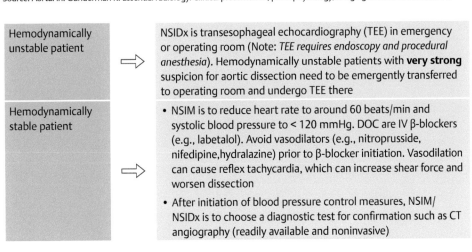

| Hemodynamically unstable patient | ⇨ | NSIDx is transesophageal echocardiography (TEE) in emergency or operating room (Note: *TEE requires endoscopy and procedural anesthesia*). Hemodynamically unstable patients with **very strong** suspicion for aortic dissection need to be emergently transferred to operating room and undergo TEE there |
| Hemodynamically stable patient | ⇨ | • NSIM is to reduce heart rate to around 60 beats/min and systolic blood pressure to < 120 mmHg. DOC are IV β-blockers (e.g., labetalol). Avoid vasodilators (e.g., nitroprusside, nifedipine,hydralazine) prior to β-blocker initiation. Vasodilation can cause reflex tachycardia, which can increase shear force and worsen dissection

• After initiation of blood pressure control measures, NSIM/NSIDx is to choose a diagnostic test for confirmation such as CT angiography (readily available and noninvasive) |

Diagnostic imaging for dissection in order of accuracy are TEE > MRI with contrast > CT scan with contrast.

171

Treatment method	Indication
Emergent surgical intervention	• All type A dissection that **involve** the ascending aorta
	• For type B dissection, indications are hemodynamically unstable patient, persistent pain/hypertension, evidence of propagation of dissection, occlusion of major aortic branch, aneurysmal expansion or rupture
	• Acute type B dissection in patients with Marfan's syndrome is also an indication for surgery
Medical management	Hemodynamically stable, uncomplicated type B aortic dissections
	• Follow-up with regular MRI or CT angiography in an outpatient basis

4.11.3 Symptomatic Abdominal Aortic Aneurysm and Ruptured Abdominal Aortic Aneurysm

Symptoms: Abdominal/back pain and/or bilateral flank ecchymosis. Patients can also present with limb ischemia secondary to thromboemboli originating from abdominal aortic aneurysm (AAA).[44]

[44]Development of symptoms in AAA implies impending rupture.

Presentation of rupture: hypotension, severe pain, and pulsatile mass.

Management step

If hemodynamically **unstable** and has a documented hx of AAA	High prediagnostic probability. NSIM is to rush to surgery for repair	In all hemodynamically unstable patients, do not forget to place large bore IV catheters and administer IV fluids.
If hemodynamically **unstable** and has no prior hx of AAA	NSIM is immediate bedside abdominal US	
Hemodynamically stable	Abdominal CT angiography with IV contrast (We have time to perform the diagnostic test)	
Surgical options are endovascular aneurysm repair (EVAR) or open surgery		

🔍 Clinical Case Scenarios

36. A 65-year-old male nonobese patient with multiple risk factors for ASCVD comes to the clinic for routine follow-up. Exam reveals pulsatile **nontender** mass above umbilicus. What is NSIDx?

    a. CT abdomen with contrast.

    b. US abdomen.

    c. MRI angiography.

37. Patient presents with severe sudden onset chest pain radiating to back. EKG shows ST-T wave elevation in II, III, AVF. CXR shows mediastinal widening. What is the diagnosis?

    a. Acute coronary syndrome.

    b. Aortic dissection.

    c. Mediastinitis.

For coarctation of Aorta: see Chapter 22, Pediatrics.

4.11.4 Peripheral Vascular Disease aka Peripheral Arterial Disease (PAD)[45]

Definition: Formation of atherosclerotic plaques in peripheral arteries leading to narrowing or occlusion and ischemic complications.

Presentation: Symptoms depend upon the location and extent of the narrowing. The most common symptom of peripheral artery disease (PAD) is intermittent claudication (pain, usually in the calf, that occurs while walking and dissipates at rest). Patients can also present with nonhealing ulcer or infectious complications (e.g., cellulitis/osteomyelitis). Severe disease can have gangrene.

Work-up: NSIDx is ankle-brachial index (ABI). It is both sensitive and specific for dx of PAD. It is calculated by dividing the systolic blood pressure at the ankle by systolic blood pressure in arm. If the ratio is <0.9, it is diagnostic of PAD. This number means that compared to the arm, there is lower blood pressure in the leg, which is an indication of macrovascular disease in the leg.[46]

General management: Use aspirin and statin. Aggressive ASCVD risk factor modification should be done. Smoking cessation has been associated with lower risk of progression and complications.

Stepwise management of claudication

- Supervised exercise program is recommended in all patients with claudication.
- If patient is still having persistent symptoms, NSIM is cilostazol[47] (phosphodiesterase inhibitor, which causes vasodilation and reversible inhibition of platelet aggregation). It has been shown to improve pain-free walking distance; however, it may take months for the benefit to be clinically evident.
- If still having persistent troublesome symptoms, NSIM is percutaneous stent placement or bypass surgery, depending upon vascular anatomy. Lower extremity CT or MR angiography is done prior to any invasive procedure.

4.11.5 Acute Limb Ischemia

Etiology

- Arterial embolism due to atrial fibrillation, post-myocardial infarction, cholesterol-emboli syndrome, thrombophilic states, heparin-induced thrombocytopenia, etc.
- In situ thrombosis in patients with peripheral vascular disease (*this is equivalent of acute coronary syndrome in coronary arteries*).

Presentation: Symptoms can progress from pain, pallor, pulselessness, paraesthesias, to paralysis (the 5 Ps of acute limb ischemia). If clot progresses, gangrene ensues.[48]

Work-up: NSIDx is doppler arteriography. (This can be deferred if diagnosis is obvious, for example, acute severe pain and absent pulse).

Treatment: Usually depends upon the source of clot.

Cardiac source: patient has recent MI or hx of chronic atrial fibrillation	NSIM is immediate anticoagulation with heparin and urgent vascular surgery consult. Angiography with percutaneous catheter embolectomy[a] is usually the treatment of choice. After acute management, do TTE to assess for presence of intracardiac thrombus and start anticoagulation
In patients with in situ thrombosis with hx of PAD	The severity is usually mild due to presence of collaterals. Heparin and urgent vascular surgery consult is needed. Arterial bypass surgery might be necessary. Angiography is done before surgery

[a]Potential complications of interventional reperfusion are compartment syndrome and myoglobinuria.

Abbreviations: PAD, peripheral artery disease; TTE, transthoracic echocardiography

[45] Screening with ankle-brachial index (ABI) at regular intervals is recommended in:
- Patients ≥ 50 years of age with risk factors for ASCVD.
- All patients ≥ 65 years of age.

[46] ABI of ≥1.4 might be due to calcified noncompressible vessel. NSIDx is toe-brachial index (*uses doppler signal for BP reading.*)

[47] Cilostazol is contraindicated in patients with chronic heart failure.

[48] As opposed to deep vein thrombosis (DVT), where clot is in the venous system, the risk of a limb loss, if not promptly treated, is high.

4.11.6 Subclavian Steal Syndrome

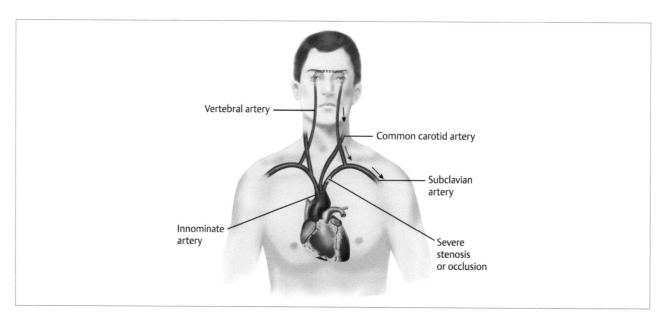

Pathophysiology: This phenomenon occurs due to stenosis in either innominate (aka brachiocephalic artery) or subclavian artery proximal to the origin of vertebral artery. When arm is exercised, reactive arterial dilatation can create almost like a negative pressure causing retrograde blood flow from the vertebral artery ("stealing" blood from the vertebral artery to supply the arm).

Etiology of stenosis: Atherosclerosis, Takayasu's arteritis, due to extrinsic arterial compression by cervical rib, etc.

Presentation: Patients may present with hx of dizziness/vertigo or ataxia precipitated by vigorous hand movement and arm/hand pain after exercise (claudication of upper extremity).

Management steps

- NSIDx blood pressure check in both arms and if different by >15 mmHg, dx is likely subclavian steal syndrome.
- NSIDx is duplex US of subclavian and carotid arteries. Carotid US may show reversal of flow in vertebral artery. Confirmatory test is MRI or CT angiography of head and neck.
- NSIM is vascular surgery evaluation.

4.11.7 Cardiac Myxoma aka Atrial Myxoma

Background: Benign tumor made up of primitive connective tissue cells, most commonly located in the left atria.

Presentation scenarios: Patient may present with any of the following:

- Hx of few months of fatigue, SOB on exertion, palpitations, fever, and weight loss.
- Valvular stenosis (tricuspid or mitral) or its complications (e.g., heart failure, arrhythmias). Exam may reveal mid-diastolic murmur.
- Cardioembolic event (hx of TIA, acute limb ischemia, ischemic colitis, or acute leg pain).
- Arrhythmias, heart block, or pericardial effusion (because of local myocardial invasion).

Management steps: NSIDx is TTE. NSIM is prompt surgical resection.

🔍 Clinical Case Scenarios

Patient presents with few months' history of SOB on exertion. He has hx of sustained ventricular tachycardia and was started on an antiarrhythmic drug. CXR done shows diffuse reticulonodular pattern.

38. What is the like drug?

39. What is the NSIM?

Answers

1. Addition of a calcium channel blocker.

2. Addition of long-acting nitrates.

3. CABG.

4. Sildenafil.

5. TTE.

6. LV aneurysm.

7. Stop ACE-i. Cutoff for stopping ACE-i or ARB is increase in creatinine more than 30% from baseline.

8. Combination of hydralazine + oral nitrate (e.g., isosorbide dinitrate or mononitrate).

9. ACE-i-induced angioedema. This can occur any time after initiation of ACE-i; even after few months-years.

10. Angiotensin receptor blockers. ARBs do not inhibit bradykinin metabolism.

11. Oral anticoagulation. CHADSVASc score is 2 for age.

12. CHADSVASc score is 1 for age. Discuss with patient regarding choices of oral anticoagulation, aspirin or none.

13. Idiopathic ventricular tachycardia. Usually it is not life threatening. If clinical symptoms are mild, NSIM is reassurance. If clinical symptoms are frequent or severe, use β-blocker or CCB. If still persistent, NSIM is either catheter ablation or antiarrhythmic agents.

14. Atropine.

15. Any of the following: transcutaneous pacemaker, dopamine drip, or isoprenaline drip.

16. Arrange for insertion of transvenous pacemaker as soon as possible. Also, consult cardiology to prepare for permanent pacemaker placement, if reversible cause is not identified.

17. Bicuspid aortic valve (MC congenital cause of AR).

18. Rheumatic heart disease is the MCC of AR in developing countries.

19. TTE (transthoracic echocardiogram).

20. Furosemide to treat heart failure.

21. B. Mitral valve repair.

22. A. CABG + aortic valve replacement.

23. No indication for surgery.

24. B. Mitral valve repair. (Note that with MR, threshold EF for surgery is <60%.)

25. Atrial septal defect. Because of the left to right shunt, the RV is thought to be continuously overloaded, hence maneuvers such as inspiration or Valsalva produces no net pressure changes. This is the reason for wide-split fixed S2 and fixed systolic murmur.

26. Mitral valve prolapse.

27. Later initiation of the click and shorter duration/intensity of systolic murmur.
    Reason: with afterload increase, less blood is pumped out of left ventricle. With increase in systolic ventricular volume, ventricle is stretched. Floppy valves become less floppy when stretched.

28. Severe myocarditis.

29. Rheumatic fever.

30. Dx is white coat HTN. NSIM is reassurance; no treatment is needed.

31. Dx is masked HTN; high home blood pressure reading with normal blood pressure in office. NSIM: treat as essential HTN (evidence suggests that cardiovascular risk is similar to essential HTN).

32. Advise patient to switch to alternative forms of birth control. Follow-up blood pressure after discontinuation.

33. Advise on reducing alcohol intake, which is directly associated with high blood pressure. (Note that smoking does not directly cause HTN, but all patients should be advised to quit smoking).

34. Initiate on double regimen of CCB and thiazides as patient has stage II HTN and advise lifestyle modification.

35. Studies suggest that CCB or ARB/ACE-i have better effect on regression of LVH than β-blockers. However, there is no clear-cut data on the choice of treatment. Better HTN control will prevent or halt LVH progression.

36. B. US of the abdomen. LOM: do not choose CT scan in asymptomatic patient, unless patient is very obese and has a poor acoustic window.

37. B. In this case, ischemia/infarction in RCA territory is a result of dissection, and not due to acute coronary artery plaque rupture.

38. Amiodarone.

39. Discontinue amiodarone.

5. Acid-Base Disorders

"An interesting fact about pH is that it is measured in log scale—meaning pH of 6 is 10 times more acidic than pH of 7 and 100 times more acidic than pH of 8."

5.1 General Principles

How to interpret arterial blood gas (ABG) to diagnose acid-base disorder?

- **Step 1**: Look at serum pH (normal pH = 7.35–7.45). If abnormal, is it acidic (low pH) or alkalotic (high pH)?
- **Step 2:** Find out which component ($PaCO_2$ or HCO_3^-) correlates with the abnormal pH, as this will point toward the primary disorder:

$$pH \propto \frac{HCO_3^-}{PaCO_2\,(H^+)}$$

- CO_2 is an acidic gas. It increases the acid content of blood by reacting with H_2O to form carbonic acid. Normal value of $PaCO_2$ (H^+) is 40 mmHg, and it is always controlled by respiratory system.
- HCO_3^- is a base and an important buffer of hydrogen ions in the blood. Normal value of HCO_3^- is 24 mEq/L +/– 3, and HCO_3^- content is always controlled by metabolic components, largely through the kidneys.

  Example: If pH is acidotic and $PaCO_2$ is elevated, then the primary disorder is respiratory acidosis. If pH is acidotic and HCO_3 is low, then the primary disorder is metabolic acidosis.
- **Step 3:** Know that compensation is almost always **never complete** (e.g., respiratory compensation of metabolic acidosis can never bring back the pH to normal). Hence the rule is that "primary disorder always reflects the pH status." And, if pH is **normal** and HCO_3^- or $PaCO_2$ is abnormal, then it should be a mixed disorder of primary acid/primary base, because "compensation is never complete."[1]

Compensation

Respiratory compensation is immediate, so most of the nonrespiratory causes of acid-base disorders will have respiratory compensation.

Metabolic compensation, which is mostly by the kidneys, is not immediate and can take 2 to 3 days to kick in. Thus, in primary respiratory acid-base disorder, metabolic compensation may not be present, especially if the respiratory pathology is acute.

- In acidosis, kidneys increase reabsorption of HCO_3^- and increase H^+ excretion.
- In alkalosis, kidneys increase excretion of HCO_3^- and increase reabsorption of H^+.

Clinical Case Scenarios

Let's play with some ABG values

Try to explain them first, and only then look at the answer.

No.	pH	PaCO₂ (H⁺)	HCO₃⁻
1.	7.29	60	25
2.	7.32	55	32
3.	7.30	29	14
4.	7.24	36	14
5.	7.10	60	14
6.	7.50	30	23
7.	7.47	30	19
8.	7.48	45	34
9.	7.40	50	35
10	7.40	33	18

If serum HCO_3^- increases, then pH increases; if $PaCO_2$ (H^+) increases, then pH decreases.

 MRS

$HCO_3 \rightarrow$ 2-3-4; the normal value is 24 +/– 3, i.e., 21–27.

[1] The only exception to this rule is high-altitude respiratory alkalosis, where compensation can be complete resulting in normal pH.

In a nutshell

- $pH \alpha \dfrac{HCO_3^-}{PaCO_2 (H^+)}$

- Normal pH = 7.35 to 7.45.

- Normal value of HCO_3^- is 24 mEq/L +/– 3.

- Normal value of $PaCO_2$ is 40 mmHg.

A simplified algorithm for diagnosis of acid-base disorders

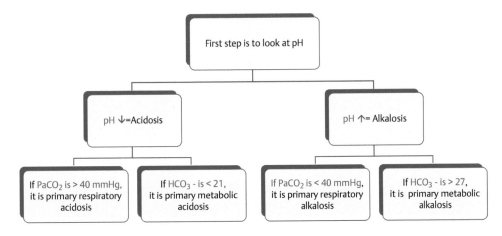

First step is to look at pH

pH ↓=Acidosis

pH ↑= Alkalosis

If $PaCO_2$ is > 40 mmHg, it is primary respiratory acidosis

If HCO_3^- is < 21, it is primary metabolic acidosis

If $PaCO_2$ is < 40 mmHg, it is primary respiratory alkalosis

If HCO_3^- is > 27, it is primary metabolic alkalosis

5.2 Respiratory Alkalosis

5.2.1 Acute Respiratory Alkalosis

Etiology

- Any cause of hypoxia (e.g., acute pulmonary embolus, asthma exacerbation, pneumonia) can lead to compensatory increase in ventilatory drive, which increases minute ventilation resulting in patients blowing off their CO_2. If hypoxemia is not corrected in time, respiratory muscle fatigue can ensue resulting in acute respiratory acidosis.
- Central nervous system pathology (e.g., intracranial or subarachnoid hemorrhage): protective mechanism of hyperventilation kicks in, which has the final effect of decreasing intracranial pressure.[2]
- Respiratory stimulation due to aspirin, caffeine abuse, high fever, etc.
- Iatrogenic: if minute ventilation in intubated patients is set too high.
- Panic/anxiety attack.

[2] Compensatory hyperventilation → decreased arterial $PaCO_2$ → arterial vasoconstriction → decreased cerebral blood flow → compensatory decrease in intracranial pressure

A Complication of Acute Respiratory Alkalosis: Acute Hypocalcemia

Mechanism: alkalosis → less H^+ ions concentration → less H^+ (positive ion) binding to albumin → more sites are available for Ca^{++} (another positive ion) to bind with albumin → low free ionized calcium → acute hypocalcemia.

Clinical features: neuromuscular excitation leading to paresthesias, hyperactive deep tendon reflexes, perioral numbness, carpopedal spasms (early tetany) and sometimes, even seizures.

Clinical Case Scenarios

A 30-year-old female patient with prior medical hx of anxiety disorder presents with sudden onset of severe shortness of breath. Exam reveals increased respiratory rate. ABG done reveals normal PaO_2 on room air, pH of 7.51, $PaCO_2$ of 30 and HCO_3^- of 23.

11. What is the likely dx?

12. What is the NSIM?

Patient develops hand and leg paraesthesias. While taking blood pressure, her wrist hand muscles go into a transient spasm.

13. What is the underlying cause?

14. Is total serum calcium affected?

5.2.2 Chronic Respiratory Alkalosis

Etiology

[3] Most common acid-base disorder in cirrhosis is chronic respiratory alkalosis.

- Pregnancy: **progesterone** is a respiratory stimulant
- Cirrhosis: due to decreased metabolism of progesterone and other endogenous respiratory stimulants[3]
- High altitude

Complication: if chronic, it can lead to renal parathyroid hormone (PTH) resistance and pseudo-hypoparathyroidism (hyperphosphatemia and hypocalcemia despite high-normal or high PTH).

5.3 Primary Metabolic Acidosis

Approach to identify the cause of metabolic acidosis

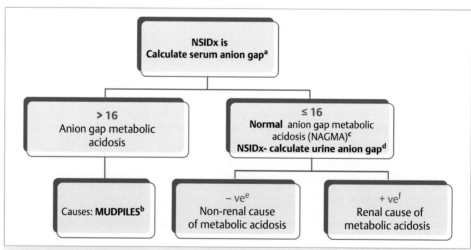

[4] If potassium is not included in this equation, then cut-off value for normal anion gap will be ≤ 12.

[a] Anion gap is the sum of all the positively charged ions **minus** sum of all negatively charged ions in serum electrolyte panel:

> **Serum anion gap = (Na⁺ + K⁺) − (Cl⁻ + HCO₃⁻)**
> If anion gap is ≤ 16,[4] then it is **normal** anion gap metabolic acidosis (NAGMA).
> If anion gap is > 16, then there are **unmeasured anions** in blood, causing acidosis. Careful history review should point to the cause, as shown below.

[b]Refer to the following table:

Methanol[5] ingestion	Methanol gets metabolized into formic acid. This leads to CNS and visual disturbances (optic neuritis). (*See emergency medicine chapter for further details.*)
Uremia (renal failure)	Inorganic acids (e.g., sulfates, phosphates, urate), which are the unmeasured anions, accumulate in advanced acute/chronic renal failure
Diabetic ketoacidosis (DKA)	Besides DKA, ketoacidosis can also occur in alcoholism and starvation
Propylene glycol[5] ingestion	Used as antifreeze and also used as a solvent for several parenteral medications including lorazepam and phenobarbital. It gets metabolized into lactic acid
Isoniazid poisoning Infection	May cause seizures resulting in lactic acidosis
Lactic acidosis (other causes)	• Severe sepsis causing lactic acidosis • Any cause of excessive anaerobic glycolysis can cause lactic acidosis shock, cyanide poisoning, carbon monoxide poisoning, transient postseizure acidosis, metformin, bowel ischemia, etc.
Ethylene glycol[5] ingestion	It gets metabolized into oxalic acid. This leads to CNS and renal toxicity. (*See emergency medicine chapter for further details.*)
Salicylates toxicity	• Anion gap is due to increased ketoacids and lactic acid • Adults usually have coexistent respiratory alkalosis (aspirin is a direct respiratory stimulant). Children might not develop respiratory alkalosis and just have pure metabolic acidosis. • In late stages of severe poisoning, as patient develops altered mental status, respiratory acidosis can ensue. (*See emergency medicine chapter for further details.*)

[c]Causes of NAGMA: **F**istula (pancreatic), **u**reteroenterostomy, **s**aline administration,[6] **e**ndocrine (hyperparathyroidism), **d**iarrhea,[7] **c**arbonic anhydrase inhibitors (acetazolamide), **a**mmonium chloride, **r**enal tubular acidosis, **s**pironolactone.

[d]The idea of **u**rinary **a**nion **g**ap (UAG) is similar to the idea of serum anion gap
UAG = (Na$^+$ + K$^+$) − (Cl$^-$)
i.e., the sum of all positively charged ions minus the sum of all negatively charged ions in urine. Urinary chloride (Cl$^-$) concentration directly correlates with urinary ammonium (NH$_4^+$) concentration, as ammonium chloride (NH$_4^+$ Cl$^-$), which is an acid, is excreted by kidney as a compound.

[e]If UAG is negative, this means urinary Cl$^-$ is high, so NH$_4^+$ must be high in urine, suggesting an appropriate increase in excretion of acid (H$^+$) in the form of NH$_4^+$ Cl$^-$ to compensate for nonrenal cause of acidosis. This can occur with conditions that result in fluid and HCO$_3^-$ loss (e.g., diarrhea, pancreaticoduodenal fistula).

[f]NAGMA due to renal causes is due to defective NH$_4^+$ production and secretion, resulting in low urine NH$_4^+$ concentration (and low urine Cl$^-$); so UAG will be positive. This can occur in renal tubular acidosis (*see below*) and renal failure (Renal failure can result in both normal anion-gap and high anion-gap metabolic acidosis).

MRS

MUDPILES

MRS

FUSEDCARS

[5] Methanol, ethylene glycol, and propylene glycol all taste very sweet and are also commonly used as antifreeze. Because of their sweet taste, children can easily ingest these in large amounts.

[6]Rapid isotonic saline (NaCl) infusion can result in hyperchloremic NAGMA. It is due to rise in plasma chloride (Cl$^-$) and subsequent effort by kidneys to keep sum total of negative ions in plasma within normal limits by eliminating bicarbonate (HCO$_3^-$).

[7]On the other hand, intestinal HCO$_3^-$ loss, which will result in metabolic acidosis. Gastric fluid is acidic; hence loss of gastric fluid results in metabolic alkalosis.

5.3.1 Types of Renal Tubular Acidosis

	Type I (distal) RTA	Type II (proximal) RTA	Type IV RTA
Pathology	Distal H⁺ ion pump is not working, so H⁺ is not secreted and K⁺ is not reabsorbed in exchange (potassium wasting)	In the proximal convoluted tubule HCO_3^- reabsorption pump is not working, resulting in bicarbonaturia	Aldosterone deficiency or resistance
Urinary pH	> 5.4 (alkaline urine) Remember that H⁺ is not secreted into urine	Initially urine pH is alkalotic (> 5.4), but after total body bicarbonate gets depleted, urine pH becomes < 5.4, since distal urine acidification is preserved	< 5.4 (acidic urine)
Cause	• Autoimmune: Sjögren's syndrome[a], rheumatoid arthritis, SLE, etc. • Hypercalciuric conditions: hyperparathyroidism, sarcoidosis, hereditary hypercalciuria, etc. • Hereditary channelopathies • Drugs (amphotericin B, lithium) • Infection (hepatitis B or C) • Cirrhosis	**Isolated** bicarbonate loss can occur in acetazolamide or topiramate treatment Other causes of RTA II may also result in loss of other functions of proximal convoluted tubule leading to Fanconi syndrome (RTA II with phosphaturia, uric aciduria, glycosuria and aminoaciduria). Etiologies include tenofovir use, amyloidosis, multiple **myeloma,** heavy metal toxicity (lead, mercury, copper), cystinosis, Wilson's disease, etc.	• MCC is diabetes mellitus (diabetic nephropathy may affect juxtaglomerular apparatus, leading to low renin-low aldosterone state) • Addison (aldosterone deficiency) • Pseudohypoaldosteronism (failure of response to aldosterone: It can be acquired or hereditary) • Aldosterone antagonist: spironolactone or eplerenone • Medications: ACE inhibitor, amiloride, triamterene, trimethoprim (*Bactrim*) • Renal failure

(Continued)

MRS

Remember 5.4 and this picture >> <<
pH is >5.4 in RTA type I, > 5.4 and then later < 5.4 in RTA II and < 5.4 in RTA IV

	Type I (distal) RTA	Type II (proximal) RTA	Type IV RTA
Important associations	Renal stones (calcium phosphate stones) and nephrocalcinosis can easily develop because of increased urine pH and decreased urinary citrate	Osteomalacia secondary to vitamin D deficiency (the other function of proximal convoluted tubule is to produce active form of vitamin D)	Features of hyperkalemia (e.g., weakness)
Serum potassium	↓	N or ↓	Increased
Management: In all cases, if applicable, remove offending agent and treat primary disorder	• Alkali replacement with sodium bicarbonate, sodium citrate and/or potassium citrate • K⁺ replacement, if needed	• Alkali replacement is preferred with potassium citrate • Thiazide diuretics[b] • K⁺ replacement, if needed	In select cases, use oral fludrocortisone (a mineralocorticoid)

[a]RTA I might be the presenting feature of Sjögren's syndrome.

[b]Thiazide-induced mild volume depletion enhances absorption of HCO3⁻ from proximal convoluted tubule.

Abbreviations: ACE, angiotensin-converting enzyme; RTA, renal tubular acidosis; SLE, systemic lupus erythematosus.

5.4 Metabolic Alkalosis

This is a very common acid-base disorder in hospitalized patients due to **diuretic use** and **gastric fluid loss** from procedures such as nasogastric tube aspiration and excessive vomiting. Compensation is immediate with respiratory hypoventilation and hypocapnia.

Approach to identify the cause of metabolic alkalosis

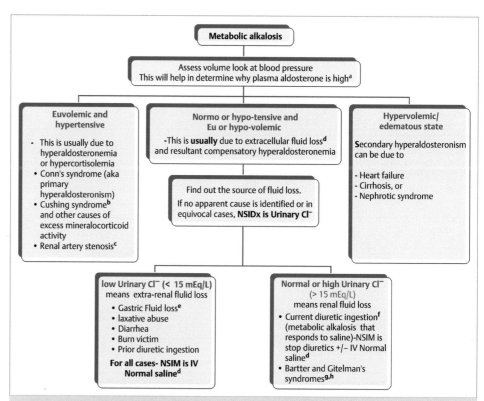

[a]High levels of aldosterone reabsorb Na^+ in exchange for K^+ and H^+, which are increasingly excreted in urine. This results in metabolic alkalosis.

[b]Glucocorticoids possess some mineralocorticoid activity and in excess, can act like its close relative aldosterone. *See endocrinology chapter for further details.*

[c]**Renal artery stenosis** results in low renal blood flow and secondary hyperaldosteronism and hypertension (HTN).

[d]Metabolic alkalosis that results from loss of extracellular fluid responds to treatment with IV normal saline. This is collectively known as contraction alkalosis or saline responsive metabolic alkalosis.

[e]**Loss of gastric fluid** as a result of excessive vomiting or nasogastric tube aspiration can result in loss of K^+, Cl^-, H^+ electrolytes and water (which are major constituents of gastric fluid) and compensatory increase in aldosterone section.

[f]Most of the diuretics result in metabolic alkalosis and volume depletion. The exceptions are acetazolamide and potassium-sparing diuretics (amiloride, triamterene spironolactone, and eplerenone) which can cause metabolic acidosis.

[g]**Bartter syndrome:** It is due to a genetic abnormality that results in loss of function of $Na^+–K^+–2Cl^-$ cotransporter in the thick ascending loop of Henle.

[h]**Gitelman syndrome:** It is due to a genetic abnormality that results in loss of function of $Na^+–Cl^-$ cotransporter in distal convoluted tubule.

Other causes of metabolic alkalosis

Hepatic encephalopathy	Hyperammonemia (NH_4^+ is a basic ion)
Citrate toxicity	It can occur in patients who have received significant amount of blood transfusion in a short period of time (e.g., in patients with major trauma and major bleeding). Citrate is used to prevent clotting of stored blood products
$Mg(OH)_2$ and $CaCO_3$ antacid overingestion	It is called the "milk-alkali syndrome," but is very rare nowadays as better medications are available for indigestion/heartburn

Clinical Case Scenarios

A young female patient with no prior medical history presents with hypokalemia and hypotension. Lab tests suggest metabolic alkalosis. Patient denies taking any medication or having any other issue. With no apparent cause identified, urinary Cl⁻ test is done. Urine Cl⁻ is 20 mEq/L.

15. What is the likely cause of metabolic alkalosis?

16. What will be the likely cause of metabolic alkalosis if urinary chloride was low?

17. What is the likely underlying diagnosis?

Answers

Number	What is the pH status?	Which value corresponds to the pH status?	Is there compensation?	Additional information
1	pH is low = acidemic	↑ $PaCO_2$; so dx is **primary respiratory acidosis**	HCO_3^- value is within the **normal** range, so metabolic compensation by the kidneys has not kicked in yet	**Etiology of acute hypoventilation:** • Due to sedative overdose, e.g., alcohol, benzodiazepines, barbiturate, and opiate intoxication/overdose • Development of respiratory muscle fatigue due to continuing acute hypoxia, e.g., severe acute asthma exacerbation, pulmonary embolus, etc. • Acute neuromuscular disorders involving respiratory muscles (e.g., Guillain–Barre syndrome or acute myasthenic crisis) **Rx:** If initial noninvasive measures fail, consider intubation
2	Acidotic	↑ $PaCO_2$ is corresponding with the acidic pH; so, the dx is **primary respiratory acidosis**	HCO_3^- is ↑, so **metabolic compensation** has already kicked in	Dx is chronic hypoventilation which can be seen in patients with chronic obstructive pulmonary disease, obesity hypoventilation syndrome, chest wall disorder such as kyphoscoliosis, etc.
3	Acidotic	↓ $PaCO_2$ does not correlate with the pH status. ↓ HCO_3^- corresponds to the pH value, therefore dx is **primary metabolic acidosis**[b]	As $PaCO_2$ is ↓↓, compensatory respiratory alkalosis is present. Exam will reveal hyperventilating patient with deep fast breathing (Kussmaul breathing)	• **Winter's formula**[b] gives expected $PaCO_2$ level (expected respiratory compensation) in patients with primary metabolic acidosis Expected $PaCO_2$ = {(1.5 × HCO_3^-) + 8} +/− 2 In this case, the expected $PaCO_2$ is 29 +/−2, which matches with patient's current $PaCO_2$ level. Patient is adequately compensating for metabolic acidosis

4	Acidotic	As above	PaCO$_2$ is ↓	If you calculate Winter's formula here, the expected PaCO$_2$ is 29 +/−2. This patient's PaCO$_2$ is 37
5	pH is acidic and quite low	Both PaCO$_2$ and HCO$_3^-$ correlate with the pH status; dx is combined respiratory and metabolic acidosis	*Not applicable*	This is seen in cardiopulmonary arrest; cardiac arrest causes systemic hypoperfusion leading to lactic acidosis and pulmonary arrest causes alveolar hypoventilation
6	pH is high = alkalemic	↓ PaCO$_2$ = primary respiratory alkalosis	HCO$_3^-$ is within normal range; hence metabolic compensation has not kicked in yet	**Etiology:** acute hyperventilation due to acute hypoxemia, panic attack, etc. (*see below in respiratory alkalosis section*)
7	Alkalotic	↓ PaCO$_2$ = primary respiratory alkalosis	↓ HCO$_3^-$ = compensatory metabolic acidosis	This is due to chronic hyperventilation of any cause (e.g., anemia, pregnancy, cirrhosis)
8	Alkalotic	↑ HCO$_3^-$ = primary metabolic alkalosis	↑ PaCO$_2$ (compensatory respiratory acidosis)	*See metabolic alkalosis section below*
9	pH is normal	PaCO$_2$ is ↑ (respiratory acidosis) and HCO$_3^-$ is ↑ (metabolic alkalosis) = mixed acid/base disorder (coexistent primary respiratory acidosis and primary metabolic alkalosis)		Can it be either primary respiratory acidosis with compensatory metabolic alkalosis or vice versa? No, it cannot; because remember that compensation is never complete (except in one instance: do you remember what it is?[c])
10	pH is normal	PaCO$_2$ is ↓ (respiratory alkalosis) and HCO$_3^-$ is ↓ (metabolic acidosis)		Example scenarios • Aspirin overdose in **adults**: aspirin stimulates respiratory center causing hyperventilation and also uncouples oxidative phosphorylation leading to excessive keto/lactic acid formation • **Acclimatization** in high altitudes: The **only** situation where compensation is complete, when primary respiratory alkalosis is fully compensated by metabolic acidosis

[a]To find out the cause, calculate serum **anion gap** (*see metabolic acidosis section below*).

[b]In exam, calculate Winter's formula only if question requires doing so. The trick is to look at the answer choices, if you see "consider intubation" as one of the options in a question about primary metabolic acidosis, only then you need to calculate Winter's formula.

An example scenario: A patient with diabetic ketoacidosis was compensating well with respiratory alkalosis (as in case 3). As patient gets tired, he is not able to compensate adequately (as in case 4). At this juncture, we must think about assisting his ventilation.

[c]High-altitude respiratory alkalosis.

11. Normal PaO$_2$ on room air with primary respiratory alkalosis points toward panic/anxiety attack.

12. NSIM: "ask the patient to breathe into a bag" (this corrects respiratory alkalosis as patient breathes in his or her own CO$_2$). If still not responding, then give diazepam.

13. Acute hypocalcemia.

14. No. Only free calcium is low.

15. Current diuretic abuse.

16. Prior diuretic or laxative abuse.

17. Always think of anorexia/bulimia nervosa and factitious disorders.

6. Nephrology

Being stranded in the middle of a vast ocean is life's biggest irony of eventual death—**being surrounded by water everywhere, but to die due to lack of water. This happens because our kidney's concentrating ability is limited. For every liter of ocean water that we drink, an additional 1/2 liter of freshwater is needed to excrete the total salt load consumed. Rodents' kidneys have more than 2 times the concentrating ability of humans', hence they can survive on salty sea water.**

6.1 Irritative and Voiding Symptoms

Irritative symptoms	Voiding symptoms
Something is irritating the bladder wall or urethra causing inflammation. This results in: • Dysuria and resulting hesitancy • Frequency, urgency (irritated smooth muscles of kidney are contracting frequently)	Something in bladder is obstructing the urinary outflow, leading to dribbling of urine, sensation of incomplete voiding, and/or needing to strain to urinate. • Additional symptoms may include incontinence and nocturia (due to full bladder and incomplete voiding)
Causes: • Stones • Infection (prostatitis, cystitis, urethritis, etc.) • Tumor in the urinary tract	Causes: • Benign prostatic hyperplasia (BPH; most common cause of voiding symptoms in male) • Prostatic carcinoma • Acute prostatitis (inflammatory swelling) • Stone that is lodged in the neck of the bladder • Tumor in the neck of the bladder
Common causes: Stone, infection and tumor (MRS ☺ SIT)[a]	
NSIDx is urinalysis (UA)	For recent onset of symptoms, NSIDx - UA. For chronic symptoms • In males, think prostate first. So NSIDx is digital rectal exam, UA and serum prostate-specific antigen • In females, consider pelvic floor dysfunction

[a]These can also cause hematuria.

 In a nutshell

Irritative and voiding symptoms are collectively called "lower urinary tract symptoms" and have significant overlap:

- Acute prostatitis can present with acute irritative and voiding symptoms.
- Tumor in the neck of bladder can present with chronic irritative and voiding symptoms.
- Patients with BPH have increased risk of urinary tract infection. In this case, a patient with longstanding hx of voiding symptoms, now presents with acute irritative symptoms due to development of cystitis or prostatitis.

6.2 Urinary Tract Infection and Prostatitis

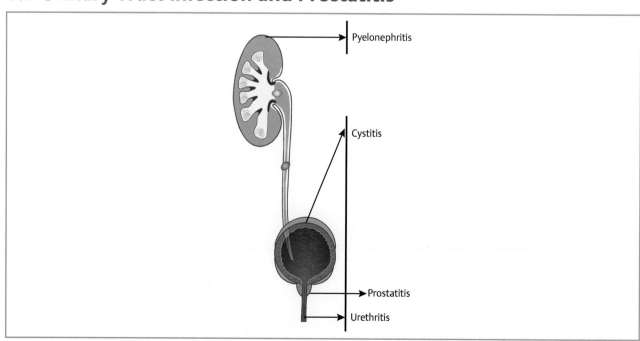

Acute onset irritative symptoms (frequency, urgency, hesitancy, and/or dysuria) +/− systemic signs of infection	Condition
+ Urethral discharge (in women also look for cervical tenderness)	Urethritis (STD)- see STD section in ID chapter
+ prostate tenderness	Prostatitis (generally patients with acute bacterial prostatitis have signs of sepsis with spiking fevers; presentation is NOT subtle)
No urethral discharge No flank pain and no costovertebral angle (renal area) tenderness	• Cystitis (look for suprapubic pain or tenderness) OR Urethritis (sometimes urethritis does not have urethral discharge)
+ renal-angle tenderness and/or flank pain	Acute pyelonephritis (generally patients have signs of sepsis)

Urinalysis

In patients presenting with acute irritative symptoms, first SIDx is always urinalysis (UA).

UA findings	Additional info
Pyuria = inflammation in the urinary tract	**Definition** WBC ≥ 3–6/hpf (high-powered field) in unspun sample WBC ≥ 10/hpf in centrifuged urine sample
Leukocyte esterase	When WBCs are present, urine leukocyte esterase will also be positive
Positive nitrites = presence of *Enterobacteriaceae* in urine	*Enterobacteriaceae* can change nitrates to nitrites (*E. coli* is the most common cause) If nitrites are negative, but patients have pyuria consider infection with *Staphylococcus epidermidis*, *enterococcus*, *S. saprophyticus*, or STD (chlamydia and gonorrhea). These organisms cannot change nitrates to nitrites

Urinary tract infection (UTI) may also cause hematuria (RBCs ≥ 3/hpf in unspun sample)

6.2.1 Acute Cystitis

Presentation: acute irritative symptoms (+/- voiding symptoms). Older patients can have mild confusion. UA will show significant pyuria.

Management

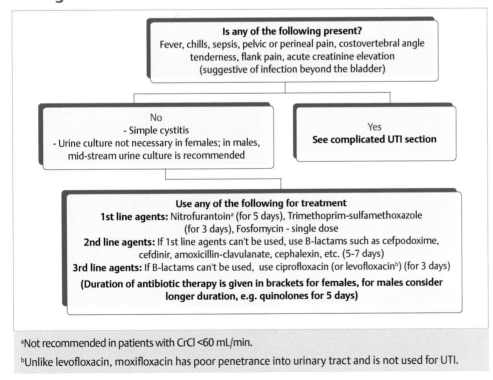

Is any of the following present?
Fever, chills, sepsis, pelvic or perineal pain, costovertebral angle tenderness, flank pain, acute creatinine elevation
(suggestive of infection beyond the bladder)

No
- Simple cystitis
- Urine culture not necessary in females; in males, mid-stream urine culture is recommended

Yes
See complicated UTI section

Use any of the following for treatment
1st line agents: Nitrofurantoin[a] (for 5 days), Trimethoprim-sulfamethoxazole (for 3 days), Fosfomycin - single dose
2nd line agents: If 1st line agents can't be used, use B-lactams such as cefpodoxime, cefdinir, amoxicillin-clavulanate, cephalexin, etc. (5-7 days)
3rd line agents: If B-lactams can't be used, use ciprofloxacin (or levofloxacin[b]) (for 3 days)
(Duration of antibiotic therapy is given in brackets for females, for males consider longer duration, e.g. quinolones for 5 days)

Clinical Tip: Urine culture should be performed in all men with suspected acute UTI, even if uncomplicated.

[a]Not recommended in patients with CrCl <60 mL/min.

[b]Unlike levofloxacin, moxifloxacin has poor penetrance into urinary tract and is not used for UTI.

Asymptomatic Bacteriuria

Definition: Significant colony counts of bacteria in urine culture (i.e., $\geq 10^5$ cfu/mL) but with no irritative bladder symptoms or systemic signs of infection.

Rx: Antibiotics are indicated only in pregnancy or in patients who are undergoing urological procedure likely to have mucosal bleeding.

6.2.2 Acute Complicated UTI (including Pyelonephritis) and Acute Prostatitis

Definition: UTI + signs of extension beyond bladder e.g., fever, chills, rigors, sepsis, costovertebral angle tenderness, flank pain, acute creatinine elevation, altered mental status.

Risk factors for extension: uncontrolled diabetes, immunosuppression, urinary stones, urinary tract abnormalities, presence of indwelling structures (e.g., Foley catheter, urinary stent), pregnancy, etc.

Management

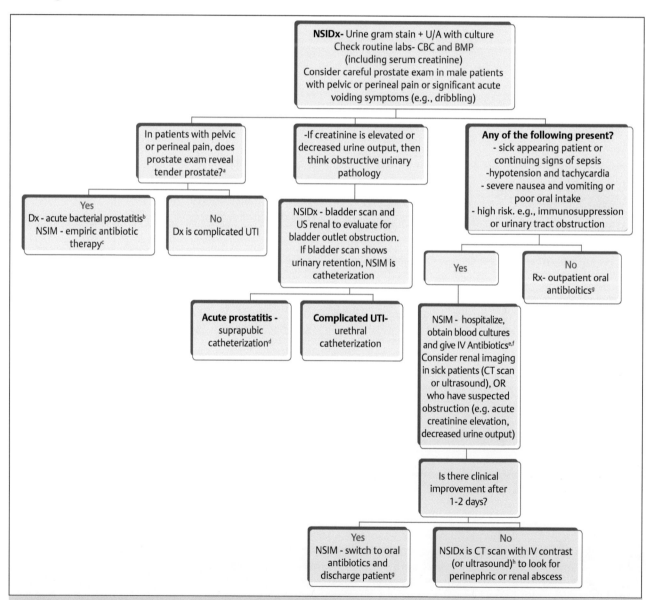

[a]Prostatic massage is contraindicated in suspected acute bacterial prostatitis, but it is ok to do a digital rectal examination to examine prostate.

[b]Acute elevation of PSA can support the dx of acute prostatitis.

[c]In patients > 35 years old AND no hx of high-risk sexual behavior, use trimethoprim-sulfamethoxazole or a fluoroquinolone for a total of 6 weeks.[1] MCC is *E. coli*. Note: trimethoprim-sulfamethoxazole and fluoroquinolones have good prostatic penetration.

[d]Urethral catheterization is contraindicated in acute bacterial prostatitis as this might lead to dissemination of infection.

[e]Choose empiric antibiotic therapy as following:

- If risk factors for pseudomonas are present (e.g., recent urological instrumentation or neutropenia), use anti-pseudomonal antibiotic (e.g., cefepime, piperacillin-tazobactam).
- If urine gram stain reveals gram positive cocci, cover for enterococcus and staphylococcus; can use piperacillin-tazobactam
- If no hx of multi-drug resistant organism (e.g., MRSA, vancomycin resistant enterococci)
- Otherwise, use IV ceftriaxone.

[f]In very sick patients (e.g., ICU or step-down unit), add antibiotics with MRSA and ESBL coverage (e.g., IV vancomycin + meropenem).

[g]Use oral ciprofloxacin, levofloxacin (5–7 days), trimethoprim-sulfamethoxazole (7–10 days) or B-lactams such as cefpodoxime, cefdinir, amoxicillin-clavulanate (10–14 days).

[h]CT scan with IV contrast is the best test. When contraindicated (e.g., in pregnancy) do renal ultrasound. Look for pyelonephritis complications such as abscess or emphysematous pyelonephritis.[2] Risk factors for development of these complications include immunosuppression or DM. Treatment for both is percutaneous or surgical drainage and IV antibiotics. Severe cases may require nephrectomy.

[1]In sexually active patients with prostatitis <35 years of age, or >35 years of age with high risk sexual behavior, MCC are gonorrhea and chlamydia. For these patients, test for STD and initiate empiric treatment that covers these organisms.

[2]In emphysematous pyelonephritis imaging will reveal air in the renal parenchyma.

6.2.3 Perinephric/renal Abscess

Source of infection: local infection (e.g., pyelonephritis), or hematogenous spread (e.g., *Staph. aureus* abscess due to infective endocarditis)

Presentation: history of pyelonephritis with no clinical improvement despite adequate treatment, with persistent flank pain and high-grade fever. Exam may reveal palpable abdominal mass. UA may reveal pyuria, but urine culture may be negative (when abscess is not communicating with urinary system).

Workup: CT scan with IV contrast is the best test. When contraindicated (e.g., in pregnancy), do renal ultrasound.

Rx: IV antibiotics (e.g., Piperacillin-tazobactam) and percutaneous drainage of abscess. Severe cases may require nephrectomy.

6.2.4 Chronic Prostatitis and its Differential Diagnosis

Presentation: chronic or recurrent irritative symptoms in males with or without voiding symptoms.[3]
Workup:

[3]In patients with hematuria, do bladder cancer workup (urine cytology, CT scan and cystoscopy)

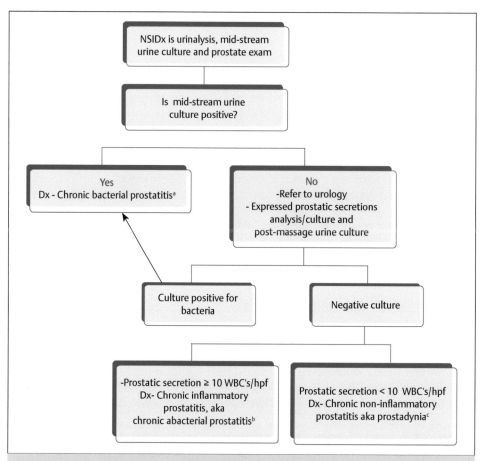

[a]Patients can also present with recurrent UTIs or recurrent bacteriuria of the same organism. Treatment is similar to acute bacterial prostatitis: use fluoroquinolone (ciprofloxacin or levofloxacin) or trimethoprim-sulfamethoxazole for total of 6 weeks.

[b]Prostate may be mildly tender. Treatment includes a **trial of empiric** antibiotic therapy (e.g. ciprofloxacin) and alpha-1 blocker (e.g., tamsulosin). In sexually active males, rule out STD prostatitis and consider infection with atypical organism (chlamydia, mycoplasma, etc.). In patients with hematuria, do further urologic workup (including cystoscopy).

[c]In patients with chronic irritative bladder symptoms of unknown cause, particularly in patients > 40 years of age, or in patients with persistent hematuria we must rule out urogenital cancer by doing cystoscopy and urine cytology.

Benign Prostatic Hyperplasia

Presentation: Older male patients presenting with chronic voiding symptoms. Patient may also have chronic mild urgency and frequency. Benign prostatic hyperplasia (BPH) alone usually does not cause dysuria.

Exam: Digital rectal examination may reveal firm, smooth enlargement of prostate gland; however, there is a poor correlation between prostate enlargement (by exam or transrectal US) and obstructive symptoms due to BPH.

Workup: NSIDx is urinalysis, serum creatinine, and prostate-specific antigen (PSA) to screen for prostate cancer.

Step-wise management

Drug of choice is alpha-1 antagonist which act on smooth muscles. Tamsulosin is preferred, because it has fewer side effects than other drugs in this group. Prazosin and doxazosin (+ azosin) can be considered when patients have coexistent hypertension

If patient continues to have symptoms, NSIM: add a 5-alpha reductase inhibitor (inhibits conversion of testosterone to dihydrotestosterone). They act on the epithelial portion of prostate, and has been shown to reduce prostatic volume. For example, finasteride and dutasteride (+terides)

Transurethral resection of prostate is indicated, if symptoms do not improve significantly with medical management or patients develop complications (e.g., hydronephrosis, renal failure, recurrent infection.)

Prostate Cancer

Background: Most common cancer in males and second Most common cause (MCC) of cancer death in males. There is a familial predisposition.

Risk factors: Black men, family hx of prostate cancer, BRCA mutation, etc.

Screening: Routine screening via **PSA** is controversial. Informed decision-making process is recommended. Patients who opt to screen for prostate cancer can begin at age 50 years.

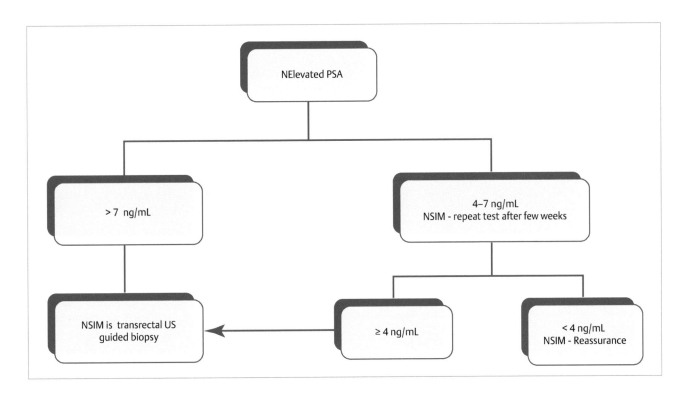

Presentation: In most patients, prostate cancer is suspected when found to have high PSA levels or abnormal digital rectal examination. Symptoms, when present, are often due to metastatic disease, such as low back pain/bone pain or pathological fracture (especially around the lumbar vertebra region).

Prostate exam: This may reveal indurated, nodular and/or irregular prostate enlargement.

Best SIDx: Prostate biopsy under trans**rectal** ultrasound guidance.

Management

Localized disease	Surveillance **or** Intervention with **either** prostate tissue ablation with radiation[a] **or** removal with surgery[b] Any of the above is acceptable. No studies have proven superiority of one over another[c]
Locally advanced disease or low-volume disseminated disease	Either prostate tissue ablation with radiation or removal with surgery + androgen depriving therapy[d]
Disseminated disease (high-volume disease)	Docetaxel (chemotherapy) + Androgen depriving therapy

[a]External beam radiation or radioactive pellets implantation into prostate.

[b]Most common side effects of surgery are erectile dysfunction and urinary incontinence.

[c]In patients with high-risk features, prostate tissue ablation or removal may be offered.

[d]Prostate cancer is an androgen-dependent cancer, so decreasing androgen production will shrink the tumor. This can be achieved by either removing both testicles (surgical orchiectomy) or by using medical therapy to decrease androgen production (as shown below).

Medical antiandrogen therapy

GnRH agonist: leuprolide, goserelin,[a] nafarelin, etc. (+ relins)	**Mechanism of action:** Continuous stimulation by GnRH paradoxically results in downregulation of androgen production • In initial phase, it may increase production of androgens, so androgen receptor antagonist, such as flutamide or bicalutamide, are used **for short term** to prevent **initial** androgen-mediated flare-up (+ tamides)
GnRH antagonist, e.g., degarelix	No increase in production of androgens in the initial phase

[a]Goserelin – Gonadotropin Inhibitor

Abbreviation: GnRH, gonadotropin-releasing hormone

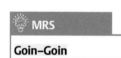

MRS

Goin–Goin

Bladder Cancer

MRS

PEE SAC cancer

Risk factors: Phenacetin-containing analgesics, **p**ioglitazone (possible), **e**thanol, **s**moking, **S**chistosoma haematobium (parasitic infection), **a**niline dyes, **a**rsenic exposure, **c**yclophosphamide (chemotherapy).

Presentation: Painless gross or microscopic hematuria. Patients may also have chronic or intermittent-and-recurrent, irritative, and/or voiding symptoms.

Screening is not recommended for bladder cancer; even in patients with risk factors.

Workup

- NSIDx is office-based cystoscopy with biopsy (most appropriate diagnostic step) + urine cytology.
- After confirming dx, NSIM is transurethral resection of bladder tumor (requires anesthesia), and CT/MRI scan with IV contrast for staging.

Treatment

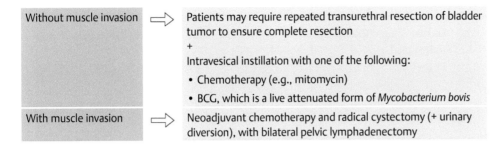

| Without muscle invasion | ⇒ | Patients may require repeated transurethral resection of bladder tumor to ensure complete resection
+
Intravesical instillation with one of the following:
• Chemotherapy (e.g., mitomycin)
• BCG, which is a live attenuated form of *Mycobacterium bovis* |
| With muscle invasion | ⇒ | Neoadjuvant chemotherapy and radical cystectomy (+ urinary diversion), with bilateral pelvic lymphadenectomy |

Urinary Tract Stones

Presentation: Depends upon location of stone and complication (stones → obstruction → urine stasis → infection).

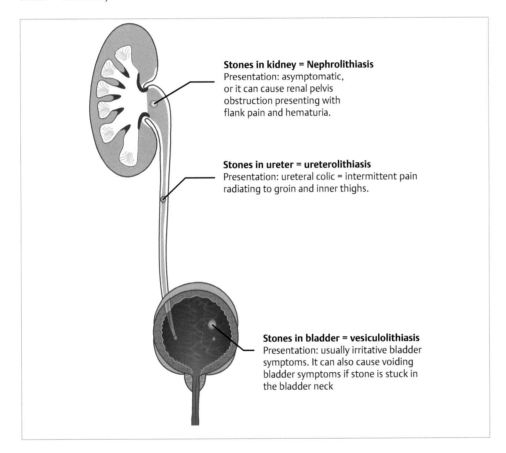

Stones in kidney = Nephrolithiasis
Presentation: asymptomatic, or it can cause renal pelvis obstruction presenting with flank pain and hematuria.

Stones in ureter = ureterolithiasis
Presentation: ureteral colic = intermittent pain radiating to groin and inner thighs.

Stones in bladder = vesiculolithiasis
Presentation: usually irritative bladder symptoms. It can also cause voiding bladder symptoms if stone is stuck in the bladder neck

Management of Suspected Urinary Tract Stone

- If patient is in pain, First SIM is adequate hydration and analgesia (the choice of analgesia is nonsteroidal anti-inflammatory drugs [NSAIDs]).[4] Opiates are given when NSAIDs fail to control pain or when NSAIDs are contraindicated (e.g., renal failure). Opiates may exacerbate nausea/vomiting, which is common in renal/ureteral colic.
- NSIM is UA (best initial test): symptomatic stones usually present with hematuria. Alkaline pH (pH > 7.5) may signal possible infection with urease-producing bacteria (e.g., *Proteus*, *Klebsiella*) and possibility of staghorn calculi. Urine pH < 5.5 may suggest uric acid stone.

[4] First step is always to control pain before doing further diagnostic test.

[5]Do not use contrast when looking for stones (or hemorrhage). Stones, blood, and contrast have similar high density appearance on CT. Using contrast will muddle the picture. For example, first diagnostic test in suspected stroke is CT scan of head without contrast.

On the other hand, when looking for malignancy or infection use IV contrast. For example, first diagnostic test in a patient with fever and a new focal neurological deficit is CT scan of head with contrast.

[6]In septic patients with obstructive uropathy, urgent urology evaluation for decompression is indicated.

- NSIDx is CT scan of abdomen and pelvis without IV contrast.[5] It has high sensitivity and specificity. In pregnant patients, do renal ultrasound, as CT scan is not desirable.
- Hospitalization and urology evaluation is indicated in following situations:
  - Persistent significant pain, nausea, or vomiting (not controlled by oral medications).
  - Solitary kidney.
  - Sepsis.[6]
  - Creatinine elevation.

These patients frequently need emergent decompression, such as percutaneous nephrostomy or ureteral stent placement.

Further management of symptomatic urinary tract stone depends upon stone size, type, and location

Size	Management (when urgent decompression is not needed)		
≤ 0.5–1 cm	Stone of this size is expected to pass through. Use tamsulosin, which can facilitate stone passage If stone does not pass spontaneously, consider intervention in patients with ongoing symptom		
1 cm–2 cm **renal** (or ureteral) stone	Extra-corporeal shock wave lithotripsy (**ECSWL**) • It is contraindicated in pregnancy and bleeding disorders • It is commonly used for **renal stones.** It can also be used as a first-line treatment for small (< 1 cm) proximal ureteral stone		
> 2 cm **renal stone**, or cystine stones, or stones in patients with urological anatomic abnormality (e.g., horse-shoe kidney)	Percutaneous nephrolithotomy (stone removal); this requires general anesthesia. • Bigger stones > 2 cm have higher risk of complications when broken down in situ with ECSWL and, cystine stones cannot be broken down by ECSWL • This can also be used for large, severely impacted proximal ureteral stones		
Middle, distal (or proximal) **ureter stone** not passing through	Laser lithotripsy + ureteroscopic stone extraction	Laser lithotripsy helps to break down large stones which makes it easier to extract	Ureteroscope and cystoscope are both inserted through urethra; difference is that ureteroscope is more flexible and longer
Bladder stone not passing through	Laser lithotripsy + cystoscopic extraction		

Always check stone composition after its removal or spontaneous passage, because it determines preventive strategies

Stone composition	Additional information

Calcium oxalate (MC type)	**Risk factors**
	• **Hypercalciuria:** due to hypercalcemia (e.g., multiple myeloma, sarcoidosis) or idiopathic renal hypercalciuria
	• **Hyperoxaluria**
	  – High oxalate food intake
	  – Increased gastrointestinal (GI) absorption of oxalate: dietary calcium combines with oxalates and forms a compound that cannot be absorbed from GI tract into the circulation. In fat malabsorption, unabsorbed fat binds with calcium leaving oxalates to be readily absorbed into circulation and then to urine
	• **Hypocitraturia:** citrate prevents calcium-oxalate stone formation
	Prevention: the following dietary modifications are recommended to prevent calcium stones formation:
	• Increase fluid intake
	• Decrease sodium, oxalate, and protein intake
	! It is not recommended to decrease dietary calcium

 MRS

Decrease **SOP** intake

(Continued)

Stone composition	Additional information
Calcium phosphate	Found in primary hyperparathyroidism, as parathyroid hormone promotes phosphaturia
Magnesium-aluminum phosphate stone (aka struvite stone or staghorn calculus)	This is the **only stone** that forms in an **alkaline** environment. Urease-producing bacterial infection predisposes to formation of this type of stones Source: Common clinical problems. In: Gunderman R. Essential radiology. Clinical presentation, pathophysiology, imaging. 3rd ed. Thieme; 2014. **Rx:** do percutaneous nephrolithotomy. These stones are frequently colonized and can predispose to recurrent infection, unless removed
Uric acid stones	Forms in low urine pH This is the **only stone** that is usually **radiolucent**. It cannot be seen on plain X-ray but can be seen by ultrasound or CT scan **Risk factors:** hyperuricosuria due to gout, hematologic malignancies, etc. **Rx:** urinary alkalization (with either oral potassium citrate or potassium bicarbonate) can dissolve the stone. Uric acid stones are most readily dissolvable. Allopurinol is indicated for recurrent uric acid stone
Cystine stones	Hereditary disorder of failure to reabsorb cystine amino acid from renal tubules, resulting in cystinuria. Cystine stones are only faintly radiodense **Lab findings:** Urine nitroprusside test will be positive and UA will show hexagonal crystals Source: Urea synthesis disorders. In: Riede U, Werner M. Color atlas of pathology: Pathologic principles, associated diseases, sequela. 1st ed. Thieme; 2004. **Rx:** alkalization of urine with potassium citrate. For stones > 1 cm, surgical extraction is done. It is not amenable to shock wave lithotripsy

MRS

Proteus MUSt kill urea.
Proteus, Morganella, Ureaplasma, SerraTia, Klebsiella, etc. produce urease (which breaks down urea)

 In a nutshell

Types of hematuria

Early/initial hematuria	Indicates urethral source, as proximal blood is flushed out by urine
Terminal hematuria	From prostate, bladder neck, or trigone area • Bladder compression of this area occurs at the end of urination
Continuous or total hematuria	Bleeding at the level of mid-bladder or higher

Clinical Case Scenarios

A 25-year-old female presents with urinary frequency, urgency, dysuria, and hesitancy for the last few days. Exam reveals suprapubic pain and mucopurulent discharge out of urethra. She has hx of multiple sexual partners. UA is leukocyte esterase positive but nitrites negative.

1. What is the likely Dx?

2. What is the treatment?

A 42-year-old male presents with few weeks hx of urinary frequency, urgency, dysuria, and dribbling of urine. For the last few days he also started noticing painful, tender, and swollen testes. Exam reveals tender testes and prostate.

3. What is the likely dx?

4. What is the MCC?

5. What is the treatment and duration?

6. Patient has bile salt deficiency due to ileitis in Crohn's disease. What type of urinary stone would you expect?

7. A 67-year-old male has few years hx of intermittent bloody urine, urinary frequency, urgency, dysuria, and dribbling of urine. He has no hx of fevers, chills, but has had significant unintentional weight loss. UA shows multiple RBCs and only few WBCs. What is the likely Dx?

8. A 45-year-old male is diagnosed with severe acute transverse myelitis and neurogenic bladder. What is an effective way to reduce risk of UTI in patients with neurogenic bladder?

A patient has ureteral colic. Urine pH is alkaline (pH> 5.4).

9. What two diagnoses should come to your mind?

10. By looking at basic metabolic profile, would you be able to differentiate in between them?

A patient has recurrent calcium oxalate stones with no obvious risk factors.

11. What is the NSIDx?

12. If urinary Ca^{2+} excretion is high and serum Ca^{2+} is normal, then what is the likely dx?

13. What adjunctive treatment would you give to prevent stone formation?

14. If both urinary Ca^{2+} and serum Ca^{2+} are high, what is the likely Dx?

A 50-year-old male presents with few months hx of bloody urine, urinary frequency, urgency, dysuria, difficulty urination, and dribbling of urine. He has no hx of fevers, chills or weight loss. UA shows multiple RBCs and only few WBCs. Prostate exam is unremarkable.

15. What is the NSIDx?

16. If that testing is unremarkable, what is the NSIDx?

6.3 Acute Renal Failure/Acute Kidney Injury

Classification

Prerenal acute kidney injury (AKI)	Due to renal hypoperfusion
Renal AKI	Due to intrinsic renal disease (e.g., acute tubular necrosis, glomerulopathies)
Postrenal AKI	Due to obstruction

General presentation

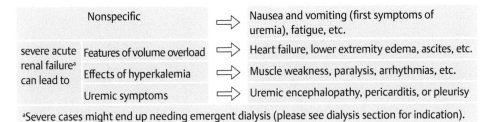

	Nonspecific	⇒	Nausea and vomiting (first symptoms of uremia), fatigue, etc.
severe acute renal failure[a] can lead to	Features of volume overload	⇒	Heart failure, lower extremity edema, ascites, etc.
	Effects of hyperkalemia	⇒	Muscle weakness, paralysis, arrhythmias, etc.
	Uremic symptoms	⇒	Uremic encephalopathy, pericarditis, or pleurisy

[a]Severe cases might end up needing emergent dialysis (please see dialysis section for indication).

Best initial test: serum creatinine and blood urea nitrogen (BUN). Creatinine is the most sensitive indicator of renal failure and is used to calculate glomerular filtration rate (GFR).

The following properties make creatinine one of the best indicators of renal function:

● It is usually produced (by breakdown of creatine in muscles) and excreted (by kidneys) in constant amounts and in a highly predictable fashion.

● It is not reabsorbed and very little is secreted into the renal tubules.

Management

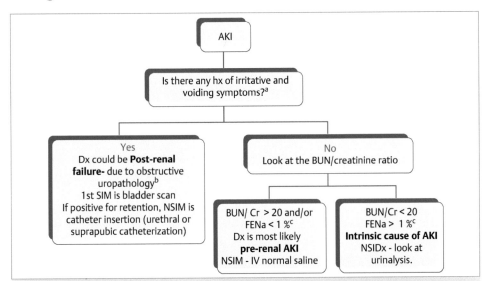

AKI

Is there any hx of irritative and voiding symptoms?[a]

Yes
Dx could be **Post-renal failure-** due to obstructive uropathology[b]
1st SIM is bladder scan
If positive for retention, NSIM is catheter insertion (urethral or suprapubic catheterization)

No
Look at the BUN/creatinine ratio

BUN/ Cr > 20 and/or FENa < 1 %[c]
Dx is most likely **pre-renal AKI**
NSIM - IV normal saline

BUN/Cr < 20
FENa > 1 %[c]
Intrinsic cause of AKI
NSIDx - look at urinalysis.

[a]If patient cannot provide good history (e.g., confused patient), first step is to rule out urinary retention by doing a simple bedside test, i.e., bladder scan.

[b]Bladder outlet obstruction is a common reason for acute renal failure in old patients. Causes include urethral stricture, prostate cancer, benign prostatic hypertrophy, cervical cancer, retroperitoneal fibrosis, stone in bladder-neck, atonic bladder, etc.

[c]Fractional excretion of sodium (FENa). In addition to serum sodium and creatinine, we need urine sodium and urine creatinine to calculate this ratio, but no need to remember the formula of FENa as it will be given in exam. A hypoperfused kidney will try to conserve Na by increasing reabsorption of Na[+].[7]

[7]**Caution:** Do not rely on FENa when patients are on diuretics or have preexisting tubular disease. In patients on diuresis, use FEUrea instead. Urea is also an osmolyte like Na, but it is not affected by diuretics.

6.3.1 Prerenal Causes of Acute Kidney Injury

Anything that can decrease renal perfusion can cause prerenal acute kidney injury (AKI).

Low circulatory volume and hypovolemic shock	Extrarenal fluid loss	Due to hemorrhage, poor oral intake, burns, dehydration, etc.	
	Renal fluid loss	DKA or HONK (osmotic diuresis), diuretic overuse, salt-wasting nephropathies, etc.	Clinical tip: FENa will be inaccurate in these cases
Cardiac cause	Congestive heart failure (known as cardiorenal syndrome[a])		
	Pericardial disease: constrictive pericarditis and pericardial tamponade		
	Cardiogenic shock		
Local decrease in renal blood flow	• **NSAIDs:** can decrease renal perfusion pressure by negating prostaglandin-mediated vasodilation of afferent (preglomerular) arterioles. • **ACE inhibitor or ARBs:** can decrease renal perfusion pressure by negating angiotensin-mediated vasoconstriction of efferent (postglomerular) arterioles		
	Hepatorenal syndrome: Typically occurs in patients with **end-stage** cirrhosis. It presents with slowly rising creatinine despite adequate fluid resuscitation. Urine electrolytes will reveal persistently low urine Na and FENa < 1. UA is typically bland (no casts). Most appropriate treatment is liver transplantation.		

[a]Best pointer to dx of cardiorenal syndrome is decreasing creatinine levels with ongoing diuresis. Other factors that contribute to cardiorenal syndrome are renal venous congestion (due to backward pressure build-up from heart) and increase in neurohormonal activation (e.g., excessive sympathetic activity).

Abbreviations: ACE, angiotensin-converting enzyme; ARB, angiotensin receptor blocker; DKA, diabetic ketoacidosis; FENa, fractional excretion of sodium; HONK, hyperglycemic hyperosmolar nonketotic coma.

6.4 Intrinsic Renal Failure

Etiology: acute tubular necrosis, allergic tubulointerstitial nephritis, thrombotic thrombocytopenic purpura/hemolytic-uremic syndrome (TTP/HUS), glomerulopathies, renal papillary necrosis, etc.

Best initial test to find the cause of intrinsic renal disease is **UA with direct microscopy.**

Look for the following:

UA findings		Cause of intrinsic renal failure
Pyuria (WBCs) and **WBC casts** with evidence of kidney infection	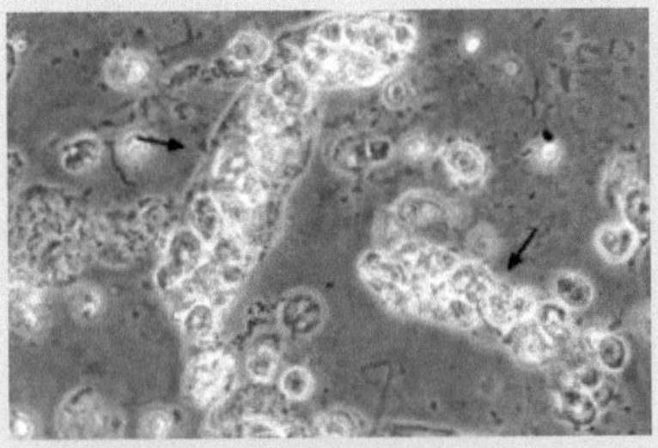	**Pyelonephritis with direct extension of infection into interstitium**
WBC casts, without evidence of kidney infection (eosinophiluria might be present)		**Allergic tubulointerstitial nephritis, cholesterol emboli**
Dysmorphic RBCs, RBC casts[1] +/− WBC casts	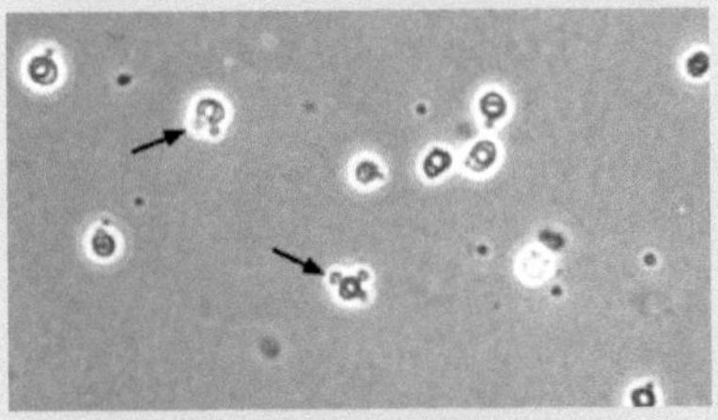 Arrows show a characteristic form of dysmorphic RBCs with ear-shaped extrusions (Mickey Mouse forms).	**Glomerulonephritis**
Muddy brown or colorless granular casts, or renal tubular epithelial cellular cast	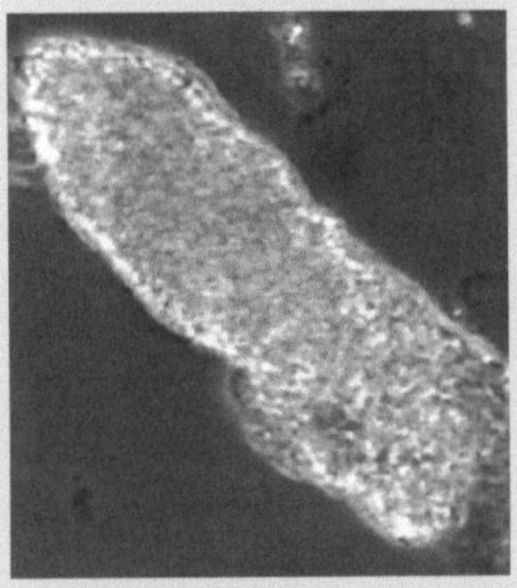 It looks granular.	**Acute tubular necrosis** Renal tubular cells necrosis and subsequent passage of necrotic cells in the urine results in urine-microscopy revealing muddy brown, granular or epithelial casts.
Oxalate crystals	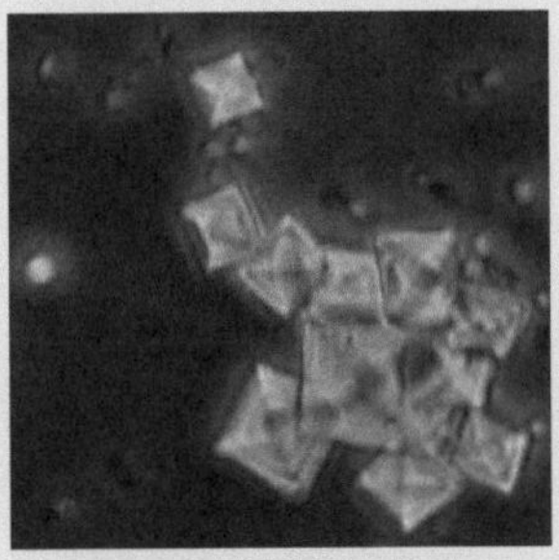 They look like an envelope under the microscope.	**Ethylene glycol ingestion**
Uric acid crystals	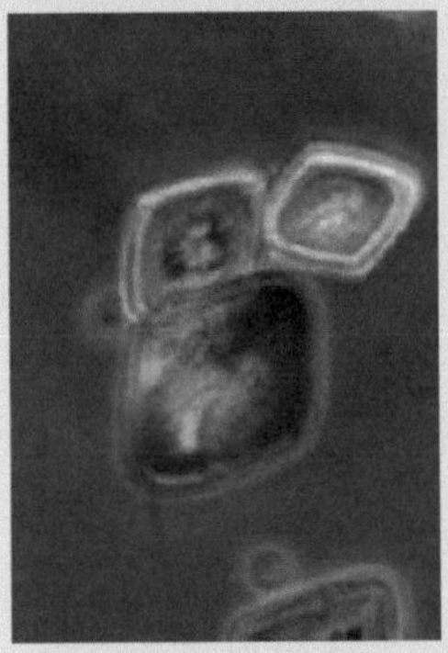 Polymorphous crystals, or Rhomboid uric acid crystals, appearing colorful under polarized light as shown above.	**Tumor lysis syndrome or overexcretion of uric acid in gout patients**

[a]Dysmorphic RBCs or RBCS casts are glomerular in origin. As opposed to dysmorphic RBCs, isomorphic RBCs are found in urinary tract bleeding (due to stones, infection, tumor, etc.).

Source: Differential diagnosis of pathologic urine findings. In: Siegenthaler W. Siegenthaler's differential diagnosis in internal medicine: from symptom to diagnosis. 1st ed. Thieme; 2007.

Broad-waxy casts are found in chronic renal failure patients.

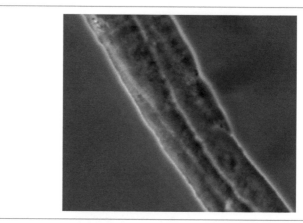

Source: Differential diagnosis of pathologic urine findings. In: Siegenthaler W. Siegenthaler's differential diagnosis in internal medicine: from symptom to diagnosis. 1st ed. Thieme; 2007.

6.4.1 Acute Tubular Necrosis

Etiology

- **Ischemic acute tubular necrosis (ATN):** Prerenal failure can progress to intrinsic renal failure as it may lead to ischemic necrosis of the renal tubular cells. Duration and severity of decreased renal blood flow is the most important factor for development of ATN.
- **Nonischemic (nephrotoxic) ATN**

Nephrotoxins	Additional points	Management
IV contrast dye used for radiological procedures (e.g., CT or MRI)	**Pathology:** contrast dyes, besides being toxic to tubules, may also induce severe renal arteriolar vasospasm, leading to avid renal sodium reabsorption. (Low FENa is present as opposed to other causes of ATN)	**Prevention:** Best method of prevention is using nonionic contrast agents, instead of ionic ones. Patients who are at higher risk (i.e., serum creatinine > 1.5) should receive periprocedural **IV normal saline.** Acetylcysteine (oral or IV) is not recommended as it is of questionable benefit and has risk of anaphylaxis
Drugs	**V**ancomycin, **c**isplatin,[a] **c**yclosporine, **am**photericin-B, **am**inoglycosides,[a] etc.	If serum creatinine rises when patients are on these drugs and clinical picture is suggestive of ATN, NSIM is to discontinue the drug. In some cases, check the serum drug level (e.g., vancomycin, cisplatin level)
Pigments • **Hemoglobinuria:** from massive intravascular hemolysis[b] • **Myoglobinuria:** from rhabdomyolysis[c] (significantly elevated CK of > **5,000** IU/L)	Dipstick is positive for blood, but microscopic examination of urine shows **normal RBCs/hpf**	IV normal saline Additionally, consider bicarbonate infusion in patients with severe rhabdomyolysis

[a]Coexistent hypomagnesemia may increase risk of cisplatin and aminoglycoside renal toxicity.

[b]Example scenario: emergency blood transfusion with ABO incompatible group.

[c]**Causes of rhabdomyolysis:** alcoholism, cocaine, hypokalemia, crush injuries, severe seizure, heat stroke, etc. Another indicator of rhabdomyolysis is disproportionally high BUN compared to creatinine.

 MRS

VCAM or Video CAM induced ATN

The combination of nephrotoxins and low blood pressure can be highly nephrotoxic (e.g., patient with rhabdomyolysis also develops hypotension). Therefore, when patients are exposed to toxic causes of ATN, administration of IV isotonic fluids is the best method of treatment. This avoids hypotension and decreases toxin concentration.

Other nephrotoxic substance includes light chains (Bence Jones protein) found in multiple myeloma.

Clinical Case Scenarios

A patient with hx of DM on oral metformin must undergo contrast study.

17. What is the NSIM?

18. Why?

19. At what level of estimated GFR (eGFR) is metformin contraindicated?

Crystal Nephropathy

Pathophysiology: Intratubular crystal formation with renal tubular obstruction and direct toxicity.

Etiology: Higher risk with IV formulation of acyclovir, sulfonamides, and methotrexate. Other causes include ethylene glycol, indinavir, atazanavir, etc.

Presentation: Flank pain; UA may reveal crystals, pyuria, and/or hematuria.

Prevention: Give IV fluids during IV administration of above agents. When on oral regimen, recommend adequate oral hydration.

6.4.2 Allergic Tubulointerstitial Nephritis aka Acute Interstitial Nephritis

Pathology: Type IV T-cell-mediated hypersensitivity reaction to the following agents:

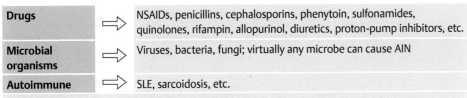

Drugs	⇒	NSAIDs, penicillins, cephalosporins, phenytoin, sulfonamides, quinolones, rifampin, allopurinol, diuretics, proton-pump inhibitors, etc.
Microbial organisms	⇒	Viruses, bacteria, fungi; virtually any microbe can cause AIN
Autoimmune	⇒	SLE, sarcoidosis, etc.

Abbreviations: AIN, acute interstitial nephritis; SLE, systemic lupus erythematosus.

> **MRS**
>
> **AIN = IV:**
> AIN is due to type **IV** hypersensitivity (T-cell-mediated reaction)

Presentation

- Acute rise in creatinine
- Peripheral eosinophilia
- **Eosinophiluria**[8]
- WBC casts in urine
- Maculopapular or morbilliform rash
- Fever

Management

- NSIM: Address the underlying cause. If drug-induced, first SIM is to stop the suspected drug immediately.
- Renal biopsy is indicated if creatinine continues to worsen. After biopsy confirmation, a trial of steroids can be considered. Histology will typically reveal marked interstitial inflammatory cell infiltrate.

[8]Urine eosinophil test is not sensitive, so negative test does not effectively rule out acute interstitial nephritis (AIN).

Differential diagnosis: other causes of eosinophilia in blood + acute renal failure + skin rash.

Cholesterol emboli syndrome	These patients will typically have multiple risk factors for atherosclerosis and they will have a recent history of intervention or manipulation of arteries (e.g., angiogram or percutaneous angioplasty). They also have a typical skin rash called livedo reticularis (purple brown mesh-work like skin rash) and may have blue toe syndrome (picture) +/– necrosis. These skin lesions can be biopsied to make the diagnosis	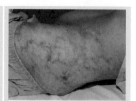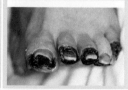
Polyarteritis nodosum	Patients have multisystem involvement. Urinalysis is typically bland in this case (no casts)	

Source: Differential diagnosis of reduced glomerular filtration rate. In: Siegenthaler W. Siegenthaler's differential diagnosis in internal medicine: from symptom to diagnosis. 1st ed. Thieme; 2007.

6.4.3 Glomerulopathies

Pathology: These are group of diseases that primarily involve glomeruli and lead to renal dysfunction. Depending on underlying pathologic process, presentation can range from mild to severe—*asymptomatic isolated recurrent hematuria, i solated proteinuria, acute renal failure that can progress on to chronic renal failure, or rapidly progressive decline in renal function.*

There are 2 group-types of glomerulopathies

	Nephrotic syndrome	**Nephritic syndrome**
Main features	• Proteinuria > 3.5 gm/day is pathognomonic[a] • Edema • Hypoalbuminemia < 3 gm/dL	• RBC casts (aka dysmorphic RBCs or acanthocytes)[b] – pathognomonic • Hypertension[c] • Oliguria (with elevated BUN and creatinine) • Proteinuria < 3.5 gm/day • Edema[c]
Best initial test (to look for pathognomonic findings)	24-hr urinary protein	UA with microscopic analysis
Best (confirmatory) test	Biopsy is usually performed for definite diagnosis	
Etiology	Can occur as a primary condition (disease originates in kidneys) or as a secondary manifestation of systemic process: • MCC of primary nephrotic syndrome in United States is focal segmental glomerulosclerosis in adults and minimal change disease in children. Other cause includes membranous nephropathy • MCC of secondary nephrotic syndrome in United States is DM	• IgA nephropathy: MCC of nephritic syndrome • Postinfectious glomerulonephritis • Rapidly progressive glomerulonephritis • Membranoproliferative glomerulonephritis • Alport syndrome • Goodpasture syndrome • Granulomatosis with polyangiitis (old name: Wegener's granulomatosis) • Henoch–Schonlein purpura

MRS

HOPE RBC casts aren't in the urine.

[a]The degree of proteinuria determines severity and management. The more severe is the proteinuria, the more aggressive is the management.

[b]RBCs are disfigured by their journey through the podocytes of glomerular capillaries into tubular lumen. If you see RBC casts, it is always due to glomerular pathology.

[c]Drug of choice for HTN management in nephritic syndrome with significant edema is oral furosemide.

Nephrotic Syndrome

Pathophysiology: Normally large molecules, such as albumin, are NOT filtered into urine. In nephrotic syndrome, due to glomerular pathology, many important proteins, such as albumin, transferrin, cholecalciferol (vitamin D)-binding protein, anticlotting factors (e.g., antithrombin III, protein C/S), gets filtered into the urine and excreted.

Disease features	Additional points
Proteinuria	ACE inhibitor or angiotensin receptor blocker are used to decrease proteinuria
Edema	Severity ranges from periorbital edema to whole body edema (anasarca). **Rx:** dietary salt restriction and diuretics
Hypercoagulability	• Due to loss of clotting factors in urine • Complications like renal venous thrombosis, arterial thromboembolic phenomenon and DVT/PE can occur
Dyslipidemia (loss of HDL and increased synthesis of LDL)	Leads to accelerated atherogenesis, hence statins are given to decrease serum cholesterol
Iron-therapy-resistant microcytic hypochromic anemia.	Due to loss of transferrin in urine
Low calcium, phosphorus, and vitamin D	Due to loss of cholecalciferol-binding protein in urine

Condition	Etiology and pathophysiology	Microscopic findings	Management
Minimal change disease	• Associated with Hodgkin's lymphoma and NSAIDs • There is a loss of **negative** charge of the glomerular basement, which functions normally to repel negatively charged proteins, e.g., albumin. This results in albuminuria	**Light microscopy:** no pathological changes are seen; therefore it is called "Nil disease" or minimal change disease **Electron microscopy:** fusion of podocytes or effacement of foot processes Source: Teoh DC, El-Modir A. Managing a locally advanced malignant thymoma complicated by nephrotic syndrome: a case report. J Med Case Reports. 2008; 2: 89. **Arrows show two normal non-fused podocytes** **Immunofluorescence:** no immune complex deposition	Responds to steroids most of the time
Focal segmental glomerulosclerosis (FSGS) (Common cause of chronic renal failure in USA)	**Risk factors:** obesity, heroine abuse, **H**IV, **A**frican American race, **s**ickle cell anemia	**Light microscopy:** • **focal** = only some of the glomeruli involved (not all) • **segmental** = only **segments** of the glomeruli are involved, and not all of the glomeruli • **sclerosis** = fibrosis There is segmental involvement of left lower glomerulus. The two glomeruli on the right look normal Source: Han MH, Kim YJ. Practical Application of Columbia Classification for Focal Segmental Glomerulosclerosis. Biomed Res Int. 2016; 2016: 9375753. **Electron microscopy picture:** effacement of podocytes (similar to minimal change disease)	Steroids for nephrotic-range proteinuria

MRS

Obese **HAS** FSGS

(Continued)

Condition	Etiology and pathophysiology	Microscopic findings	Management
Membranous nephropathy (aka membranous glomerulonephritis)	Antibody against phospholipase A2 receptor is commonly found. This is an immune complex disease associated with the following conditions: • Infections: Hep B, Hep C, syphilis, etc. • Drugs: NSAIDs, penicillamine, etc. • Solid tumors: lung cancer, colon cancer, etc. • Systemic lupus erythematosus	**Light microscopy picture:** • membranous = only membrane thickening (glomerular basement membrane and capillary membrane thickening), with normal mesangium **Electron microscopy picture:** subepithelial deposits along the glomerular basement membrane (GBM) and thickening of GBM Source: Differential diagnosis of nephrologic syndromes. In: Siegenthaler W, ed. Siegenthaler's differential diagnosis in internal medicine: from symptom to diagnosis. 1st ed. Thieme; 2007. Typical subepithelial electron dense deposits (humps) **Immunofluorescence:** IgG and C3 deposits	For moderate to high risk disease, start immunosuppressive therapy with steroids+ one of the following- cyclophosphamide (preferred), chlorambucil, cyclosporine or tacrolimus. • Disease can be rapidly progressive.

Nephritic Syndrome

Condition	Etiology and pathophysiology	Microscopic findings	Management
Rapidly progressive glomerulonephritis (RPGN) Severe condition that can lead to progressive rapid decline in renal function resulting in need for hemodialysis within weeks or months	Can be caused by any glomerulopathy when inciting condition is very aggressive. Common etiologies include the following: • Goodpasture syndrome= anti-GBM (anti-glomerular basement membrane antibody) disease • Pauci-immune glomerulonephritis due to ANCA associated conditions: microscopic polyangiitis, granulomatosis with polyangiitis (old name: Wegener's granulomatosis) and Churg–Strauss syndrome • Immune complex glomerulonephritis (postinfectious glomerulonephritis, IgA nephropathy, SLE, etc.)	**Light microscopy:** crescent formation in glomeruli Source: Adnan MM, Morton J, Hashmi S, Abdul Mujeeb S, Kern W, Cowley BJ. Anti-GBM of pregnancy: acute renal failure resolved after spontaneous abortion, plasma exchange, hemodialysis, and steroids. Case Rep Nephrol. 2014; 2014: 243746.	• Empiric treatment is with steroids + cyclophosphamide • Plasmapheresis is indicated in anti-GBM disease (remove antibodies from blood)

Condition	Etiology and pathophysiology	Microscopic findings	Management
Membranoproliferative glomerulonephritis (MPGN)	**Autoimmune:** SLE, rheumatoid arthritis, etc. **Chronic infection:** Hep C > Hep B, cryoglobulinemia, infective endocarditis, osteomyelitis, etc. **Liquid tumors:** lymphoma, leukemia, and lymphoproliferative disorders (e.g., multiple myeloma, Waldenstrom's macroglobulinemia)	**Light microscopy:** reveals mesangial **proliferation** and glomerular basement **membrane** thickening (hence called MPGN) Type I MPGN (primary immune complex-mediated disease)[a] As opposed to subepithelial deposits, these do not look like humps Source: Differential diagnosis of nephrologic syndromes. In: Siegenthaler W, ed. Siegenthaler's differential diagnosis in internal medicine: from symptom to diagnosis. 1st ed. Thieme; 2007. Type II MPGN (primary auto-antibody-mediated disease) A unique pathology is presence of **C3 nephritic factor**, which is an antibody that leads to activation of complement factors and subsequent deposition of immune complexes. Serum complement level is typically very low Source: Cook HT. C3 glomerulopathy. Version 1. F1000Res. 2017; 6: 248. **Electron microscopy:** dense deposits within the GBM (hence, type II MPGN is also known as dense deposit disease)[b]	Treat underlying cause For idiopathic disease, use prednisone. Add cyclophosphamide for severe disease
Goodpasture syndrome	Production of autoantibody against components of basement membrane in lungs and kidney (type II hypersensitivity). This leads to hemoptysis and nephritic syndrome which frequently manifests as RPGN Screening test is anti-GBM-antibody, which is pathognomonic of Goodpasture syndrome[c]	**Light microscopy:** diffuse membrane-like thickening of capillary walls **Electron microscopy:** subepithelial deposits[d] along the basement membrane **Immunofluorescence:** linear deposition of IgG along the basement membrane[e] Source: Differential diagnosis of nephrologic syndromes. In: Siegenthaler W, ed. Siegenthaler's differential diagnosis in internal medicine: from symptom to diagnosis. 1st ed. Thieme; 2007.	For active disease, use prednisone, cyclophosphamide, and plasmapheresis (remove antibodies from blood)

(Continued)

Condition	Etiology and pathophysiology	Microscopic findings	Management
Postinfectious glomerulonephritis (PIGN) - one-subtype is post-streptococcal glomerulonephritis (PSGN)	Autoimmune immune-complex-mediated disease incited by group A streptococcus infection (skin or throat infection), or other infections (e.g., staphylococcus or gram-negative bacterial infection) • Look for low C3 and C4 If PSGN is suspected, NSIDx is documentation of strep infection with either • throat or skin culture OR • ASO titer or streptozyme test	**Light microscopy:** findings are nonspecific **Electron microscopy:** subepithelial deposits[d] of immune complex **Immunofluorescence:** granular IgG and C3 deposition	• Usually self-limiting • Supportive treatment

MRS

[a]The only one with sub**en**dothelial deposits is **M**PGN type I (**MEN I**).

[b]MPGN's basement membrane is **TOO** dense to **C** through: Too = type 2: Dense= dense deposit disease: C through= C three= C3 nephritic factor.

[c]GPS is anti-GBM: GPS= Goodpasture syndrome

[d]Subepithelial deposits in electron microscopy is nonspecific. It can be found in GPS, postinfectious GN, and membranous nephropathy.

[e]Basement membrane is linear.

Abbreviations: ANCA, antineutrophil cytoplasmic antibody; SLE, systemic lupus erythematosus.

6.5 Henoch–Schonlein Purpura and IgA Nephropathy

Background: These two conditions are closely related.[9] Common pathology is autoimmune production of antibody against IgA.

IgA nephropathy	**Pathophysiology:** Immune complexes of IgA and anti-IgA antibody are deposited in the mesangium **Presentation:** can vary from recurrent isolated hematuria to fatal RPGN. It is usually associated with concurrent upper respiratory tract symptoms of sore throat and flu-like syndrome	
Henoch–Schonlein purpura	IgA nephropathy + extrarenal manifestations occurring primarily in children (due to development of leukocytoclastic vasculitis with IgA immune complexes) • Palpable purpura to ecchymosis, especially in area below the trunk • Abdominal pain and blood in stool (due to submucosal hemorrhage and edema) • Arthralgia or arthritis	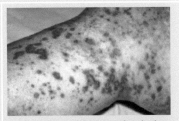 Source: Differential diagnosis of nephrologic syndromes. In: Siegenthaler W, ed. Siegenthaler's differential diagnosis in internal medicine: from symptom to diagnosis. 1st ed. Thieme; 2007.

Abbreviations: IgA, immunoglobulin A; RPGN, rapidly progressive glomerulonephritis.

 In a nutshell

Nephritic and Nephrotic Syndrome Made Easy

Clinical conditions	Most likely Dx
Nephritic syndrome + hearing loss and visual defects	**Alport syndrome** (hereditary disorder of basement membrane collagen biosynthesis) NSIDx is skin biopsy to check for absence of a specific type of collagen
Nephritic syndrome + lung and/or sinus problem	Granulomatosis with polyangiitis (old name: Wegener's granulomatosis)
Nephritic syndrome + only lung problem	Goodpasture syndrome
Nephritic syndrome + hx of upper respiratory tract symptoms or skin infection more than 10 days ago	Poststreptococcal glomerulonephritis
Nephritic syndrome + coexistent or recent (< 5 days ago) hx of upper respiratory tract symptoms	IgA nephropathy (aka Buerger's disease, aka synpharyngitic nephropathy)
Rheumatoid arthritis or multiple myeloma + nephrotic syndrome	Amyloidosis
Rheumatoid arthritis or multiple myeloma + nephritic syndrome	MPGN
Hep B + nephrotic syndrome	Membranous glomerulonephritis
Hep C + nephritic syndrome (no skin rash)	MPGN
Hep C + nephritic syndrome+ skin rash	Cryoglobulinemic vasculitis-associated MPGN
SLE + nephrotic syndrome	Membranous glomerulonephritis
SLE + nephritic syndrome	MPGN (I or II), RPGN or diffuse proliferative glomerulonephritis

Abbreviations: IgA, immunoglobulin A; MPGN, membranoproliferative glomerulonephritis; RPGN, rapidly progressive glomerulonephritis, SLE, systemic lupus erythematosus

[9]**Dermatitis herpetiformis** and **celiac sprue** are also closely associated with these two conditions. Sometimes all can occur in the same patient. For example, a child with past hx of IgA nephropathy develops celiac sprue and dermatitis herpetiformis.

Membranoproliferative glomerulonephritis (MPGN)	VS	Membranous glomerulonephritis (aka membranous nephropathy)
MRS ☺ see liquid proliferating in red sea		MRS ☺ If it is not that, then it should be this
See = C= Hep C[a]		**Hep B**[a]
Liquid tumors: leukemia, leukemic phase of lymphoma, multiple myeloma, etc.		**Solid** tumors like colon and pancreatic cancer
Proliferating = membrano**proliferative** glomerulonephritis		Only membranous glomerulonephritis
RED= Red blood cell cast = nephritic syndrome		**No RBC cast** = nephrotic syndrome
Sea = C= C3 nephritic factor		Phospholipase A2 receptor antibody

[a]Hep B is also associated with MPGN, and Hep C is associated membranous nephropathy, but incidence is lower. For example, in a question with chronic hepatitis and MPGN, Hep C infection is more likely than Hep B.

Clinical Case Scenarios

An adult patient with severe nephrotic syndrome now develops acute abdominal pain, fever, and hematuria.

20. What is the likely dx?

21. Which glomerulopathy is most associated with this condition?

22. Nephrotic or nephritic syndrome with risk factors for STD. What is the NSIDx?

6.6 Renal Papillary Disorders

Background: Renal papilla is a relatively low oxygenated area; thus, it is very vulnerable to decrease in blood supply and arteriopathies.

Etiology: Renal papillary necrosis can occur in the following conditions:

	Underlying mechanism
Diabetes mellitus (DM)	Atherosclerosis and hyaline arteriosclerosis decrease arterial lumen, reducing blood flow
NSAID abuse	Patients with underlying arteriopathy (e.g., patients with DM) with chronically decreased renal blood flow depend on prostaglandin synthesis to maintain normal renal perfusion. NSAIDs, by blocking prostaglandin production, eliminate this compensatory mechanism leading to renal injury
Sickle cell anemia and trait	Low oxygenation state in renal papilla predisposes to sickling in this area, leading to infarction
Chronic pyelonephritis	Direct infection and necrosis

Abbreviation: NSAID, nonsteroidal anti-inflammatory drug.

Presentation: Can vary from sterile pyuria, asymptomatic micro- or macrohematuria (little amount of necrosis) to macroscopic hematuria, abdominal pain, and right flank pain (massive necrosis of papillae with obstruction of urine outflow). Another interesting presentation is polyuria due to decreased concentrating ability of kidney.

Rx: Supportive treatment and address underlying etiology.

Renal Problems Associated with NSAIDs

Condition	Presentation
Chronic tubulointerstitial nephritis	Look for WBC casts and creatinine elevation. It can progress to chronic renal failure
Papillary necrosis	Sterile pyuria, asymptomatic micro- to macrohematuria, or acute right flank pain
Nephrotic syndrome	Minimal change disease or membranous nephropathy
Prerenal kidney injury	Usually presents with isolated BUN and creatinine elevation
Increased risk for **urinary tract cancers**	Patient on chronic NSAIDs develops chronic irritative and voiding symptoms. UA reveals hematuria. Cytology is positive for urothelial cancer

Abbreviations: BUN, blood urea nitrogen; NSAIDs, nonsteroidal anti-inflammatory drugs; UA, urinalysis.

6.7 Chronic Kidney Disease aka Chronic Renal Failure

Functions of kidney	Clinical effect in chronic renal failure	Supportive treatment in advanced CKD patients
Excrete **water soluble** by-products of metabolism. For example, creatinine and **BUN**	Uremia[a] and elevated creatinine	Hemodialysis
Maintain electrolyte levels within normal range by increasing or decreasing excretion	Hyperkalemia, hyperphosphatemia[b] due to decreased excretion	Target phosphorus is • < 5.5 in hemodialysis patients • < 3.5 in patients not on hemodialysis First SIM is dietary phosphate restriction. If still elevated, add phosphate binders, either calcium containing or noncalcium ones • In patients with hypercalcemia, vascular calcifications or adynamic bone disease,[c] use sevelamer and lanthanum which do not contain calcium • In patients with hypocalcemia, use calcium carbonate or calcium acetate
Maintain volume status	Increased risk of volume overload	Use oral diuretics. Patients with significant volume overload resistance to diuretic treatment may need hemodialysis to remove extra volume
Synthesizes erythropoietin to stimulate RBC production in bone marrow	Normocytic anemia with decreased reticulocyte count	In patients with Hb < 10, iron replacement therapy is indicated if low ferritin or iron saturation. Erythropoietin stimulating agents are given (e.g., darbepoetin) only after ensuring adequate iron stores[d]

(Continued)

Functions of kidney	Clinical effect in chronic renal failure	Supportive treatment in advanced CKD patients
Activates vitamin D	Vitamin D deficiency[b]	Vitamin D (calcitriol) supplementation, if found to have low levels
Maintenance of pH (kidneys excrete excess acid load)	Acidosis[e]	Oral bicarbonate or hemodialysis

HTN and accelerated atherosclerosis commonly develops

- MC cause of death in CKD is **coronary artery disease**

[a]**Urea** is toxic in high amounts and can cause uremic encephalopathy, uremic pericarditis, and uremic coagulopathy (platelet dysfunction).

[b]Hyperphosphatemia, can lead to increased calcium chelation causing hypocalcemia. In patients with chronic renal failure, the hypocalcemia is compounded by decreased Vit D levels. This hypocalcemia can then lead to secondary hyperparathyroidism, renal osteodystrophy, and osteomalacia. Secondary hyperparathyroidism is treated with combination of phosphate binders and vitamin D supplementation. These help to normalize calcium and decrease parathyroid hormone (PTH) secretion. Calcimimetics, like cinacalcet, are also used to decrease PTH secretion.

[c]In advanced CKD patients, adynamic bone disease occurs because of decreased bone turnover due to suppressed PTH and/or PTH resistance. Features include bone pain, fractures, vascular calcifications and hypercalcemia.

[d]Anemia of chronic inflammation is also treated similarly, but with different cut-offs of ferritin and iron (transferrin) saturation.

[e]Acidosis also occurs due to retention of inorganic acid ions—sulfates and phosphates (anion gap metabolic acidosis).

Abbreviations: BUN, blood urea nitrogen; CKD, chronic kidney disease; HTN, hypertension.

Interventions that may slow down progression of CKD are the following: oral bicarbonate therapy, smoking cessation, dietary protein restriction, ACE inhibitors or angiotensin receptor blockers therapy, tight blood sugar and blood pressure control.

6.7.1 Uremic Coagulopathy

Background: High urea leads to platelet degranulation defect.

Coagulation tests profile: normal prothrombin time (PT), activated partial thromboplastin time (APTT), and platelet count, but prolonged bleeding time.

Rx: In patients with active bleeding, use desmopressin (aka DDAVP). Platelet transfusion is usually not helpful, as platelets become dysfunctional once they are in uremic blood.

6.8 End-Stage Renal Disease

Renal replacement therapy (renal transplant or dialysis): It is generally indicated when creatinine clearance is < 5 mL/minute. It can be considered in patients with GFR < 15 mL/minute. When feasible, kidney transplant is preferred over long-term dialysis, because it has better prognosis and increased chance of survival. Dialysis patients with end-stage renal disease (ESRD) continue to have issues with anemia, bone disease, and hypertension.

6.8.1 Kidney Transplant

Type of organ transplant is given below in the order of preference:
- Kidney transplant from a living related donor.
- Kidney transplant from a living unrelated donor.
- Transplant with a cadaver kidney.

If kidney transplant is not feasible, then only chronic dialysis is preferred.

Post-transplant complications

Presentation (common presenting features are rising creatinine, proteinuria, and worsening HTN)	Diagnosis and workup		Additional notes
When the donor kidney is vascularly connected during surgery, it becomes white and pale	**Hyperacute rejection**		Recipient has pre-existing antibodies against donor antigens ABO isoagglutinins, antiendothelial antibodies, and anti-human leukocyte antigen antibodies (type II hypersensitivity). It is rare as it is prevented by doing pretransplant cross-matching
Oliguria/anuria within 1 week of surgery	NSIM is to check Foley catheter function and do fluid challenge. Also check donor-specific antibodies. Do renal US with doppler and radionuclide renal scan to rule out obstruction, vascular thrombosis, and urine leak If all above tests are unremarkable, dx is likely ischemic acute tubular necrosis		
Persistent rise in creatinine between 2 week to 3 months after transplant	Check the following • compliance to immunosuppressive regimen • serum cyclosporine or tacrolimus levels if patients are on it • blood BK virus (polyomavirus) and CMV viral load • donor-specific antibodies titer • US renal with doppler If all above test unremarkable, do biopsy of transplanted kidney.	In **acute rejection,** biopsy will show lymphocytic infiltration.[a] Even though termed acute, it can also occur months to years later	Acute rejection is due to mismatched HLA antigen and cytotoxic T-cell-mediated type IV hypersensitivity NSIM: IV steroids
Persistent rise in creatinine more than 3 months after transplant		In **chronic rejection** biopsy will show vascular fibrosis. Cause is not well known, but prognosis is very poor as it does not respond well to treatment	**Commonly tried treatment is** escalation of immunosuppressive regimen

[a]If biopsy shows intracellular inclusion body, think of CMV infection. NSIM is valganciclovir or ganciclovir. Look for coexistent pneumonitis or retinitis that suggests disseminated CMV infection.

Abbreviations: CMV, cytomegalovirus; HLA, human leukocyte antigen.

[10] When patients on dialysis develop these symptoms, assess dialysis compliance. If compliant, it is a signal for intensification of dialysis.

 MRS

I **HAVE** pericarditis/pleurisy, that is why I need hemodialysis.

6.8.2 Dialysis for End-Stage Renal Disease

Indications: Following are the indications for emergent dialysis in acute or chronic renal failure[10]:

- **H**yperkalemia refractory to medical treatment.
- **A**cidosis refractory to medical treatment.
- **V**olume overload refractory to diuretics.
- **E**ncephalopathy + altered mental status due to uremia.
- **P**ericarditis or pleurisy due to uremia.

Type of dialysis	Access
Peritoneal dialysis	Intraperitoneal catheter
Hemodialysis	Intravenous dialysis catheter or arteriovenous shunt/graft

6.8.3 Peritoneal Dialysis

Usually done at home overnight by patient, so compliance and ability to perform it at home is important. Dialysate fluid is infused intraperitoneally through a peritoneal catheter.

Complication: Increased risk of peritonitis with gram-positive cocci organisms such as *S. aureus* or *S. epidermidis*. It can present with abdominal pain, ileus, and fever.

NSIDx is peritoneal fluid analysis and gram staining.

Rx: Intraperitoneal empiric antibiotic therapy to cover:

- Gram-positive cocci (vancomycin in patients with MRSA risk factors, or first-generation cephalosporin) +
- Gram negatives (e.g., third-generation cephalosporin).

6.9 Cystic Diseases of Kidney

6.9.1 Autosomal Dominant Polycystic Kidney Disease (ADPKD)

[11] **Conditions with bilateral renal enlargement**
- Bilateral hydronephrosis due to obstruction of urine outflow below the neck of bladder (e.g., prostatic hyperplasia, posterior urethral stricture).
- Bilateral renal cell carcinoma in Von Hippel–Lindau syndrome.
- Autosomal dominant polycystic kidney disease (ADPKD).
- Amyloidosis.

[12] MCC of death in ADPKD is cardiovascular cause.

Pathology: Inherited mutation in polycystic kidney disease-1 (PKD1) or PKD2 gene. PKD1 mutation is more common and more severe.

Presentation: May present with following progression—asymptomatic micro/macrohematuria, chronic flank pain, bilateral flank mass (due to bilateral kidney enlargement)[11] and chronic kidney disease (CKD). Patients may ultimately need dialysis or renal transplantation.[12]

Extrarenal manifestations of ADPKD	Clinical presentation
Intracranial Berry aneurysms that can rupture	Sudden thunder clap headache due to subarachnoid hemorrhage
Extrarenal cysts (e.g., liver cysts, pancreatic cysts)	Liver enlargement and pain
Colonic diverticula	Alternating constipation-diarrhea, or acute diverticulitis
HTN due to high renin-angiotensin-aldosterone	Drug of choice is ACE inhibitor or ARB to slow progression of renal disease
Mitral valve prolapse	Chest pain, syncope, etc.
Abbreviations: ACE, angiotensin-converting enzyme; ARB, angiotensin receptor blocker; HTN, hypertension.	

[13] Renal US is also used to screen asymptomatic family members. LOM: do not choose CT scan.

NSIDx: Ultrasonography (best test)[13]

Management: supportive. Provide genetic counseling to patient and family members.

6.9.2 Other Types of Cystic Kidney Disease

Condition	Disease features
Autosomal recessive polycystic kidney disease (aka infantile polycystic kidney disease)	• Presents in infancy • Associated with liver duct pathology and cirrhosis • Very poor prognosis
Medullary cystic kidney disease (aka autosomal dominant tubulointerstitial kidney disease)	• Early onset • Slowly progressive disease with development of ESRD between 20–60 years of age
Medullary sponge kidneys	• **Presentation:** can present with features of urinary tract stone or UTI • **Dx** is usually suspected with incidental findings in radiological imaging. CT abdomen typically reveals multiple calcifications in renal parenchyma (nephrocalcinosis). But note that nephrocalcinosis can also be seen in other causes (e.g., conditions with hypercalciuria). Dx can be confirmed by IVP or CT with contrast, but is usually not necessary as this condition is benign with good prognosis • Main management issue is prevention of stones
Dialysis-associated cyst	• Multiple small cysts

Abbreviations: ESRD, end-stage renal disease; IVP, intravenous pyelogram; UTI, urinary tract infection.

6.9.3 Isolated Cysts in Kidney

Presentation: Usually asymptomatic and typically detected incidentally.
Management: First differentiate benign-looking cyst from malignant cyst.

Benign cysts	Malignant cysts
Regular **smooth** borders	**Irregular** borders
One cavity (**uniloculated**)	Multiple cavities (**multiloculated**)
Cystic cavity is usually filled with watery material; no echogenic materials inside	Echogenic materials within cystic cavity
NSIM is reassurance	NSIM is biopsy

Clinical Case Scenarios

A patient with eGFR of 12 mL/minute presents with sharp chest pain that gets worse with lying flat and inspiration. Electrocardiogram (EKG) shows diffuse ST wave elevation.

23. What is the likely dx?

24. What is best NSIM?

25. A 35-year-old African American woman presents with long-standing history of asymptomatic macrohematuria with NO history of chronic NSAID ingestion, recent infection or other risk factors. What dx should you think of?

26. A woman with hx of osteoarthritis, using over-the-counter pain medications, presents with asymptomatic macroscopic hematuria. What is the likely dx?

Six months after renal transplantation, patient's creatinine is normal, but patient has hypercalcemia, hypophosphatemia, and elevated parathyroid hormone.

27. What is the likely Dx?

28. What is the mechanism?

Answers

1. Acute irritative symptoms due to gonococcal urethritis and cystitis. Presence of mucopurulent discharge points toward gonococcus.

2. Single dose oral azithromycin and intramuscular ceftriaxone.

3. Acute prostatitis (irritative and voiding symptoms) with epididymitis (tender and swollen testes).

4. MCC is *E. coli* in this age group.

5. Trimethoprim-sulfamethoxazole or a fluoroquinolone (ciprofloxacin or levofloxacin) for total of 6 weeks.

6. Calcium oxalate stone.

7. Few years of mild irritative and voiding symptoms, along with hematuria and weight loss suggests bladder cancer in the neck area. FYI-*voiding symptoms in bladder cancer can be due to involvement of trigone, bladder neck or urethra, or due to decrease in bladder capacity, or detrusor overactivity.*

8. Intermittent catheterization.

9. Struvite stone due to infection with urease producing organism or RTA type I.

10. If serum bicarbonate is low think of RTA type I.

11. Check serum calcium, phosphorus, vitamin D and 24-hour urinary calcium, oxalate, citrate excretion.

12. Dx is idiopathic renal hypercalciuria.

13. For idiopathic renal hypercalciuria, use thiazide diuretic, which stimulates reabsorption of Ca^{2+} from urinary tubules, and thus decreases urine Ca^{2+}.

14. Primary hyperparathyroidism. NSIDx: check PTH level.

15. CT abdomen and pelvis without contrast to rule out urinary tract stone. Think of MRS SIT: stone, infection, or tumor.

16. NSIDx is office-based cystoscopy + urine cytology.

17. Stop metformin.

18. There is risk of contrast-induced nephropathy and subsequent development of severe lactic acidosis.

19. Discontinue metformin if eGFR < 30 mL/minute. Do not start a new metformin regimen if eGFR is < 45 mL/minute.

20. Renal vein thrombosis.

21. Membranous glomerulonephritis.

22. Check hepatitis serology and HIV antigen–antibody assay.

23. Uremic pericarditis.

24. Dialysis.

25. Sickle cell trait. Sickle cell disease would have presented with features of sickling crises.

26. NSAID-induced papillary necrosis.

27. Tertiary hyperparathyroidism.

28. Development of parathyroid hyperplasia after prolonged secondary hyperparathyroidism prior to transplantation.

7. Hematology

> *"There are about 25 trillion red blood cells* **packed** *inside a single human body—line them side by side and they will circle the earth 15 times. This astoundingly large surface area was created to deliver what each cell in our body needs: oxygen."*

7.1 Anemia

Anemia is the state of reduced hemoglobin in blood.

Clinical pathophysiology: Presentation can vary with the degree of anemia—from exercise intolerance and easy fatigability to shortness of breath at rest. Also, with decrease in oxygen delivery to tissues, the body signals the heart to pump more blood, so there is increase in heart rate (palpitations) and increase in stroke volume (physical exam may reveal high flow midsystolic murmur in aortic area, known as a functional murmur). Additional exam findings includes scleral pallor.

- Cardiac ischemia can develop due to increased work load (tachycardia) and increased demand for O_2, while O_2 content in blood is low.[1]
- In long-standing severe anemia, high output heart failure can ensue.

> [1] MCC of death in anemia is myocardial infarction.

Work-up of Anemia

Legend: 1st SIDx, first step in Dx; NSIDx, next step in dx; MCV, mean cell volume.

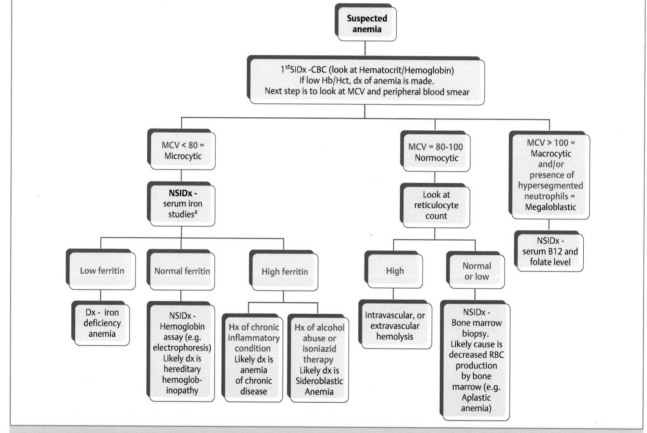

[a] Serum iron studies: ferritin, iron level, iron saturation, and total iron binding capacity. MCC of low MCV anemia is iron deficiency, so 1st SIDx is iron studies.

7.1.1 Microcytic Anemias (MCV < 80)

> [2] Hemoglobin = heme + globin
> Heme = iron + protoporphyrin
> - hemoglobin
> - heme

Low mean cell volume (MCV) means there is a problem with production of hemoglobin component of red blood cell (RBC).[2]

Problem in production of		Due to
The heme part (which is made up of iron and protoporphyrin)	⟹	Iron deficiency anemia, anemia of chronic disease, and sideroblastic anemia
The globin part: α and β protein	⟹	Alpha and beta thalassemias

Iron Deficiency Anemia

What happens to serum iron studies in iron deficiency state?

- Ferritin is the storage form of iron. When the body iron stores are low, serum ferritin is low.
- Low iron stores result in compensatory increase in synthesis of transferrin. (Transferrin is a serum protein that binds and transports iron to various tissues.)
- Increase in transferrin means increase in **serum iron binding capacity**.
- As serum iron is low, the iron saturation is low. Iron saturation refers to the number of iron molecules that are bound to transferrin molecule.

Serum iron studies cofirms iron defeciency state. NSIM is to treat the iron deficiency and find the cause.

Rx: Iron replacement therapy (IV or oral) and supportive transfusion as needed. Follow-up response with reticulocyte count and iron studies.[3]

Etiology

- Main etiology is bleeding.
  - Less than 50 years: likely etiology in this age group is menorrhagia in females, and peptic ulcer disease in males.
  - More than 50 years: consider colon cancer. Check fecal occult blood test and do colonoscopy.
- Prematurity: most of the iron stores in the newborns is acquired from mother during third trimester of pregnancy.
- In children, there is increased demand for iron, thus decreased intake of iron can easily result in iron deficiency.[4] In children, if there is no response to iron supplementation, gastrointestinal bleeding due to Meckel's diverticulum is the potential cause.
- Chronic mechanical hemolysis (e.g., in mechanical heart valve).
- Increased demand after erythropoietin treatment in end-stage renal disease (ESRD) patients.

[3] If there is no response to iron supplementation, 1st SIM is to check for compliance and ask for side effects. Main reason patients do not take iron pills is because of GI upset.

[4] Cow milk is low in iron.

In a nutshell

	Iron deficiency anemia
Serum ferritin	Low
Transferrin and total iron binding capacity	↑
Serum iron	Low
% saturation	Low

Clinical Case Scenarios

Iron deficiency anemia in a patient > 50 years of age.

1. What is the 1st SIDx?

2. What is the best SIDx?

Anemia of Chronic Disease

Etiology: Any cause of chronic inflammation such as collagen vascular diseases, active malignancy, chronic infection (e.g., chronic osteomyelitis), etc.

Pathphysiology: Increase in inflammatory mediators signal liver to produce hepcidin that blocks the release of iron from its storage form. Increased iron stores mean high serum ferritin[5] leading to negative feedback for transferrin synthesis (low total iron binding capacity [TIBC]). As iron is not released from its storage form, serum iron and iron saturation is low.

[5] Ferritin is also a marker of inflammation. It can be high in patients with ongoing infection and/or inflammation.

Management: Treat underlying cause.

Supportive Rx: In patients with Hb < 10 g/dL, iron replacement therapy is indicated if ferritin < 100 ng/mL OR iron (transferrin) saturation < 20%. Erythropoietin-stimulating agents are given (e.g., darbepoetin) after ensuring adequate iron stores.

 In a nutshell

	Anemia of chronic disease
Serum ferritin	↑
Transferrin and total iron binding capacity	Low
Serum iron	Low
% saturation	Low

Sideroblastic Anemia

Pathophysiology: Inadequate or abnormal synthesis of protoporphyrin to make heme. This will result in idle iron not being used for hemoglobin synthesis (so serum ferritin, serum iron, and iron saturation is high).

Etiology:

- Hereditary (congenital)
- Alcohol
- Vit B$_6$ (pyridoxine) deficiency: it can be hereditary or acquired (e.g., due to isoniazid use)
- Copper or lead poisoning
- Clonal sideroblastosis, likely due to underlying myelodysplastic syndrome

Diagnostic evaluation: usually history and iron study point toward the diagnosis.

	Sideroblastic anemia
Serum ferritin	↑
Transferrin and TIBC	Low
Serum iron	↑
% saturation	↑

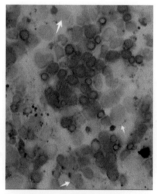

Source: Microcytic hypochromic anemia. In: Siegenthaler W. Siegenthaler's differential diagnosis in internal medicine: from symptom to diagnosis. 1st ed. Thieme; 2007.

The most specific test is bone marrow biopsy with iron staining (Prussian blue stain) of specimen. In absence of protoporphyrin to complete the hemoglobin synthesis, iron dedicated for heme synthesis becomes trapped in mitochondria of erythrocyte precursors (mitochondria is where heme biosynthesis begins). This shows up like an apparent ring around the nucleus, hence called ringed sideroblasts (white arrows). Sometimes you can see stippled RBCs (basophilic stippling) on peripheral blood smear.

Some types of **refractory** sideroblastic anemia are associated with **myelodysplastic syndrome** and development of leukemia. Presence of sideroblasts along with high MCV points toward this development.

Management: Treat underlying cause.

Thalassemia

Definition: Abnormal production of globin protein (of hemoglobin) due to hereditary genetic defect.

α thalassemia is genetic defect in production of α-globin protein	β thalassemia is genetic defect in production of β-globin protein
Four genes are responsible for production of α-globin, so there are four levels of severity: • 1 gene deleted—asymptomatic • 2 genes deleted—mild anemia • 3 genes deleted—moderate to severe anemia, usually requiring blood transfusions • 4 genes deleted—incompatible with life and fetuses die in utero	There are two genes responsible for production of β-globin: • 1 gene deleted—minor degree of anemia • 2 gene deleted—β-thalassemia major (aka Cooley's anemia). Severe symptoms develop **6 months** after birth[a]

[a] Fetal hemoglobin does not have β-globin protein, so fetuses and newborns are not affected. After 6 months, adult hemoglobin replaces fetal hemoglobin.

Diagnostic evaluation:

- **When to suspect**: Microcytic anemia with normal iron panel, and normal red cell distribution width (RDW). Peripheral blood smear shows homogenous hypochromic cells and target,[6] or tear drop cells(see '1' on the right image).
- NSIDx is **hemoglobin assay**[7]
- Confirmatory testing includes DNA-based methods (e.g., PCR).

Hemoglobin Assay

To undestand hemoglobin assays, we need to know about different types of hemoglobin.

Hb A	⇒	Two alpha (α) chains and two beta (β) chains	The main adult hemoglobin
Hb A$_2$	⇒	Two alpha (α) and two delta (δ) chains	It constitues approximately 2% of adult hemoglobin
Hb F	⇒	Two alpha (α) and two gamma (γ) chains	This is the primary hemoglobin produced by fetus during gestation. Its production usually falls to a low level after birth

- In alpha thalassemias, there is reduced synthesis of all forms of hemoglobin. Four gamma (γ) chains can fuse to form Bart's hemoblogin, and percentage of Bart's hemoblogin corresponds with severity of alpha thalassemia. In 3 or 4 genes-deleted severe alpha thalassemias, excess of β chains can fuse to form β-globin tetramer (HbH).
- In beta thalassemia, there can be compensatory increase in Hb A$_2$ or HbF.

Management

- Severe anemia is treated with regular blood transfusion.[8]
- Splenectomy can decrease the need for transfusion. Spleen is where donor erythrocytes are naturally destroyed.

Prenatal Screening for Thalassemias

Indication: pregnant patients with abnormal screening complete blood count (CBC) (low MCV with normal RDW), or in couples with positive family hx.

Test of choice is hemoglobin assay of both parents.[9] If hemoglobin assay is negative in at least one parent, the risk of clinically important disease is low. Reassure the parents-to-be. If both are carriers, only then there is a risk of clinically important disease in the baby. Offer counseling and further prenatal diagnostic options.

[6] When "target cells" (2) are mentioned in a test question, think of the following conditions: Hemoglobinopathies (hemoglobin C, sickle cell disease, thalassemias, etc.) Liver disease Splenectomy

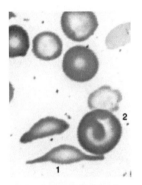

Source: Cytomorphological anemias with erythrocyte anomalies. In: Theml H, Diem H, Haferlach T. Color atlas of hematology: Practical microscopic and clinical diagnosis. 2nd ed. Thieme; 2004.

[7] FYI, Hb assaying methods include high-performance liquid chromatography, capillary electrophoresis, and isoelectric fusing. These newer methods are preferred over traditional gel electrophoresis.

[8] This can lead to secondary hemochromatosis (iron overload) later in life. Now serum iron panel will show elevated ferritin and increased iron saturation.

[9] In patients with family hx of thalassemias, screening starts with CBC and peripheral blood smear.

Clinical Case Scenarios

3. Patient has hx of multiple RBC transfusions in the past. Hemoglobin assay shows increased HbA2 and HbF. What is the likely dx?

4. Patient with history of hypertension, dyslipidemia, diabetes, and rheumatoid arthritis is found to have anemia. TIBC and iron saturation is low and serum ferritin is high. What is the likely cause of anemia?

7.1.2 Macrocytic (MCV > 100) or Megaloblastic Anemias

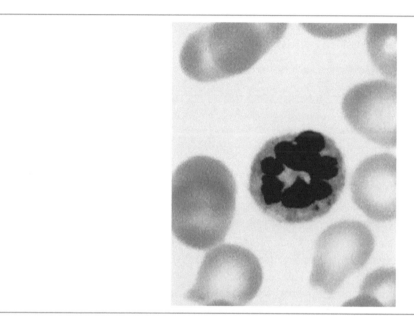

Source: Cell degradation, special granulations, and nuclear appendages in neutrophilic granulocytes and nuclear anomalies. In: Theml H, Diem H, Haferlach T. Color atlas of hematology: Practical microscopic and clinical diagnosis. 2nd ed. Thieme; 2004.

Background: Bone marrow stem cells require vitamin B_{12} (cobalamin) and folic acid for DNA synthesis. Deficiency of either can result in abnormal DNA synthesis and formation of large RBCs (macroytic anemia). Antimetabolite medications, such as methotrexate, phenytoin, trimethoprim, 6-mercaptopurine, can also impair DNA synthesis resulting in macrocytosis.

Work-up: If macrocytosis is seen, NSIDx is peripheral blood smear and serum folate and vitamin B_{12} level. Presence of hypersegmented neutrophils ($\geq$ 5 lobes in nucleus) is pathognomonic of megaloblastic anemia.

Other notable causes of macrocytosis:

Without megaloblastosis, or hypersegmented neutrophils	Can have hypersegmented neutrophils, or megaloblastosis
• Alcoholism	• Myelodysplastic syndrome can present with macrocytosis
• Liver disease	• HIV
• Hypothyroidism	• Antimetabolites

Vitamin B_{12} Deficiency

Mechanism of vitamin B_{12} absorption: Vitamin B_{12} is released from food in presence of gastric acid. It then binds with intrinsic factor (secreted from gastric parietal cells) in the duodenum, which requires presence of pancreatic enzymes. This vitamin B_{12}–intrinsic factor complex is absorbed by ileum into the circulation.

Etiology of vitamin B12 deficiency:

Pernicious anemia (autoimmune destruction of gastric parietal cells) • The MCC of vitamin B_{12} deficiency	• It can be associated with other autoimmune diseases. • Pernicious anemia can lead to development of atrophic gastritis (loss of gastric rugae/folds and achlorhydria) and compensatory increase in gastrin level; hence it is associated with an increased risk of gastric cancer
Chronic pancreatitis with exocrine pancreatic deficiency	Decreased binding of intrinsic factor to vitamin B_{12}
Conditions with ileal involvement	Ilectomy, Crohn's disease, tropical sprue, etc.
Strict vegan diet for more than 3 years	Vitamin B_{12} deficiency can develop in a completely vegetarian patient (no dairy products or eggs); but note that it takes at least few years for the body stores of vitamin B_{12} to be depleted
No gastric acid (achlorhydria)	Gastrectomy or long history of proton pump inhibitors use (> 3 years)
Fish tapeworm (*Diphyllobothrium latum*) **infection**	Risk factor: people who consume raw fish (including sushi and sashimi)

Additonal manifestation (neurological symptoms): Vitamin B_{12} deficiency can result in excessive production of methylmalonic acid, which is toxic to myelin sheath leading to demyelination. Patients may develop decreased position and vibratory sense. Glove stocking peripheral neuropathy is common, but note that any nervous system can be involved (autonomic neuropathy, motor paralysis, cranial nerves involvement, dementia, etc.)

Diagnostic Evaluation

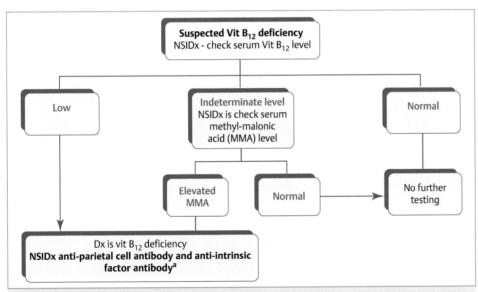

[a]If patient does not have an obvious cause of deficiency such as hx of ilectomy or being a complete vegeterian for > 3 years.

Treatment: Oral or intramuscular vitamin B_{12} supplementation. In patients with significant anemia, neurological symptoms, or pernicious anemia, start intramuscular vitamin B_{12} injections.[10] Otherwise, oral vit B12 can be given.

[10]Parenteral vitamin B_{12} treatment can result in hypokalemia due to rapid uptake of potassium by newly forming hematopoietic cells.

Schilling Test

Even though it is not used for diagnosis nowadays, it is asked on exam, as it requires knowledge of mechanism of vitamin B_{12} absorption.

How it is performed: Intramuscular vitamin B_{12} is first given to saturate all the serum vitamin B_{12} receptors. Next step is oral administration of radiolabeled (RL) vitamin B_{12}. If absorption is intact, the absorbed RL vitamin B_{12} will be directly excreted with urine (as there are no seats left to bind in receptors).

- If urinary excretion of RL (radio-labeled) vitamin B_{12} is high, then the deficiency is related to poor intake.
- If urinary excretion of RL vitamin B_{12} is low, then NSIDx is to add intrinsic factor to oral RL vitamin B_{12}.
  - If urinary excretion is high, dx of intrinsic factor deficiency is made.
  - If urinary excretion is still low, then other dx that can be considered are pancreatitis (test normalizes after pancreatic enzyme supplementation), bacterial overgrowth (normalizes when the test is repeated after a trial period of empiric antibiotic therapy), etc.

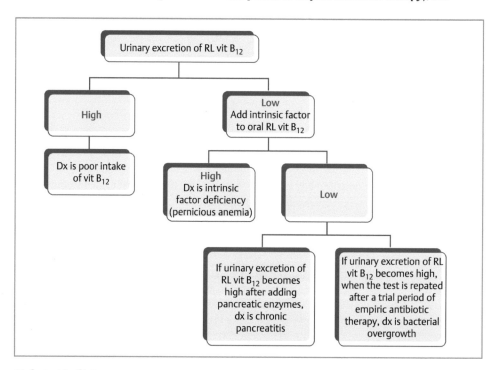

Folate Deficiency

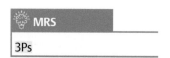

MRS

3Ps

Etiology:	Additional info
Alcoholism (MCC in the United States)	Alcohol blocks absorption of folate
Antiepileptics (phenytoin, primidone and phenobarbital, carbamazepine)	These drugs block absorption of folate from GI tract.
Methotrexate, trimethoprim, pyrimethamine	**Mechanism:** inhibits dihydrofolate reductase • Patients taking one of these medication for long term need leucovorin (aka folinic acid, which is reduced folate) for prophylaxis
Chronic hemolysis	Body's folate stores can be readily depleted (e.g., in sickle cell anemia, spherocytosis)
Increased requirements	For example in pregnancy
Low dietary intake	• Infants fed with goat milk which is low in folate • Diet low in fresh vegetables, fruits, or meat (e.g., tea-and-toast diet, typically elderly or psychiatric patients)

Treatment: Replace folate (almost always **orally**, because the MCC of folate deficiency is due to decreased intake or absorption).

In a nutshell

Vitamin B$_{12}$ and Folate Deficiency
- Homocysteine can be elevated in both.
- Both can cause mild hemolysis (elevated lactate dehydrogenase [LDH] and elevated bilirubin) and pancytopenia, if severe. (The abnormally large blood cells get destroyed).
- Only vitamin B$_{12}$ deficiency can have elevated methymalonic acid level and neurological manifestation.

7.1.3 Normocytic Anemia (MCV 80–100)

Normal MCV means that there is no problem in hemoglobin or DNA synthesis. This anemia can be due to the following:
- Increased **destruction** of RBCs (hemolytic anemias): look for high peripheral reticulocyte count (there is compensatory increased RBC production).
- Decreased **production** of RBCs (primary bone marrow pathology): low reticulocyte count.

7.1.4 Hemolytic Anemia

Intravascular hemolysis	Extravascular hemolysis
Etiology	**Etiology**
• Production of IgM antibody against RBC, aka cold agglutinins. IgM antibodies are potent activators of the complement system, so destruction occurs inside blood vessels	RBCs are being gobbled up by the splenic macrophages, but why?
• Physical destruction of RBCs moving past calcified aortic valves, metallic prosthetic valves, or thrombi	• The RBCs with attached IgG (in warm autoimmune hemolytic anemia) activate phagocytic process of macrophages. IgG are less potent activators of complement system so there is no intravascular hemolysis, but macrophages in splenic sinusoids have IgG receptors which will recognize it and destroy the RBC
- Acute process occurs in states of generalized clot formation, for example, *TTP/HUS* or *DIC*	
- Chronic process (e.g., metallic prosthetic valves) may lead to chronic hemolysis and chronic hemoglobinuria. This may lead to iron deficiency or folate deficiency anemia	• The RBCs cannot enter the narrow splenic sinusoids because their biconcave shape to squeeze in is lost, such as in hereditary spherocytosis, hereditary elliptocytosis
• Hereditary deficiency in one of the enzymes involved in glycolytic pathway leads to increased sensitivity of RBCs to oxidative stress (e.g., pyruvate kinase or glucose-6-phosphate dehydrogenase deficiency)	• Physiologic: old RBCs, usually after about 3 months, start losing their membrane flexibility, hence they cannot squeeze in through the splenic sinusoids and are subsequently eaten up by splenic macrophages
• Paroxysmal nocturnal hemoglobinuria	

Abbreviations: DIC, disseminated intravascular coagulation; HUS, hemolytic uremic syndrome; IgM, immunoglobulin M; RBC, red blood cells; TTP, thrombotic thrombocytopenic purpura.

Diagnostic work-up: To find out whether RBCs are being destroyed in the blood vessels (intravascular hemolysis) or the spleen (extravascular hemolysis), do the following tests: peripheral blood smear, Coomb's test, serum LDH, haptoglobin, and bilirubin levels.

	Intravascular	Extravascular
Haptoglobin[a]	Low[a]	Normal or low
Hemoglobinuria	Can be present[a]	Absent
LDH (spill over of LDH from RBCs)	↑	Normal or ↑
Indirect bilirubin[b]	↑	↑
Splenomegaly	No	Yes

[a]When RBCs are destroyed intravascularly, hemoglobin is released directly into blood stream. There is a protein named haptoglobin that binds to free hemoglobin in blood and transports it to spleen. Low haptoglobin levels are indicative of intravascular hemolysis. In severe acute hemolysis, there is not enough haptoglobin to sequester excessive hemoglogbin, which ends up being filtered by kidneys (hemoglobinuria). This can be toxic to renal tubular cells, causing acute tubular necrosis and renal failure. Moreover, some of this hemoglobin gets oxidized to hemosiderin resulting in hemosiderinuria. Patients may have gross red-/tea-/cola-colored urine. Urine dipstick test is positive for blood but no RBCs are seen in microscopy.[11]

[b]Patients with chronic hemolysis have increased risk of calcium bilirubinate gallstones formation.

Abbreviation: LDH, lactate dehydrogenase.

[11]Urine dipstick test detects globin protein—hemoglobin (either free or inside RBCs) or myoglobin.

Autoimmune Hemolytic Anemia

MRS

CHIMP queen has SLE

Type	Cold autoimmune hemolytic anemia (IgM antibody)	Warm autoimmune hemolytic anemia (IgG antibody)
Etiology	• *Mycoplasma pneumonia* • EBV infection (infectious mononucleosis) • Isoagglutinins: people with blood type O have IgM antibody against A and B antigens; transfusion of type A, B, or AB to type O patient will cause intravascular hemolysis. Likewise, people with blood type B have IgM antibody against A, and blood type A have IgM antibody against B • Quinidine—an antiarrhythmic drug • Lymphomas • Waldenstrom's macroglobunemia	• Causes: • SLE • Drugs that can induce SLE-like condition: • **C**hlorpropamide, **H**ydralazine, **I**soniazid, **M**ethyldopa, **P**rocainamide, **Quin**idine, etc. • Hemolytic disease of the newborn (only IgG can cross the placental barrier; IgM cannot) • Chronic lymphocytic leukemia • Lymphomas
Direct Coomb's test is positive with following reagent[a]	Anti-C3b[b]	Anti-IgG
Additional test	Cold agglutinin titer is the most accurate test	• Peripheral blood smear may show presence of spherocytes • The spherocytes have increased osmotic fragility (splenic macrophages bite off pieces of RBC membrane, resulting in loss of its surface area)
Management	• Avoidance of cold temperature • May use rituximab +/− fludarabine[c] • If severe and acute, plasmapheresis can be done	• Corticosteroids and if refractory, splenectomy[d] • If severe and acute, IVIG can be given[e]

[a]Direct and indirect Coomb's (antiglobulin) agglutination test.[12]

[b]IgM antibodies are powerful activators of complement. In cold auto-immune hemolytic anemia, complement proteins are bound to RBCs.

[c]Other immunosuppressive agents that can be used are azathioprine, cyclosporine, and cyclophosphamide.

[d]In IgG-type autoimmune condition, blood cell destruction takes place in spleen.

[e]Treatment is similar to other IgG-mediated diseases (e.g., immune thrombocytopenia).

Abbreviations: EBV, Epstein–Barr virus; IgG, immunoglobulin G; IgM, immunoglobulin M; IVIG, intravenous immunoglobulin; SLE, systemic lupus erythematosus.

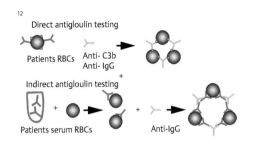

Hereditary Spherocytosis

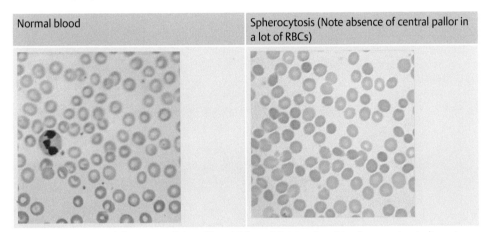

Normal blood	Spherocytosis (Note absence of central pallor in a lot of RBCs)

Source: Anemia. In: Siegenthaler W. Siegenthaler's differential diagnosis in internal medicine: from symptom to diagnosis. 1st ed. Thieme; 2007.

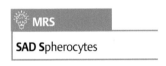

MRS

SAD Spherocytes

Background: It is mostly of **a**utosomal **d**ominant inheritance. It is due to genetic defect of structural proteins that are involved in giving the biconcave shape to RBCs. One of the commonly involved protein is called **s**pectrin.

Pathophysiology: RBCs in this disorder are spherocytic, they cannot squeeze through the splenic sinusoids and are subsequently eaten up by splenic macrophages. These patients have chronically elevated bilirubin (due to chronic hemolysis), which in turn increases the risk of calcium bilirubinate gallbladder stones formation.

When to suspect: Features of extravascular hemolytic anemia with positive family hx, +/− biliary colic. Spherocytes are seen in peripheral blood smear and direct Coomb's test is negative.

Work-up: Best screening test is eosin-5-maleimide binding test (a flow cytometric test). If this is not available, other tests that can be done are osmotic fragility test, acidified glycerol lysis time test, or the cryohemolysis test.

Management: Oral folate replacement and transfusions as required. If moderate to severe anemia, splenectomy can be done (remove the organ where the RBCs are being destroyed).

How to differentiate between autoimmune IgG hemolytic anemia and hereditary spherocytosis?

	Autoimmune IgG type	Hereditary spherocytosis
Extravascular hemolysis	Yes	Yes
Spherocytes in peripheral blood smear	Yes	Yes
Osmotic fragility (RBCs are more fragile to osmotic swelling)	↑	↑
Positive Coomb's test	Yes	No
Family hx	No	Yes

Glucose-6-Phosphate Dehydrogenase Deficiency

Background: This is an X-linked recessive[13] hereditary disorder with deficiency of glucose-6-phosphate dehydrogenase (G6PD), which is a powerful antioxidant in RBCs. In patients of African American descent, it usually presents in a milder form, whereas patients of Mediterranean descent have more severe form.

Precipitating factors: Acute intravenous hemolysis occurs whenever there is an increased oxidative stress:

- Any infection (MC precipitaing factor).
- Drugs: sulfamethoxazole, primaquine, quinine, dapsone, isoniazid,[14] nitrofurantoin, etc.
- Fava beans.

Work-up:

During an acute episode	Peripheral blood smear with Heinz stain (methylene blue stain): This will show Heinz bodies +/− bite cells. • Heinz bodies are oxidized hemoglobin in in RBCs. These can get bitten off by splenic macrophages, leaving behind bite cells. 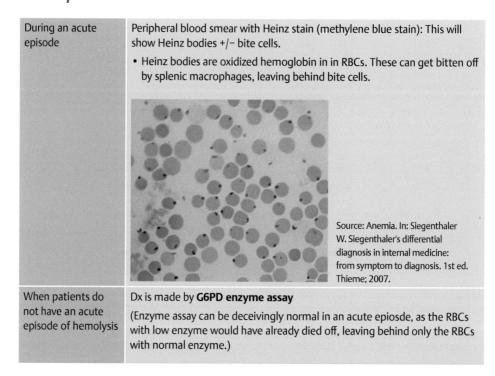 Source: Anemia. In: Siegenthaler W. Siegenthaler's differential diagnosis in internal medicine: from symptom to diagnosis. 1st ed. Thieme; 2007.
When patients do not have an acute episode of hemolysis	Dx is made by **G6PD enzyme assay** (Enzyme assay can be deceivingly normal in an acute epiosde, as the RBCs with low enzyme would have already died off, leaving behind only the RBCs with normal enzyme.)

Rx: Supportive transfusion during an acute episode, treat underlying problem and avoid oxidant stress.

Paroxysmal Nocturnal Hemoglobinuria

Background: It is due to hereditary genetic defect in red cell membrane protein—phosphatidylinositol glycan (PIG-A), aka decay-accelerating factor (proteins CD55 and CD59). This leads to easy binding of complement system to the red cell causing intravascular lysis of RBC, especially in acidic environment. This disorder is also associated with increased risk of varying degree of bone marrow failure (causing pancytopenia) and myelodysplastic syndrome.

Clinical pathophysiology: Nocturnal hemolysis can occur due to development of mild acidosis related to sleep-induced hypoventilation. Patients may present with early morning red urine. Hemolysis can also develop after exercise.

Along with acute hemolysis, patients also have increased risk of venous thrombosis, especially in uncommon locations such as hepatic vein or cerebral vein. Arterial thombosis has also been reported.

[13] X-linked recessive disorders manifest in male patients. Females are carriers.

[14] Isoniazid + anemia: think of G6PD deficiency (when acute) or sideroblastic anemia (when presentation is insidious)

Thrombosis is the MCC of death in paroxysmal nocturnal hemoglobinuria (PNH).

Work-up: NSIDx is flow cytometry, which will show absent or reduced expression of *CD55/CD99*. Older methods of detection are acidified hemolysis test (Ham's test) and sugar water test (sugar is metabolized by RBCs into lactic acid).

Management

- Supportive: Blood transfusion as needed and iron/folate supplementation.
- For ongoing hemolysis, prednisone (steroids) might be helpful.
- For patients with significant disease, give eculizumab (monoclonal antibody that inhibits complement activation).
- In patients with severe disease, bone marrow transplantation can be done.

> **MRS**
>
> **Peculi**ar **P**NH can cause venous and arterial thrombosis and is treated with **eculi**zumab.

7.1.5 Sickle Cell Anemia

Background: It occurs due to single nucleotide (point) mutation in β-globin gene. This mutation replaces the amino acid glutamate (which is hydrophilic) with valine (which is hydrophobic) in the sixth position of β-globin protein. This change of a single amino acid increases risk of change in RBC shape, from biconcave to sickle shaped, whenever the hemoglobin is relatively desaturated. These sickled cells can clump together and easily get stuck in the vessels, obstructing the blood flow, thus causing infarction in various organs.

Factors that promote sickling and precipitate sickle cell crisis	Example clinical scenario where it occurs
Relatively higher concentration of sickle cells promotes sickling of RBCs	Dehydration
Low oxygen saturation due to hypoxia	Pneumonia, pulmonary embolus, exposure to high altitude, etc.
Any condition that decreases the affinity of hemoglobin for oxygen (conditions that cause right shift in Hb-O$_2$ dissociation curve)	• Acidosis • CO2 elevated—hypercarbia increases acid (H+) content in blood • Temperature elevation (fever) • Elevated Diphosphoglycerate (2,3-DPG)

> **MRS**
>
> He **ACTED RIGHT**

Diagnosis

For acute presentation, NSIDx is peripheral blood smear to look for sickled cells.
To make the definitive diagnosis, use **hemoglobin assay.**[15]

[15] Hb assay is also used for screening relatives of the patient.

Hb assay	Diagnosis
> 40% HbS	Sickle cell **disease**
< 40% HbS	Sickle cell **trait**[a]

[a] Most of the time, patients with sickle cell **trait** are asymptomatic or can have minor renal manifestations such as microscopic or macroscopic hematuria and/or isosthenuria.[16]

Abbreviation: Hbs, hemoglobin sickle.

[16] Isosthenuria is loss of concentrating or diluting ability of kidney that results in urine having the same specific gravity as plasma. (Iso = same)

Acute presentation of sickle cell disease (acute anemia and acute painful crises)

7.1.6 Acute Anemia in Sickle Cell Disease

NSIDx is CBC, reticulocyte count and peripheral blood smear.

High reticulocyte count	**Splenic sequestration crisis:** Sickled cells are stuck and pooled in spleen. *This doesn't occur in patients who have fibrotic spleen.*
	Look for sudden splenomegaly, abdominal pain +/− systemic hypotension (not only the RBCs, the whole blood pools in spleen)
	Hemolytic crisis with component of both intravascular and extravascular hemolysis. This can occur in conjunction with acute painful crisis
Low reticulocyte count	There are two possible causes: • Parvovirus B19 infection (acute aplastic crisis or pure red cell aplasia) • Folate deficiency

Rx: is supportive with RBC transfusion as needed and treatment of underlying cause.

Acute vaso-occlusive sickling crisis

Acute clumping of sickled RBCs in the arteries and arterioles can cause ischemia/infarction. Depending on location, it can present with the following:

Acute chest syndrome	Chest pain, fever, leukocytosis, hypoxia, and infiltrates on chest X-ray. It is clinically indistinguishable from pneumonia
Priapism	Painful prolonged erection +/− penile infarction
Dactylitis	Sickling in vessels of the hands and feet can cause, severe pain in distal extremities, i.e., painful hand and foot syndrome (infarction in the hands and toes)
Visual problems	Sickling in the retinal vessels causing retinal artery occlusion
Stroke (ischemic or hemorrhagic)	Acute focal neurological deficits
Renal infarction	Hematuria, acute renal failure, etc.
Avascular necrosis of femoral head	Hip pain

Stepwise management of acute vaso-occlusive sickling crisis

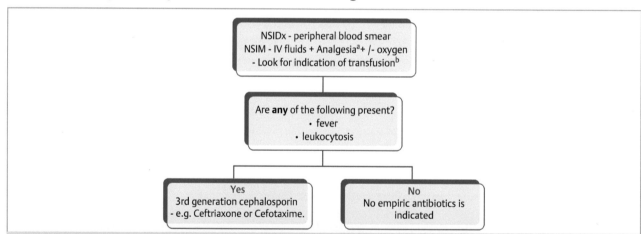

[a]Pain management with opioid analgesics is an important part of management.

[b]Transfusion can be either simple RBC transfusion or exchange transfusion. Exchange transfusion is when sickle cells are filtered out and normal RBCs are transfused in exchange (*remove blood and then give blood back*).

Exchange transfusion indications	RBC transfusion
• Multiorgan failure • CNS abnormalities like confusion (altered mental status) and focal neurological deficits • Moderate to severe acute chest syndrome • Acute cardiac manifestations • Refractory priapism	Only preferred in patients with severe **symptomatic** anemia (Hb < 5)
• This decreases sickle cell concentration without increasing blood viscosity	Does not decrease sickle cell concentration by that much and can actually increase blood viscosity in patients with baseline hemoglobin levels.

Other Presentations of Sickle Cell Disease

- Calcium bilirubinate gallstones.
- Osteomyelitis—MCC is *Staphylococcus aureus* (!).
- Pulmonary hypertension.
- Nephrogenic diabetes insipidus.

Chronic/Preventive management of patients with sickle cell disease

- Within the first 3 months of age, prophylactic penicillin is initiated and continued until age 5. After this, decision to continue prophylaxis is made on a case-by-case basis.
- All patients with underlying chronic hemolysis should be on oral **folate** therapy.
- In symptomatic patients, **hydroxyurea** is recommended. Hydroxyurea increases production of HbF and decreases production of HbS, thus decreasing risk of sickling crisis.
- **Functional asplenia:** By the time patients reach late childhood, they usually have fibrosed spleen due to recurrent splenic infarction (rightly called autosplenectomy). So, all patients with sickle cell disease should receive prophylaxis indicated in asplenia.

⚠ **Caution**

(!) *Do not choose Salmonella typhimurium as the MCC of osteomyelitis in sickle cell disease. This is however more commonly seen in patients with sickle cell disease than in general population.*

In a nutshell

Vaccination and antibiotic prophylaxis for patients with splenectomy or functional asplenia

Vaccination: Spleen plays important role in immune defense against encapsulated microorganisms. Patients undergoing splenectomy, or with functional asplenia should be vaccinated against the following organisms:

Streptococcus pneumoniae	• First dose: PCV13 once, followed by PPSV 23 • Second dose: Repeat PPSV23 after 5 years of first dose • Third dose: PPSV23 at age 65 or more (always maintain 5-year interval)
Neisseria meningitidis	Booster dose q5 years
Haemophilus influenzae	One dose

In patients underoing splenectomy, administer vaccination either 2 weeks prior to surgery (preferred), or 2 weeks after the surgery

Antibiotic prophylaxis:

- Asplenic children receive daily oral penicillin prophylaxis for at least 1 year or until age of 5, whichever is later. Elective splenectomy (e.g., for treatment of hereditary spherocytosis) is usually deferred until age 6, but if needed due to severe anemia, partial splenectomy can be done earlier.

- In **adults,** antibiotic prophylaxis is not recommended.

Peripheral blood smear findings in asplenia:

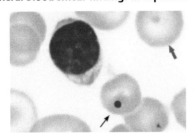

Source: Erythrocyte inclusions. In: Theml H, Diem H, Haferlach T. Color atlas of hematology: Practical microscopic and clinical diagnosis. 2nd ed. Thieme; 2004.

- Howell–Jolly bodies are remnants of nuclear material inside of RBCs *(black arrow).*

- Target cells *(red arrow)*

Clinical Case Scenarios

5. Patient with hx of intermittent cola-colored urine presents with history of right upper quadrant (RUQ) pain usually after eating. What is the likely dx?

6. Patient develops abdominal pain and jaundice in the setting of 3-day history of fever and increased frequency of urination. CBC reveals acute anemia and elevated bilirubin. Urine analysis (UA) is positive for dipstick blood but no RBCs are seen microsopically. What are the differential dx?

7. African American man presents with hx of long-standing asymptomatic gross and microscopic hematuria. CT abdomen reveals no renal or urologic issues. What is the NSIDx?

In a nutshell

In all chronic hemolytic anemias (i.e., sickle cell disease, thalassemias, chronic autoimmune hemolytic anemia, hereditary spherocytosis, etc.), if there is *acute anemia with low reticulocyte count,* think of the following:

- **Acute folate deficiency:** all patients with chronic hemolysis should be on oral folate replacement.

- **Parvovirus B$_{19}$ infection:** can cause acute aplastic crisis (pancytopenia) or pure red cell aplasia (only anemia).

Work-up: If folate is normal, consider testing for parvovirus B$_{19}$ IgM antibody and PCR.

[17] Normocytic anemia with reduced reticulocyte count can develop due to following conditions:
- Advanced chronic kidney disease leads to erythropoietin (epo) deficiency. (Epo stimulates marrow stem cells to produce RBCs.)
- Advanced age.
- Anemia of chronic disease.
- Severe medical illness (e.g., severe alcoholism, endocrine disease, infection, etc.).
- Deficiency of raw materials needed to make RBCs (iron, folate, or vitamin B$_{12}$ deficiency).
In these cases, if no other features of bone marrow disorder are present, bone marrow biopsy can be deferred.

7.1.7 Normocytic Anemia with Zero or Low Reticulocytic Count

In this case, bone marrow is not producing new RBCs. In anemic patients with low reticulocyte count and no obvious cause,[17] or in patients with features worrisome for bone marrow disorder (e.g., pancytopenia or increased blasts in peripheral blood smear), NSIDx is **bone marrow biopsy**.

Bone marrow biopsy findings	Diagnosis
Absent or reduced stem cells in the marrow which involves all cell lineage	Aplastic anemia
Only RBC stem cells are absent or reduced	Pure red cell aplasia[a]
Overcrowding of bone marrow space with dysplastic or cancerous malignant cells	Myelodysplastic syndrome, leukemias, etc.

[a]This is associated with parvovirus infection and thymoma. Congenital form of pure cell aplasia is Blackfan–Diamond syndrome (look for skeletal abnormalities).

7.1.8 Aplastic Anemia

Etiology[18]:

[18] Pure red cell aplasia has similar etiology.

Drugs	Anticonvulsants (e.g., carbamazepine), NSAIDs, antithyroid medications, etc.
Infection	HIV, EBV, parvo-virus B19, etc.
Others	SLE, paroxysmal nocturnal hemoglobinuria, thymoma, etc.

Abbreviations: EBV, Epstein–Barr virus; HIV, human immunodeficiency virus; NSAIDS, nonsteroidal anti-inflammatory drugs; SLE, systemic lupus erythematosus.

Presentation: Any feature of pancytopenia; features of anemia (fatigue), thrombocytopenia (purpura, ecchymosis), and leukopenia (infection).

Work-up:

	Findings
1st SIDx is CBC , reticulocyte count, and peripheral blood smear	• Normocytic anemia, leukopenia, thrombocytopenia, and no blast cells • Low or zero retic count
NSIDx is bone marrow biopsy	The marrow has reduced or absent stem cell population of all types and is hypoplastic, filled with fat/stromal cells. 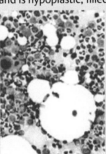 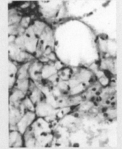 Bone marrow cytology with normal cell density. Source: Bone marrow: Cell composition and principles of analysis. In: Theml H, Diem H, Haferlach T. Color atlas of hematology: Practical microscopic and clinical diagnosis. 2nd ed. Thieme; 2004. Bone marrow cytology with decreased cell density in aplastic anemia. Source: Pure red cell aplasia (PRCA, erythroblastopenia). In: Theml H, Diem H, Haferlach T. Color atlas of hematology: Practical microscopic and clinical diagnosis. 2nd ed. Thieme; 2004.

Management

- Supportive with transfusions as needed.
- Remove offending agent and treat underlying condition whenever possible.
- For severe cases of aplastic anemia, specific treatment is indicated as below:
  - If patient is < 50 years of age AND has human leukocyte antigen (HLA)-matched sibling donor available, hematopoietic stem cell transplant is the treatment of choice. Bone marrow is the preferred source of hematopoietic stem cell transplant. Other sources of stem cells are peripheral blood or umbilical cord blood bank.
  - In absence of available donor, or in patients older than 50 years,[19] immunosuppression is indicated. Combination of antithymocyte globulin, cyclosporine, and prednisone is commonly used. (Aplastic anemia is due to T cell-mediated autoimmune destruction of bone marrow stem cells, hence treatments like antithymocyte globulin work.)

[19] In this age-group, there is higher risk of graft-versus-host disease and increased morbidity with stem cell transplant.

 Clinical Case Scenarios

8. Patient presents with dry cough and noisy breathing. Chest X-ray (CXR) reveals mass in the thymic area. Blood work reveals normocytic normochromic anemia with low retic count. What is the likely dx?

7.1.9 Packed Red Blood Cell Transfusion

Indications:

- Severe anemia—Hb < 7–8.
- Evidence of active cardiac ischemia with Hb < 8 to 10.[20]
- Symptomatic anemia.
- Acute bleeding.

[20] Example CCS: a patient with hx of diabetes presents with recurrent chest pain and has active EKG changes. CBC reveals Hb of 8.5. His baseline is around 11.
NSIM: consider transfusion in this case.

Different types of reaction with transfusion of blood products (RBC, platelets, FFP, etc.)

Reaction type	Clinical features		Mechanism	NSIM
Febrile nonhemolytic reaction (MC reaction)	• Fever, chills, no rash • Usually occurs within few hours of transfusion		During blood storage, cytokines released by WBC got accumulated	Supportive (e.g., antipyretics). This can be prevented by use of leukoreduced blood
Allergic/urticarial reaction	• Urticaria, itching, or angioedema • Occurs within few hours of transfusion		Patient's IgE antibodies reacted to allergens in donor plasma causing mast cell activation	Supportive (antihistamines)
Anaphylactic shock	• Angioedema, wheezing, or stridor + acute respiratory failure or shock • +/− urticaria, itching • Occurs within few minutes of transfusion		• Occurs in patients who have IgA deficiency and, hence may have anti-IgA antibodies • Patient's anti-IgA antibodies react against donor IgA	Stop transfusion and supportive care
Acute hemolytic reaction	• Fever, flank pain, red urine, +/− acute renal failure. Severe forms may lead to DIC • Occur within few hours • Positive direct Coomb's test		ABO incompatibility! mistake by blood bank	Stop transfusion and supportive care
Delayed hemolytic reaction	• Occurs **few days** after transfusion • Fever, hemolytic anemia • Positive direct Coomb's test		Patient was sensitized to RBC antigen in the past, and the antibody was undetectable during cross-matching process. Exposure to antigen stimulates specific antibody production (anamnestic response)	Usually no treatment needed
Transfusion associated circulatory overload (TACO)	• Acute dyspnea • CXR reveals bilateral opacities	Elevated BNP, JVP • hx of CHF	Rapid transfusion of large volume of blood	Diuretics
Transfusion associated Acute Lung Injury (TRALI)		Absence of signs of volume overload	Inflammatory reaction caused by donor antileukocyte antibodies • Similar in pathophysiology to ARDS and acute lung injury	Supportive care. Severe cases may require mechanical ventilation

Abbreviations: CHF, congestive heart failure; CXR, chest X-ray; DIC, disseminated intravascular coagulation; JVP, jugular venous pressure.

7.2 Clonal Bone Marrow Disorders

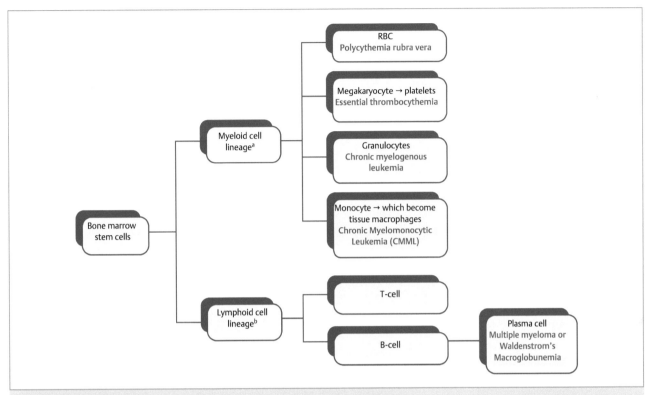

^aDisorders related to this lineage are AML, CML, and myeloproliferative syndromes.

^aDisorder related to this lineage are ALL, CLL, and plasma cell disorders.

Abbreviations: ALL, acute lymphoblastic leukemia; AML, acute myelogenous leukemia; CLL, chronic lymphoblastic leukemia; CML, chronic myelogenous leukemia.

7.2.1 Myeloproliferative Syndromes

Background: In these disorders, there is an overproduction of cells of **myeloid** lineage due to clonal neoplastic proliferation of stem cells (RBC, platelets, granulocytes; either alone or in various combinations).

Chronic myelogenous leukemia (CML)	Proliferation of all **myeloid** lineage cells, with predominant proliferation of granulocytes
Essential thrombocythemia	Predominant proliferation of platelets
Polycythemia rubra vera	Predominant proliferation of RBCs
Myelofibrosis with myeloid metaplasia (primary myelofibrosis)	The bone marrow is replaced with fibrous tissue (myelofibrosis) and proliferation of myeloid cells occurs outside the marrow. Myeloid stem cells migrate to another place (myeloid metaplasia); most commonly to spleen (massive splenomegaly can develop)

All forms of myeloproliferative syndromes have the following common characteristics:
- Elevated cell count in blood may lead to increased blood viscosity and hyperviscosity syndrome.
- Increase in basophils and eosinophils.
- May have splenomegaly.
- May result in development of secondary myelofibrosis (this is called the spent phase of myeloproliferative syndromes).
- May transform into acute leukemia.
- Presence of *JAK2* mutation (highly specific test).
- Bone marrow biopsy is the definitive test.

MRS

- Philadelphia chromosome (t 9;22)
- P = 9 (looks geometrically similar)
- "Philadelphia chromosome" has 22 alphabets if you count it.

Chronic Myelogenous Leukemia

Background: This condition is due to translocation of C-abl oncogene on chromosome 9 to break-point cluster region in chromosome 22. These genes fuse to form the Philadelphia chromosome (t 9;22). This fusion gene codes for a new protein with increased tyrosine kinase activity, which promotes proliferation of myeloid cells.

Presentation: MC presentation is chronic asymptomatic leukocytosis with nonspecific symptoms such as fatigue. Blood smear will reveal increased immature granulocytes (with increase in basophils and eosinophils just like in other myeloproliferative syndromes).

Management steps:

- NSIDx is bone marrow biopsy and cytogenetic analysis for Philadelphia chromosome (best test).
- NSIM is **t**yrosine kinase **inhib**itors (e.g., ima**tinib**, bosu**tinib**, pona**tinib,** etc.).
- If no response to one tyrosine kinase inhibitor, use alternative tyrosine kinase inhibitor or consider hematopoietic cell transplant.

Complication: Chronic myelogenous leukemia (CML) can progress to an accelerated phase or blast crisis, which can mimic acute myelogenous leukemia (AML)/acute lymphoblastic leukemia (ALL).

Differential diagnosis: Leukemoid reaction

[21] LAP score high or normal = leukemoid reaction. Low LAP score = CML.

Sometimes infection can induce florid leukocytosis with prominent white blood cell (WBC) elevation and left shift. Sometimes this can mimic CML, hence called leukemoid.

To distinguish between the two, use leukocyte alkaline phosphatase (LAP) score. LAP is present in normal leukocytes but not in clonal leukocytes.[21]

If distinction cannot be made, testing for Philadelphia chromosome or *JAK2* mutation can also be done.

Essential Thrombocythemia

Background: There is a predominant increase in abnormal platelets (usually > 450,000) with increase in basophils and eosinophils.

Clinical pathophysiology: The clonal platelets-
- May be too sticky, leading to increased risk of vascular thrombosis and its complications (major issue with this disorder).
- Maybe not sticky at all, leading to increased risk of bleeding.

Peripheral blood smear may reveal large immature platelets and platelet aggregates (sticky platelets).

Rx: All patients need to be treated with aspirin. Add hydroxyurea to high-risk patients (age ≥ 60, or prior hx of thrombosis). Hydroxyurea reduces platelet count.

Differential dx: Reactive thrombocytosis, which can be due to:
- Iron deficiency anemia (iron deficiency should be ruled out in essential thrombocythemia).
- Any form of inflammation, e.g., Crohn's disease flare-up, tuberculosis, etc.
- Malignancy.

Polycythemia (Rubra) Vera aka Primary Polycythemia

Background: Predominant increase in clonal RBC production. There is also increase in basophil and eosinophil production, just like in other forms of myeloproliferative syndromes.

Clinical presentation: Itching while taking hot shower can be very bothersome to patients. It happens due to histamine release from abnormal mast cell degranulation.[22] These patients also have increased facial redness (facial plethora).

[22] Itching (particularly after shower) can be seen in other myeloproliferative disorders as well.

Management steps:

- NSIDx is erythropoietin level (typically low or low normal), and test for *JAK2* mutation.
- Treat all patients with phlebotomy at regular intervals and low dose aspirin. Add hydroxyurea to high-risk patients (age ≥ 60, or prior hx of thrombosis).

Polycythemia Vera versus Relative and Secondary Polycythemia

Polycythemia is elevated hematocrit (Hct) or hemoglobin.

There is a difference between relative polycythemia and absolute polycythemia. To understand relative polycythemia, look at the formula below:

- Hb % = Hb in gm/dL
- Hct % = RBC volume/dL

If plasma volume (dL) is decreased, then hemoglobin (measured as ratio) will be high. This is called **relative polycythemia**. This can happen in loss of extracellular fluid without loss of RBCs (e.g., severe diarrhea).[23] This is usually transient and resolves after volume repletion.

In **absolute polycythemia**, there is an actual increase in RBC total mass.

[23] On the other hand, in early stage of acute hemorrhage, Hb/Hct level can be falsely normal due to loss of equal parts of RBC and plasma. After replacing volume deficit with normal saline, the Hb deficit becomes apparent.

	Relative polycythemia	Primary polycythemia[a]	Secondary polycythemia[a]
Hct/Hb	↑	↑	↑
Total RBC mass	N	↑	↑
Urinary erythropoietin level	N	Undetectable or low	↑
Cause	Loss of extracellular fluid volume	Primary myeloproliferative disorder	• Erythropoietin-secreting tumor (e.g., renal cell cancer) • Any condition that causes chronic hypoxia leads to compensatory increase in erythropoietin[b]

[a]Severe forms of both primary and secondary polycythemia are treated with regular interval phlebotomies (drainage of venous blood).

[b]For example, chronic obstructive pulmonary disease, pulmonary arteriovenous malformation, obesity hypoventilation syndrome, obstructive sleep apnea chronic carboxyhemoglobinemia, etc.

In a nutshell

Common features of polycythemia vera and essential thrombocythemia:

- Both can present with severe pain, redness, and swelling in hands and feet. This is called erythromelalgia. Treatment is aspirin.

- There is increased risk of thrombosis and all patients should be on aspirin.

- Patients aged ≥ 60 years or with hx of prior thrombosis are treated with hydroxyurea.

Myelofibrosis with Myeloid Metaplasia

Background/presentation: Abnormal clonal proliferation of myeloid stem cells may lead to increased fibrosis in bone marrow. Bone marrow may get replaced with fibrous tissue (bone marrow aspiration reveals nothing, "dry tap"), and stem cells migrate to another place to produce blood cells; usually to spleen (massive splenomegaly). Peripheral blood smear shows immature cells and tear drop cells. **Rx:** In symptomatic young patients (< 45 years) allogeneic hematopoietic stem cell transplant can be curative. Older symptomatic patients can be managed with hydroxyurea, thalidomide, or lenalidomide.

 In a nutshell

What is Myelophthisic process

- Bone marrow is displaced by either abnormal hematopoietic cells (e.g., due to multiple myeloma) or other processes, such as myelofibrosis, hereditary storage disease, lymphoma, prostate cancer, etc.

- Peripheral blood smear may reveal immature red cells (including reticulocytes), immature WBCs/platelets, and cells with different shapes. Extra-bone marrow hematopoiesis occurs in spleen, hence splenomegaly is usually present.

- Note that myelofibrosis and myleophthisic process from other causes have similar blood smear findings and associated splenomegaly.

7.2.2 Leukemias

Acute leukemias	Chronic leukemias[a]
Faster course	Slower course
Florid production of abnormal cells—increased blasts are seen in peripheral blood smear and bone marrow biopsy	Less production of abnormal cells
"Overcrowding" of bone marrow by the abnormal cells leads to decrease in production of normal cells	Milder symptoms and severity
More than 20% blasts in peripheral blood smear or bone marrow biopsy	Less than 20% blasts in bone marrow biopsy
[a]Note that all form of chronic leukemia can progress on to acute leukemia, which is called blast crisis.	

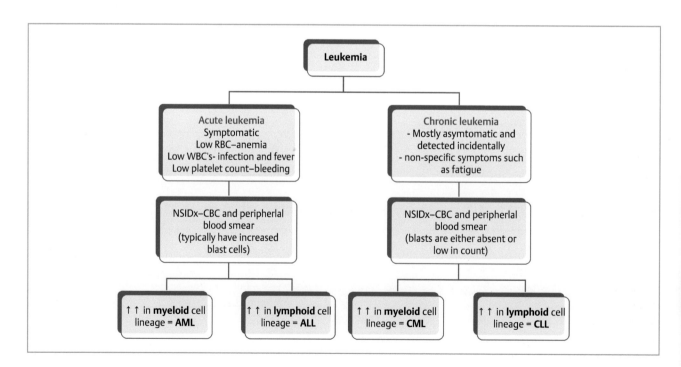

Flow cytometry is commonly used to detect expression of specific CD antigens in leukemic cells, which helps to determine the exact type of leukemia.

Acute Leukemia

Acute leukemia is of two types: AML that commonly occurs in adults and acute lymphoblastic leukemia (ALL) that occurs in children.

Acute Myelogenous Leukemia

Few notes on specific subtypes of AML:
- **P**romyelocytic **l**eukemia (PML)—the M3 subtype of AML has three unique features:
  - **D**isseminated intravascular coagulation (DIC) can occur.
  - **A**uer rods are present.[24]
  - **T**reatment includes vitamin **A** (retinoic acid). In PML, genetic translocation (t15:17) results in formation of abnormal **retinoic acid receptor** which promotes myeloid cell proliferation.
- Monocytic variants of AML can invade tissues and form tissue collections, known as chloromas or myeloid sarcoma.[25] This can occur in virtually any organ or tissue (e.g., chloromas in gums causes gum hypertrophy and bleeding).
- Platelet origin leukemia (i.e., megakaryoblastic leukemia) can cause bone marrow fibrosis due to increased production of platelet-derived growth factor (PDGF), which is a profibroblast.

General management of acute leukemia (AML or ALL)

- For all the acute leukemias (AML or ALL), treatment starts with combination chemotherapy targeted at killing abnormal blasts cells (induction chemotherapy). Additionally for ALL, intrathecal methotrexate is routinely indicated for prophylaxis of meningeal leukemia.
- Remission is a state when most blasts are killed and are no longer detectable. If combination chemotherapy fails to induce remission OR if leukemia is positive for high risk cytogenetic abnormalities, bone marrow transplant is recommended.

Complications: Hyperviscosity syndrome and tumor lysis syndrome.

Hyperviscosity Syndrome

Etiology:

- Conditions with high cellular count such as acute leukemia and myeloproliferative disorders.
- Conditions with high numbers of large proteins such as IgM antibody in Waldenstrom's macroglobulinemia.

Clinical pathophysiology: Blood is highly viscous and thick which leads to relative stasis and easy clot formation in multiple vessels. This can present with blurry vision, confusion/headache, stroke, etc. Fundoscopy may reveal dilated segmented tortuous retinal veins.

Rx: Plasmapheresis if underlying condition is due to increased protein, and leukapheresis if due to increased leukocytes.

Tumor Lysis Syndrome

Etiology: Tumor lysis syndrome can occur with chemotherapy in any malignancy, but is more common in cancers with high cellular count (e.g., AML, ALL, lymphoma with bulky disease).

Clinical pathophysiology: In this syndrome, as cells are killed rapidly by chemotherapy, intracellular contents are spilled into extracellular space, which results in:
- High K^+.[26]
- High PO_4^-: This leads to chelation of free Ca^{2+} leading to hypocalcemia.

MRS

- AML = M for middle age
- ALL = All children are beautiful

MRS

1. PML = 3 words = M3 subtype
2. DATA of M3
- D = DIC
- A = Auer rods
- TA = Treatment of PML includes vitamin A

MRS

Additionally, in AML leukemic cells may be positive for **A**uer rods, **M**yeloperoxidase, and/or **L**eukoesterase.

[24] Auer rods (*white arrow*)

Source: Acute myeloid leukemias (AML). In: Theml H, Diem H, Haferlach T. Color atlas of hematology: Practical microscopic and clinical diagnosis. 2nd ed. Thieme; 2004.

[25] Monocytes are cells that normally enter tissues and change into tissue macrophages.

[26] Remember cells are full of potassium phosphate.

- Spillover of nucleic acids that are later metabolized into uric acid. This leads to hyperuricemia that can cause acute gouty arthritis and increased risk of uric acid stones in kidney.
- Acute tubular necrosis and acute renal failure can occur due to deposition of calcium phosphate and/or uric acid crystals in the renal tubule.

Prevention: In at-risk cases, use prechemotherapy rasburicase[27] or allopurinol and hydration.

Treatment of established cases: Aggressive supportive monitoring, +/− rasburicase.

Chronic Lymphocytic Leukemia

Presentation: Most commonly presents as chronic leukocytosis.

Lab feature:

Smudge cells can be seen in peripheral blood smear (these are fragile cells that easily rupture during smear preparation).

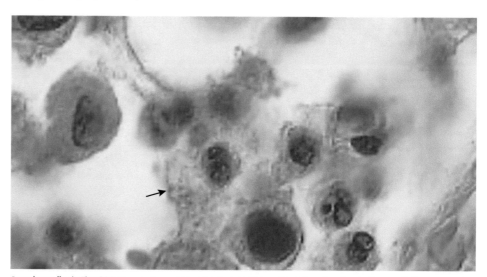

Smudge cells. (HE) × 800. Source: Parvoviridae. In: Riede U, Werner M. Color atlas of pathology: Pathologic principles, associated diseases, sequela. 1st ed. Thieme; 2004.

Dx: Confirmed with peripheral blood **flow cytometry**. Bone marrow biopsy is not needed for confirmation.

Treatment depends upon **staging**:

Stage[a]		Treatment
0	Asymptomatic (lymphocytosis alone)	No treatment needed
I	Lymphadenopathy	If localized, radiation treatment to involved area
II	Splenomegaly	Chemotherapy[c]
III	Anemia[b]	
IV	Thrombocytopenia[b]	

[a]The higher the stage the poorer the prognosis. Development of anemia or thrombocytopenia heralds poor prognosis.

[b]Prednisone is indicated for autoimmune anemia or thrombocytopenia associated with CLL.

[c]For patients aged > 65–70 yrs or with del (17p), use ibrutinib[28]-based regimen. For younger patients without del (17p), use fludarabine-based chemotherapy regimen.

🔆 MRS

ALL SATurday **I CaLL** old people to get their **Ibrutinib** shots, instead of **flu** shots.
Call = CLL; **Old** = typical patient age group
older patients get ibrutinib-based regimen.

28 Ibrutinib = Bruton tyrosine kinase inhibitors
It is also used in other B cell cancers.

9. A 72-year-old male presents with non-specific symptoms of fatigue for the last few months. CBC reveals leukocytosis, with normal hemoglobin and platelet count. Flow cytometry reveals CLL. What is the NSIM?

10. A 76-year-old male diagnosed with CLL now develops splenomegaly. What is the NSIM?

11. A 60-year-old male diagnosed with CLL 4 years ago, now develops significant anemia and thrombocytopenia. LDH and bilirubin is elevated. Direct Coomb's test is positive. Bone marrow aspiration reveals increased megakaryocytes, RBC precursors, and 5% blast cells. What is the NSIM?

Hairy Cell Leukemia

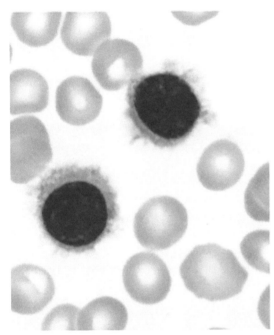

Leukemic cells have hairy projections. Source: Lymphoma, usually with splenomegaly In: Theml H, Diem H, Haferlach T. Color atlas of hematology: Practical microscopic and clinical diagnosis. 2nd ed. Thieme; 2004.

Background: It is a unique form of B cell leukemia.
Presentation: Nonspecific symptoms, such as fatigue. Exam typically reveals splenomegaly.

Work-up:

- CBC may reveal pancytopenia and blood smear may reveal "hairy" cells, which are positive for tartaric resistant acid phosphatase (TRAP).
- Flow cytometry is positive for CD11 and CD22.
- Bone aspiration reveals a dry tap and absent/reduced hematopoietic cells.

Rx: DOC is Cladribine (purine analog).

 MRS

Hairy **lad**'s **double trap:**
- One can see **11** in **H. Double** of 11= 11X 2 = 22; so CD 11 and CD 22 is positive.
- **Lad** = c**LAD**ribine
- TRAP = tartaric resistant acid phosphatase

In a nutshell

Differential diagnosis of dry bone marrow aspirate

Condition	Splenomegaly	Blast cells and immature cells in peripheral blood smear	Pancytopenia
Aplastic anemia	No	No	Yes
Myelofibrosis and other myeloproliferative disorders	Yes	Yes	Usually no (they have increased number of specific types of hematopoietic cells)
Hairy cell leukemia	Yes	Occasional	Yes

 Clinical Case Scenarios

12. Old person presents with pancytopenia in CBC and there is no splenomegaly on exam. Bone marrow aspirate is dry. What is the likely dx?

Myelodysplastic Syndrome

Background: It is a preleukemic disorder, and in certain cases can progress to AML.

Presentation: Hallmark of presentation is unexplained decrease in production of one or more marrow elements (e.g., unexplained anemia or pancytopenia).

Lab findings:

- Blood smear might reveal macrocytosis and small number of dysplastic or blasts cells.
- Bone marrow biopsy will reveal hypercellular and dysplastic marrow +/− blast cells (which should be < 20%).
- Other pathological findings may include ringed sideroblasts and Pelger–Huët cells (bilobed nucleated cells).
- Cytogenetic analysis may reveal 5q deletion, which carries better prognosis.

Treatment: supportive treatment (e.g., for anemia, give transfusion and erythropoietin as needed). Lenalidomide is indicated for RBC transfusion dependent patients with 5q deletion.

 Clinical Case Scenarios

13. A patient with hx of chronic myeloid leukemia, presents with acute symptoms of fatigue and petechial eruption. Peripheral blood smear shows 25% blast cells. What is the likely dx?

    a) ALL.

    b) Blast crisis with conversion to AML.

    c) Myeloid metaplasia.

7.2.3 Plasma Cell Disorders

Background: It is unchecked proliferation of a single clone of plasma cells, which goes on to secrete one type of monoclonal antibody, leading to monoclonal spike (M-spike) in protein electrophoresis.

Protein electrophoresis:

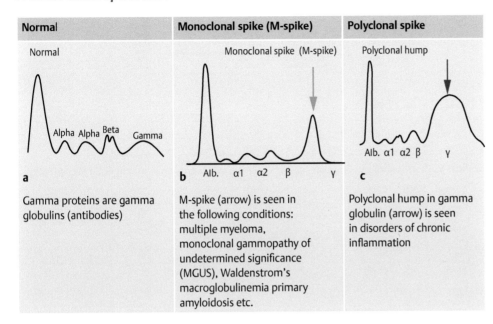

Normal	Monoclonal spike (M-spike)	Polyclonal spike

a Gamma proteins are gamma globulins (antibodies)

b M-spike (arrow) is seen in the following conditions: multiple myeloma, monoclonal gammopathy of undetermined significance (MGUS), Waldenstrom's macroglobulinemia primary amyloidosis etc.

c Polyclonal hump in gamma globulin (arrow) is seen in disorders of chronic inflammation

Types of Plasma Cell Disorders

Plasma cells disorders	Waldenstrom's macroglobinemia[a]	Multiple myeloma (MM)	Monoclonal gammopathy of undetermined significance (MGUS)[b]
Monoclonal antibody type	IgM antibody	IgG antibody (MC type). *Other types include IgA, light chain only, IgD, etc.*	IgG (MC type)
Additional info	–	• M-protein ≥ 3 g/dL • ≥ 10% plasma cells in bone marrow	• M-protein < 3 g/dL • < 10% plasma cells in bone marrow
Elevated β-2 microglobulin[c]	Present	Present	Rare
Anemia	Present[d]	Present	Absent
Hyperviscosity syndrome	Common[e]	Rare	Never present

> **MRS**
>
> M sideways is 3.

[a]FYI- Waldenstrom's macroglobulinemia is a type of non-Hodgkin lymphoma. It is also called lymphoplasmacytic lymphoma. The clonal B cells start secreting large amounts of IgM. Long-term treatment is directed against B cells and is similar to cold autoimmune hemolysis, with rituximab or cyclophosphamide.

[b]MGUS is totally asymptomatic; all lab values are normal except high protein and M-spike in protein electrophoresis. NSIDx is a whole-body low dose computed tomography (CT) without contrast to look for bone lesions. Bone marrow biopsy should also be done. If there is no hypercalcemia, bone lesions and anemia, the M-spike is due to MGUS. Treatment is not necessary. Periodic follow-up of protein electrophoresis is recommended. Some patients may go on to develop myeloma or other lymphoproliferative disorder.

[c]β-2 microglobulin level corresponds to disease severity.

[d]Usually due to IgM-mediated cold autoimmune hemolysis. Bone marrow infiltration can also occur.

[e]IgM (with its pentamer form) is a very large protein. Increased IgM can lead to hyperviscosity syndrome.

In all the above plasma cell disorders, increased monoclonal protein makes the RBCs stick together, giving them the "stacked tires (rouleaux)" appearance.

Multiple Myeloma

Background: Multiple myeloma is a malignancy with unchecked proliferation of a single clone of plasma cells, which secretes one type of monoclonal antibody (MC type is IgG).

Clinical pathophysiology: The excessive proliferation of plasma cell has the following effects:

Hypercalcemia	Plasma cells secrete interleukin-1 which activates osteoclasts, causing bone resorption. This leads to bone pain (commonly back pain) and hypercalcemia. X-ray typically reveals punched-out lytic lesions	
Renal failure and proteinuria	Due to nephrotoxic effect of excessive light chains and hypercalcemia. Filtered light chains in urine are called Bence-Jones protein, which can be detected by urine protein electrophoresis and immunofixation. (This protein is not detected on a routine urinalysis.)	
Anemia	Abnormal plasma cells infiltrate and overcrowd the bone marrow leading to normochromic normocytic anemia	
Increased risk of infection	Particularly with encapsulated organisms such as *Haemophilus influenzae* and *Pneumococcus*. Abnormal plasma cells are using up all resources, so normal plasma cells cannot function and produce effective antibodies	MCC of death in multiple myeloma is infection

Work-up:

- Screening test is serum protein electrophoresis (SPEP) with immunofixation and serum-free light chain assay. For screening purposes, instead of free light chain assay, we can also do 24-hour urine protein electrophoresis (UPEP) and immunofixation.
- After protein electrophoresis shows M-spike and M-protein, NSIDx is bone marrow biopsy (≥ 10% of clonal plasma cells is diagnostic).
- For risk stratification and prognosis, do genetic testing, check β-2 microglobulin levels, C-reactive protein, and plasma cells labelling index: increased levels signal poor prognosis.
- Do whole-body low-dose CT, positron emission tomography (PET)-CT, or MRI. Traditional method of whole-body X-ray is less sensitive.

Management: Depends upon risk stratification, but generally, hematopoietic stem cell transplant is the treatment of choice[29] along with pretransplant chemotherapeutic regimen as follows:
- **B**ortezomib, or **C**arfilzomib +
- **L**enalidomide +
- **D**examethasone

7.3 Lymphomas (Non-Hodgkin Lymphoma and Hodgkin Lymphoma)

These are cancers arising from lymphocytes (mostly B cells or T cells).

	HL	NHL
Etiology	Not clear	• **Infectious**: HIV[a], EBV[a], HTLV[b], *Helicobacter pylori*, etc. • Associated with **autoimmune** condition such as Sjogren's and Hashimoto's disorders • Lymphoma that develops after chemotherapy is likely NHL
Presentation	• Both can present with painless lymphadenopathy with or without constitutional symptoms of fever, drenching night sweats, and weight loss (called B symptoms)[c] • In most patients, the presence of B symptoms signifies advanced stage or bulky disease. In HL, it is a clear negative prognostic marker. In NHL, the relevance is less clear	
	Usually localized at presentation (stage I or II)	More likely to have extranodal involvement and be disseminated at presentation (stage III or IV): • Blood and bone marrow involvement (this is called leukemic phase of lymphoma) • Extralymphatic site (e.g., skin, stomach, liver, etc.)
Best SIDx	Excisional lymph node biopsy • FNAB is not acceptable, as diagnosis requires complete lymph node assessment	
	Presence of R–S cells (binucleated cells) which are positive for CD15 and 30 Source: Hodgkin's lymphomas. In: Riede U, Werner M. Color atlas of pathology: Pathologic principles, associated diseases, sequela. 1st ed. Thieme; 2004.	R–S cells are not present
Prognosis	• Lymphocyte dominant–best prognosis • Lymphocyte depleted–worse prognosis	Burkitt's and immunoblastic have the worst prognosis
Staging	Integrated PET/CT scan of chest, abdomen, and pelvis is usually needed for staging in HL and NHL	
		• Bone marrow biopsy is usually recommended for staging in NHL but is not recommended in HL • Lumbar puncture is also recommended for NHL staging in certain subset of patients with highly aggressive forms[1] or in patients with advance stage

[a]**Burkitt's lymphoma** (NHL) is associated with HIV and EBV infection. HIV is also associated with immunoblastic **lymphoma (NHL).** These types of NHL are highly aggressive.

[b]HTLV-1 = Human T cell lymphocytotrophic virus.

[c]*Although pruritus is relatively common in lymphomas, it is not considered a B symptom.*

Abbreviations: EBV, Epstein–Barr virus; FNAB, fine needle aspiration biopsy; HIV, human immunodeficiency virus; HL, Hodgkin lymphoma; NHL, Non-Hodgkin lymphoma; PET, positron emission tomography; R–S, Reed–Sternberg.

Staging of NHL/HL and treatment

Stage	Definition	Treatment
I	**One** lymphatic group involvement[a] or single lymphoid structure (e.g., spleen, thymus, or Waldeyer's ring)	Chemotherapy[b] plus radiation therapy
II	**Two or more** lymphatic group **on the same side of diaphragm** (e.g., cervical and axillary), or with limited involvement of contiguous lymphoid structure	Cancer is localized enough to be contained within one radiation field
III	Involvement of lymphatic groups or lymphoid structure on **both side of the diaphragm**	Chemotherapy[c] Radiation therapy may be used for selected patients with bulky disease
IV	Widespread involvement[d]	

[a]For example, cervical lymph node group only.

[b]Exception is asymptomatic follicular lymphoma (excluding pathologic grade 3b)[30] which is treated by radiation alone. Follicular lymphoma is usually an indolent disease with good prognosis, where chemo-treatment is not curative anyways.

[c]Exception is **asymptomatic** follicular lymphoma (excluding pathologic grade 3b), where wait and watch is recommended.

[d]Bone marrow involvement is stage IV.

[30]Pathologic grade 3b follicular lymphomas are treated like other NHL with chemoradiation.

MRS

Hodgkin is Very BAD Non-CHOP Rita

Choice of chemotherapy depends on type of lymphoma

	Hodgkin lymphoma	Non-Hodgkin lymphoma
Chemotherapy regimen	**V**inblastine, **B**leomycin, **A**driamycin (**d**oxorubicin), **D**acarbazine[a]	For diffuse large B cell lymphoma (MC form of **Non-**Hodgkin)[b] **C**yclophosphamide, **H**ydroxydaunomycin (doxorubicin), **O**ncovin (vincristine), **P**rednisone, **Rit**uximab[c]
		• For grade 3b follicular lymphoma, use R-CHOP regimen
		• For **symptomatic** follicular lymphoma (excluding grade 3b) use rituximab +/− bendamustine

[a]It is commonly known as AVBD regimen.

[b]It is commonly known as R-CHOP regimen.

[c]Rituximab is a monoclonal antibody to CD20—a common B cell antigen (it is practically an anti-B-cell antibody). It is also used for other B cell-mediated conditions (e.g., granulomatosis with polyangiitis, rheumatoid arthritis, autoimmune hemolytic anemia).

Common adverse effects or sequelae of lymphoma treatment

MRS

Bleo blows lungs

Radiation	Increases risk of thyroid, breast, and lung cancer
Cyclophosphamide	Hemorrhagic cystitis and increased risk of bladder cancer
Doxorubicin	Cardiotoxicity
Vincristine	Neuropathy
Bleomycin	Lung fibrosis
Cisplatin	Renal toxicity

Note: Lymphoma chemotherapy regimens increase risk of secondary leukemias and NHL.

Lymph node enlargement

CCS	NSIM
Rubbery, mobile, and small (< 1 cm) lymph nodes with no hx of fever or weight loss	Observation
Fluctuant lymph node/s that is painful and/or tender	Empiric antibiotics +/− incision and drainage (this is likely infectious)
Immobile, > 2 cm, hard, firm, unilateral lymph nodes	Further investigation: these features are suggestive of malignancy

Clinical Case Scenarios

A 56-year-old female presents with history of multiple enlarged cervical lymph nodes > 2 cm in size for the last few months. She denies any symptoms. CBC is unremarkable.

14. What is the best SIDx?

15. Biopsy reveals pathologic grade 2 follicular lymphoma. What is the NSIDx for staging?

16. Is bone marrow biopsy required?

17. Bone marrow is positive for follicular lymphoma cells. Is chemotherapy recommended?

18. If it was grade 3b follicular lymphoma, what chemotherapy would you give?

7.4 Bleeding Disorders

Platelet disorders generally present with superficial or mucosal bleeding	Clotting factor deficiency generally presents with deep tissue bleeding
Petechiae and purpura	Hemarthrosis (bleeding into the joints)
Epistaxis and menorrhagia	Hematomas (bleeding into the tissues)
Early gum bleeding	Late bleeding (example scenario: immediately after dental surgery, there is no bleeding, but as soon as patient gargles his mouth, bleeding begins)
Gastrointestinal, urinary tract, or CNS bleeding can occur in any type of bleeding.	
Best NSIDx is to check **platelet count.** If normal platelet count, NSIDx is bleeding time and then platelet function study	Best NSIDx is to check **PT/APTT**; if either of them is prolonged, NSIDx is mixing study (discussed below)
Abbreviations: APTT, activated partial thromboplastin time; CNS, central nervous system; PT, prothrombin time.	

Mixing Study

In mixing study, the first step is to mix patient's serum with normal serum.
- If there is a factor deficiency in patient's serum, then mixing would correct PT or APTT. NSIDx is specific factor assay.
- If patient's serum has an inhibitory factor, then mixing study would not correct the abnormality (the inhibitor will block the factor activity in the control serum too). NSIDx specific antibody assay.

For example, in a patient with factor VIII deficiency, APTT would be prolonged and with mixing study APTT would normalize. In a patient with acquired bleeding disorder due to anti-factor VIII antibody (autoimmune disorder), APTT would not normalize with mixing.

7.4.1 Process of Clot Formation after Endothelial Injury

1. Process of temporary platelet plug formation after endothelial injury and its testing

2. Formation of a Stronger Stable Platelet Plug: The Coagulation Cascade and its testing

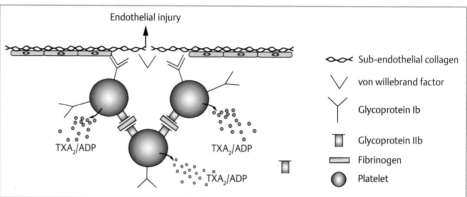

Process of temporary platelet plug formation[a]	Diagnostic assay	Clinical problem (All of the following cause platelet-type bleeding and increased bleeding time)
Step 1: Endothelial injury exposes highly thrombogenic subendothelial collagen, to which **vWF** binds	Ristocetin-induced platelet aggregation test[b]	vWF deficiency (It may also have prolonged APTT due to coexistent factor VIII deficiency)
Step 2: Platelets then bind with vWF via **glycoprotein Ib**		Congenital glycoprotein **Ib** deficiency = **B**ernard–Soulier syndrome. Other features of this syndrome include thrombocytopenia and macrothrombocytes (big platelets)
Step 3: After binding with vWF, platelets get activated and secrete chemical messengers, such as • **TxA2**, which activates other platelets and constricts blood vessels, thereby decreasing blood flow, making it easier for platelets to clog up together • **ADP**, which activates other platelets	ADP/epinephrine-induced platelet aggregation	• Decreased TxA$_2$ synthesis (NSAIDs causes reversible inhibition; aspirin causes irreversible inhibition) • ADP receptor blockers: ticlopidine, prasugrel, ticagrelor, and clopidogrel • Disorders related to platelet storage pool deficiency
Step 4: These activated platelets then attach to other activated platelets using **glycoprotein IIb/IIIa** receptors and through **fibrinogen** bridge		• Glycoprotein IIb/IIIa deficiency (Glanzmann's thrombasthenia) • Glycoprotein IIb/IIIa blockers (abciximab or tirofiban)

[a]The time from initial injury to temporary unstable platelet plug formation is called bleeding time.

[b]Ristocetin closely resembles subendothelial collagen. This test is different from ristocetin cofactor assay (see table below).

Abbreviations: ADP, adenosine diphosphate; APTT, activated partial thromboplastin time; NSAIDs, nonsteroidal anti-inflammatory drugs; TxA2, thromboxane A2; vWF, von Willebrand factor.

	Patient's sample	What lab reagents are used	Test for
Ristocetin-induced platelet aggregation test	Blood (has vWF + platelets)	Ristocetin	vWF and glycoprotein Ib
Ristocetin cofactor assay	Plasma (has vWF but no platelets)	Ristocetin + exogenous platelets	vWF factor only

In vitro platelet aggregation tests in various disorders

Bleeding disorder	Ristocetin	ADP or norepinephrine + collagen	Other associated findings
Bernard–Soulier syndrome	0	Normal	PT/APTT normal Big platelets
von Willebrand disease	variable[a]	Normal	APTT may be elevated
Glanzmann thrombasthenia	Normal	0	PT/APTT normal Normal looking platelets

[a]FYI 4 out of 6 types of vWD have decreased or no aggregation.

Other causes of prolonged bleeding time

- Advanced chronic renal failure leads to platelet dysfunction. Treat active bleeding with DDAVP (vasopressin analogue).
- Platelet deficiency (thrombocytopenia) (discussed later).

Formation of a Stronger Stable Platelet Plug: The Coagulation Cascade and its Testing

With initial endothelial injury and subendothelial collagen exposure, in addition to the platelet cascade, the coagulation cascade gets activated.

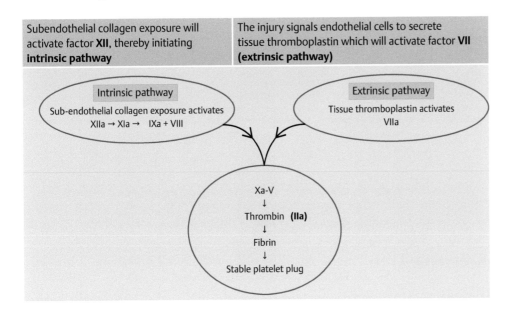

Subendothelial collagen exposure will activate factor **XII**, thereby initiating **intrinsic pathway**

The injury signals endothelial cells to secrete tissue thromboplastin which will activate factor **VII** (**extrinsic pathway**)

These pathways will finally converge to change fibrinogen into fibrin, which will then form a **stable** platelet plug.

Intrinsic pathway
Sub-endothelial collagen exposure activates
XIIa → XIa → IXa + VIII

Extrinsic pathway
Tissue thromboplastin activates
VIIa

Xa-V
↓
Thrombin **(IIa)**
↓
Fibrin
↓
Stable platelet plug

Coagulation Cascade Testing

PT measures the speed of clot formation via **extrinsic** pathway system	⇨	**7 PETs** Factor 7 is the unique factor of the extrinsic pathway
APTT measures the speed of clot formation via **intrinsic** pathway system Remember the factors that are unique to APTT	⇨	**8, 9....11,12** (note:10 is missing)
If both PT and APTT are prolonged, think of factors 2, 5, 10 or fibrinogen deficiency (factor 1)	⇨	**2 × 5 = 10** Factor II is prothrombin, which gets activated to form thrombin (IIa)

Abbreviations: APTT, activated partial thromboplastin time; PT, prothrombin time.

7.5 Lab Parameters in Various Bleeding Disorders

Diagnosis	PT	APTT (PTT)	Platelet count	Bleeding time	Additional diagnostic test or findings
Thrombocytopenia For example, due to ITP or TTP/HUS *Bernard–Soulier syndrome can also have low platelet count*	N	N	Low	↑	– TTP/HUS has schistocytes and increased creatinine – ITP has isolated thrombocytopenia
von Willebrand disease	N	↑ or N	N	↑	NSIDx: plasma vWF antigen, vWF activity and factor VIII activity
Nonthrombocytopenic causes of increased bleeding time	N	N	N	↑	If patient does not have obvious cause, such as hx of antiplatelet agent use (e.g., aspirin) or advanced CKD, NSIDx is platelet aggregation test
Factor 13 deficiency (Note: Factor 13 is a cross linker of fibrin)	N	N	N	N	NSIDx: assessment of clot stability
DIC	↑	↑	Low	↑	Low fibrinogen, elevated D-dimer and schistocytes
• Warfarin intake[a], liver failure, or vitamin K deficiency • Direct thrombin inhibitors such as argatroban/dabigatran • Factor 1 (fibrinogen), 2 (prothrombin), 5, 10 deficiency, or presence of their inhibitors	↑	↑	N	–	If no obvious cause, NSIDx is mixing study
• Unfractionated heparin (PT might be slightly elevated) • Factor 8, 9, or 11 deficiency, or presence of inhibitors[b]	N	↑	N	N	– If no heparin use as the obvious cause, NSIDx is mixing study – In hemophilia, patient will have family hx of affected male relatives

[a]In patients taking warfarin with therapeutic international normalized ratio, APTT might be marginally elevated.

[b]Interestingly factor 12 (aka Hageman factor) deficiency is associated with increased risk of thrombosis rather than bleeding. Factor 12 plays a role in activation of fibrinolysis.

Abbreviations: APTT, activated partial thromboplastin time; CKD, chronic kidney disease; DIC, disseminated intravascular coagulation; HUS, hemolytic uremic syndrome; ITP, immune thrombocytopenic purpura; PT, prothrombin time; TTP, thrombotic thrombocytopenic purpura.

7.5.1 Causes of Thrombocytopenia

Decreased production	Aplastic anemia and bone marrow crowding by leukemic cells
Increased destruction	Autoantibodies against platelets (ITP and other autoimmune disorders like SLE)
Increased consumption	Due to multiple clot formation (DIC and TTP/HUS)

Abbreviations: DIC, disseminated intravascular coagulation; ITP, immune thrombocytopenic purpura; HUS, hemolytic uremic syndrome; SLE, systemic lupus erythematosus; TTP, thrombotic thrombocytopenic purpura.

7.5.2 Immune-Mediated or Idiopathic Thrombocytopenic Purpura

Background: Autoimmune disease with formation of autoantibodies against platelets.

Presentation: Platelet-type bleeding with isolated thrombocytopenia.

Work-up: This is a diagnosis of exclusion. Following causes need to be ruled out:

- Drugs: Antibiotics (β-lactams, linezolid, sulfonamides, vancomycin, etc.), antiepileptics (carbamazepine, phenytoin), heparin, etc.
- In acute cases, peripheral blood smear and creatinine should be done to exclude conditions such as thrombotic thrombocytopenic purpura (TTP) and hemolytic uremic syndrome (HUS). Megathrombocytes (large platelets) are commonly seen in immune thrombocytopenic purpura (ITP).
- Presence of the following points toward an alternate diagnosis: lymphadenopathy, splenomegaly,[31] hepatomegaly, or systemic symptoms (e.g., fever, joint pain, or weight loss).[32]
- Screen for HIV and hepatitis C virus (HCV) infection.

Bone marrow biopsy is usually not needed for dx. It can, however, be done if platelet counts do not respond to initial therapy. Bone marrow will reveal **megakaryocytes** and no other abnormalities.

Management of ITP

It depends on platelet count and presence of bleeding.

```
                        ┌─────────────────┐
                        │ ITP management  │
                        └─────────────────┘

┌──────────────────┐   ┌──────────────────┐   ┌──────────────────┐
│ <10 K platelet   │   │ < 20 K–30K       │   │ > 30 K platelet  │
│ count,           │   │ platelet count,  │   │ count            │
│ OR               │   │ OR               │   │ AND              │
│ Serious CNS or   │   │ Non-serious      │   │ no bleeding      │
│ GI bleeding      │   │ bleeding         │   │                  │
└──────────────────┘   └──────────────────┘   └──────────────────┘

┌──────────────────┐   ┌──────────────────┐   ┌──────────────────┐
│ NSIM             │   │ NSIM             │   │ NSIM             │
│ Platelet         │   │ Steroids         │   │ Observation      │
│ tranfusion +     │   │                  │   │ No treatment     │
│ IV immunoglobulin│   │                  │   │ indicated        │
│ therapy^a or     │   │                  │   │                  │
│ RHO-gam^b +      │   │                  │   │                  │
│ Steroids         │   │                  │   │                  │
└──────────────────┘   └──────────────────┘   └──────────────────┘

        ┌──────────────────┐   ┌──────────────────┐
        │ If platelet      │   │ Platelet count   │
        │ count is still   │   │ > 20–30 K        │
        │ < 20 K–30 K,     │   │ AND              │
        │ OR               │   │ no bleeding      │
        │ has continuing   │   │                  │
        │ issues with      │   │                  │
        │ bleeding         │   │                  │
        └──────────────────┘   └──────────────────┘

        ┌──────────────────┐
        │ NSIM splenectomy │
        │ or rituximab     │
        └──────────────────┘

        ┌──────────────────┐
        │ If above         │
        │ treatment-steps  │
        │ fail to control  │
        │ ITP, NSIM is TPO │
        │ receptor agonist^c│
        └──────────────────┘
```

Legend: K = 1000/µL, so 30 K = 30,000 µL

[a]Splenic macrophages recognize IgG-coated platelets via their IgG receptors and destroy them. Now if we saturate these IgG receptors with immunoglobulins, platelet destruction will slow down.

[b]Rho-Gam (anti-Rh D) can only be given to patients who are Rh(D) positive. It decreases splenic platelet destruction by saturating splenic macrophage receptors with anti-D coated RBCs. Some amount of hemolysis is to be expected.

[c]Thrombopoietin receptor agonist—eltrombopag or romiplostim.

[31] Large splenomegaly points toward hypersplenism (e.g., in chronic liver disease).

[32] If patient has features suggestive of SLE, ANA screening needs to be done, but routine testing with ANA is not recommended.

Antiplatelet antibodies are not used for dx or management of ITP.

Indications for platelet transfusion

Platelet count < 10 K

Platelet count < 50 K with active bleeding

Platelet count < 100 K with serious bleeding (e.g., CNS or ocular bleeding)

 MRS

Romi**plostim** = **PL**atelet **STIM**ulator

7.5.3 Thrombotic Thrombocytopenic Purpura and Hemolytic Uremic syndrome

	TTP	HUS
Background	• Both disorders are associated with generalized clot formation due platelet activation. • Clot formation occurs primarily in small vessels, hence the name "microangiopathic"—similar to DIC. • These clots are platelet rich and do not activate coagulation pathway hence PT/APTT are usually normal.	
Etiology	ADAMTS13 is a protease that normally cleaves large vWF molecule into smaller units. TTP occurs due to reduced activity of this protease, which results in larger vWF molecules circulating and activating platelets. • Autoimmune: involves production of anti-ADAMTS13 antibody. Patients may have underlying autoimmune condition such as SLE • Hereditary (inherited dysfunction of ADAMTS13 protein)	• *E. Coli* O7: H157 serotype infection (commonly found in undercooked hamburgers) and Shigella dysentery • Uninhibited complement activation (hereditary or acquired antibody-mediated defect in complement downregulation)
Presentation	• Thrombocytopenia with platelet-type bleeding—purpura, ecchymosis, gum bleeding, etc. • Microangiopathic hemolytic anemia[a]: RBCs collide with thrombus in arterioles and get damaged, forming fragmented RBCs **(schistocytes)**. These are seen in peripheral blood smear. As in other causes of intravascular hemolysis, elevated LDH, bilirubin, and low haptoglobin are present • +/− fever Source: Normochromic hemolytic anemias. In: Theml H, Diem H, Haferlach T. Color atlas of hematology: Practical microscopic and clinical diagnosis. 2nd ed. 2004. **Schistocytes** (1), target cell (2)	
	More likely to have CNS manifestations, such as confusion (due to clots formation in the small arteries of brain). There is usually minimal creatinine elevation	Predominant manifestation in HUS is renal failure, and this is also more likely to occur in children (clot formation in the arterioles of kidney decreases glomerular blood flow). History of bloody diarrhea points toward HUS, but note that bloody diarrhea may also be seen in TTP
Work-up	ADAMTS13 activity • Low ADAMTS13 activity without presence of inhibitor suggests hereditary cause • Presence of inhibitor suggests acquired autoimmune TTP	Stool culture or PCR, serum antibodies against Shiga-producing organisms, etc.
Management (including supportive treatment)	**Initial treatment for autoimmune TTP:** • Plasma exchange to remove toxins or antibodies that promote clot production • Glucocorticoids • Rituximab If not responding, second-line treatments are high-dose steroids, and/or twice daily plasma exchange **For hereditary TTP**, use plasma infusion instead of exchange (give ADAMTS 13 protein)	• Plasmapheresis + eculizumab (monoclonal antibody to complement protein) • Antibiotics are contraindicated in HUS because dying bacteria release more endotoxin, aggravating the condition

7.5.4 Disseminated Intravascular Coagulation

Definition: This condition is due to generalized platelets and fibrin-rich clot formation.
Etiology: Virtually any condition that can result in severe cellular destruction and massive release of tissue factor can activate the clotting system resulting in disseminated intravascular coagulation (DIC).

- Severe: burns, acute pancreatitis, rhabdomyolysis, etc.
- Obstetrical complications such as abruptio placenta, intrauterine fetal death, amniotic fluid embolism, etc.
- Massive trauma.
- Promyelocytic leukemia.

Clinical pathophysiology	Additional info	
Microangiopathic hemolytic anemia	**Lab findings:**	Schistocyte in peripheral blood smear
		Elevated LDH, bilirubin, and low haptoglobin
Increased clot destruction		Elevated fibrin-degradation products and D-dimer
Increased clot formation[a] leads to increased consumption of factors that form clots		Low platelet, low plasma fibrinogen
		Increased PT/APTT
Increased risk of bleeding[a]	**Reasons are two-fold:**	
Blood oozing out of the venipuncture sites can be an early sign of DIC	Fibrinolytic pathway activation (increased plasmin activity) that occurs in response to increased clot formation[b]	
	Deficiency of platelets, coagulation factors, and fibrinogen due to increased consumption	

[a]DIC is a dual thrombotic and bleeding disorder.

[b]Also, antithrombin III levels are decreased due to increased consumption. Markedly reduced ATIII levels are associated with poor prognosis in patients with DIC and sepsis.

Management:

- Address the underlying cause.
- Supportive transfusion of following products may be needed:
  - Fresh frozen plasma (has coagulation factors as well as fibrinogen).
  - Cryoprecipitate (mostly used to replenish fibrinogen).
  - Platelet, or blood transfusion, as needed.
- If patient develops severe complication related to thrombosis, then anticoagulation (e.g., heparin) can be given.

 In a nutshell

How to differentiate between ITP, TTP/HUS, and DIC *(Cover the last column and try to make the dx in each case)*

PT/APTT (coagulation panel)	Anemia and hemolysis (schistocytes)	Platelet count	Dx
Normal	No	Low	**ITP**
↑	Yes	Low	**DIC**
Normal	Yes	Low	**TTP/HUS**

7.5.5 von Willebrand Disease

Background: It is the MC hereditary bleeding disorder. It is due to deficient or defective production of von Willebrand factor (vWF). There are different subtypes of von Willebrand disease (VWD) and inheritance patterns can be varied. Also, depending upon VWD subtype, APTT may be normal or markedly elevated due to coexistent factor VIII (8) deficiency. Normal vWF prevents degradation of factor 8.

Presentation: Platelet-type **and/or** clotting-factor-deficiency-type bleeding, usually with family hx of bleeding.

- Prothrombin time and platelet count are usually normal.
- Bleeding time is prolonged, but also can be normal in mild disease.

Work-up: When suspected, NSIDx is plasma vWF antigen, vWF activity, and factor VIII activity.

Management:

Other adjunctive treatment options include estrogen and antifibrinolytic agents (aminocaproic acid or tranexamic acid). Antifibrinolytics are effective for mucosal bleeding (gum or nasal bleeding).

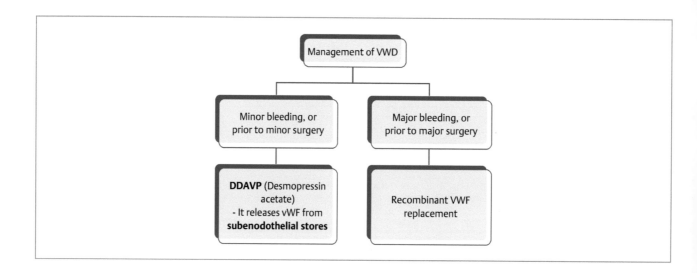

7.5.6 Hemophilia (A, B, and C)

Background: Hemophilia A (factor 8 deficiency) and B (factor 9 deficiency) mostly affect males because they are X-linked recessive disorders. Hemophilia C (factor 11) deficiency can affect both males and females as it is an autosomal recessive disorder.

 Caution

Remember: factors 8, 9, 11 & 12 (not including factor 10) is the intrinsic pathway. What does factor 12 deficiency cause?

Presentation: Clotting-factor-deficiency-type bleeding in a pediatric patient with history of affected relatives.

Work-up: NSIDx is APTT/PT. If APTT is high, NSIDx is mixing study. If mixing study corrects APTT, then NSIDx is specific factor assay and activity.

Factor deficiency	Diagnosis
8	Hemophilia A (MC hemophilia)
9	Hemophilia B
11	Hemophilia C

Management:

Factor 8 deficiency (hemophilia A)	Factor 9 or 11 deficiency
Note that treatment of hemophilia **A** and VWD is similar.	• For bleeding patients, or undergoing surgery, give recombinant factor 9 or 11, or FFP
• May use DDAVP alone for minor bleeding, or minor procedures in mild hemophiliacs (who have acceptable factor 8 activity). DDAVP releases factor VIII from subendothelial stores	
• For major bleeding or surgery, recombinant factor VIII is recommended	

Antifibrinolytic agents (aminocaproic acid or tranexamic acid) are used for mucosal bleeding, as an adjunctive or stand-alone treatment for lower-risk dental procedure, or minor mucosal bleeding.

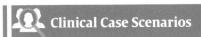 **Clinical Case Scenarios**

19. If mother is a carrier of hemophilia A, what are the chances of her **child** having hemophilia?

20. What are the chances of her **male** baby having hemophilia?

7.5.7 Vitamin K Deficiency

Background: Vitamin **K** is a fat-soluble vitamin. It functions as a cofactor in production of clotting factors 2, 7, 9, and 10 in the liver. Vitamin K is acquired through food and from de novo production by intestinal bacterial flora. Its deficiency can be seen in following situations:

● Babies born at home may not have received vitamin K injection.[33]

● Use of broad-spectrum antibiotics (which decreases bacterial gut flora).

● Patient with hx of fat malabsorption (e.g., chronic pancreatitis). They usually have coexistent vitamin **A, D,** and **E** deficiency.

Lab findings: Elevated prothrombin time (PT)/international normalized ratio (INR); APTT is not as elevated.

Management: Patients with acute bleeding should receive fresh frozen plasma (FFP) or prothrombin complex concentrate along with parenteral vitamin K. In patients without bleeding (elevated INR only), give vitamin K.

7.5.8 Liver Disease and Coagulopathy

Liver produces all clotting factors, except factor VIII and vWF. It also produces anticlotting factors. So in liver failure, elevated INR/APTT do not necessarily correlate with the risk of bleeding as there is concomitant decrease in production of anticlotting factors. Clinical bleeding should be taken into account. Coexistent thrombocytopenia and nutritional vitamin K deficiency may also be present.

[33]All newborn babies should receive vit K, as intestinal bacterial colonization hasn't taken place yet.

 MRS

Fat soluble vitamins are **DrAKE.** Dr DrAKE has malabsorption.

21. A patient with advanced liver disease presents with ongoing gastrointestinal bleeding. INR is 4 and platelet count is 40,000. What is the NSIM, regarding factors and platelet replacement?

7.6 Anticoagulation Agents

7.6.1 Unfractionated Heparin and Low-Molecular-Weight Heparin

UFH	LMWH
Pharmacology: Both types of heparin form a complex with antithrombin III. This complex inactivates factor Xa	
• Used as intravenous infusion for therapeutic purposes • Used subcutaneously for thromboprophylaxis	Subcutaneous form only
Needs monitoring with APTT	• Usually does not need monitoring, as there is a predictable dose response • If needed, can be monitored with antifactor Xa activity (e.g., in a patient with high risk of bleeding) • Has minimal effect on APTT
Antidote—protamine sulfate	Protamine sulfate is less effective but may be used, as it partially reverses LMWH effect
Higher risk of HIT	Lower risk of HIT
Abbreviations: HIT, heparin-induced thrombocytopenia; LMWH, low-molecular-weight heparin; UFH, unfractionated heparin.	

FYI - LMWH dosage needs to be adjusted in patients with GFR of < 30 mL/minute.

Heparin-Induced Thrombocytopenia (HIT)

In some individuals, heparin exposure results in formation of IgG antibodies that bind to heparin/platelet factor 4 complexes, which in turn activate platelets and produce a hypercoagulable state. This can cause generalized (arterial and venous) clot formation. This is called type II heparin-induced thrombocytopenia (HIT). There is Type I HIT, but is benign.

MRS

HIT type II (two) – too dangerous; 5 is an important number here.

	Type I (non-immune mediated-unknown etiology)	Type II (immune-mediated)
Onset after heparin exposure	1–4 days	• 5–15 days • Rarely, it occurs within < 24 hours after heparin exposure[a]
Typical decrease in platelet count	Less severe	More than 50% decrease from baseline platelet levels
Clinical outcome	Benign, and resolves after discontinuation of heparin. No clinical thrombosis	Increased risk of thrombosis and its complication

[a]This can be seen if patient has been exposed to heparin recently and has circulating HIT antibodies.

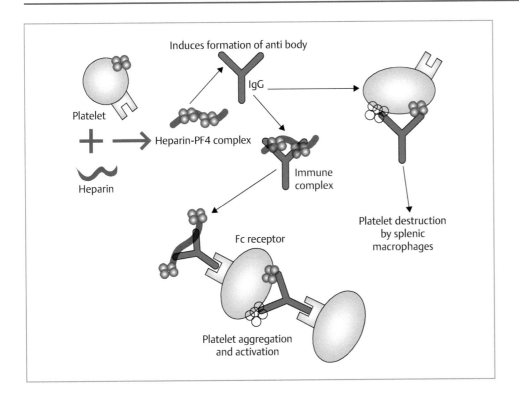

Management of suspected HIT type II

- First SIM: Stop heparin.
- NSIDx: Screening test with ELISA for HIT antibody (anti-PF4 antibody). If patient has high titers with clinically compatible scenario, dx is confirmed.
- If dx is not yet clear (e.g., low or intermediate titers of HIT antibody), NSIDx is functional platelet assay for HIT. This tests the ability of the HIT antibody from patient's serum to activate platelets in vitro (confirmatory test). There are two types—serotonin release assay and heparin-induced platelet aggregation test.

Rx: Anticoagulation is started as soon as diagnosis is made. Use any of the following:

Argatroban or bivalirudin	⇨	Direct thrombin antagonist
Danaparoid	⇨	Recommended in pregnant patients
Fondaparinux	⇨	Recommend in patients with hepatic impairment

Warfarin is initiated after platelet count returns to normal (i.e., > 150,000). There is not much clinical experience of novel oral anticoagulants with HIT, hence not commonly used.

7.6.2 Warfarin

Pharmacology: Warfarin inhibits vitamin K carboxylation and production of coagulation factors 2, 7, 9, and 10 in liver. It also inhibits the carboxylation of anticoagulant proteins C and S.

Dose monitoring:

- All patients on chronic warfarin therapy are regularly monitored with INR.[34]
- For most clinical situations target INR range is 2 to 3 (except in mechanical mitral valve, where therapeutic INR range is 2.5 to 3.5).

[34]INR is a ratio created to standardize prothrombin time (PT) values obtained from various laboratory methods that are commercially available.

Management of supratherapeutic INR

INR	What to do?
> 3 but < 5, with no significant bleeding	• Omit a dose
≥ 5–9, with no significant bleeding	• Omit 1–2 doses, **OR** • Omit a dose **and** give small dose **oral** vitamin K (1–2.5 mg). This is preferred in patients with high risk of bleeding (e.g., patient with severe HTN)
≥ 9; with no significant bleeding	• Hold warfarin, **AND** give higher dose vitamin K (> 2.5–5 mg). Monitor INR frequently and give vitamin K as needed
≥ 20 **OR** serious or life-threatening bleeding at any INR level	• Hold warfarin **AND** give intravenous vitamin K (which takes time to reverse INR) + fresh frozen plasma or prothrombin complex concentrates (which has immediate effect on INR)
In patients with life-threatening or serious bleeding, assess risks and benefits of continuing anticoagultaion	

Drugs Interactions of Warfarin (High Yield)

Reduces effect	Potentiates effect
Cholecystyramine and colestipol decrease absorption of warfarin	Almost all antibiotics may potentiate warfarin effect by decreasing gut flora that produces vitamin K. Note: Narrow-spectrum antibiotics not directed against gram-negative rods have less or no effect. For example, first-generation cephalosporin—cephalexin, have no effect on INR
Hepatic cytochrome p450 inducers increase warfarin metabolism For example, antiepileptics (barbituarates, carbamazepine), St. John's wort, rifampin, etc.	Hepatic cytochrome p450 inhibitors increase warfarin levels • **I**—**i**soniazid, **i**ndinavir • **C**iprofloxacin and other quinolones • **A**ntidepressants (SSRI) • **A**—**a**zole antifungals, **a**miodarone, **a**ntacid (cimetidine, ranitidine, and omeprazole). Note: famotidine has no effect on warfarin • **M**acrolides, except azithromycin • **E**thanol (**a**cute ingestion). Note: chronic ingestion of alcohol induces cyto-p450 system
Diet: increased vitamin K intake, commonly found in green leafy vegetables	Almost all NSAIDs and aspirin may potentiate effect through different mechanisms. Even acetaminophen can do it, but is considered more safe
	Phenytoin, **a**spirin, **d**oxycycline, and **s**ulfonamides can displace warfarin from plasma-binding proteins
	Coadministration of vitamin E, which also inihibits vitamin K-dependent carboxylase, may potentiate effect of warfarin
	Propranolol increases warfarin bioavailability. Other beta-blockers usually do not have this effect

🔍 Clinical Case Scenarios

Patient recently started on warfarin **without** coadministration of heparin develops sharply demarcated erythematosus rash, which progresses to hemorrhagic bullae.

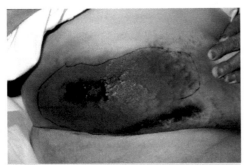

Source: Skin. In: Siegenthaler W. Siegenthaler's differential diagnosis in internal medicine: From symptom to diagnosis. 1st ed. Thieme; 2007.

22. What is the Dx?

23. What is the mechanism?

24. What protein is the patient most likely deficient in?

7.6.3 Novel Oral Anticoagulants (aka Direct Oral Anticoagulants)

- Direct thrombin inhibitor (dabig**atran**)
- Factor Xa inhibitor (api**xaban**, rivaro**xaban**, edo**xaban**)

Advantage of the direct oral anticoagulants over warfarin include no need to monitor INR and is not affected by diet.

 MRS

– Thrombin **an**tagonist
– **Xa Ban** (i.e., Xa is banned)

What is the likely diagnosis in each of the following scenario?

Question	Clinical presentation	PT	APTT	Bleeding time
25.	Found to have deep venous thrombosis	N	↑	N
26.		↑	N	N
27.	Hx of recurrent bleeding with no obvious cause (e.g., no liver/renal disease or anticoagulation therapy)	N	N	N
28.		N	↑	↑ (however patient has normal platelet count)
29.		N	N	↑ (Platelet count is found be low and big platelets are seen in blood smear)

Answers

1. Fecal occult blood test.

2. Colonoscopy. It is also the most appropriate step in management.
   For "exam" purpose, noninvasive tests are usually the 1st SIDx or the 1st SIM. The invasive tests are usually the best SIDx or the best SIM.
   (Invasive tests are more likely to give you the definite answer, but noninvasive testing should be done first).

3. β-thalassemia major.

4. Anemia of chronic disease due to rheumatoid arthritis.

5. Biliary colic, in a patient with chronic hemolysis, likely due to formation of calcium bilirubinate stone.

6. This is intravascular hemolysis in the setting of acute infection (likely urinary tract infection). Abdominal pain can occur due to intravascular hemolysis. This could be G6PD deficiency or sickle cell anemia.

7. Hemoglobin assay to look for sickle cell trait.

8. Thymoma with pure red cell aplasia.

9. Regular follow-up.

10. Ibrutinib-based chemotherapy.

11. Initiate treatment with steroids before initiating treatment of CLL. Clinical picture is suggestive of autoimmune process.

12. Hairy cell leukemia.

13. (**b**) Blast crisis with conversion to AML.

14. Excisional lymph node biopsy.

15. PET/CT scan of chest, abdomen, and pelvis.

16. Yes; bone marrow biopsy is recommended for staging in NHL.

17. For asymptomatic follicular lymphoma that is not grade 3b, wait and watch approach can be done.

18. R-CHOP regimen.

19. 1/4 (25%).

20. 1/2 (50%)

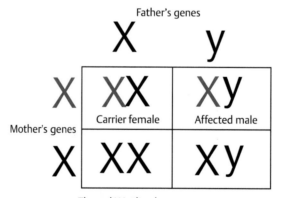

The red X is the chromosome carrying homophillia

21. Give FFP +/− vitamin K. Platelet transfusion is also indicated.

22. Warfarin-induced skin necrosis.

23. Warfarin also inhibits carboxylation of anticoagulant protein C and S. In patients with inherited heterozygote deficiency of proteins C or S, warfarin initiation can lead to transient hypercoagulable state with subsequent development of superficial clotting in dermal vessels and necrosis. Note: as this is a relatively rare condition, bridging with heparin while initiating warfarin is not routinely indicated.

24. Protein C or S

25. Antiphospholipid antibody syndrome can present with hx of recurrent abortions in second trimester and recurrent venous or arterial thrombosis. NSIDx: anticardiolipin antibody and lupus anticoagulant (*note, anticoagulant is a misnomer*).

26. Factor 7 deficiency.

27. Factor 13 deficiency (cross-linker of fibrin).

28. vWF deficiency.

29. Bernard–Soulier syndrome.

8. Infectious Disease

"Bacteria, just like any other life form, need energy to survive, multiply, and colonize.
Patients with uncontrolled diabetes have high sugar content in their sweat and connective tissues, which can become a perfect energy source for bacterial colonization and subsequent infection. To make matters worse, diabetic patients also frequently have immunosuppression and microvasculopathy."

8.1 Infection and Sepsis

Systemic infection with any microbe can present with nonspecific features of fever, tachycardia, leukocytosis, altered mental status, etc. As infection progresses, patients can start looking sicker, and develop decompensation in various organ systems, as following:

Circulatory	Persistent hypotension, despite adequate IV fluids resuscitation → vasopressor requirement
	Lactic acidosis
Kidney	Oliguria or anuria (renal failure), acute tubular necrosis
Lung	Tachypnea → acute lung injury → acute respiratory distress syndrome
CNS	Agitation, confusion, coma
Hematologic	Anemia, thrombocytopenia, DIC, etc.
Liver	Ischemic or septic liver injury
To prevent this, prompt diagnosis and aggressive treatment are of utmost **urgency**.	

Abbreviations: CNS, central nervous system; DIC, disseminated intravascular coagulation.

Clinical pearl: any patient who presents with fever of unknown source, think of an infectious source from head to toe: CNS → upper respiratory tract → lower respiratory tract → heart → GI → urinary tract → joints → skin. This helps in history taking and to make the diagnosis.

8.2 A Simplified Approach to Antibiotics for Empiric Therapy

Antibiotics	Gram positive (staphylococcus/ streptococcus, except MRSA)	Gram negatives	Anaerobes	Pseudomonas
• B-lactamase resistant narrow spectrum penicillins (oxacillin, cloxacillin, dicloxacillin, nafcillin)[a] • First generation cephalosporins[b]	■			
• Third generation cephalosporin[c]	■	■		
• Ciprofloxacin (IV, PO) • Aztreonam (IV) • Ceftazidime (IV) • Amikacin, Gentamicin, Tobramycin[d]		■		■
• Metronidazole			■	
• Cefepime (IV)	■	■		■
• Amoxicillin-clavulanate (oral) • Ampicillin-sulbactam (IV)	■	■	■	
• Piperacillin- tazobactam (IV) • Ticarcillin-clavulanate (IV)	■	■	■	■
• (IV Meropenem, IV Doripenem)[e]	■	■	■	■
• Clindamycin[f]	■		■	

[a]Other penicillins (such as Penicillin V or G, amoxicillin, ampicillin) are good against the Streptococcus group (*S. viridans, S. pneumoniae, S. pyogenes*) but not against staph, as staph usually have B-lactamases which deactivate penicillins.
[b]For example, oral cephalexin, IV cefazolin.[1]
[c]IV forms are ceftriaxone, cefotaxime, and ceftazidime. Oral forms are cefpodoxime and cefdinir. These drugs have good Streptococcus/Staphylococcus coverage as well, but not as good as 1st generation cephalosporins or B-lactamase resistant narrow-spectrum penicillins.[1]
[d]Aminoglycosides for pseudomonas is usually not used as monotherapy, but as an adjunctive treatment for serious infections.

[1]Cephalosporins can be given in patients with mild penicillin allergy (e.g., rash), but are contraindicated in patients with severe penicillin allergy (e.g., anaphylaxis, Stevens–Johnson syndrome, allergic interstitial nephritis).

[e]Unlike piperacillin-tazobactam, carbapenems cover extended spectrum beta-lactamase (ESBL)-producing superbugs, such as *Acinetobacter baumannii* or ESBL *E. coli/Klebsiella*.[2]

[f]The old dictum of treating above-diaphragm infection (e.g., lung abscess) with clindamycin and below-diaphragm infection (e.g., intestinal infection or perforation) with metronidazole no longer applies. Clindamycin is no longer preferred due to increased risk of *C. difficile*. The preferred antibiotics for treatment of aspiration pneumonia now are amoxicillin-clavulanate, or third-generation cephalosporin + metronidazole.

Abbreviations: IV, intravenous; MRSA, methicillin-resistant Staphylococcus aureus

[2]Meropenem or imipenem may be the right answer in a patient with prolonged hospitalization and evidence of active gram-negative infection who does not improve despite adequate antibiotic therapy.

The only difference of coverage in between (meropenem, doripenem, imipenem) and ertapenem, is that ertapenem does not cover *Pseudomonas*.

8.2.1 Other Bacteria and Their Antibiotic Coverage

Bacteria	Antibiotic coverage	
MRSA (methicillin-resistant *Staphylococcus aureus*)	**Intravenous agents:** vancomycin (DOC) Second line—daptomycin (IV only), linezolid (oral or IV), IV ceftaroline (fifth-generation cephalosporin), IV quinupristin, or IV dalfopristin. **Oral agents:** doxycycline, clindamycin, and sulfamethoxazole-trimethoprim.	All MRSA antibiotics have good gram-positive coverage, except doxycycline which does not have good Streptococcus coverage.
Atypical bacteria (*Legionella, Chlamydia, Mycoplasma, Coxiella,* **etc.**)	Macrolides (azithromycin) Doxycycline Respiratory fluoroquinolones (levofloxacin)	
Listeria monocytogenes	Ampicillin	
Bacillus Anthracis	**C**iprofloxacin or **D**oxycycline ☺**MRS ABCD**	
Syphilis	Penicillin or doxycycline	

Abbreviations: DOC, drug of choice; IV, intravenous.

☺ **MRS**

Cephalosporins are LAME because they do not cover:
- Listeria
- Atypicals
- Mycobacteria
- Enterococcus

Clinical pearl: Do not use ceftriaxone or cephalexin to treat UTI caused by Enterococcus.

8.2.2 Example Clinical Cases

Condition	Coverage needed for	Examples of empiric coverage
Cellulitis without MRSA risk factors[a]	Gram positives (staph and strep)	Cephalexin or IV cefazolin or nafcillin
• Diverticulitis • Fistulating Crohn's disease	GI flora (anaerobes and gram negatives)	Ceftriaxone[b] + metronidazole or Ampicillin-sulbactam
Infections with risk factor for Pseudomonas[c]	Pseudomonas	IV cefepime or IV piperacillin-tazobactam
Hospital-acquired catheter infection	MRSA	IV vancomycin
Community-acquired pneumonia requiring hospitalization	Streptococcus spp., gram negatives (Moraxella catarrhalis, Haemophilus influenzae), and atypicals.	Ceftriaxone + azithromycin or Cefpodoxime + doxycycline

[a]**MRSA risk factors:** IVDA (intravenous drug abuse), human immunodeficiency virus (HIV) positive, recent prior antimicrobial therapy, hemodialysis, recent hospitalization, residence in long-term care facility such as nursing homes, etc.

[b]Nowadays third-generation cephalosporins are preferred over quinolones (e.g., ciprofloxacin), because quinolones are associated with higher risk of *C. difficile and other side effects.*

[c]Risk factors for *Pseudomonas* infection include the following:

Abbreviations: GI, gastrointestinal; IV, intravenous; MRSA, methicillin-resistant *Staphylococcus* aureus.

- Neutropenic fever (*always look at WBC count in a question about empiric antibiotic therapy*)
- Burns
- Hospital-acquired pneumonia, especially in intubated patient
- Chronic granulomatous disease
- Severe pulmonary infection in a patient with cystic fibrosis
- Diabetes mellitus with certain infections such as malignant otitis externa
- Cellulitis and osteomyelitis associated with a punctured sole wound

8.2.3 Indications for Antibiotic Prophylaxis in Adults

Clinical situation	Drug of choice
Close contacts of patients with *Neisseria meningitidis*	Rifampin or fluoroquinolone
Significant bite wounds	(Ampicillin-sulbactam) or (amoxicillin-clavulanate)
High-risk cardiac defects undergoing high-risk procedures require endocarditis prophylaxis	Amoxicillin

8.2.4 Notable Side Effects of Antibiotics

Antibiotic	Notable side effects	
Penicillin	All types of hypersensitivity reaction (type I, II, III, and IV)	An uncommon but unique side effect of oral pen-VK is black hairy tongue
Trimethoprim-sulfamethoxazole	• Rash, angioedema, allergic interstitial nephritis, serum sickness, etc.	• Folate deficiency • Hyperkalemia • Hemolysis (in patients with G6PD deficiency)
Doxycycline	Pill esophagitis, tooth discoloration in children	
Linezolid	Thrombocytopenia, serotonin syndrome	
Fluoroquinolones	Tendinitis, Achilles tendon rupture, irreversible neuropathy, and bony growth abnormalities (use with caution in children)	
Cefotetan (second-generation cephalosporin with anaerobic coverage) and metronidazole	Disulfiram-like effect (with alcohol)	
Vancomycin	• Renal toxicity • **Red man syndrome**: itching and erythematous flushing reaction during infusion due to histamine release. In rare situation chest pain and hypotension can occur. This is not an allergic reaction and is related to rate of infusion. **Rx:** use antihistamines (diphenhydramine + ranitidine), and slow down the infusion rate.	

8.3 Skin Infections

Condition (given below in order of severity from superficial to deep infection)	Presentation	Microbial cause	Empiric therapy
Infection of epidermis = **Impetigo**[a] Source: Impetigo. In: Laskaris G, ed. Color Atlas of Oral Diseases. Diagnosis and Treatment. 4th ed. Thieme; 2017.	Papules, vesicles, pustules and/or bullae containing yellow fluid, surrounded by erythema. When pustules/bullae break, they form a honey-colored crust. (Look for weepy, oozy, crusty, dirty looking skin rash)	Staph. aureus or B-hemolytic streptococcus	• If mild and localized, use topical mupirocin or retapamulin. • If severe or widespread, use oral semi-synthetic penicillins (e.g., cloxacillin) or cephalexin[b]
Infection of dermis and epidermis = **Erysipelas** Source: Erysipelas. In: Sterry W, Paus R, Burgdorf W, ed. Thieme Clinical Companions - Dermatology. 1st ed. Thieme; 2006.	Shiny red, edematous, patch found particularly on face, arms or legs. May be painful. (Look for raised, clearly demarcated borders)	B-hemolytic streptococcus	• If mild, use oral amoxicillin or penicillin (usually staph coverage isn't required). • If severe, use IV ceftriaxone or cefazolin.
Infection of dermis and subcutaneous tissue = **Cellulitis** **Footnote:** Facial cellulitis on the right side due to dental abscess. Source: Cellulitis. In: Laskaris G, ed. Color Atlas of Oral Diseases. Diagnosis and Treatment. 4th ed. Thieme; 2017.	Redness, swelling, increased temperature and tenderness over the involved skin area. Borders are not raised or clearly demarcated	S. aureus or B-hemolytic Streptococcus	• Management is discussed on next page

[a]This is contagious, and outbreaks can occur.[3]

[b]In culture proven S. pyogenes, penicillin or amoxicillin alone should suffice.

*In patients with immunosuppression, morbid obesity, or uncontrolled diabetics, soft-tissue infection can cross the fascial planes and involve muscles causing necrosis = **necrotizing fasciitis**.*

Abbreviations: IV, intravenous; MRSA, methicillin-resistant *Staphylococcus* aureus.

Impetigo and erysipelas can progress to lymphangitis or cellulitis.

Potential autoimmune complication of strep infection (e.g., erysipelas, cellulitis, strep throat) is Rheumatic fever and postinfectious glomerulonephritis (glomerulonephritis can also occur with staph infection).

[3]D/Dx (differential dx) of impetigo is **eczema herpeticum**
Causative organism: HSV infection
Presentation: Painful rash with clear vesicles with underlying erythematous area. When the vesicles rupture, they leave behind punched-out ulcers. Vesicles might be hemorrhagic, which form dark red crusting after rupture.
Rx: Systemic acyclovir

Cellulitis management depends on the type of cellulitis:

1. Management of non-purulent cellulitis

Severity	MRSA risk factor[a]	Empiric therapy
Cellulitis with signs of severe infection (e.g., fever, tachycardia) - requires hospitalization. NSIM is blood culture and IV antibiotics	Present	IV vancomycin or ceftaroline - If no improvement, initiate gram-negative coverage
	Absent	IV cefazolin - If no improvement, initiate MRSA and/or gram-negative coverage
Mild (outpatient treatment)	present	• Trimethoprim-sulfamethoxazole, or • Amoxicillin (for strep) + doxycycline or minocycline[b], or • Oral clindamycin (last choice)
	Absent	Cephalexin or dicloxacillin

[a]Risk factors for MRSA include - IVDA (intravenous drug abuse), HIV positive status, recent prior antimicrobial therapy, hemodialysis, recent hospitalization, residence in long-term facilities such as nursing homes, etc.

[b]Unlike clindamycin or trimethoprim-sulfamethoxazole, doxycycline doesn't have good streptococcus coverage (hence it is combined with amoxicillin or cephalexin).

Clindamycin is increasingly falling out of favor due to increased risk of C difficile infection.

2. Management of - Purulent Cellulitis or - abscess with significant cellulitis, systemic symptoms or immunosuppression

These cases are almost always due to Staph and MRSA coverage is needed.

- Send wound cultures
- I&D if there is an abscess

High risk population for Infective endocarditis[a]	Empiric therapy
YES (patient needs strep coverage)	Severe infection: IV Vancomycin or Daptomycin Mild infection : doxycycline + amoxicillin or sulfamethoxazole-trimethoprim
NO (doesn't warrant strep coverage)	Doxycycline alone should suffice.

[a]Examples of high risk conditions include prosthetic cardiac valve (including bioprosthetic heart valve), previous infective endocarditis, unrepaired cyanotic congenital heart disease, etc. Please refer to infective endocarditis section discussed later in this chapter.

Clinical tip : Note in all the above situations if Cellulitis is associated with periodontal disease, perirectal location, pressure ulcer or with prominent necrosis , it warrants anaerobic coverage.

8.3.1 Necrotizing Fasciitis and Differential Diagnoses

The following severe soft tissue infections usually have signs of systemic toxicity (Toxic shock syndrome is included in this table as sometimes cellulitis can lead to toxic shock syndrome and cause severe systemic toxicity).

	Necrotizing fasciitis	Gas gangrene	Toxic shock syndrome
Causative organism	Polymicrobial (gram positive, gram negative, anaerobes, MRSA, etc.) -or Group A ß-hemolytic streptococci	*Clostridium perfringens* or *Clostridium histolyticum* *(gram positive bacilli)*	*Staph. aureus*[a]
History	May not have bacterial point of entry at all, or may have coexistent groin ulcer or colonic fistula.	More likely to have hx of trauma. Trauma can be as minor as intramuscular injection, or as major as surgery.	Look for foreign body in situ (tampons or prosthesis), or an active site of *Staph.* infection, (e.g., osteomyelitis, or even cellulitis)
Clinical feature	They do have overlapping features – Crepitus (more prominent in gas gangrene) – Gas in tissue seen in imaging (mostly along fascial planes in Necrotizing fasciitis) – Skin is dark blue to black necrotic – Severe pain out of proportion to clinical exam findings – Elevated creatine kinase		• Sick looking patient with severe systemic features (as in necrotizing fasciitis and gas gangrene) • **Generalized red sunburn like rash** (diffuse erythroderma) involving palms and soles and/or maculopapular rash • This rash can later desquamate after about a week or so (shown below in hands)
	 Source: Necrotizing Fasciitis. In: Sterry W, Paus R, Burgdorf W, ed. Thieme Clinical Companions - Dermatology. 1st ed. Thieme; 2006.	 Footnote: multiple lucent gas collections deep to the deltoid muscle. Source: Pathology. In: Gunderman R, ed. Essential Radiology. Clinical Presentation, Pathophysiology, Imaging. 2nd ed. Thieme; 2000.	 Source: Toxic Shock Syndrome Caused by Methicillin-Resistant Staphylococcus aureus (MRSA) After Expander-Based Breast Reconstruction. In: Suga H, Shiraishi T, Takushima A, Harii K. Eplasty; 2016.
Treatment of choice	Surgical exploration. Surgical specimens' wound gram stain/culture can differentiate in between them.		Removal of foreign body
Adjunctive empiric antibiotic treatment (Intravenous immunoglobulin, which neutralizes toxins, can be tried in severe cases.)	One broad spectrum antibiotic (meropenem or piperacillin/tazobactam or ampicillin-sulbactam) + Clindamycin[b] + MRSA coverage- Vancomycin or daptomycin	Penicillin + clindamycin[b] +/- hyperbaric oxygen therapy	Clindamycin[b] + Oxacillin, or vancomycin (if MRSA suspected)

[a]This is due to colonization or infection with *Staph. aureus* that produces toxic-shock-syndrome-toxin (TSST). This toxin is unique in that it non-specifically activates T-helper cells, which release excess inflammatory mediators into the bloodstream causing SIRS, sepsis and even death.

[b]Clindamycin also decreases exotoxin production

8.3.2 Diabetic Foot Ulcer Infection

Type	Features	Treat
Nonlimb-threatening mild infection	Minimal cellulitis (erythema) that extends not more than 2 cm from a superficial ulcer that does not go beyond superficial fascia and lacks systemic toxicity	**Treat as cellulitis (as above)** • No risk factor for MRSA, use any one of the following: cephalexin, dicloxacillin, amoxicillin-clavulanate, or clindamycin • If risk factor for MRSA present, use either clindamycin, or trimethoprim-sulfamethoxazole alone or combination of cephalexin + doxycycline
Moderate infection	Any one of the following present: erythema extends >2 cm, lymphangitic streaking or infection goes beyond superficial fascia (to involve muscle, tendon, etc.)	Mostly this requires coverage for staph, strep, gram negatives, and anaerobes. Use antibiotics that cover MRSA, if risk factors present, e.g., Amoxicllin-clavulanate (covers anaerobes, GNR, gram positives) + trimethoprim-sulfamethoxazole (covers MRSA)
Severe infection	Infection with systemic toxicity or limb-threatening infection	NSIM is to admit the patient, do careful wound debridement, and start broad-spectrum IV antibiotic that covers gram-negative bacilli, anaerobes, and MRSA. Urgent consultation and a multidisciplinary approach are needed.

aCiprofloxacin and levofloxacin have good pseudomonal coverage. Use them if macerated looking wound or hx of significant water exposure.

Abbreviations: IV, intravenous; MRSA, methicillin-resistant Staphylococcus aureus.

In patients with diabetic foot ulcer infection, workup for osteomyelitis is recommended if one or more of the following are present:

- Elevated ESR > 70 mm/h.
- Bone exposure or probe to bone positive.
- Ulcer size > 2 cm².
- Duration of ulcer >1–2 weeks.

Clinical Case Scenarios

24 y/o F with history of diabetes presents with raised, erythematous, weepy rash with clear border on her face. Patient reports of malaise.

1. What is the likely diagnosis?
2. What is the likely causative organism?
3. How do you treat it?

8.4 CNS Infections

In a nutshell: clinical presentation and likely Dx

Fever + headache ± seizures +	Likely Dx
+ Stiff neck or other signs of meningismus[a]	Meningitis
+ Focal neurological deficit (e.g., right lower extremity weakness)	Brain abscess or toxoplasmosis
+ Altered mental status ± personality change	Encephalitis[b]

[a]Signs of meningeal inflammation include photophobia, Kernig's sign (inability to straighten the leg when hip is flexed), and Brudzinski's sign (neck flexion causes reflexive flexion of hips and knees).[4]

[b]Viral causes of encephalitis include:

- HSV-1.[5]
- Arboviruses: western equine encephalitis, eastern equine encephalitis, Japanese encephalitis, West Nile virus, Venezuelan encephalitis, St. Louis encephalitis, California encephalitis, etc.
- Enteroviruses.

Encephalitis can also be associated with **S**ystemic **L**upus **E**rythematosus (SLE), acute disseminated encephalomyelitis, etc.

[4]Remember that subarachnoid hemorrhage can present similarly with signs of meningeal inflammation and fever.

[5]HSV-2 does not cause encephalitis, but may cause meningitis.

8.4.1 General Management of Suspected CNS Infection

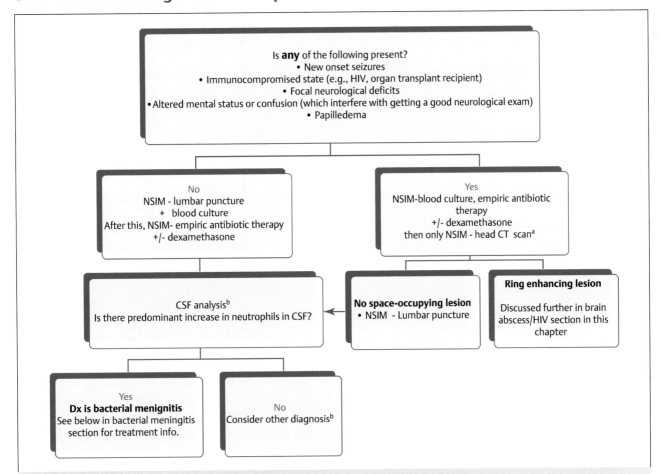

[a]If there is a suspicion for space-occupying lesion, perform computed tomography (CT) scan prior to lumbar puncture as lumbar puncture can precipitate brainstem herniation in patients with elevated intracranial pressure (ICP). Also give antibiotics, as diagnostic workup should not delay life-saving antibiotic therapy.

[b]**CSF analysis table**

Abbreviation: CSF, cerebrospinal fluid.

	Bacterial	Viral	Fungal or Lyme/rickettsia	Tuberculosis
Cell count	↑↑↑↑	↑↑	↑↑	↑↑
Differential	Neutrophils	Lymphocytes	Lymphocytes	Lymphocytes
Protein	↑↑	↑	↑	Can be ↑↑↑↑
Glucose	Low	Normal[a]	Normal or low	Low

[a]As opposed to viruses, organisms like bacteria, fungi, and mycobacteria directly use glucose for energy production.

8.4.2 Bacterial Meningitis

Microbiology[6]:

Age	MCC in this age group
Neonate (<1 month)	*Streptococcus agalactiae* • 2nd MCC is *E. coli*.
1 month to 2 years	*S. pneumoniae*
2 years to 18–21 years, adults in military, or living in dormitories	*N. meningitidis* 2nd MCC is *S. pneumoniae*
>18–21 years (after one leaves college or dormitories)	*S. pneumoniae*
Other groups:	
HIV	MCC is *Streptococcus* (NOT *Cryptococcus*)
Ventriculoperitoneal shunt	MCC is coagulase-negative Staph (*S. epidermidis*)

Empiric Treatment of Bacterial Meningitis

Age group	Empiric IV antibiotics of choice[a]
< 7 days of age	Gentamicin (or some-other aminoglycoside). **Ampicillin[b]** + Cefotaxime[c]
7 days to < 1 month	Community-acquired Meningitis - as above Gentamicin (or some-other aminoglycoside) + ampicillin[a] + cefotaxime[c] If neonate never left the hospital, consider this hospital acquired - vancomycin + aminoglycoside+ cefotaxime[c]
1 month to 50 years old (immunocompetent)	**Vancomycin[d]** + Ceftriaxone or cefotaxime
> 50 years of age, **or** patients with alcoholism, diabetes mellitus (DM) or pregnancy	**Vancomycin[d]** + **Ampicillin[b]** + ceftriaxone or cefotaxime
Community-acquired meningitis with risk factor for Pseudomonas, such as neutropenia, severe immunocompromised state (e.g., lymphoma, high-dose steroids, chemotherapy	**Vancomycin[d]** + **ampicillin[b]** + antipseudomonal cephalosporin (e.g., cefepime) or meropenem
Hospital acquired meningitis (penetrating trauma or postsurgery meningitis)	**Vancomycin[d]** + ceftazidime/cefepime[e]

[a]Consider adding dexamethasone (except in neonates < 6 weeks old). In children, the greatest benefit of dexamethasone is in suspected *H. influenzae* meningitis; in adults in pneumococcal meningitis. It should be given concurrently with or immediately before the first dose of antibiotics, there's probably no benefit if the corticosteroid is given after antibiotics are initiated. It reduces inflammation and decreases risk of neurologic complications, such as hearing loss.[7]

[b]Ampicillin covers Listeria.

[c]Ceftriaxone is contraindicated in this age group because of increased risk of biliary stasis.

[d]Vancomycin is added in countries where pneumococcal resistance rate to ceftriaxone is > 1% e.g., USA, Canada.

[e]No reason to cover Listeria, if not community-acquired.

[6]Know the MCC (most common cause) of bacterial meningitis in each age group.

MRS

The first exposure of a baby is to maternal vaginal flora, which may include *S. agalactiae* and *E. coli*.

In infants, community-acquired *Streptococcus* is most prevalent.

When a child starts attending day care, kindergarten and then school, there is increased crowding and hence increased risk of *Neisseria*.

As one becomes an adult and is no longer living in dorms or exposed to classmates, the incidence of Neisseria decreases, and community-acquired *Streptococcus* again becomes more prevalent.

MRS

GAC= Gentamicin + Ampicillin+ Cefotaxime

Coverage for vancomycin-resistant *S. pneumoniae* is not needed.

VCS: S = steroids

VACS

Age > 50, or with risk factors, give **VACS** therapy: **V**ancomycin, **A**mpicillin, **C**ephalosporin, and **S**teroids (dexamethasone)

[7]MC sequela of untreated bacterial meningitis is eighth cranial nerve palsy.

Additional notes on *N. meningitis*

- Additional unique clinical features include:
  - Petechia and <u>purpura.</u>
  - It can also cause hemorrhagic infarction of adrenal glands leading to acute adrenal crisis (severe hypotension).
- *N. meningitis* prophylaxis is indicated (with either rifampin or ciprofloxacin) in the following situations:
  - Close contacts of *N. meningitis* patients—all household members, childcare center, military recruits in training center, and roommates/dorm mates. (Note: classmates or coworkers are not automatically considered as close contact.)
  - Health care providers who were exposed to respiratory secretions of patients with *N. meningitis*, e.g., a clinician who performed endotracheal intubation.

8.4.3 Lymphocytic Meningitis

Meningitis + lymphocytosis in CSF +	Causative organism	NSIM	Treatment of choice
+ Hx of camping trip in endemic areas	Lyme disease due to *Borrelia burgdorferi*	• Serology for Lyme disease • CSF for Lyme antibody and PCR	Ceftriaxone
	Rickettsia causing Rocky Mountain spotted fever (RMSF)[a]	Serology and CSF PCR	Doxycycline
+ Hx of or risk factors for HIV	*Cryptococcus neoformans*	If India ink test is negative in a HIV-positive patient with lymphocytic meningitis, NSIDx is cryptococcal antigen test in CSF	Amphotericin B + flucytosine
+ Hx of tuberculosis	TB meningitis	AFB stain of spinal fluid obtained daily for 3 days, and CSF nucleic acid testing.	Anti TB regimen + **steroids**
Viral meningitis Enteroviruses are the most common viral cause of meningitis.	• Dx of exclusion • In patients with coexistent genital lesions, suspect HSV-2 meningitis. Consider IV acyclovir therapy and send CSF for HSV PCR. • Symptomatic treatment is the mainstay and hospitalization is not routinely required unless patient has defective humoral immunity or overwhelming infection.		
Early bacterial meningitis or partially treated bacterial meningitis	Consider empiric antibiotics, especially in very young, elderly, or immunocompromised patients, or who have received antibiotics prior to presentation.		
Hx of over-the-counter medication (NSAIDs) overuse	NSAID-induced aseptic meningitis		

[a]Unlike lyme meningitis, RMSF may have neutrophilic predominant CSF, but cell count is usually below <100 cells/μL. Differential diagnosis of RMSF is *N. meningitis*:

Abbreviations: CSF, cerebrospinal fluid; HSV, herpes simplex virus; NSAIDs, nonsteroidal anti-inflammatory drugs; PCR, polymerized chain reaction.

Meningitis + petechia + **purpura** = *N. meningitidis*	Meningitis-like symptoms (fever, headache) + ONLY **petechiae** = also suspect Rocky Mountain spotted fever

8.4.4 HSV-1 Meningoencephalitis

Background: This can be due to primary infection or latent reactivation of HSV-1. (This is the same virus that causes cold sores)

Presentation: Affects predominantly temporal lobes, hence patients may present with symptoms of visual, auditory, or olfactory hallucinations or even seizures.

Workup/Management:

- Usually presents with acute confusion and personality changes, thus CT scan is done prior to lumbar puncture. CT scan **may** reveal unilateral or bitemporal lobe abnormalities or hemorrhage. With clinical and/or CT findings suggestive of HSV-1; NSIM is IV acyclovir.[8]
- NSIM is lumbar puncture with HSV-1 PCR (most accurate test). CSF fluid typically shows increased lymphocytes + increased RBCs. After that, brain magnetic resonance imaging (MRI) is recommended to assess temporal lobe involvement.[9]

[8]This can be life-saving; do not wait for further diagnostic procedures if HSV CNS infection is suspected.

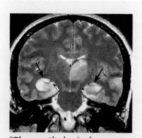

[9]The pathological process also extends into the left thalamic area.
Source: Functions of the Limbic System. In: Bähr M, Frotscher M, ed. Duus' Topical Diagnosis in Neurology: Anatomy, Physiology, Signs, Symptoms. 5th ed. Thieme; 2012.

⚕ Clinical Case Scenarios

A 25-year-old male presents to the hospital with fever and seizures. Patient is diagnosed with herpes viral encephalitis. After few days, patient develops hypersexuality and is seemingly very apathetic to other issues. He is also found to be putting things in his mouth a lot (hyperorality, which is tendency to examine objects by mouth).

4. What is the likely dx?

5. What specific brain structure is involved?

8.5 Upper Respiratory Tract Infection (URTI)

8.5.1 Acute Exudative Pharyngitis or Tonsillitis

[10]Most common etiology of **nonexudative** pharyngitis/tonsillitis, however, is viral.

Background: Two most common causes of **exudative** pharyngitis/tonsillitis are Epstein–Barr virus (EBV) and strep.[10] Ruling out *S. pyogenes* infection is important because if not treated promptly, it carries an increased risk of rheumatic fever or glomerulonephritis.

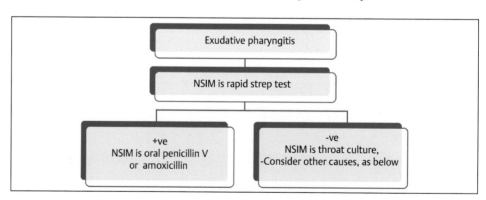

	Streptococcal pharyngitis	EBV	Acute HIV syndrome	Viral
Tonsillar exudate	Present	Present	Usually absent	Usually absent[a]
Upper respiratory symptoms	−ve	May be present	Usually absent	Present[b]
Generalized lymphadenopathy	−ve[c]	May be present	Present	−ve[c]
Hepatosplenomegaly	−ve	Present	Present	−ve
Rash	−ve	May be present[d]	May be present[e]	−ve

[a]However, adenovirus or herpes virus pharyngitis may have exudates.

[b]Coexistent symptoms such as nasal congestion, dry cough, conjunctivitis pointing toward viral origin.

[c]Usually associated with local cervical lymphadenopathy, but not generalized.

[d]Maculopapular rash, if present, signifies that patient might have been exposed to antibiotics (e.g., amoxicillin) prior to presentation.

[e]Patients with acute retroviral syndrome may have painful mucocutaneous ulcerations (oral, esophageal, penile, etc.) and generalized well-circumscribed salmon-colored macules or papules.

Other causes of sore throat include the following:

- Mononucleosis-like illness; see below.
- *Corynebacterium diphtheriae*: sticky dense gray pseudomembrane covering tonsils.
- Gonococcal pharyngitis: due to oral sex.

8.5.2 Infectious Mononucleosis

Background: EBV is transmitted by salivary secretions, e.g., during kissing (hence, especially prevalent in college students) .

Diagnostic evaluation:

- NSIM/NSIDx is rapid strep throat test. If negative, NSIDx is CBC with peripheral blood smear, and heterophile antibody test (a.k.a. monospot test).[11]
- If monospot test is negative, NSIDx is either repeating monospot test or serologic testing for <u>antibodies</u> against EBV-specific proteins (viral-capsid antigen or early nuclear antigen). [12]
- Peripheral smear may reveal atypical lymphocytes.

Treatment: Supportive (acetaminophen ± NSAIDs).

Consider steroids if any of the following is present:

- Impending airway obstruction
- Liver failure
- Aplastic anemia
- Significant autoimmune hemolytic anemia or thrombocytopenia.

Complication: Splenic rupture (patients are advised to avoid non-contact sports for 3 weeks and contact sports for at least 4 weeks).

🔍 Clinical Case Scenarios

A 24 y/o college-going male patient presents with exudative pharyngitis, posterior cervical lymphadenopathy, and fatigue for the last 10 days.

6. What is the immediate NSIDx?

7. If rapid strep test is negative, what test should be done next?

8. What test would likely confirm the dx?

9. Heterophile antibody test comes back positive. CBC reveals platelet count of 18,000. What treatment would you consider?

[11]Monospot test detects the presence of antibody against RBC antigen of sheep and horse. This test is both very sensitive and specific; however, it can be negative in early infection.

[12]If both monospot test and antibodies against EBV-specific proteins are negative, then consider the following causes:
- **C**MV: Known as heterophile-negative infectious mononucleosis
- **H**IV: **A**cute retroviral syndrome
- **T**oxoplasmosis

💡 MRS

They **CHAT** like EBV. They can also have atypical lymphocytes. CHAT or EBV infection can cause Glandular fever syndrome = triad of fever, pharyngitis, and generalized lymphadenopathy.

8.5.3 Influenza

Presentation: Fever, myalgias (generalized muscle pain), headache, and upper respiratory symptoms, such as runny nose and nonproductive cough (due to the postnasal drip). Chest X-ray (CXR) may show increased interstitial marking due to viral bronchitis.

Workup: Rapid molecular DNA-based testing is preferred (e.g., RT-PCR). Antigen-based detection has lower sensitivity, but can also be used.

Rx: Antivirals (Oseltamivir or Zanamivir). Indication for antiviral treatment has been broadened. The only group that might not be treated is healthy patients < 65 years of age with uncomplicated influenza who present after >48 hours of symptoms, or who are already feeling better or pediatric population.

Complications: Adult respiratory distress syndrome, severe necrotizing pneumonia due to *S. Aureus*.

In a patient presenting with fever and cough +/- CXR infiltrates, order rapid COVID-19 PCR.

8.6 Lower Respiratory Tract Infection

Common differential dignosis of "fever + cough" are acute bacterial sinusitis with postnasal drip, bronchitis, pneumonia, and lung abscess.

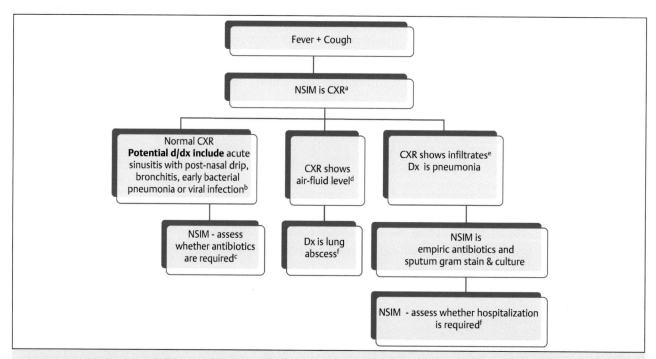

[a]Do not choose CBC as the NSIM, because it does not help to make diagnosis.

[b]In hospitalized patients with hx of sick contacts or coexistent upper respiratory tract symptoms, a PCR testing that detects common viruses (e.g., RSV, parainfluenza, influenza) can be done.

[c]Young patients without comorbid conditions and low-grade fever may not need antibiotics.

Empiric antibiotics used for treatment of bronchitis are similar to sinusitis (same microbiologic cause): amoxicillin-clavulanate or doxycycline.

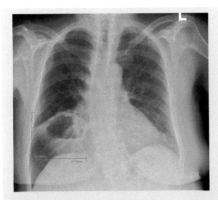

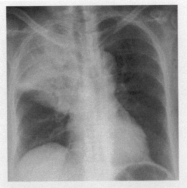

[d]CXR above shows air-fluid level (lung abscess).

[e]Lobar pneumonia with multiple air bronchograms and absence of significant tracheal deviation (If there was lung opacity similar to this but with tracheal deviation to the same side and no air bronchogram, the diagnosis would be more likely atelectasis).
Source: Imaging. In: Gunderman R, ed. Essential Radiology. Clinical Presentation, Pathophysiology, Imaging. 2nd ed. Thieme; 2000.

[f]Lung abscess is commonly a sequelae of aspiration (look for risk factors of aspiration, e.g., advanced dementia, alcoholism). NSIM is sputum gram stain/culture and CT thorax to rule out obstructive pathology. Empiric antibiotics should cover anaerobes (e.g., amoxicilin-clavulanate). Antibiotics is continued until chest imaging is clear (might take weeks).

[g]If you think the patient is sick (e.g., septic, hypoxemic, and/or immunocompromised), then NSIM is to hospitalize the patient and give IV antibiotics (after taking blood cultures). There is a CURB-65 criteria to help you make that decision too.

If any of the following present, consider hospitalization:

- **C**onfusion
- **U**rea ≥ 20 mg/dL
- **R**espiratory rate ≥ 30/min
- **B**lood pressure—systolic BP < 90 mmHg
- **65** or older aged patient (particularly if patient lives alone).

MRS

CURB-65

8.6.1 Pneumonia

Classification of pneumonia	Definition	Likely organism
Community-acquired pneumonia	Patient living in community and with no risk factor for infection with multidrug-resistant organisms	Streptococcus, *H. influenzae*, mycoplasma, etc. (see table below for empiric therapy)
Hospital-acquired pneumonia[a]	Patient develops pneumonia after more than 48 hours of hospitalization	Empiric treatment: • Cover gram-negative organisms and *Pseudomonas*, e.g., cefepime, or piperacillin-tazobactam.[b]
Ventilator-associated pneumonia	Intubated patient develops new-onset fever and has increased secretions, more than 48 hours after intubation.	• If facility has higher rates of MRSA, add coverage with IV vancomycin or linezolid. • No need to routinely cover atypical organisms.

[a]Health care-associated pneumonia (HCAP) is no longer included in recent guidelines. Treatment depends upon individual risk factors.

[b]Consider double pseudomonal coverage in very sick patients (e.g., Tobramycin + cefepime).

Empiric Antibiotic Treatment for Community-Acquired Pneumonia

Test commonly done for hospitalized patients with pneumonia
1. Sputum gram stain and culture
2. Chest X-ray
3. Respiratory pathogen panel (a DNA/RNA based PCR test) which detects multiple respiratory pathogens including influenza, RSV, chlamydia and mycoplasma pneumonia.
4. Urine legionella and streptococcal antigen

No recent antibiotic use, CURB-65 is absent, AND patient has no comorbidities	Hospitalized patient, recent antibiotic use, OR presence of comorbidities (e.g., diabetes, alcoholism, chronic liver disease, immunosuppression)
• Azithromycin or clarithromycin (DOC) or • Doxycycline	• A third-generation cephalosporin + either doxycycline or macrolides. OR • β-Lactam + β-lactamase (e.g., amoxicillin-clavulanate) + either doxycycline or macrolides. OR • New-generation quinolones like moxifloxacin or levofloxacin.[a]

[a]Older generation quinolones like ciprofloxacin, norfloxacin, or ofloxacin do not cover Streptococcus.

Specific Clinical Situations Involving Pneumonia

Streptococcus pneumonia is the MCC of pneumonia.

Community-acquired pneumonia +	Causative organism	Additional points
Lobar pneumonia (CXR reveals infiltrates **localized** to a specific region)	*S. pneumoniae*	• Rusty colored sputum. • Urine *Streptococcus* antigen testing
	Klebsiella (**gram-negative bacteria**)	• **Risk factors:** alcoholism, advanced age, significant comorbid conditions (e.g., ESRD, chronic liver disease), etc. • *Klebsiella* has a very thick sputum which is classically called currant jelly sputum. • Culture of sputum may show **mucoid** colonies.
Presence of the following co-existent features: • Symptoms of upper respiratory tract infection—pharyngitis, rhinitis, and/or bullous otitis media. • Intravascular immunoglobulin M (IgM)-mediated hemolysis. • Target-like skin rash (erythema multiforme).	**Mycoplasma pneumonia**	**CXR** usually shows diffuse bilateral streaky interstitial infiltrates Source: Clinical Aspects. In: Galanski M, Dettmer S, Keberle M et al., eds. Direct Diagnosis in Radiology. Thoracic Imaging. 1st ed. Thieme; 2010. Most patients are treated empirically with antibiotics that cover atypical organisms (e.g., azithromycin). If diagnosis is sought, may use PCR of respiratory secretions or serum antimycoplasma antibody (Note: Cold agglutinins are neither sensitive nor specific).

Community-acquired pneumonia +	Causative organism	Additional points
Presence of the following co-existent features: • Confusion, headache • **Diarrhea**, abdominal pain • LFT abnormalities • Hx of going to a cruise or attending a convention (*Legionella* is frequently found in infected water resources such as in air-conditioning systems) • Hyponatremia (due to SIADH)	*Legionella pneumonia*	**Risk factors:** smokers, alcoholics, old age **CXR:** single or multifocal infiltrates (usually involving bilateral lower lung fields) **NSIM/NSIDx:** urine Legionella antigen test or sputum PCR. Sputum culture on special media is the most specific test. **Rx:** DOC is respiratory quinolone (e.g., levofloxacin) or azithromycin.
Recent hx suggestive of influenza; now patient feels sicker and is having high fever.	*S. aureus pneumonia*	Chest imaging may reveal nodular cavities and pneumatoceles (multiple thin-walled cavities). Source: Differential Diagnosis. In: Galanski M, Dettmer S, Keberle M et al., eds. Direct Diagnosis in Radiology. Thoracic Imaging. 1st ed. Thieme; 2010.
		Other causes of post-flu pneumonia include Streptococcus pneumonia and H. influenzae.
• Recurrent pneumonia in the same lobe or segment • Pneumonia that fails to respond to adequate antibiotic therapy	**Postobstructive pneumonia.**	NSIM is Chest CT scan to rule out obstructive mass.
Hx of bird exposure	*Chlamydia psittaci*	DOC is doxycycline
Hx of animal exposure (e.g., sheep, cattle)	*Coxiella burnetii*	DOC is doxycycline

Abbreviation: LFT, liver function test.

MRS

Think of old drunk smoking legionnaires

Clinical Case Scenarios

10. A 65-year-old alcoholic, active smoker patient who recently went to a convention has pneumonia. What is the likely cause?
1. Strep. pneumonia
2. Legionella
3. Klebsiella

Additional Clinical Pointers

Cavitary pneumonia	⇒	Pneumonia due to Streptococcus, Klebsiella, Staphylococcus, etc.
Sick, septic patient	⇒	Patients with Staphylococcus or Legionella pneumonia are typically sicker than other forms of pneumonia.
Cough + foul smelling sputum	⇒	The foul-smelling sputum is a very important clue for the following conditions: • Aspiration pneumonia • Lung abscess • Bronchiectasis

8.6.2 Aspiration Pneumonia/Pneumonitis

	Pathophysiology	Typical clinical case progression
Aspiration **pneumonitis**	Aspiration of sterile gastric acid contents and subsequent transient inflammatory response, without development of infection	25 y/o M presents with acute gastroenteritis and significant vomiting. Day 2, he develops low-grade fever and has small new infiltrates on CXR. Day 4, patient feels great and wants to go home.
Aspiration **pneumonia**	Aspiration of oropharyngeal contents with accompanying anaerobic flora of oral cavity, resulting in infection of lung parenchyma	65 y/o M, day 2 after surgery, develops productive cough and fever. CXR shows lobar opacity. Day 4, he still looks sick and is continued on IV antibiotics.

Conditions that can predispose to aspiration:

Impaired swallowing and epiglottic reflex lead to increased risk of aspiration of oropharyngeal and gastric contents into the lung

Altered consciousness	⟹	Seizures, alcoholism, sedative drugs, anesthesia, etc.
Oropharyngeal dysphagia	⟹	Zenker's diverticulum and bulbar/pseudobulbar palsy
Neurologic disorders	⟹	Dementia, Parkinson's disease
Surgical procedures	⟹	Endoscopy and anesthetic surgery

Periodontal disease and gingivitis increase bacterial load of aspirated material

 MRS

PS RULe out aspiration in this lobe.
FYI: The right main bronchus is wider, shorter, and more vertical than the left main bronchus.

When aspiration occurs in supine position, the most commonly affected lobe is **P**ost-**S**egment of **R**ight **u**pper **l**obe, because it is directly connected with main right bronchus.
Treatment: (Amoxicillin-clavulanate), or (cefdinir + metronidazole).

 In a nutshell

Empiric treatment for Pneumonia

Empiric antibiotic choice should cover...

Pneumonia Type	Typical organisms[a]	Atypicals[b]	MRSA	Pseudomonas	Anaerobes	Example empiric antibiotic therapy
CAP	✓	✓	Depends[c]	Depends[d]	✗	In patients without risk factor for MRSA or pseudomonas: Ceftriaxone + azithromycin, or Cefdinir + Doxycycline
HAP/VAP	✓	✗	✓	✓	✗	Vancomycin + Cefepime
ASP	✓	✗	Depends[c]	✗	✓	Amoxicillin-clavulanate in patients without risk-factor for MRSA

[a]Covered by antibiotics such as 3rd or 4th generation cephalosporins, β-Lactam + β-Lactamase combination, newer generation quinolones, etc.

[b]Atypicals (Chlamydia, legionella, mycoplasma, etc.) are covered by azithromycin, doxycycline or newer generation quinolones

[c]In patients who have risk factor for MRSA- Hx of MRSA colonization, IVDA (intravenous drug abuse), HIV positive, recent prior antimicrobial therapy (particularly fluoroquinolone), prisoners, hemodialysis, recent hospitalization, etc.

[d]In patients who have risk factor for pseudomonas infection: -immunosuppression, significant pulmonary comorbidity (cystic fibrosis, bronchiectasis, or repeated exacerbations of chronic obstructive pulmonary disease that require frequent glucocorticoid and/or antibiotic use), previous antibiotic therapies or recent hospitalizations, etc.

Abbreviations: ASP, aspiration pneumonia; CAP, community-acquired pneumonia; HAP, hospital-acquired pneumonia; VAP, ventilator-associated pneumonia.

8.7 Infective Endocarditis

Definition: Microbial infection with formation of bacterial vegetation in the endocardium (heart valves, mural endocardium, septum, etc.)

Risk factors

- Underlying heart disease (e.g., high-risk congenital heart defects).
- Foreign body (cardiac devices such as pacemakers, mechanical heart valve, etc.).
- Bacteremia with highly virulent pathogen, e.g., *S. aureus*.

Microbiology

Clinical scenario	Likely pathogen
Hx of dental extraction or dental surgery	*S. viridans*[a]
Hx of lower gastrointestinal or urinary tract manipulation	*Enterococcus faecalis*
Within 2 months of surgery for prosthetic device or valve replacement	*S. epidermidis*[b]
After 2 months of surgery for prosthetic device placement	*S. viridans*[a]
Intravenous drug abuse	*S. aureus*[c]
Culture negative endocarditis	Consider fastidious organisms—such as the HACEK group[d]
Colon cancer or liver disease	Group D *Streptococcus* (e.g., *Streptococcus bovis*)[e]

[a]*Streptococcus* (strep) *viridans* group is the normal flora of oral cavity. This group includes *Strep mutans, Strep sanguis, Strep mitis, Strep salivarius*, etc.

[b]*Staph epidermidis* is frequently resistant to penicillin and nafcillin.

[c]IVDA is associated with higher risk of MRSA infection.

[d]HACEK group is also oral flora (*Haemophilus, Actinobacillus, Cardiobacterium, Eikenella, and Kingella species*).

[e]All patients with group D Streptococcus bacteremia should undergo colonoscopy.

Clinical classification:

Acute endocarditis	Course of illness is over a few days and is likely due to virulent pathogens such as *S. aureus*.
Subacute endocarditis	Course of illness is over a couple of weeks and is likely due to other microbial causes.

Pathophysiology/presentation

Heart valve infection	⇒	Acute valvular insufficiencies may cause congestive heart failure.	In a patient presenting with **new** heart murmur + constitutional signs and symptoms of fever, headache, and myalgia—the diagnosis is IE, unless proven otherwise.	MC murmur in IE is of mitral regurgitation. In patients with IV drug abuse, MC murmur is of tricuspid regurgitation.
Direct contiguous spread of infection within heart structures	⇒	• Heart blocks • Myo/pericarditis		
Immune-complex formation and deposition	⇒	In glomeruli	Acute glomerulonephritis: RBC casts in urine with proteinuria	
		In retina	Roth spots: it requires fundoscopy to visualize	
		In subcutaneous tissue	Can lead to formation of painful nodules (Osler's nodes)	
Septic emboli	⇒	Right-sided endocarditis can lead to septic pulmonary emboli		
		Left-sided endocarditis can lead to infarction and infection anywhere.		
		• Small emboli in skin can present as painless flat lesion and is known as Janeway lesions (can be of any color; from red to black necrotic)		
		• Emboli to brain can result in ischemic stroke, infectious intracranial aneurysms (old name: mycotic aneurysm), brain abscess, etc.		

Management steps

First SIM is blood culture, followed by empiric IV antibiotic therapy. This should include vancomycin. In patients with prosthetic valve, add gentamicin + antipseudomonal cefepime or meropenem. Then only do transthoracic echocardiogram (TTE). Transesophageal echocardiogram (TEE) can be done if TTE is nondiagnostic, as it is more sensitive.[13]

[13]Do simple things first, then only, do more sophisticated invasive procedure.

Treatment:

Organism		Native valve	Prosthetic valve
S. aureus	MRSA	Vancomycin or linezolid	Vancomycin + gentamicin + rifampin[a]
	MSSA (methicillin-sensitive S. aureus)	Nafcillin or cefazolin	Nafcillin or cefazolin + gentamicin + rifampin[a]
Streptococcus spp[b]		Penicillin or ceftriaxone	Penicillin ± gentamicin

[a]S. aureus is known to produce biofilms on surfaces of foreign bodies (e.g., prosthetic valve). Addition of gentamicin and rifampin is done to achieve better penetration through biofilms and to eradicate infection.

[b]Streptococcus is less virulent than S. aureus.

Indications for surgery

- Progressive congestive heart failure unresponsive to medical measures.
- Recurrent systemic emboli.
- Fungal etiology: due to lack of effective microbicidal treatment. Use amphotericin as an adjunctive treatment.
- Extravalvular manifestation, e.g., high grade AV block and purulent pericarditis.
- Prosthetic valve dehiscence.
- Persistent bacteremia despite adequate treatment for > 72 hours.

Infective endocarditis prophylaxis

Only required in patients with high-risk condition undergoing high-risk procedures

High-risk condition	High-risk procedure
• Prosthetic cardiac valve (including bioprosthetic heart valve) • Previous infective endocarditis • Valvular heart disease in a cardiac transplant patient • Unrepaired cyanotic congenital heart disease • Repaired congenital heart disease with prosthetic patch or device, during the first 6 months of surgery • Repaired congenital heart disease with residual defect at or near the site of prosthetic patch or device	• Dental procedures that involve manipulation of the gingival or the periapical region of teeth, or perforation of oral mucosa. This includes routine dental cleaning and tooth extraction. • Incision or biopsy of respiratory tract mucosa • Genitourinary or gastrointestinal procedure in patients with ongoing infection • Procedures on infected skin or musculoskeletal structures

Differential diagnosis: Atrial myxoma can present with systemic symptoms, such as fever, weight loss, and cardiac murmur (mid-diastolic murmur similar to one heard in mitral stenosis). Echo will show mass in the left atrium.

Clinical Case Scenarios

A patient presents with acute fever. He vehemently denies IVDA. Exam reveals a new pan-systolic murmur and track-marks are seen in both arms. CT scan as pictured shows bilateral nodules, some with cavitation.

11. What is the likely dx?

12. What is the NSIM?

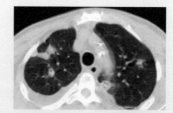

Source: Lung. In: Gunderman R, ed. Essential Radiology. Clinical Presentation, Pathophysiology, Imaging. 3rd ed. Thieme; 2014.

8.8 Infectious Diarrhea[14]

8.8.1 Community-Acquired Diarrhea

[14]Diarrhea of less than 1-week duration is infectious unless proven otherwise.
New-onset diarrhea in an ill-appearing patient, hospitalized patients, nursing home residents, or with hx of recent antibiotic use—always rule out *C. difficile infection.*

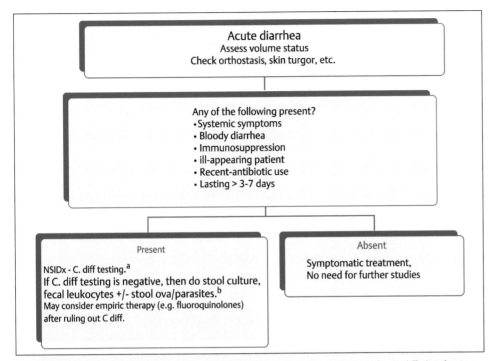

Acute diarrhea
Assess volume status
Check orthostasis, skin turgor, etc.

Any of the following present?
• Systemic symptoms
• Bloody diarrhea
• Immunosuppression
• ill-appearing patient
• Recent-antibiotic use
• Lasting > 3-7 days

Present

NSIDx - C. diff testing.[a]
If C. diff testing is negative, then do stool culture, fecal leukocytes +/- stool ova/parasites.[b]
May consider empiric therapy (e.g. fluoroquinolones) after ruling out C diff.

Absent

Symptomatic treatment, No need for further studies

[a]Community-acquired diarrhea in an ill-appearing patient should be ruled out for *C. difficile* infection, even without history of recent hospitalization or antibiotic use.

[b]In sick patients with persistent nonresolving diarrhea, nucleic-acid-based GI pathogen panel that detects multiple microbes can be done (this testing includes detection of *C. jejuni, E. coli,* norovirus, *Cyclospora,* and many more).

8.8.2 Classification of Infectious Diarrhea

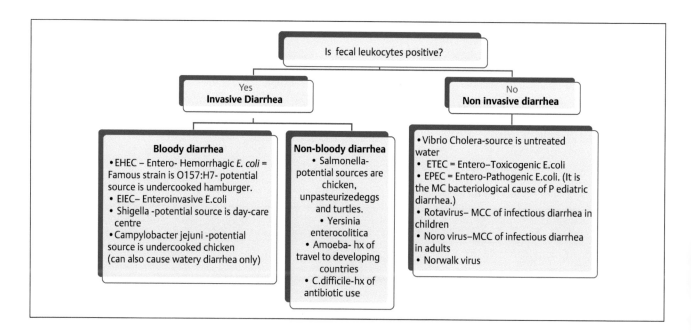

Clinical Scenarios Involving Infectious Diarrhea

History	Most likely Dx	Additional points
• Close contact with domestic animals like cats and dogs • Ingestion of poorly cooked chicken	*Campylobacter jejuni*[a]	Stool culture will confirm the diagnosis. **Rx:** azithromycin or quinolones (e.g., ciprofloxacin)
Exam scenario: new onset diarrhea with hx of recent travel to developing countries	ETEC (enterotoxigenic *E. coli*)	Look for high-volume watery diarrhea. **Rx:** ciprofloxacin or TMP/SMX may be considered in cases with severe, persistent diarrhea (particularly in children or immunocompromised hosts).
	Amebiasis	• Bloody-mucoid diarrhea ± fever[b] • Can have liver abscess (single or multiple) • **Dx:** stool microscopy, PCR or antigen dectection. • **Rx:** Metronidazole or tinidazole + paromomycin to eliminate intraluminal cysts
	Giardiasis	Usually have upper GI symptoms like flatulence/bloating[c] • **Dx:** stool microscopy, antigen or PCR[d] **Rx:** depends on age: • > 3 yrs of age- tinidazole (single dose) • 1-2 yrs of age- nitazoxanide • < 1 year of age - metronidazole • For pregnant patients in their 1st trimester, if treatment is deemed necessary, paromomycin is preferred. In 2nd or 3rd trimester, any of the medication mentioned here can be given.

History	Most likely Dx	Additional points
	Cryptosporidium, Cyclospora, and microsporidia	> 2 weeks of watery diarrhea (discussed further in HIV section)[d]
New onset voluminous watery diarrhea with hx of travel to endemic area or outbreaks	Vibrio Cholera	**Rx:** aggressive hydration is mainstay. Antibiotics might be considered in moderate to severe cases or in epidemics (doxycycline, macrolides)
Sudden-onset vomiting + crampy upper abdominal pain ± diarrhea = food poisoning due to ingestion of preformed toxins.	*Bacillus cereus*	Usually acquired from fried rice ingestion
	S. aureus	Hx of mustard, custard, or potato salad ingestion[e]
Hx of fish ingestion, followed by development of diarrhea, rash, vomiting, and wheezing. (sounds like carcinoid syndrome)	Dx is scombroid fish poisoning.	It occurs after eating spoiled or decayed fish (e.g., *tuna, mahi-mahi, mackerels*). Histamine is formed during decay process. **Rx:** antihistamines.
Hx of shellfish ingestion	Vibrio parahaemolyticus or Vibrio vulnificus infection—they are motile, comma-shaped, gram-negative bacteria.	• *Vibrio vulnificus*[f] causes severe disease with septicemia and blisters/bulla formation, particularly in patients with hemochromatosis or liver disease. • *Vibrio parahaemolyticus* infection is usually self-limiting.

[a]*Campylobacter jejuni* is the MCC of bacterial food-borne illness in the United States. Features are abdominal pain and **watery or hemorrhagic** diarrhea. Remember two potential complications—**reactive arthritis** and **Guillain–Barre syndrome.**

[b]Think of dysentery-like presentation. Can cause intestinal perforation, too.

[c]Also, look for history of camping trips to mountains. It might be acquired through drinking water from streams or wells. Remember giardiasis infects the upper gastrointestinal tract, specifically the duodenum, affecting its absorptive function, so it usually causes symptoms of malabsorption. Chronic giardiasis can cause chronic malabsorption syndrome with weight loss.

[d]Favorite red herring for exam is stool exam unremarkable, as stool exam may not show these organisms. It might require special stains to visualize the parasites.

[e]Food workers with active staph infection (e.g., in hands) can inoculate food with *St. aureus*, which multiplies in food and secretes exotoxin. A group of people who ingested the contaminated food can be infected.

[f]Soft tissue infection with *Vibrio vulnificus* can occur due to salt water exposure or in shell-fish handlers. This can have severe presentation with myositis and necrotizing fasciitis.

 In a nutshell

Most abscesses need to be drained and treated with antibiotics, but there are certain exceptions, where surgical drainage might not be necessary—as shown below.

Condition	NSIM
Amebic liver abscess	Oral metronidazole
Lung abscess	Amoxicillin-clavulanate
Cervicofacial actinomycosis—"lumpy bumpy" swelling in the neck region	Oral penicillin

8.8.3 *Clostridium Difficile*-Associated Diarrhea

C. difficile is acquired through ingestion of spores and can be community-acquired or healthcare facility acquired (e.g., nursing homes, hospital). MC risk factor is recent antibiotic use, but can occur without it (e.g., in alcoholics, immunosuppressed, or elderly patients).

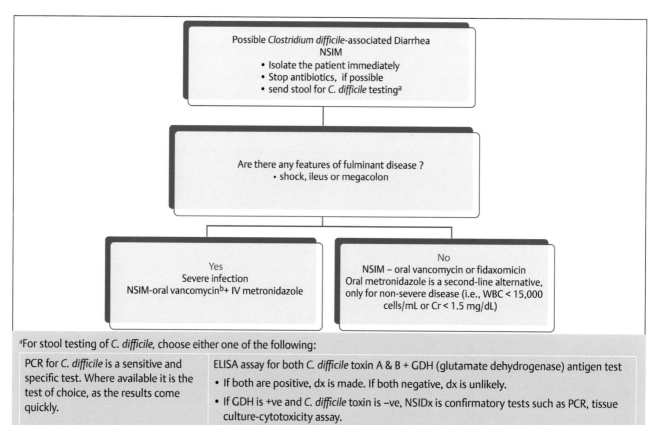

Possible *Clostridium difficile*-associated Diarrhea
NSIM
• Isolate the patient immediately
• Stop antibiotics, if possible
• send stool for *C. difficile* testing[a]

Are there any features of fulminant disease ?
• shock, ileus or megacolon

Yes
Severe infection
NSIM-oral vancomycin[b] + IV metronidazole

No
NSIM – oral vancomycin or fidaxomicin
Oral metronidazole is a second-line alternative, only for non-severe disease (i.e., WBC < 15,000 cells/mL or Cr < 1.5 mg/dL)

[a]For stool testing of *C. difficile*, choose either one of the following:

PCR for *C. difficile* is a sensitive and specific test. Where available it is the test of choice, as the results come quickly.	ELISA assay for both *C. difficile* toxin A & B + GDH (glutamate dehydrogenase) antigen test • If both are positive, dx is made. If both negative, dx is unlikely. • If GDH is +ve and *C. difficile* toxin is –ve, NSIDx is confirmatory tests such as PCR, tissue culture-cytotoxicity assay. *Note: GDH test is sensitive but not specific.*

• Most sensitive test for *C. difficile*-associated diarrhea is stool culture.
• Most specific tests are tissue culture cytotoxicity assay, enzyme-linked assay for *C. difficile* toxin A & B and presence of pseudomembrane on endoscopy. PCR can detect *C. difficile* colonization without infection.

[b]If a patient has features suggestive of ileus or megacolon, oral vancomycin might not reach the infected area of colon. Use vancomycin enema or colonic instillation in place of oral vancomycin or, as an adjunct (in partial ileus).

Management of Recurrent *C. difficile* Infection

● For first recurrence, if metronidazole or fidaxomicin was used in the first episode, use oral vancomycin. If vancomycin was used in the first episode, use a long course of tapered oral vancomycin regimen (lasting 6–12 weeks). Alternatively, fidaxomicin can be used.
● For the third episode, consider fecal microbiota transplantation in addition to anti-*C. difficile* therapy.

8.9 STD (Sexually Transmitted Diseases)

● Chlamydial and gonococcal infection
● Ulcerative STD
   – Painful ulcers (herpes simplex virus and *Haemophilus ducreyi*)
   – Painless ulcers (syphilis, lymphogranuloma venereum, granuloma inguinale)
● HIV
● Hep B, C
● Human papilloma virus (genital warts)

8.9.1 STD Screening—High Yield

HIV	All patients who are sexually active should be offered regular HIV screening
Chlamydia trachomatis and gonococcal screening	• Yearly screening in all sexually active women <25 and in older women with risk factors for STD. • In men, screening is only done for at-risk patients.
Syphilis	Screen only in patients with risk factor

8.9.2 Urethritis and Cervicitis

Etiology : Chlamydia trachomatis and Neisseria gonorrhoeae.

	Clinical presentation
Men	Urethral discharge and dysuria (pathognomonic of urethritis). • Irritative and voiding symptoms (prostatitis) • Acute tender testes (epididymitis)
Women	Urethral discharge and dysuria (pathognomonic of urethritis).
	Vaginal or cervical discharge with erythematous and tender cervix on exam (cervicitis)
	Lower abdominal pain and fever (pelvic inflammatory disease)

Differentiating points

Chlamydia	Gonorrhea
Patients with chlamydia are more likely to remain asymptomatic for a long period of time	Sore throat due to gonococcal transmission during oral sex can occur
Chlamydia infection is less likely to have purulent discharge	• Acute frank purulent discharge is more likely due to gonorrhea. • Intracellular gram-negative diplococci can be seen in gram stain of discharge.

Workup

gram stain of urethral/cervical secretions. If patient has no urethral/cervical discharge, check urinalysis and nucleic acid amplification testing (NAAT) for chlamydia and gonorrhea (most sensitive and specific test).

Management Algorithm

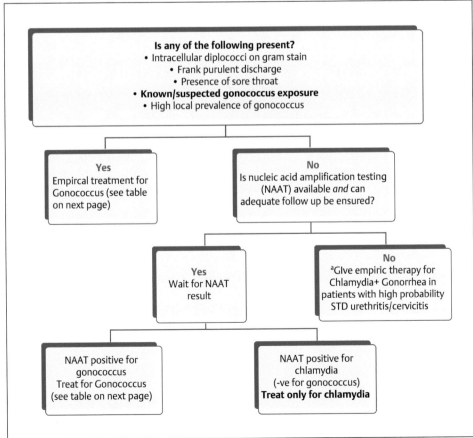

If patient still has persistent symptoms after receiving proper treatment of urethritis/cervicitis, think of infection with *Trichomonas*, resistant *Gonococcus*, or reinfection. NSIDx is urine nucleic acid testing for *Trichomonas* and chlamydia/gonorrhea. *Trichomonas* is treated with metronidazole.

For treatment of pelvic inflammatory disease, please see the gynecology chapter.

Empiric treatment

	Treatment	How to address treatment for partners?[a]	Patient presents to your clinic with hx of specific exposure[b]
Gonococcus	A single IM dose of Ceftriaxone + single 1 g dose of azithromycin (or doxycycline)[c]	Oral cefixime + azithromycin	Empiric therapy with ceftriaxone + azithromycin, along with NAAT testing
Chlamydia	Single 1 g dose of azithromycin in uncomplicated urethritis/cervicitis[d] • Alternative treatment for chlamydia is doxycycline for 7 days (pregnancy test should be done prior to giving doxycycline). • Test of cure is recommended for pregnant patients with chlamydia.	Azithromycin	Empiric treatment for chlamydia (with azithromycin), along with NAAT

[a]All sexual partners should be evaluated. If no follow-up can be ensured, expedited partner therapy is recommended with the following agents.

[b]For example, CCS: patient comes into your clinic and reports that her sexual partner was recently diagnosed with Gonococcus infection.

[c]Dual therapy is recommended for all gonococcal infection (regardless of chlamydial coinfection), as there has been an increase in gonococcal resistance to ceftriaxone or cefixime.

[d]In patients with proctitis and ependymitis, dual therapy with coverage of Gonococcus is recommended.

Complications of Urethritis:

[15]**Prostatitis and epididymitis**
- Most likely microbiological cause in a sexually active patient is *Gonococcus* or *Chlamydia*.
- In older patients who are not sexually active *E. coli* is the leading cause.

 MRS

When Gonococcus goes FAR

In males	• **Prostatitis**[15]: irritative and voiding symptoms • **Epididymitis**[15]: acute tender testes
In females	• **Cervicitis:** red friable cervix • **Cystitis:** irritative and voiding symptoms • **Pelvic inflammatory disease** and possible subsequent development of infertility
Proctitis	• Pain with defecation and sensation of incomplete voiding (tenesmus)
Disseminated gonococcal syndrome[a]	• **F**ever + **A**rthralgias (poly) + **R**ash (pustules) or • Mono/oligoarticular septic arthritis
Reactive arthritis (associated with chlamydial infection)[a]	Oligoarthritis + extra-articular manifestations (conjunctivitis, uveitis, keratoderma blennorrhagica—may involve palms and soles, genital lesions, etc.)

[a]Think of these two diagnoses when a patient presents with acute joint pain and urethritis/cervicitis. As reactive arthritis is a form of seronegative arthritis, it is more likely to present with back pain and sausage-shaped digits. Reactive arthritis can also be associated with rash in palms and soles.

8.9.3 Ulcerative STD

Background: Any patient that comes to your clinic with an ulcer in vulvar or penile region has STD unless proven otherwise. Major differentiating feature is painless versus painful.

Painful	Herpes simplex virus and H. ducreyi
Painless	Syphilis, lymphogranuloma venereum, granuloma inguinale

 MRS

You do cry with ducreyi

Painful genital ulcer

Caused by two "**H**", i.e., **H**SV-2 and H. ducreyi.

	HSV-2 (MC ulcerative STD in the United States)	Chancroid caused by H. ducreyi
Presentation	• Multiple vesicles on erythematous base (classic presentation). As vesicles rupture, they leave behind a denuded skin ulcer, which can coalesce to form a big tender ulcer. • Look for hx of recurrent vesicles. • Can also present with urethritis symptoms	• Small, painful **papule/s** that develop into single or **multiple** shallow ulcer/s. Ulcers can later coalesce into a **big ulcer**. • Inguinal lymph node enlargement Chancroid on the penis. Source: Chancroid. In: Laskaris G, ed. Color Atlas of Oral Diseases. Diagnosis and Treatment. 4th ed. Thieme; 2017.
Management steps	In patients with classic presentation, no need to do diagnostic testing. Treat with acyclovir, valacyclovir, or famciclovir. If vesicles are not present (atypical presentation—as in inset picture), confirm dx with viral culture or PCR first. **Tzanck** smear to look for multinucleated giant cells can also be done as an initial test.	Dx can be made by clinical picture in classical cases, but HSV and syphilis can also present with ulcerative disease, so testing for herpes virus (PCR or culture) and syphilis (dark-field microscopy or serology) should be done. Perform H. ducreyi -specific gram stain and special culture or nucleic acid testing when available. **Rx:** azithromycin (oral) or ceftriaxone (IM), both single dose.[MRS-1]

MRS

• HSV-1 = 1 affects the topmost part of your body (head), including herpes labialis and can also cause meningoencephalitis.

• HSV-2 affects lower body parts (STD), and can also cause meningitis[a] (but not encephalitis).

• Papules → ulcer = chancroid.

• Vesicles → ulcer = HSV infection.

MRS

[MRS-1]Treatment is like urethritis

[a]HSV-2 infection has been implicated in recurrent aseptic meningitis (known as Mollaret's meningitis).

Other causes of painful ulcers in the genital area (low yield)

Behcet's disease	It is a rare autoimmune small-vessel vasculitis. Patient may have history of recurrent oral or perineal area ulcerations. Look for other organ involvement (e.g., lung, gastrointestinal).
Circinate balanitis	– Dermatological manifestation of reactive arthritis – Ring-shaped dermatitis of the glans penis

Painless Genital Ulcer

	Syphilis	Lymphogranuloma venereum	Granuloma inguinale a.k.a. donovanosis
Causative organism	*Treponema pallidum* (a spirochete bacteria)	*Chlamydia trachomatis*	*Klebsiella* granulomatis
Clinical exam findings All have inguinal lymphadenopathy	Indurated ulcer	Small painless ulcer, with later involvement of inguinal lymph nodes. Lymph nodes are usually tender or painful, and may form abscess(es) which later ulcerate and drain[MRS-2]	Nodules that ulcerate and slowly enlarge to form a big beefy-red ulcer
Picture	 Hard chancre (black arrow) with spirochetes (white arrow) on dark field microscopy. Source: Treponema pallidum. In: Riede U, Werner M, eds. Color Atlas of Pathology: Pathologic Principles, Associated Diseases, Sequela. 1st ed. Thieme; 2004.	Massive inguinal lymphadenopathy Source: Lymphogranuloma Venereum. In: Sterry W, Paus R, Burgdorf W, eds. Thieme Clinical Companions - Dermatology. 1st ed. Thieme; 2006.	Early stage ulcerative donovanosis Source: Granuloma Inguinale. In: Sterry W, Paus R, Burgdorf W, eds. Thieme Clinical Companions - Dermatology. 1st ed. Thieme; 2006.
Dx	Dark field microscopy will reveal spirochetes.	Dx is often made clinically, supported by serological testing. Nucleic acid testing on swab can also be done.	Dx is based on clinical findings (regional lymphadenopathy is typically absent). Biopsy may show Donovan bodies (rod-shaped organism inside phagocytes).
Treatment	A single dose of IM penicillin	Use doxycycline or azithromycin (atypical bacterial coverage). Buboes may require aspiration or incision and drainage.	Use doxycycline or azithromycin (atypical bacterial coverage)
Complications	Secondary and tertiary syphilis, if not treated. (See table below.)	Lymph node involvement and suppuration may lead to the following: – abscesses or fistula formation (e.g., rectovaginal fistula)[MRS-3] – Proctocolitis[MRS-3] – Rectal stricture[MRS-3]	Scarring

MRS

[MRS-2]Lymphogranuloma = lymph node granulomas and suppuration lead to many problems. The ulcer is not painful, but lymph node involvement can be.

MRS

[MRS-3]Lymphogranuloma acts like rectal Crohn's disease.

8.9.4 Stage of Syphilis

Clinical presentation	Stage		Dx	Treatment[a]
Primary syphilis	Painless indurated punched-out ulcer with inguinal lymphadenopathy		**NSIDx**—take sample from ulcer and do dark field microscopy to visualize filamentous motile spirochetes or do direct fluorescent antibody test on the sample.	
Secondary syphilis	Generalized maculopapular rash also involving palms and soles.	 Source: Secondary Syphilis. In: Sterry W, Paus R, Burgdorf W, eds. Thieme Clinical Companions - Dermatology. 1st ed. Thieme; 2006.	**Dark field microscopy of skin lesion can be done.** Either of the following test can be used: – **Nontreponemal serology:** RPR (rapid plasma reagin test) or VDRL test.[b] – **Specific-treponemal serology:** FTA-ABS (fluorescent treponemal antibody-absorbed), TPHA (T. pallidum hemagglutination), EIAs (syphilis enzyme immunoassays).[MRS-4] – If any of the above tests is positive, NSIDx is to do the other class of tests. For example, if TPHA is +ve, NSIDx is VDRL or RPR.	Benzathine penicillin IM (single dose) In patients with penicillin allergy, use oral tetracycline or doxycycline
	Exophytic, fleshy wart-like lesions in the anogenital perineal region = condylomata lata	Source: Secondary Syphilis. In: Sterry W, Paus R, Burgdorf W, eds. Thieme Clinical Companions - Dermatology. 1st ed. Thieme; 2006.		

MRS

[MRS-4]The tests with letter "R" are nontreponemal syphilis tests. The tests with letter "A" are the specific tests.

After initiation of treatment for syphilis, some patients may develop general malaise, fever, headache, sweating, rigors, and exacerbation of syphilitic lesions. This is called **Jarisch–Herxheimer reaction.**

Penicillin allergic patients with neurosyphilis, cardiovascular manifestations of late syphilis, and/or treatment failure, should undergo penicillin challenge or desensitization, instead of alternate therapy.

Clinical presentation	Stage	Dx	Treatment[a]
Tertiary syphilis (this stage is symptomatic but **NOT** contagious.)	• Generalized nodule formation that can ulcerate (**gummas**) or • CNS infection (neurosyphilis) or tabes dorsalis (posterior column neural involvement) or • Aortitis (ascending aortic aneurysm)	First SIDx is specific-treponemal serology.[c] **For suspected neurosyphilis or tabes dorsalis,** NSIDx is CSF VDRL (it is specific but not sensitive). If negative, consider CSF FTA-ABS (most sensitive test for neurosyphilis, but not specific).	For neurosyphilis, penicillin G IV for 10 -14 days is recommended. For other cases of tertiary syphilis, IM penicillin can be given for once weekly for 3 weeks.

[a]In all pregnant patients who are penicillin-allergic, NSIM is penicillin desensitization and treat as per respective stage. Data are insufficient to recommend ceftriaxone.

[b]False-positive VDRL test can occur in patients with HIV, IVDA, advance age, autoimmune disorders (such as SLE or rheumatoid arthritis), etc.

[c]In tertiary syphilis, start with specific treponemal serology as it has more sensitivity. Nontreponemal serology can become negative in later stages of syphilis.

Clinical Case Scenarios

13. A 35 y/o M with hx of STD wants to get screened for syphilis. He has no prior hx of syphilis. What test can you use?

14. TPHA is +ve. What is the NSIDx?

15. VDRL is negative. What is the NSIDx?

MRS

CARS of palms/soles—Coxsackie A, RMSF, and syphilis are common causes

Rash in "palms and soles"—think of the following conditions:

• Coxsackie A virus infection: hand, foot, and mouth disease

• Rocky Mountain spotted fever and typhus

• Meningococcemia: petechiae on the palms and soles

• Kawasaki, measles, or toxic shock syndrome: peeling rash

• Keratoderma blennorrhagica (in Reiter's syndrome): rash that looks like psoriasis (hyperkeratotic rash in palms and soles)

• Graft versus host disease

• Secondary and congenital syphilis: in contrast to most conditions mentioned above, patients with syphilitic rash are not toxic-looking.

8.10 Joint and Bone infection

8.10.1 Acute Monoarticular Arthritis

For acute single-joint swelling, tenderness, and redness, **NSIM** is immediate **arthrocentesis**.

Arthrocentesis should be done even in a patient with clear hx of rheumatoid arthritis or gout, if clinical presentation is suggestive of septic arthritis. Septic arthritis is a highly destructive process and early diagnosis is very important.

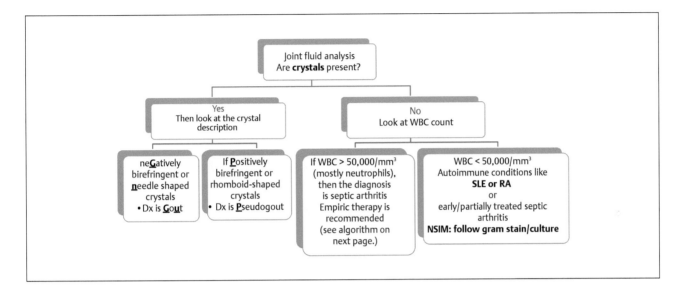

8.10.2 Septic Arthritis

- MCC in young, healthy sexually active individual is Gonococcus.
- MCC in general population is *S. aureus*.
- MCC in IV drug users is *S. aureus*. Pseudomonas is also common in this patient group.
- MC way of bacterial seeding into the joint is hematogenous spread.
- MC joint involved is knee.

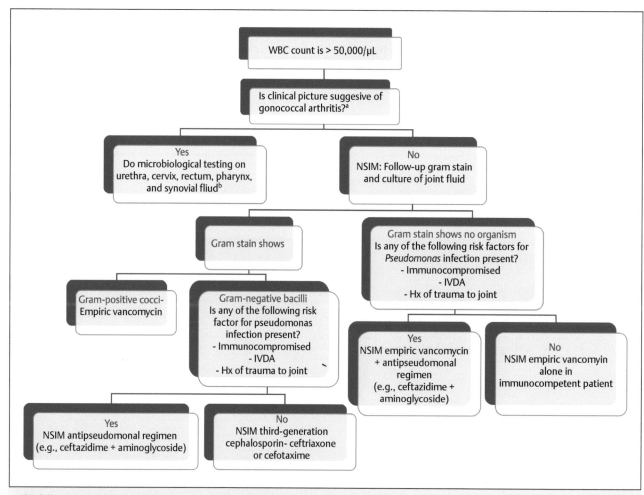

^aThe following are suggestive of gonococcal arthritis:

• Septic arthritis in a young healthy patient, who has risk factors for STD and no hx of IVDA.

• Presence of pustular skin rash, or symptoms suggestive of urethritis/cervicitis.

^bUse NAAT (nucleic acid amplification test) when available. Also do gram stain and culture. Note: synovial fluid or blood culture is less likely to be positive in gonococcal arthritis.

Joint debridement: Along with antibiotics, surgical or arthroscopic joint drainage is recommended in most patients with confirmed septic arthritis (i.e., joint fluid is positive for gram stain or culture).

Patients with prosthetic joint infection will require surgery.

For hip, shoulder, or difficult-to-access joints (such as the sternoclavicular joint)	Arthroscopic drainage – Open surgical drainage with arthrotomy may be necessary, especially in infants and children
For knee, elbow, ankle, or wrist	Needle aspiration or arthroscopy
For others	Repeated needle aspirations can be done

8.10.3 Osteomyelitis

Pathophysiology: Bone infection leads to a localized collection of necrotic bone tissue called sequestrum. There is surrounding reactive periosteal inflammation and subsequent mineralization, i.e., bone formation in periosteum (called involucrum).

So how do bacteria reach the bone?

Direct inoculation	Puncture wound with nail
Hematogenous spread	Bacteremia due to other causes – Infection due to hematogenous spread usually seed in **metaphysis** of long bones.
Contiguous spread	Risk factors for contiguous spread of infection into bones are underlying DM, vascular disease, and immunosuppression.[16] – In patients with skin ulcer which probes to bone, osteomyelitis is likely present.

[16]MC scenario of osteomyelitis is an adult patient with long-standing diabetic foot ulcer with intermittent drainage and poor vascular perfusion. Such patients require multidisciplinary approach with podiatry, infectious disease and vascular surgery consultation.

Presentation: Think of osteomyelitis when patient presents with fever + bone pain.
Exam can reveal bony point tenderness and erythema/warmth overlying the involved bone.

Diagnostic steps:

Best initial test	X-ray, as it is a simple test. If it is positive for osteomyelitis, MRI or bone scan may not be needed.
Best step in diagnosis	Definitive test such as MRI of the bone with contrast is done next. If patient has hardware (e.g., pacemaker), MRI cannot be done; bone scan is done in these situations.
Most specific test	Bone biopsy with histology and culture should be done to direct antibiotic therapy and to confirm diagnosis. It may not be needed in patients with suspected hematogenous osteomyelitis with positive blood culture and who have classic radiological findings.

Treatment: combination of surgical debridement (of necrotic bone and tissue), followed by empiric antibiotic therapy (e.g., IV vancomycin + IV antibiotic that covers gram-negative organisms, e.g., cefepime)
Response to treatment can be monitored by following inflammatory markers (erythrocyte sedimentation rate and C-reactive protein).

8.11 Immunodeficiency and Opportunistic Pathogens

8.11.1 How to Recognize Immunodeficiency Disorders with History of Recurrent Infections:

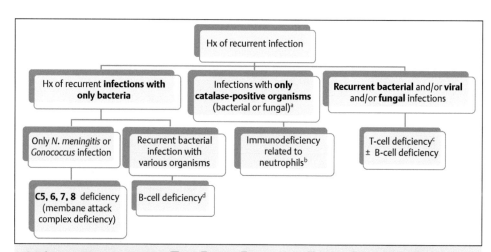

^aCatalase-positive organisms are **E.** coli, **S**erratia, **P**seudomonas, **N**ocardia, **L**isteria, **A**spergillus, **C**andida, **K**lebsiella, **S.** aureus, etc.

^bNeutropenia, leukocyte-adhesion deficiency, chronic granulomatous disease, Chediak–Higashi syndrome, etc.[17]

^c HIV (will be discussed in next section), Adenosine-deaminase deficiency,, DiGeorge syndrome, Wiskott–Aldrich syndrome, etc.[17]

^dFor example, Bruton's agammaglobulinemia, common-variable immunodeficiency syndrome, hyper IgM syndrome, etc.[17]

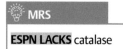

MRS

ESPN LACKS catalase

[17]Note that these genetic immunodeficiency disorders are discussed further in Chapter 12, Allergy and Clinical Immunology.

8.11.2 HIV (Human Immunodeficiency Virus)

Background: HIV is acquired through sexual transmission or infected blood products. Once inside the body, HIV invades and kills CD4+ T-helper cells that normally orchestrate the immune system battle against microbes and cancer. Decline in CD4+ cells is associated with recurrent infections with viral, bacterial and/or fungal organisms, emergence of various opportunistic and atypical pathogens. Also, CD4+ cell decline is associated with increased risk of various malignancies. This stage of low CD4 count with emergence of various opportunistic/atypical pathogens and/or atypical malignancies is known as acquired immunodeficiency syndrome.

Risk factors

- Men who have sex with men
- IVDA (intravenous drug abuse)
- Multiple sexual partners
- Hemophiliacs (high risk with older generation clotting factor replacements)

Confirming diagnosis

Presenting scenarios	NSIDx
26 y/o M presents with diarrhea, abdominal discomfort, weight loss, rash, sore throat, and generalized lymphadenopathy of few weeks' duration (**Dx—acute retroviral syndrome**).	HIV-1/2 immunoassay[a] and HIV RNA RT-PCR[b] (reverse transcriptase PCR)
Recent high-risk exposure, or a newborn to a HIV-positive mother	HIV-1/2 immunoassay[a] and HIV RNA RT-PCR[b] – If both are negative, repeat in few weeks. It might take some time for the test to become positive.
54 y/o with hx of high-risk sexual behavior presents with acute-onset dyspnea and dry cough. CXR shows bilateral pulmonary infiltrates. (Dx is likely PCP, which is the MC AIDS defining condition.)	HIV-1/2 immunoassay. – If positive, next step is HIV-1/HIV-2 antibody differentiation immunoassay. (This is a confirmatory test[c] and differentiates serotypes of HIV.)

[a]Test that detects both HIV antigen and antibody.

[b]In early infection, immunoassay might be negative, and PCR might be positive.

[c]Some laboratories still use western blot to confirm immunoassay testing.

Abbreviations: RT-PCR, reverse transcriptase polymerase chain reaction; PCP, pneumocystis pneumonia; MC, most common, AIDS, acquired immunodeficiency syndrome.

General management of HIV

- Check CD4$^+$ count, PCR viral load, and drug sensitivity-resistance profile of the virus.
- Perform the following additional screening test at the time of diagnosis:

Screen for	Test with	Additional points
Syphilis	VDRL, RPR or TPHA, FTA-ABS, EIA	If positive, NSIDx is to choose other class of syphilis test.
Toxoplasmosis	Anti-toxoplasma antibody IgG	If positive, give antibiotic prophylaxis when CD4 count falls below 100
Hep A	Anti-Hep A antibody	If negative antibody, NSIM is immunization with Hep A regardless of CD4 count.
Hep B	HBsAg, HBsAb, anti-HBc antibody	If –ve for HBsAb, NSIM is Hep B immunization regardless of CD4 count
Tuberculosis	Purified protein derivative (PPD) or interferon-gamma release assay (IGRA)	If PPD ≥ 5 mm or +ve IGRA, NSIM—CXR. If CXR negative, treat for latent TB with isoniazid + vitamin B6.
Hep C	Anti-HCV antibody	Screening test

- Other routine vaccinations in HIV:
- HPV (11–26 years of age), H. influenzae, meningococcus (2 months or older), PCV 13 followed by PPSV 23 (defer PPSV until CD4 count is ≥200, but PCV-13 can be given with any CD4 count), TDaP once and TDq10 yrs.
- If CD4 count ≥200, live vaccines like MMR and varicella zoster vaccine can be given, if no evidence of immunity.
- BCG vaccine is not recommended in HIV as there is risk for dissemination.

HAART (Highly Active Antiretroviral Treatment)

Goal of HAART is to maintain CD4$^+$ count and keep viral load undetectable. Usual regimen consists of two nucleoside or nucleotide reverse transcriptase inhibitors AND a third drug (e.g., protease inhibitor or non-nucleoside reverse transcriptase inhibitor). A 50% reduction in viral load is expected after the first month of therapy. If no such decrease, then NSIM is to check viral drug sensitivity profile.

MRS

NRTIs end with + INE

MRS

NNRTIs are the words that contain "vir"

MRS

Protease inhibitors mostly end with + NAVIR

	Nucleoside/nucleotide reverse transcriptase inhibitors (NRTIs) and their notable side effects	Non-nucleoside reverse transcriptase inhibitors (NNRTIs) and their notable side effects	Protease inhibitors and their notable side effects
	• Zidovud**ine**, a.k.a. azidothymid**ine**—bone marrow suppression, e.g., leukopenia or anemia • Stavud**ine**—peripheral neuropathy • Didanos**ine**—pancreatitis • Lamivud**ine** • Zalcitab**ine**—pancreatitis • Emtricitab**ine** • Abacavir • Tenofovir	• Efa**vir**enz—confusion • Ne**vir**apine—liver failure • Dela**vir**dine • Rilpi**vir**ine • Etra**vir**ine • Dora**vir**ine	• Nelfi**navir** • Indi**navir**—crystalluria or flank pain due to development of renal stones. • Rito**navir** • Saqui**navir** • Ampre**navir**
Side effects common to all in this group	Lactic acidosis	• Stevens–Johnson syndrome • Most can cause hepatotoxicity, but ne**vir**apine is more frequent and severe.	Cushing-like syndrome (central obesity, hyperlipidemia, and hyperglycemia; ritonavir is the most commonly implicated drug)

Specific Situations and HAART

Pregnancy	• In pregnant patients with > 1,000 copies/mL of HIV RNA, or unknown viral load at the time of delivery, give IV zidovudine to the mother to reduce perinatal transmission. • Efavirenz is contraindicated in pregnancy.
Infants born to HIV +ve mother	• All infants born to HIV +ve mother should receive postexposure prophylaxis with zidovudine.
Postexposure prophylaxis (needle stick injury)	• NSIM: clean wound thoroughly, test for HIV-1/2 immunoassay, HIV RNA RT-PCR, and start triple HAART for a total of 4 weeks (regardless of test results). • If both immunoassay and RT-PCR are negative, repeat in few weeks. It might take some time for the test to become positive.

Clinical Case Scenarios

A 35 y/o M with newly diagnosed HIV (CD4 count of 200) and TB gets started on HAART and anti-TB therapy. After 2 weeks, patient develops worsening chest symptoms and CXR reveals worsening chest infiltrate + bigger lymphadenopathy. What is happening?

IRIS (immune reconstitution inflammatory syndrome) presents with paradoxical worsening of an existing infection or disease process or, unmasking of previously occult infection/disease process soon after initiation of HAART therapy. This may be due to unbalanced recovery of various types of T-cells, leading to exuberant inflammatory response in patients with recovering CD4 count (starting CD4 count is usually < 100, except for TB).

Another CCS example—patient develops CMV retinitis after initiation of HAART (unmasking of pre-existing CMV infection).

Management: Treat underlying condition if disease was unmasked, or continue current therapy for worsening of known disease.

CD4 Count, Opportunistic Pathogens and Their Prophylaxis

CD4 count per µL (mm³)	emergence of following opportunistic pathogens at this level of CD4 count	What to do when CD4 count falls below this range	MRS
> 500	Normal		
≤ 200	• PCP (Pneumocystis pneumonia) a.k.a. *Pneumocystis jirovecii* pneumonia	• Start prophylaxis with Sulfamethoxazole-trimethoprim • Second-line agents for PCP prophylaxis are Dapsone, inhaled Pentamidine, and Atovaquone.	Name giveth all: PcP – "c" looks like 2 and there are 2 "p" letters. P's head looks like a zero(0). So, CD4 count ≤ 200
≤ 100	• Toxoplasmosis • Cryptococcosis • Cryptosporidiosis	• Continue prophylaxis with sulfamethoxazole-trimethoprim which will cover both PCP and toxoplasmosis • Second line for toxoplasmosis prophylaxis: Dapsone + pyrimethamine-leucovorin, OR Atovaquone ± pyrimethamine-leucovorin	**Toxo- cryptoco-cryptospo-** all got oo and hence 100. Toxo- looks like 100: T = 1
≤50	• CMV = cytomegalovirus • MAC = mycobacterium avium complex	• For prophylaxis of MAC, use weekly azithromycin. Second-line agents are clarithromycin and rifabutin.	• MAC: A for Azithromycin and C for Clarithromycin • For CD4 count ≤ 50: think of diseases with three-letter acronyms—MAC, CMV, PML (progressive multifocal leukoencephalopathy)

> **MRS**
>
> PADS save us from PCP

As the CD4 count increases after initiation of HAART, prophylaxis can be discontinued.

Different clinical case scenarios in HIV patients[18]

Legend: D/Dx = differential diagnosis: CNS, central nervous system

HIV with CNS Involvement

D/Dx of HIV with brain involvement; all of the following can present with seizures, focal neurological deficits, headache, etc. Look for the following differentiating feature:	Additional info: (preferred imaging modality for all of the following is MRI)		Dx and management
• Chorioretinitis (eye <u>pain</u> + blurry vision) • Features of increased ICP (intracranial pressure)	• Brain imaging shows ring-enhancing lesion (single or multiple). • Look for CD4 count ≤ 100.	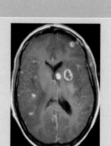 Multiple small contrast-enhancing lesions Source: Brain Tumors. In: Eastman G, Wald C, Crossin J, eds. Getting Started in Clinical Radiology. From Image to Diagnosis. 1st ed. Thieme; 2005.	**Dx: Toxoplasmosis** (Hint: In HIV patients with CNS involvement, presence of chorioretinitis points towards this diagnosis) **Rx:** Sulfadiazine + pyrimethamine.
• Personality changes and dementia • Can be chronic • Usually there is no fever • Can have <u>painless</u> visual symptoms	• Brain imaging shows <u>multiple</u> nonenhancing lesion or plaques in white matter. These are demyelinating lesions and not space-occupying, so features of increased ICP are not present. • Look for CD4 count ≤ 50.	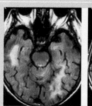 Source: Progressive Multifocal Leukoencephalopathy (PML). In: Sartor K, Hähnel S, Kress B, eds. Direct Diagnosis in Radiology. Brain Imaging. 1st ed. Thieme; 2007.	**NSIDx:** PCR of CSF fluid for JC virus. Positive PCR confirms the diagnosis. **Dx: Progressive multifocal leukoencephalopathy (PML),** caused by reactivation of **polyoma JC virus** in immunosuppressed individuals. **Rx:** HAART with goal of raising CD4 count
• Can have painless visual problems • Features of increased ICP	• Usually solitary nonhemorrhagic mass (but can be multiple too). Sometimes it can be seen as a weakly ring-enhancing lesion.	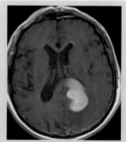 Source: Primary CNS Lymphoma. In: Sartor K, Hähnel S, Kress B, eds. Direct Diagnosis in Radiology. Brain Imaging. 1st ed. Thieme; 2007.	**Dx: Primary CNS lymphoma** NSIDx is Lumbar puncture (CSF analysis for lymphoma cells) and slit lamp exam (lymphoma involvement in posterior part of eye is common). In male patients, rule out brain metastasis due to testicular cancer by doing testicular exam and ultrasound. **Rx:** Chemotherapy (high-dose methotrexate-based regimen) ± radiation or stem cell transplant.

Note: PML is also associated with immunosuppressive therapy such as natalizumab.

HIV with Eye Involvement

D/Dx of HIV patient presenting with visual symptoms	Dx and additional info	Management
Visual disturbances with fundoscopic abnormalities • Usually painless	• **CMV retinitis** • Dx usually requires ophthalmologist assessment. • Look for CD4 count ≤ 50.	**If sight-threatening infection—** intravitreal ganciclovir or foscarnet + oral valganciclovir. **If non-sight threatening infection**—use oral valganciclovir (preferred). **Note:** systemic ganciclovir can cause neutropenia, and foscarnet can cause renal failure.
Visual disturbances with fundoscopic abnormalities + • Additionally, patient has CNS manifestations (e.g., focal neurological deficit) • May have eye pain	• **Toxoplasmosis retinitis** • Look for CD4 count ≤ 100	CT scan shows single or multiple ring-enhancing lesions. **Rx:** sulfadiazine + pyrimethamine.
• Visual disturbances with fundoscopic abnormalities + • keratitis and corneal opacification • Look for vesicles and eye pain	• **Herpes simplex virus** or • **Varicella zoster virus:** presence of extraocular vesicles in dermatomal distribution points towards this.	Dx is made by viral culture of vesicle fluid or PCR (PCR is faster). Tzanck smear can be done. **Rx:** severe cases require IV acyclovir followed by oral valacyclovir.

HIV with Pneumonia

D/Dx of HIV patient presenting with pneumonia	Likely Dx	Management
• Productive cough + lobar or lobular infiltrate in CXR	MCC of pneumonia in HIV patients is *S. pneumoniae*	**Rx:** Empiric treatment with ceftriaxone + azithromycin
• Dry cough + dyspnea + CXR reveals bilateral diffuse interstitial opacity in a perihilar distribution	PCP (PneumoCystis pneumonia) a.k.a. P. jirovecii pneumonia • Look for CD4 count ≤ 200.	**Rx:** Trimethoprim-sulfamethoxazole. Steroid is indicated if PaO2 ≤ 70 mmHg, or A-a gradient ≥35.

HIV with Skin Involvement

D/Dx of HIV patient presenting with skin rash	Additional pointers to diagnosis	Diagnosis/ Treatment

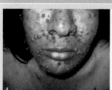 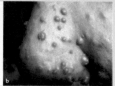
 	
Source: Mejía F, Seas C. Bacillary angiomatosis. Am J Trop Med Hyg. 2014.
	• Rash morphology
	  – Comes in various numbers, colors and forms (purplish black to flesh colored; nonfriable to red-pink friable looking)
	  – Round, exophytic
	  – Can have ulceration
	  – Can have visceral lesions (e.g. liver angiomas)
	• Associated with systemic flu-like syndrome (e.g. fever, malaise)
	• Biopsy will show vascular proliferation with neutrophilic infiltrate.
		Dx: Bacillary angiomatosis—due to infection with Bartonella henselae.
		
		Rx: Erythromycin or doxycycline (atypical bacterial coverage)

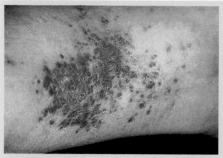 Source: Vascular Tissue. In: Laskaris G, ed. Color Atlas of Oral Diseases. Diagnosis and Treatment. 4th ed. Thieme; 2017. 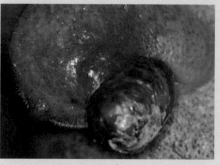 Source: Kaposi Sarcoma. In: Laskaris G, ed. Pocket Atlas of Oral Diseases. 2nd ed. Thieme; 2005.	• Similar to bacillary angiomatosis, this can be variable in color and forms (e.g., patches, plaques, papules, nodules) • Absence of systemic flu-like syndrome helps to differentiate from bacillary angiomatosis • Biopsy will show neoplastic vascular proliferation with lymphocytic infiltrate 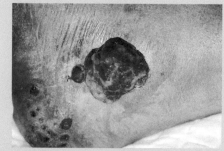 Source: Vascular Tissue. In: Laskaris G, ed. Color Atlas of Oral Diseases. Diagnosis and Treatment. 4th ed. Thieme; 2017.	**Dx: Kaposi sarcoma** due to Human herpesvirus-8 (HHV-8) infection **Rx:** HAART therapy to raise CD4 count is the best treatment. May use Intralesional chemotherapy for localized disease. Consider systemic chemotherapy for severe disease or visceral involvement.

 MRS

MRS = Kaput–Kap =
Kaposi: Ut = 8 (HHV-8)

Source: Molluscum Contagiosum. In: Laskaris G, ed. Color Atlas of Oral Diseases. Diagnosis and Treatment. 4th ed. Thieme; 2017.

- **Umbilicated** papule or nodule
- Almost flesh-colored

Dx: Molluscum contagiosum infection.

Rx: Various options—curettage, cryotherapy, podophyllotoxin, or cantharidin (cantharidin is avoided in genital areas). After initiating HAART, lesions may improve.

Miscellaneous conditions : HIV+ve patient presenting with		
Chronic progressive bilateral lower extremity weakness and numbness-Exam reveals bilateral lower extremity spasticity and hyperreflexia. • Presentation is similar to subacute to chronic transverse myelitis, or severe vitamin vitB$_{12}$ deficiency.	If MRI of spine is negative and serum Vit B12 is normal, likely Dx is **HIV-associated vacuolar myelopathy.**	Pathologically there is vacuolization of dorsal column and corticospinal tract.
Slowly progressive dementia	Rule out PML by doing MRI with contrast and neurosyphilis by doing CSF VDRL-TPHA test.	If both are negative, then the Dx is **HIV-related dementia** (HIV encephalitis).

Brain abscess and HIV

Etiology:

Spread from local contiguous sites (sinusitis, mastoiditis, otitis media, oral infection). Likely causative organisms are *S. viridans* and mixed anaerobes in this case.
Spread from a distant site. Example: Infective endocarditis, or infection with atypical organisms in immunocompromised patients (nocardiosis, toxoplasmosis)

Presentation: Seizures, focal neurological deficits, headache, features of increased ICP, etc.

Diagnostic evaluation and management

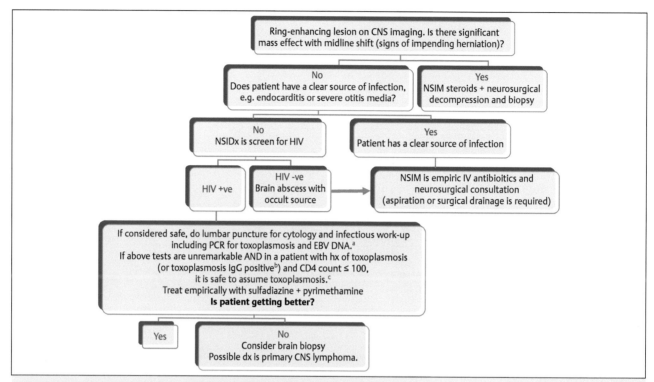

[a]EBV in CSF is associated with primary CNS lymphoma; also look for lymphoma cells in CSF.

[b]If no prior hx of documented toxoplasmosis antibody, NSIM is to check toxoplasma IgG antibody.

[c]If toxoplasmosis antibody is negative and CSF tests are unrevealing, only then do brain biopsy.

Clinical Case Scenarios

Patient with HIV and hx of medical noncompliance presents with chronic expressive aphasia and left-sided weakness. There is no hx of fever. Exam reveals hyperreflexia in left side. MRI with and without contrast shows multiple hypodense nonenhancing lesions. Toxoplasma IgG antibody is positive.

16. What is the like Dx?

    a) Testicular cancer with metastasis

    b) Progressive multifocal leukoencephalopathy

    c) Toxoplasmosis

    d) Primary CNS lymphoma

17. What is the patient's expected CD4 count?

    a) 400–500

    b) 300–400

    c) 200–300

    d) < 50

Differential diagnosis and management of HIV patients with odynophagia

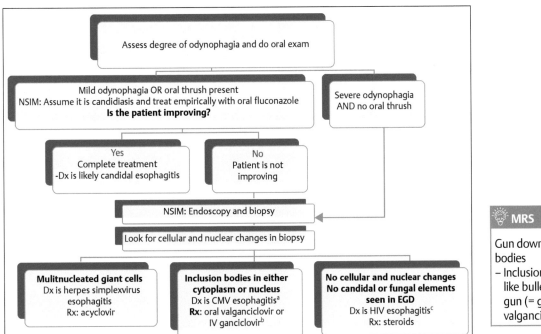

^aPatients might have coexistent retinitis or colitis.

^bIn patients who cannot tolerate oral medication, give IV ganciclovir.

^cDiagnosis of exclusion.

Differential diagnosis and management of HIV patients with diarrhea

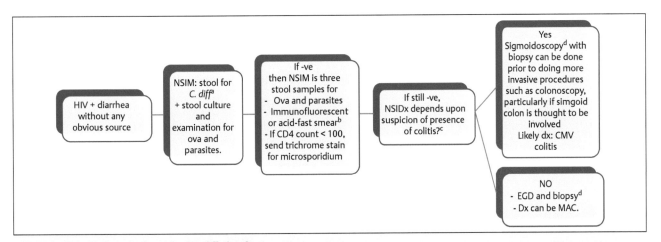

^aPatients with HIV have higher risk of *C. difficile* infection.

^bCryptosporidiosis, Isospora, and Cyclospora require acid-fast staining for diagnosis.

^cAbdominal tenderness and bloody diarrhea point toward colitis.

^dEarly invasive diagnostic procedures may be warranted in patients with low CD4 count and severe presentation.

In a nutshell

Diarrhea		Likely dx	Management
Subacute or chronic watery diarrhea	**Additional features:** fever, lymphadenopathy, night sweats, abdominal pain, malabsorption syndrome (weight loss), etc.	Disseminated mycobacterium avium complex (MAC) infection	• Blood culture and/or culture from lymph node. • If nondiagnostic, NSIDx is EGD with biopsy **Rx:** **E**thambutol + **R**ifabutin + **A**zithromycin (or other macrolides) for 6 months.
	Only watery diarrhea	Cryptosporidiosis, *Isospora*, and *Cyclospora*	NSIDx is stool ova and parasites, with modified acid-fast staining. **Rx:** Best step in treatment is HAART to raise CD4 count. Nitazoxanide can be used if persistent.
Acute or chronic **bloody** diarrhea • Can cause toxic megacolon		CMV colitis	NSIDx is sigmoidoscopy with biopsy. **Rx:** Oral valganciclovir or IV ganciclovir

[19]This CXR shows patchy, confluent infiltrates in the left upper lung zone.

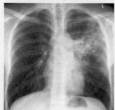

Source: Imaging Signs. In: Galanski M, Dettmer S, Keberle M et al., eds. Direct Diagnosis in Radiology. Thoracic Imaging. 1st ed. Thieme; 2010.

8.11.3 Tuberculosis (TB)

Background: TB is caused by *Mycobacterium tuberculosis* bacilli and is transmitted through aerosol secretions. After initial exposure to TB, our immune system effectively imprisons it by creating a granuloma (dormant T.B. bacilli in our lung). But anytime we become immunosuppressed, these bacilli can get reactivated and cause active infection. Nowadays, TB is resurging as an important cause of morbidity and mortality due to increasing prevalence of HIV. Monoclonal antibodies (e.g. *infliximab, adalimumab, golimumab*) also increase risk for reactivation of TB.

Presentation: chronic cough, fever, night sweats, and weight loss.

Evaluation and management of suspected active TB:

● In suspected case of active TB, NSIDx is CXR, which will classically show infiltrates or areas of consolidation or cavitary lesion typically in the apical region.[19]

● NSIM is airborne isolation, three morning sputum samples for acid-fast bacilli (**AFB**), AFB culture, check for HIV, and in high-probability cases, initiate empiric anti-TB therapy.

● If three AFB samples are negative, isolation can be discontinued. This rules out infectious TB.

Pharmacotherapy of TB

First-line TB drugs	Side effects
Rifampin	Red/orange color of body secretions (might permanently stain contact lens)
Isoniazid	• It can cause pyridoxine (Vit B$_6$) deficiency, which leads to neuritis (paresthesia, ataxia, etc.) • May also cause drug-induced lupus: eosinophilia, lymphadenopathy, and leukopenia/anemia, etc. • Isoniazid toxicity can lead to confusion and seizures.
Pyrazinamide	Hyperuricemia
Ethambutol	Optic neuritis and optic nerve atrophy • So all patients should be regularly screened with eye exam.

Hepatotoxicity: **R**ifampin, **I**soniazid, and **p**yrazinamide may be hepatotoxic.

If AST/ALT remains in the <100 range, we usually can continue RIP treatment without any issue.

Treatment options and duration:

- For uncomplicated TB, RIPE is given for 2 months. Then PE is discontinued, and RI is continued for 4 more months. Total duration is at least 6 months.
- Longer treatment is required for TB meningitis, pregnancy, and TB osteomyelitis.
- Steroids may also be indicated for TB meningitis and pericarditis.

Screening for TB

Either purified protein derivative (PPD) or interferon-gamma release assay (IGRA) can be used. PPD includes intradermal injection of tuberculin protein and assessing area of induration 48–72 hours later. IGRA includes exposing patient's blood sample to TB antigen and **quanti**fying T-cell-mediated inter**feron**-gamma release. IGRA is preferred in patients with hx of BCG vaccination or who are at risk of loss to follow-up.

Risk category for development to active TB	Clinical condition	PPD induration[a] considered positive
High risk	• Close contact of active TB cases • HIV • Abnormal CXR that is consistent past TB (e.g., apical fibronodular changes) • Organ transplant • Suppressed immune system—steroid use (steroid dose of ≥ 15 mg/day for ≥1 month), or immunosuppressive therapy (TNF-alpha inhibitors)	≥ 5 mm
Intermediate risk	• ESRD, silicosis, other malignancies (head/neck cancer, leukemia, etc.) • Patients with other conditions that increase risk for reactivation, e.g. diabetes, IVDA, underweight (BMI ≤ 20). • People who live or work in homeless shelter, prison, nursing home, or hospital (e.g., health care workers) • Recent immigrants from a country with high TB prevalence (e.g., Nepal, Mexico,) • Children < 4 years of age	≥ 10 mm
Low risk	Healthy population aged 4 years or older • Screening is not recommended and is usually done for credentialing or official requirements	≥ 15 mm

[a]LOM: remember that size of erythema does not matter; it is the induration size that matters.

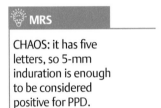

MRS

CHAOS: it has five letters, so 5-mm induration is enough to be considered positive for PPD.

What to do when PPD or IGRA comes back positive?

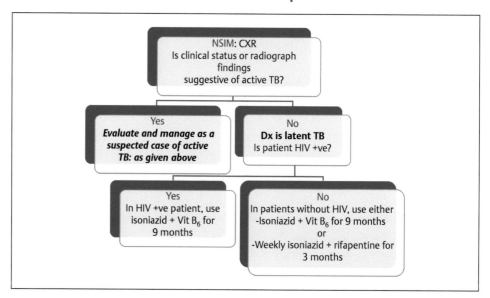

Management of Exposure to TB

[20]IGRA= Interferon-gamma release assay

The algorithm below might look confusing. The following info might help to simplify it:

- If you have a patient < 5 years of age or immunosuppressed, initial workup should include PPD (or IGRA[20]) and a CXR. If PPD is < 5 mm and 8 weeks has not passed since exposure, then start isoniazid prophylactically until repeat PPD (or IGRA) 8 weeks after exposure is negative. (better to be safe than sorry in this patient group).

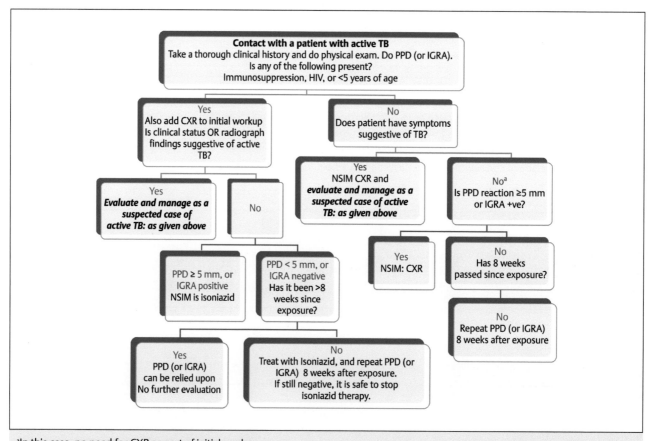

[a]In this case, no need for CXR as part of initial workup.

Clinical Case Scenarios

18. A 45 Y/O M recently had a close contact with a TB patient. He has no hx of immunosuppression and is asymptomatic. PPD is 6 mm. NSIM?

19. Perfectly healthy nurse with no hx of exposure to TB, has work-related PPD screening, with erythema of 20 mm and induration of 8 mm. NSIM?

20. What if the nurse in case 2 had induration of 10 mm. NSIM?

21. Patient recently started on adalimumab for rheumatoid arthritis develops symptoms suggestive of TB. CXR shows classical apical opacities suggestive of TB. What is the most appropriate NSIM?

22. Patient is recently started on isoniazid for latent TB. Later, patient develops rash, leukopenia, and lymphadenopathy. NSIM?

23. Patient on RIPE treatment for active TB develops red urine. NSIM?

24. Patient on RIPE treatment develops pain behind eye and some blurry vision. What medication can cause this?

25. Patient is getting treated for active TB, but he reports not feeling better. He reports of dizziness, fatigue, and skin getting darker for the last few weeks. BMP reveals metabolic acidosis. What is the likely dx?

26. A 4-year-old child's father was recently diagnosed with TB 1 week ago. His father started having cough 3 weeks ago. The child is asymptomatic and physical exam is unremarkable. What is the NSIM?

    a) PPD

    b) PPD + CXR

    c) CXR

27. The child's PPD induration is 3 mm. CXR is negative. What is the NSIM?

    a) Reassurance

    b) Repeat PPD 8 weeks after exposure

    c) Start isoniazid + repeat PPD 8 weeks after exposure

8.11.4 Opportunistic Pathogens

The following group is considered **highly immunocompromised**:
- Chronic use of high-dose steroids, or immunosuppressive medications
- HIV with low CD4 count
- Organ-transplant recipient
- Patients undergoing active chemotherapy
- Hematologic malignancy

They are more likely to get opportunistic infections with CMV, PCP, aspergillosis, and nocardiosis. All of these can present with lung involvement. The following table helps to differentiate between them:

 MRS

This is similar to the CHAOS group who are considered to have +ve PPD if induration is ≥ 5 mm.

Organism	PCP (pneumocystis pneumonia)	CMV (cytomegalovirus)	Invasive aspergillosis	Nocardiosis
Predominant clinical features	Nonproductive cough and SOB	Nonproductive cough and SOB • Can hav e coexistent diarrhea, abdominal pain (CMV colitis), and/or odynophagia (CMV esophagitis)	Cough and hemoptysis	Cough, night sweats, fever, weight loss (sounds like TB)
Radiological findings	Bilateral diffuse interstitial infiltrates CT chest—ground glass attenuation with many small nodules Above patient had pneumocystis pneumonia. Source: Imaging. In: Gunderman R, ed. Essential Radiology. Clinical Presentation, Pathophysiology, Imaging. 2nd ed. Thieme; 2000.		Depending upon stage of infection and underlying severity, it can have various radiological pictures. Classic signs include nodules with surrounding ground glass infiltrates (halo sign) These nodules can later cavitate, producing air-crescent sign (shown below) Source: Clinical Aspects. In: Galanski M, Dettmer S, Keberle M et al., eds. Direct Diagnosis in Radiology. Thoracic Imaging. 1st ed. Thieme; 2010.	Nodules, cavitation, or abscess (similar to TB)
Diagnostic workup	• Following tests are done on a sputum sample: microscopy with special staining, direct fluorescence antibody ± PCR. PCR is particularly helpful in patients without HIV. • If negative, bronchoalveolar lavage should be done for diagnosis.	• Peripheral blood CMV- PCR or antigen testing • Bronchoscopy+ bronchoalveolar lavage and transbronchial lung biopsy are the test of choice. Look for inclusion bodies in histopathological specimen. Also, do CMV PCR and culture on these specimens. • Do not use CMV antibody testing for diagnosis.	• Biomarkers of the fungus (galactomannan and beta-D-glucan, which are fungal cell-wall components[a]) can be detected in **serum.** • Obtain sputum for fungal staining and culture. • If nondiagnostic, bronchoscopy + bronchoalveolar lavage ± transbronchial lung biopsy or CT-guided nodule biopsy can be done.	Brain imaging should be performed in all patients with suspected pulmonary nocardiosis; as MC extrathoracic site involved is the brain. Gram stain of sputum or biopsy specimen may reveal branching, filamentous rod-shaped bacteria that look like fungi (picture A) and are partially acid-fast (red rods in picture B). Source: Toyomitsu S, Takumi N, Shota Y, et al. Detection of high serum levels of β -D-Glucan in disseminated nocardial infection: a case report. BMC Infect Dis. 2017.

Organism	PCP (pneumocystis pneumonia)	CMV (cytomegalovirus)	Invasive aspergillosis	Nocardiosis
Treatment	Trimethoprim-sulfamethoxazole[b,c] • **Steroid** is indicated if PaO2 ≤ 70 mmHg Or, A-a gradient ≥ 35.	• Mild disease—oral valganciclovir • Severe disease—IV ganciclovir • If resistant to ganciclovir, use foscarnet.	Use voriconazole. For severe disease, add an echinocandin (e.g., micafungin, caspofungin). **Second line:** amphotericin B (if voriconazole causes hepatotoxicity)	Trimethoprim-sulfamethoxazole

[a]Galactomannan is relatively specific for aspergillosis. Serum beta-D-glucan is not specific and can also be positive in other fungal infections (including PCP).

[b]If sulfa allergic, second line depends upon severity:

• If severe, use IV pentamidine.

• If mild to moderate—use oral atovaquone.

[c]PCP prophylaxis with trimethoprim-sulfamethoxazole is indicated in patients with solid-organ transplant and undergoing high-dose immunosuppressive therapy.

Abbreviation: SOB, shortness of breath.

8.11.5 Systemic Fungal Infections

- All of the following systemic fungal infections can cause lung infection with features of cough and TB-like symptoms with fever, night sweats, and chills.
- CXR may reveal pulmonary infiltrates, lymphadenopathy, nodules, consolidation, or cavitation. Most patients are initially treated for community-acquired pneumonia, with no improvement.

	Histoplasmosis	Blastomyces dermatitidis	Coccidioidomycosis	Cryptococcus neoformans and other cryptococcus spp.
Location where the fungus is endemic[a]	Missouri and Mississippi river valleys[b]	Missouri river valleys	Desert and dry lands (Arizona, Texas, California, New Mexico, etc.)	Nonspecific[b]
Other findings that point to diagnosis • **These** systemic fungi can disseminate anywhere—joints, bone, bone marrow, skin, meninges, lymph nodes, etc.	• Hepatosplenomegaly and lymphadenopathy (histoplasmosis involves the reticuloendothelial system as it prefers invasion of phagocytic cells such as histiocytes and macrophages)	• Warty, ulcerative skin lesions, or subcutaneous lesions • CXR may show upper lobe cavitation. • Osteolytic lesion/s in bone can be seen.	• Presence of desert bumps—red, painful subcutaneous nodule in patient with lung symptoms. These subcutaneous nodules are histologically similar to rheumatoid nodules and are due to allergic reactions. Allergic morbilliform rash may also develop. • Self-limiting pneumonia in majority of patients (known as valley fever)	• Can cause meningitis ± encephalitis • Pulmonary infection • Just like other systemic fungi, can also disseminate anywhere—eye, joints, bone, skin, lymph nodes, etc. • Can cause skin lesions—plaques, papules that look like molluscum contagiosum.

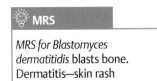

MRS

MRS for Blastomyces dermatitidis blasts bone. Dermatitis—skin rash

	Histoplasmosis	Blastomyces dermatitidis	Coccidioidomycosis	Cryptococcus neoformans and other cryptococcus spp.
Use a combination of the following tests for diagnosis	• Urine or serum histoplasma or *Blastomyces* antigen • Serum antibody • Fungal stain/culture and microscopic visualization in specimen obtained from tissue biopsy, sputum, or lavage.		• Serum IgM and IgG antibody. If positive, do immunodiffusion testing. • Serum coccidioidal antigen test is not sensitive. • May need to obtain specimen from tissue biopsy, sputum, or lavage—use fungal stain (KOH preparation) and if culture is obtained, needs biocontainment to prevent infection of lab personnel.	• Serum cryptococcal antigen • Lumbar puncture in patients with neurologic symptoms • Culture of infected tissue sample (sputum, bronchial lavage, CSF, etc.)
Form of yeast seen	Yeast cells are seen inside human histiocytes (hence called histoplasmosis) and macrophages.[c]	• Broad-based budding yeast (*Blastomyces*)	Multiple endospores within spherules[c]	Source: Candica albicans. In: Riede U, Werner M, eds. Color Atlas of Pathology: Pathologic Principles, Associated Diseases, Sequela. 1st ed. Thieme; 2004.
Treatment	• For acute mild infection, no evidence of dissemination[d] and immunocompetent patients—observation (expect spontaneous recovery). • Moderate or chronic infection, or immunocompromised host—oral itraconazole • Severe infection -use amphotericin B, followed by itraconazole	• For mild to moderate disease and no evidence of dissemination,[d] use itraconazole. • For severe disease, use amphotericin B, followed by itraconazole.	• Mild infection, no evidence of dissemination[d] and immunocompetent—observation • Moderate to severe infection, immunocompromised host, or pregnant patient—oral itraconazole or fluconazole	• For mild infection, no evidence of dissemination and no meningoencephalitis, use fluconazole • For severe pulmonary infection, disseminated disease, or meningoencephalitis, use amphotericin B + flucytosine, followed by fluconazole for at least 1 year.

	Histoplasmosis	Blastomyces dermatitidis	Coccidioidomycosis	Cryptococcus neoformans and other cryptococcus spp.
In HIV patients with hx of prior fungal infection, treatment with oral antifungal is continued until CD4 count (cells/µL) is persistently above[e]	> 150	> 150	> 250	> 100

[a]Exam Tip- If question specifies a location with lung problem think of these infections.[21]

[b]Cave exploring (spelunking) or exposure to bird droppings are risk factors. Decaying **bat** guano or bird droppings can be a perfect growth medium for fungi such as histoplasma, Cryptococcus, Aspergillus, etc.

[21]Patients living in this area can also present with asymptomatic lung nodule.

[c]

In histoplasmosis, there are multiple fungal bodies inside a nucleated cell.	In coccidioidomycosis there are multiple fungal bodies inside a nonnucleated compartment (i.e., a spherule)
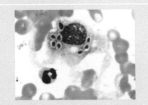	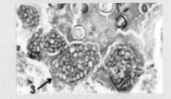
Source: Yang B, Lu L, Li D, et al. Colonic involvement in disseminated histoplasmosis of an immunocompetent adult: case report and literature review. BMC Infect Dis. 2013.	Source: Muñoz-Hernández B, Palma-Cortés G, Cabello-Gutiérrez C, Martínez-Rivera MA. Parasitic polymorphism of Coccidioides spp. BMC Infect Dis. 2014.

[d]Skin rash is not considered disseminated if it is due to allergic reactions (e.g., urticaria or morbilliform rash).

[e]Routine prophylaxis for primary fungal infection is not recommended in HIV patients, unless patient lives in a hyperendemic area.

Patient presents with few weeks' history of a painless papule that has morphed into an ulcer in left hand. Exam reveals linear arrangement of palpable nontender healing lesions distally from the primary lesion seen in left hand (inset picture). Patient regularly works in the yard.

28. What is the next step to confirm diagnosis?

29. What is likely diagnosis?

30. What is the treatment?

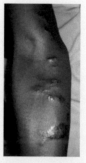

Chain of healed lesions in a lymphocutaneous distribution
Source: Govender NP, Maphanga TG, Zulu TG, et al. An Outbreak of Lymphocutaneous Sporotrichosis among Mine-Workers in South Africa. PLoS Negl Trop Dis. 2015.

FYI: Histoplasma, Blastomyces, Coccidioides, Sporothrix, and Candida are dimorphic fungi.
They are "mold in cold and yeast in the heat," except Candida, which means mycelial forms in the environment, but yeast forms in the human body.

8.12 Superficial Fungal Infections

8.12.1 Superficial Candida Infection

Predisposing conditions:

- Immunosuppressive conditions like DM, HIV, chemotherapy, or steroid use,[22] etc.
- Pregnancy and infant population
- Antibiotic use[22]
- Debilitating disease

[22] Hospitalized patients usually have multiple risk factors for Candida

Location	Presentation	Treatment
Skin infection	Erythematous area in skin fold areas	Nystatin or topical azoles (e.g. clotrimazole, ketoconazole)
Mucosal infection	• Thick white curd-like plaques in mouth or vagina, which are easily removable, and the underlying erythematous area is uncovered or • Diffuse erythematous atrophic tongue/vagina (curd-like plaques may be absent) or • Combination of the two	For oral cavity infection (oral thrush), use nystatin swish and spit or clotrimazole douche. In patients with HIV and low CD4 count, use oral fluconazole. For candidal vaginitis • In nonpregnant patients, use oral fluconazole—150 mg single dose (DOC), or topical antifungals (miconazole/clotrimazole). • In pregnant patients, topical is preferred.
Pharynx and esophagus	Sore throat and odynophagia	Empiric nystatin swish and swallow ± oral fluconazole.
Colon	Loose stools with negative *C. diff* testing and stool cultures revealing candidal overgrowth	

Febrile Neutropenia with Absolute Neutrophil Count <500/μL[23]

Risk factor: Chemotherapy and/or hematological malignancy

Management: For high-risk patients, NSIM is hospital admission, blood culture, and initiation of broad-spectrum antibiotics that cover Pseudomonas (e.g. cefepime, piperacillin-tazobactam, meropenem, etc.)

If patient has any of the following, add MRSA coverage with vancomycin or linezolid:

- Hypotension
- Evidence of pneumonia, skin or catheter-related infection
- Hx of prophylaxis with ciprofloxacin

If fever persists for > 4 days despite adequate antibiotic coverage, consider the following:

- In patients with no obvious source, add Candida coverage with caspofungin.
- In patients with pulmonary nodular infiltrates, cover Aspergillus with voriconazole or amphotericin-B.

[23]CCS
- Patient on chemotherapy presents with fever. Temperature is 38.4 °C. Lab shows WBC count of 2,000/mm^3 with 10% neutrophils.
- Here absolute neutrophil count = 200 cells/μL (10% of 2,000)

8.12.2 Other Fungal Skin Infections

Condition	Causative agent	Clinical findings	KOH preparation findings[a]
Tinea versicolor	*Malassezia furfur* a.k.a. *Pityrosporum orbiculare* Source: Tinea Versicolor. In: Sterry W, Paus R, Burgdorf W, eds. Thieme Clinical Companions - Dermatology. 1st ed. Thieme; 2006.	• *T. versicolor* = versatile color—that means macules and patches can be of various color (erythematous, hyperpigmented, or hypopigmented) • Asymptomatic (there is no itching)	Round and filamentous forms of fungi ("spaghetti with meatballs" appearance) Source: Tinea Versicolor. In: Sterry W, Paus R, Burgdorf W, eds. Thieme Clinical Companions - Dermatology. 1st ed. Thieme; 2006.
Tinea cruris/corporis	*T. rubrum* Source: Tinea manuum. In: Sterry W, Paus R, Burgdorf W, eds. Thieme Clinical Companions - Dermatology. 1st ed. Thieme; 2006.	• **Location:** Can be found throughout the body, but is less common in scalp, interdigital areas, and sole of feet. • Classically called round worm because there is a round rash with central clearing and it is very **itchy.**	Segmented hyphae
Tinea pedis[b]	*T. rubrum* and *T. interdigitale* Source: Tinea Pedis. In: Sterry W, Paus R, Burgdorf W, eds. Thieme Clinical Companions - Dermatology. 1st ed. Thieme; 2006.	• **Location:** interdigital areas, or in soles of feet. • Excoriations, fissures, hyperkeratotic lesions; even vesiculobullous lesions can occur. • Also called "swim mer's itch," as it causes significant pruritus • *T. rubrum* can have nail involvement causing *Tinea unguium.*	Segmented hyphae

Condition	Causative agent	Clinical findings	KOH preparation findings[a]
Tinea capitis	*Trichophyton* and *Microsporum* Source: Tinea Capitis. In: Sterry W, Paus R, Burgdorf W, eds. Thieme Clinical Companions - Dermatology. 1st ed. Thieme; 2006.	• Scaly semi-bald patches, with black dots representing broken hair. (Presence of the black dots is the differentiating feature from alopecia.) • Risk of permanent hair loss.	Fungal spores are found

[a]For all suspected cases of cutaneous fungal infection, NSIDx is scraping and KOH preparation of the scrapings. Visualize the fungi in a microscope and confirm the diagnosis before treating.

[b]The most common (MC) complication of *T. pedis* is cellulitis and lymphangitis. **Example CCS:** patient with *T. pedis* presents with new-onset rash with red linear streaks that goes up from the toe (lymphangitis) and redness and tenderness in the calf region (cellulitis).

Treatment: Use topical meds (topical azoles, tolnaftate, etc.). In patients with hair or nail involvement, infection refractory to topical medications, OR involving extensive areas, use oral antifungals (e.g. oral fluconazole, itraconazole, or terbinafine).

8.13 Tick-Borne Illness

[24]In the United States, disease-carrying ticks are found in many states.

Major risk factor: tick bite, history of camping, or living/traveling to endemic nonmetropolitan areas of the United States.[24]

Tick-borne illness	Lyme	Human monocytic ehrlichiosis	Human granulocytic anaplasmosis	Babesiosis	Rocky Mountain spotted fever (RMSF)
Tick vector	*Ixodes* • Reservoir is white tailed deer	*Amblyomma* spp.	*Ixodes* • Reservoir is white-tailed deer	*Ixodes* • Reservoir is white-tailed deer	*Dermacentor* spp.
Causative organism	*B. burgdorferi*	*Ehrlichia* spp.	*Anaplasma* spp.	*Babesia microti* (protozoa)	*Rickettsia rickettsii*
Clinical features (All may have flu-like syndrome with fever, malaise, headache, etc.)	• Erythematous lesion with central clearing—bull's-eye lesion (pathognomonic) • Can later disseminate to heart, nerves, joint, brain, etc.	Fever, malaise, headache, chills • Thrombocytopenia, leucopenia, and elevated liver function test[a]		• Severe infection occurs in old, immune-compromised or asplenic patients • Presents like malaria with fever, chills, rigors, and hemolysis. • Can cause disseminated intravascular coagulation	Name giveth all: it is **spotted** (**petechia** and maculopapular rash), and has fever. • Malaise, headache, chills, arthralgia, etc. • Can present with meningitis-like features

Tick-borne illness	Lyme	Human monocytic ehrlichiosis	Human granulocytic anaplasmosis	Babesiosis	Rocky Mountain spotted fever (RMSF)
Diagnostic evaluation	No need for diagnostic testing in patients *from Lyme-endemic area or hx of tick bite*, and classic bull's-eye skin rash (Lyme serology may be negative in the early stage) Source: Skin. In: Siegenthaler W, ed. Siegenthaler's Differential Diagnosis in Internal Medicine: From Symptom to Diagnosis. 1st ed. Thieme; 2007. • In all other cases, confirm dx with ELISA antibody with reflex confirmatory western blot testing.	• Best initial test is peripheral blood smear or buffy coat microscopic examination: may show intracytoplasmic inclusions (called morulae) in **leukocytes.** A morula (group of bacterial cells) seen inside a granulocyte Source: Fever with Multiple Organ Involvement. In: Siegenthaler W, ed. Siegenthaler's Differential Diagnosis in Internal Medicine: From Symptom to Diagnosis. 1st ed. Thieme; 2007. • **Serology for antibody ± serum PCR**[25]		• Best initial test is peripheral blood smear—may reveal intra**erythrocytic** trophozoites. The white arrow shows a ring-like structure which may represent an early form of malaria parasite, but the Maltese-cross like structure (black arrow) is pathognomonic of Babesia. Source: Tobler WD, Cotton D, Lepore T, Agarwal S, Mahoney EJ. Case Report: Successful non-operative management of spontaneous splenic rupture in a patient with babesiosis. World J Emerg Surg. 2011. **Serum PCR for babesiosis**[25]	Serology antibody testing can be done to confirm diagnosis; but do not wait for the serology to start, empiric treatment with doxycycline in suspected cases.
Treatment	• If < 8 years or pregnant, treat with amoxicillin or cefuroxime. • If ≥ 8 years, doxycycline is DOC[b]	Doxycycline		• **Mild infection:** atovaquone + azithromycin • **Severe infection:** clindamycin + quinine\	Doxycycline

[a]Presence of these lab abnormalities will point toward ehrlichiosis/anaplasmosis in a clinical-case scenario involving tick bite or camping trip.

[b]Indication for intravenous **ceftriaxone** for Lyme treatment

• Second- or third-degree AV block
• Myopericarditis
• Recurrent Lyme arthritis despite adequate prior oral treatment.
• Meningitis or encephalitis[26]
• Polyneuropathy

[25]As sensitivity of blood smear isn't that great for Babesiosis, Anaplasmosis, or Ehrlichiosis, do antibody or PCR panel for suspected cases when smear is negative.

MRS

Think of an antimalarial + a macrolide.

[26]A simple rule is if heart or brain is involved, give IV ceftriaxone.

Clinical Case Scenarios

Patient presents to your clinic with tick attached to skin.

31. What is the NSIM?

32. When is Lyme prophylaxis indicated in such scenarios?

33. A 35 y/o M living in Rhode Island presents with migratory arthralgia and arthritis. There is no risk factor for STD. Lyme serology is found to be positive. NSIM?

34. A 35 y/o F with a recent hx of bull's-eye skin rash, now presents with isolated facial nerve palsy. NSIM?

35. A 45 y/o M from rural Connecticut presents with second-degree heart block. Lyme serology is positive?

8.13.1 Parasitology

MRS

ENTER YOUR PIN number

Parasite and condition	Mode of infection	Presentation	NSIDx	Treatment
Enterobius vermicularis (**pin**worm) infection	Orofecal route	• Itchy perianal region, especially at night • Can also occur in vulva or scrotum	Do a scotch tape test (place a scotch tape in the anal orifice at night and as the pinworms come out and lay their eggs, they get stuck on the scotch tape. It can be viewed under microscope the next day.)	DOC is albendazole or mebendazole. • Treatment of entire household is recommended
Cutaneous larva migrans due to *Ancylostoma* spp.	Larvae are found in sandy beaches contaminated with animal (dog or cat) feces. Larva can penetrate through skin upon contact with contaminated sand.	• Pruritic erythematous rash that is serpiginous • Can occur in hands, body, or feet.	Dx is made clinically	Ivermectin (DOC) or albendazole
Visceral and ocular larva migrans due to *Toxocara canis*	Larvae are found in sand or playground contaminated with animal (dog or cat) feces. It is acquired through ingestion of larvae, hence occurs primarily in children.	**Visceral larva migrans:** fever, hepatomegaly pneumonitis, rash, etc. Can also disseminate to brain, eye, muscles, heart, etc. **Ocular larva migrans:** infection localized in the eye (vision loss, eye pain, uveitis, etc.).	• Peripheral eosinophilia • Antibody serology assay (e.g., ELISA) • Radiological imaging	Albendazole

Necator americanus (hookworm) infection	Mainly **acquired** by walking barefoot on contaminated soil.	The nectar it sucks is our blood, causing iron deficiency—anemia.	Stool exam	Albendazole
Trichinellosis	Acquired from consumption of raw or undercooked meat (pork)	• Abdominal pain, nausea and vomiting, and diarrhea • Fever with muscle pain/tenderness, periorbital edema, and splinter hemorrhages (*! Makes you think of endocarditis*)	• Peripheral eosinophilia • Elevated creatine kinase • Serology (it can be negative in early infection) • If needed, muscle biopsy can be done	Albendazole

MRS

Hooks and sucks the nectar out of us.

8.13.2 Taenia solium

Pathophysiology/life cycle: the parasite has the following life cycle: eggs → larva → adults. Disease presentation depends upon whether the infected person ingested the egg or larva form.

- Viable larva can be ingested by humans with uncooked/poorly cooked pork. The ingested larva changes into the adult form in human intestine (noninvasive infectious stage) and stays there, which keeps on laying eggs that can be found in the stool.
- When eggs are ingested (with contaminated water, food, etc.), they turn into larvae, which now become invasive and can travel to other organs (e.g. muscles or brain[27]) and form cysts.

Treatment: albendazole.

[27]FLAIR demonstrating the scolex (arrow), which is the anterior end of a tapeworm, bearing suckers and hooks for attachment.

Source: Parasites. In: Borsody M, ed. Comprehensive Board Review in Neurology. 2nd ed. Thieme; 2009.

8.13.3 Hydatid Cyst

Risk factors: close contact with sheep or dogs.

Causative organism: *Echinococcus* spp.

Presentation: right upper quadrant discomfort + hepatomegaly, or incidental finding in imaging of liver.

Diagnosis: made with combination of radiological findings and serology (antibody assay). Ultrasound of liver[28] reveals smooth round big cysts with daughter cysts within it, ± eggshell calcification. Pulmonary cysts might also be present.

Rx: Albendazole +/- percutaneous aspiration-&-injections or surgery. Potential complications of procedure include secondary seeding of infection and/or anaphylaxis.

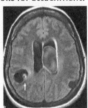

[28]

Source: Special Differential Diagnosis of Jaundice. In: Siegenthaler W, ed. Siegenthaler's Differential Diagnosis in Internal Medicine: From Symptom to Diagnosis. 1st ed. Thieme; 2007.

8.13.4 Malaria

Risk factor: travel/living in endemic areas.

Causative organism: Plasmodium spp.

Presentation: fever, chills, and rigors with associated flu-like syndrome. Dark urine might also be present. Exam may reveal pallor and splenomegaly.

Dx: made by peripheral blood smear (visualization of parasite) or malarial antigen assay.

Rx: empiric therapy depends upon travel history, as discussed on next page.

Clinical Case Scenarios

36. A 35 y/o M pig farmer presents with acute onset seizures. CT scan reveals hypodense cystic non-calcified lesions. What is the treatment of choice?

a) Albendazole
b) Albendazole + praziquantel
c) Albendazole + praziquantel+ steroids
d) Albendazole + praziquantel+ steroids + anti-seizure therapy

MRS

You get MAD when malaria is chloroquine-resistant

Travel history to	Areas	Empiric therapy
Chloroquine-sensitive areas	Dominican Republic, Haiti, etc.	Chloroquine
Chloroquine-resistant areas	Sub-Saharan African continent, the Sub-Himalayan Indo-Nepal territory, and the upper regions of South America	**M**efloquine, **A**tovaquone-Proguanil, **Arte**misinin derivatives (e.g., **arte**mether or **arte**sunate) or, **D**oxycycline + quinine.

8.14 Miscellaneous

	Causative organism	Risk factor	Presentation	Treatment
Cat scratch disease	*Bartonella henselae* (the same microbe that causes bacillary angiomatosis in patients with HIV)	Cat exposure	Linear papule or vesicle that can progress onto ulcer, and/or Isolated enlarged lymph node with history of cat exposure • In children can rarely cause encephalitis and seizures.	Nowadays all suspected cases receive a short course of macrolides (e.g., azithromycin).
Ulceroglandular disease	*Francisella tularensis*	Exposure to rabbits	Necrotic ulcer with central eschar and tender lymphadenopathy	Ciprofloxacin or doxycycline

8.15 Miscellaneous CCS for Practice

What empiric antibiotic therapy would you give in each case?

CCS	Empiric therapy	
A 25-year-old male patient with no comorbidity presents with features of pneumonia with right lower lobe opacity seen on CXR.	Macrolides (Dx is uncomplicated community-acquired pneumonia)	
A 60-year-old male with prosthetic valve MRSA endocarditis.	Vancomycin + gentamicin + rifampin	
A 50-year-old male with native valve MRSA endocarditis	Vancomycin	
A 20-year-old male: urethral gram stain is positive for intracellular diplococci.	Single IM dose of ceftriaxone + single oral 2 g dose of azithromycin	
A 45-year-old male with classic bacterial meningitis (no hx of DM or immunosuppression).	VCS	• V = vancomycin
A 60-year-old male with hx of DM with classic bacterial meningitis.	VACS	• A = ampicillin • G = gentamicin or other aminoglycosides
A 2-week-old neonate with classic bacterial meningitis.	GAC	• C = ceftriaxone or cefotaxime
A 4-month-old infant with meningitis.	VC ± steroids	• S = steroids (IV dexamethasone)

Answers

1. Erysipelas.

2. Group A **ß-hemolytic** *Streptococcus*.

3. Penicillin or amoxicillin.

4. Kluver–Bucy syndrome due to herpes encephalitis.

5. Loss of amygdala function. Kluver–Bucy syndrome can also occur after brain surgery, stroke, or trauma involving the amygdala.

6. Rapid strep test.

7. Throat culture, CBC with peripheral smear, complete metabolic profile (serum electrolytes + LFT), and heterophile antibody test.

8. Heterophile antibody test a.k.a. monospot test.

9. Steroids.

10. MCC of lobar pneumonia is S. pneumoniae, regardless of risk factors (e.g., alcoholic, HIV-positive patient, patient who went to a convention, nursing home resident). Other causes of lobar pneumonia include aspiration pneumonia, Legionella and M. tuberculosis infection.

11. Dx is septic pulmonary emboli likely due to right-sided endocarditis.

12. Blood cultures, empiric IV antibiotics, and TTE.

13. Any syphilis serology test can be used; either nontreponemal tests or specific treponemal serology.

14. Do the other class of syphilis testing: here it would be nontreponemal serology test (e.g., VDRL or RPR)

15. Do another type of specific treponemal serology. Here TPHA was used first, so do FTA-ABS. If FTA-ABS is negative, then TPHA might have been a false-positive test.

16. b: Progressive multifocal leukoencephalopathy. Positive toxoplasma antibody, which is common in general population and is a common red herring in exam questions.

17. d: CD4 count is likely < 50.

18. Chest X-ray. PPD is positive, as patient is a close contact of active TB case.

19. No further steps needed. PPD is negative.

20. Chest X-ray.

21. Stop adalimumab and evaluate as per active TB (airborne isolation, sputum AFB times 3, and culture and empiric initiation of RIPE).

22. Stop isoniazid and change to **rifampin**.

23. Urinalysis, because know that renal tuberculosis can also present with red urine due to hematuria. If urinalysis is negative for RBCs, it is likely related to rifampin (Red).

24. Ethambutol (optic neuritis).

25. Adrenal insufficiency (Addison's disease), due to TB adrenalitis.

26. b: Do PPD + CXR.

27. c: Start isoniazid + repeat PPD 8 weeks after exposure.

28. Fungal culture of lesion.

29. Sporotrichosis a.k.a. Rose-Gardner's disease.

30. Oral itraconazole or potassium iodide.

31. Remove with tweezers.

32. Consider prophylaxis for Lyme if <u>all</u> the following criteria are met:
    - Tick identified as "deer" tick
    - Estimated exposure/attachment ≥36 hours or, tick is engorged
    - High local rates of infection
    - Should be within the window of 72 hours of tick removal.

33. Doxycycline. Arthritis is the most likely sequela of untreated Lyme.

34. Pregnancy test and Lyme titer. If pregnancy test is negative, start doxycycline (no need to wait for Lyme titer results).

35. IV ceftriaxone. Once high-grade AV block has resolved and PR interval is <300 milliseconds, patient can be discharged with oral antibiotics.

36. c) For > 2 viable cyst, Albendazole + praziquantel combination therapy is recommended. For 2 or less viable cyst, use albendazole alone. Concurrent steroids is recommended ,to prevent cerebral edema , with anti-parasitic therapy. As patient had seizures, anti-seizure medication is also added.

COVID-19 (corona - virus induced disease)

Background: highly contagious viral infection caused by severe acute respiratory syndrome coronavirus 2 (SARS-CoV-2), an RNA virus of family corona viridae. It can cause viral pneumonia and in some cases, severe systemic inflammatory response, acute respiratory distress syndrome, particularly in elderly population or in immunosuppressed patients.

Presentation: fever, myalgias, headhache, cough, pneumonia, loss of sense of taste, smell and GI upset (nausea, vomiting, or diarrhea).

Diagnosis: Rapid molecular DNA-based testing is preferred (e.g. RT-PCR). Antigen-based detection has lower sensitivity, but can also be used.

Management: low dose dexamethasone (6mg daily for 10 days) is indicated for hypoxic patients on supplemental oxygen (shown to improve mortality). Remdesivir (antiviral agent) indicated for oxygen saturation ≤94 percent on room air but not on supplemental oxygen. Monoclonal antibodies has been shown to reduce hospitalization in non-hospitalized patients.

DVT Prophylaxis is indicated in all hospitalized patients and in non-hospitalized patients with high-risk feature include prior VTE, recent surgery or trauma, immobilization, or obesity.

9. Gastroenterology

It is estimated that the population of human gut microbiome is around 100 trillion bacterial cells. That would mean there are more bacterial cells inside us than our own human cells.

This gut microbiome is considered not only a passive synergistic system but also an active system with its own signaling chemicals that has a positive and protective effect on the human body. To this gut microbiome, broad-spectrum antibiotics, sadly, are nuclear bomb equivalent. So, even though antibiotics can be life-saving, be aware of its effect on our friendly and beneficial gut microbiome. Dictum is to give as narrowest spectrum antibiotics as possible, for the shortest period of time as permitted.

9.1 Esophageal Pathology Based on Location

Part of esophagus	Type of muscle	Pathology	Additional points
Upper one-third	Skeletal muscles only, which are innervated by somatic (voluntary) nervous system.	Diseases that primarily affect – Skeletal muscles (e.g., myasthenia gravis, myositis syndromes) – Somatic nerves (e.g., motor nerve palsy)	Squamous cell carcinoma usually occurs in upper or middle part of esophagus. Its major risk factors are alcohol, smoking, achalasia, lye ingestion, etc.
Middle third	Upper part of middle esophagus is mostly skeletal muscles and lower part is mostly smooth muscle cells.		
		Diseases that primarily affect – Smooth muscles (e.g., scleroderma)	
Lower third	Smooth muscle cells only, which are innervated by autonomic nervous system.	– Autonomic nerves (e.g., achalasia cardia)	Adenocarcinoma usually occurs in the lower third. Its major risk factor is chronic gastroesophageal reflux disease.

9.2 Dysphagia (Difficulty in Swallowing)—Mechanical and Neuromuscular

9.2.1 Mechanical Dysphagia

Definition: Dysphagia for solids, progressing on to dysphagia of liquids can be defined as mechanical dysphagia. Patients presenting with such history usually have a structural lesion that is progressively obstructing the lumen of the esophagus. MCC is esophageal stricture.

Workup: In patients with prior hx of conditions that are associated with complex esophageal anatomy (e.g., hx of radiation, caustic injury, surgery for esophageal or laryngeal cancer), do barium swallow prior to endoscopy (It provides a road map for endoscopy and makes it safer.). Otherwise, go directly for upper gastrointestinal (GI) endoscopy, a.k.a. esophagogastroduodenoscopy (EGD). If structural lesion is found, do biopsy.

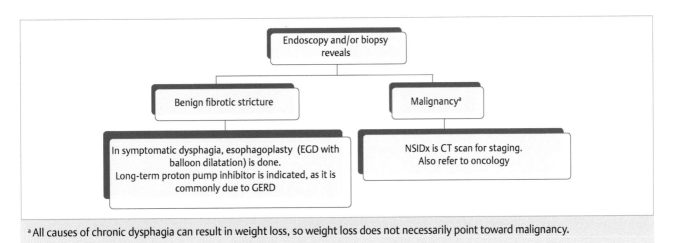

[a] All causes of chronic dysphagia can result in weight loss, so weight loss does not necessarily point toward malignancy.

9.2.2 Lower Neuromuscular Dysphagia

Definition: It can be defined as difficulty in swallowing both liquids and solids that starts simultaneously. This kind of dysphagia is most likely due to esophageal motility problems.

Etiology: Achalasia-pseudoachalasia (problem with esophageal smooth muscle innervation), scleroderma (esophageal smooth muscle itself is replaced by fibrous tissue), and other esophageal motility disorders (e.g., diffuse esophageal spasm).

Workup: EGD followed by manometry. Manometry is the most accurate test.

9.2.3 Achalasia and Pseudoachalasia

Background: After food ingestion, the autonomic nervous system signals esophageal peristalsis to propel food downward and when food reaches the lower part of esophagus, it signals the lower esophageal sphincter (LES) to relax. This relaxation is very important for food to pass into the stomach. Loss of autonomic innervation results in inadequate peristalsis and inability of LES to relax, resulting in dysphagia for both solids and liquids.

	Achalasia cardia (idiopathic achalasia)	Pseudoachalasia (a.k.a. secondary achalasia)
Primary pathology	Idiopathic destruction of myenteric (Auerbach's) plexus	Denervation/destruction of myenteric plexus by: – **Tumor** (esophageal or gastric adenocarcinoma, lymphoma, etc.): presence of hx of long-standing GERD features may point toward adenocarcinoma of lower esophagus – **Vagal nerve denervation** (e.g., surgical vagotomy) – **Infection** (e.g., Chagas disease which can cause megaesophagus)
Barium swallow appearance	Smooth distal esophageal narrowing or tapering (called "bird beak's appearance"). Proximal esophageal dilation signals advanced disease. Proximal esophagus Source: In: Michael J, Sircar S, eds. Fundamentals of Medical Physiology. 1st ed. Thieme; 2010.	In malignancy, the tapering is **usually NOT smooth**; proximal esophagus may or may not be dilated. Note the irregular proximal contour (arrow) and the distal margin of the stenosis.
EGD and biopsy	Primary destruction of the neural plexus in absence of other pathologic features[a]	Usually reveals the underlying disorder, e.g., lymphoma cells in myenteric plexuses
Treatment	– In low-surgical-risk patients, do pneumatic dilation[b] or surgery[c] (pyloromyotomy) – In patients with high risk of complication with invasive procedures (e.g., advanced age), give botulinum toxin injection into lower esophageal sphincter via EGD. It usually requires retreatment. If it fails, use nitrates and calcium channel blockers	Treat underlying disorder

[a]Never miss the chance of detecting malignancy in its earliest stage. Endoscopy and biopsy are mandatory even in apparent achalasia cardia.
[b]Potential complication includes esophageal perforation.
[c]In patients younger than 40 years of age who are low risk for surgery, surgical approach may be preferred over pneumatic dilatation, as risk of recurrence in pneumatic dilatation is higher.

9.2.4 Other Esophageal Motility Disorders (Esophageal Spasm)

Presentation:

- Intermittent crushing substernal chest pain unrelated to exertion, which is sometimes aggravated by hot or cold liquids.
- Intermittent feeling of food (solids or liquids) getting stuck in esophagus.
- Intermittent heart burn or food regurgitation.

Workup:

- In patients presenting with chest pain, always do electrocardiogram (EKG) first. In patients with dysphagia, do endoscopy first. In patients with prominent heart burn symptoms, if patient fails high-dose proton pump inhibitor (PPI) therapy, do esophageal pH and impedance testing to rule out gastroesophageal reflux disease (GERD).
- If above test is inconclusive, NSIDx is manometry, which can show typical high-pressure episodic contractions.
  - If contractions are **diffuse**, diagnosis is **diffuse esophageal spasm.**[1]
  - If contractions are **localized** to a specific area of esophagus, diagnosis is "nutcracker" esophagus (aka hypertensive peristalsis). (They say the pressure is so high, it can even crack a nut.)
  - If patient has high LES (lower-esophageal sphincter) resting tone, dx is hypertensive LES.

Rx: Calcium channel blockers (diltiazem, nifedipine) or tricyclic antidepressants such as imipramine (M-antagonist effect). Sublingual nitroglycerin can relieve the pain/spasm.

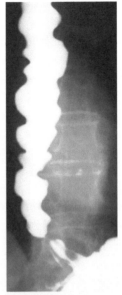

[1]Corkscrew esophagus pattern in barium swallow.
Source: Siegenthaler W, ed. Siegenthaler's Differential Diagnosis in Internal Medicine: From Symptom to Diagnosis. 1st ed. Thieme; 2007.

9.2.5 Esophageal Manometry

Test description: A thin flexible plastic tube is inserted (e.g., a nasogastric feeding tube) and pressures are monitored by this tube while swallowing.

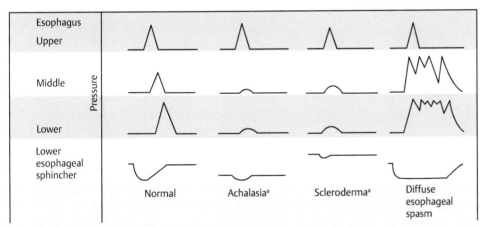

[a]LES **resting pressure** is **high** in achalasia cardia and **low** in scleroderma.[2] Both can present as neuromuscular dysphagia.

[2]Also, scleroderma can present with mechanical and/or neuromuscular dysphagia
- Poor LES tone → GERD → peptic stricture → mechanical dysphagia
- Smooth muscles of lower half of esophagus gets replaced by fibrous tissue → diminishing peristalsis → neuromuscular dysphagia

9.2.6 Upper Neuromuscular Dysphagia

Definition: It refers to difficulty initiating swallowing, nasal regurgitation, and choking or coughing while eating.

Etiology: Dementia[3] and bulbar/pseudobulbar palsy.

[3]This form of neuromuscular dysphagia is common in elderly patients with advanced dementia. They forget how to swallow.

	Pseudobulbar palsy	Bulbar palsy
9, 10, 11, 12 cranial nerve involvement	Upper motor neuron palsy	Lower motor neuron palsy
Causes	Stroke (MCC), multiple sclerosis	Guillain–Barre syndrome, syringobulbia, myasthenia gravis, lower motor neuron disease, etc.

Workup: Videofluoroscopy (modified barium swallow under fluoroscopic surveillance).

Rx: Usually supportive. Address underlying cause.

In a nutshell

Type of dysphagia	Etiology	Clinical history	Steps in diagnosis
Mechanical dysphagia	Peptic stricture, malignancy, etc.	Dysphagia for solids, progressing on to dysphagia of liquids	EGD (+/− pre-EGD barium swallow[a])
Lower neuromuscular dysphagia	Achalasia and pseudoachalasia	Dysphagia with difficulty swallowing both liquids and solids simultaneously	EGD (+/− pre-EGD barium swallow[a]), followed by manometry
Upper neuromuscular dysphagia (aka oropharyngeal dysphagia)	Dementia and bulbar/pseudobulbar palsy	Difficulty initiating swallowing, nasal regurgitation, and/or choking or coughing while eating	Videofluoroscopy

[a]In patients with prior hx of conditions that are associated with complex esophageal anatomy (e.g., hx of radiation, caustic injury, surgery for esophageal or laryngeal cancer), do barium swallow prior to endoscopy.

9.3 Other Esophageal Disorders Related to Dysphagia Disorders

Condition	Pathophysiology	Presentation	Management
Esophageal rings	Development of soft mucosal concentric rings in esophagus, therefore, only food with a certain diameter gets stuck – Schatzki's ring is one subtype and associated with hiatal hernia – Rings due to eosinophilic esophagitis are associated with other findings suggestive of this disorder	Nonprogressive episodic dysphagia, particularly with larger-size food chunks	Dx is made by barium swallow, or EGD and biopsy. **Rx:** EGD with pneumatic dilatation, followed by PPI therapy
Esophageal webs	Formation of thin mucosal eccentric fold that protrudes into esophageal lumen, which typically occurs in upper cervical area of esophagus – When it occurs with iron deficiency anemia, it is called **Plummer–Vinson syndrome**. It has higher risk of squamous esophageal carcinoma – Other associated conditions include pemphigus disorders, chronic graft versus host disease, etc.	Can present similar to esophageal rings. Patient complains of difficulty swallowing, particularly in the **cervical zone of esophagus**. Lab test may reveal iron deficiency anemia	Dx is made by barium swallow, or EGD and biopsy. For Plummer–Vinson syndrome, NSIM is iron replacement (it may lead to resolution of dysphagia). In patients with significant symptoms, EGD +/− dilatation might be needed. Usually webs are easily ruptured by the endoscope itself
Zenker's diverticulum	Motor dysfunction and weakness of esophageal muscles can lead to development of diverticular pouch in the upper part of posterior esophagus.	Dysphagia, foul breath, regurgitation of previously eaten food – High risk of aspiration pneumonia	**NSIDx:** barium contrast esophagogram. **Rx:** endoscopic or surgical correction

Source: Steffers G, Credner S, eds. General Pathology and Internal Medicine for Physical Therapists. 1st ed. Thieme; 2012.

Condition	Pathophysiology	Presentation	Management
Esophagitis	**Etiology** **Drugs:** tetracycline, doxycycline, aspirin, NSAIDs, alendronate (bisphosphonates), oral potassium/iron supplements, etc. **Other causes:** infectious esophagitis (candida, CMV, HIV, HSV), eosinophilic esophagitis, etc.	Acute onset painful swallowing (odynophagia) + difficulty swallowing (dysphagia) +/- vague to sharp persistent central chest pain	If dx is not apparent or if severe, NSIDx is **EGD** **Rx:** supportive (may use acid suppression). If medication that caused esophagitis cannot be discontinued, use its liquid formulation, which has less risk.

Abbreviations: CMV, cytomegalovirus; EGD, esophagogastroduodenoscopy; HIV, human immunodeficiency virus; HSV, Herpes simplex virus; NSAIDs, nonsteroidal anti-inflammatory drugs.

9.4 Gastroesophageal Reflux Disease

Background:

Reflux of gastric contents and acid into esophagus can occur either due to	Underlying cause
Increased intra-abdominal pressure	Obesity, pregnancy, delayed stomach emptying (gastroparesis), etc.
Decreased contraction of lower esophageal sphincter	Scleroderma, smoking, etc.

Clinical pathophysiology: Patients can present with various symptoms such as chest pain, "heartburn," hoarse voice, cough, etc. Physical exam may reveal inflamed pharynx and larynx.

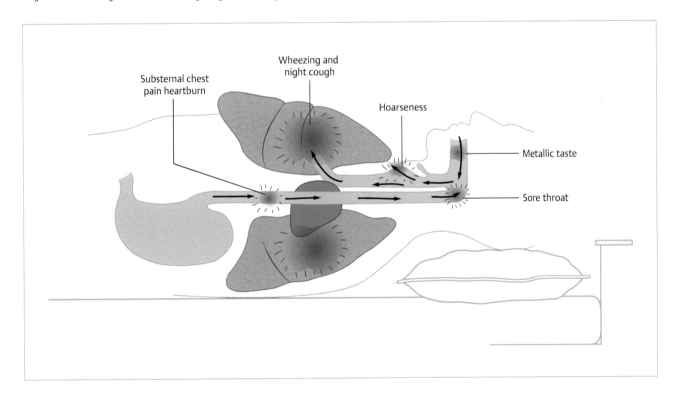

Management:

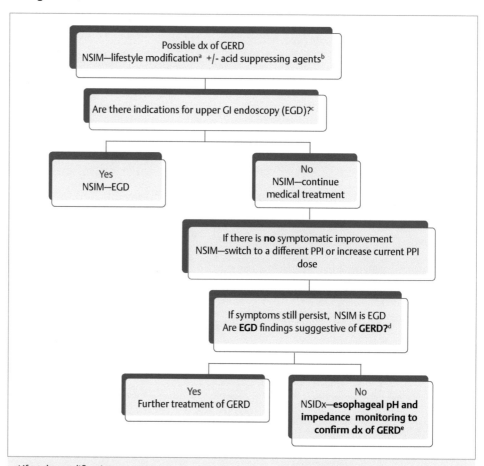

ᵃLifestyle modifications:

– Avoid smooth muscle relaxants (which can relax the lower esophageal sphincter) such as calcium channel blockers, nitrates, chocolate, peppermint (commonly found in chewing gums).

– Weight loss is recommended in obese patients.

– Elevate head of the bed at night; use more pillows.

ᵇPPI[4] is generally added when lifestyle modifications fail to improve symptoms or when symptoms are moderate to severe. In mild GERD, histamine-2 receptor antagonists (e.g., famotidine, ranitidine) can be used.

ᶜIndications for EGD in GERD include presence of any of the following alarm features:

– New-onset dyspepsia at age ≥ 60 years.

– Recurrent or persistent nausea and vomiting.

– Weight loss or anorexia.

– Odynophagia or dysphagia.

– Any evidence of GI bleeding: positive fecal occult blood test, melena (hx of black tarry stool), or microcytic iron deficiency anemia.

– Family hx of gastrointestinal cancer in a first-degree relative.

ᵈEGD findings suggestive of GERD include peptic stricture, reflux esophagitis, and Barrett's esophagus.

ᵉEsophageal pH and impedance monitoring is a highly sensitive and specific test for GERD, but is a cumbersome study that takes 24 hours to perform. Impedance detects movement of intraluminal contents. Combined with pH monitoring, it can differentiate between acid and nonacid reflux.

Surgical treatment for GERD: Patients who require high doses of PPI to control symptoms can be offered surgery (e.g., Nissen fundoplication), particularly in young patients. Before doing surgery for intractable GERD, multiple tests as given below need to be done to confirm the diagnosis and make sure that the surgery will benefit the patient:

– Esophageal pH and impedance monitoring.

– Upper gastrointestinal (UGI) endoscopy (EGD).

⁴ Most drugs ending with "prazole" are PPIs: omeprazole, lansoprazole, pantoprazole, etc.

- Esophageal manometry.
- Gastric emptying study to make sure that the stomach is emptying properly, and gastroparesis is not contributing to refractory GERD.

9.4.1 Complications of Untreated or Uncontrolled GERD

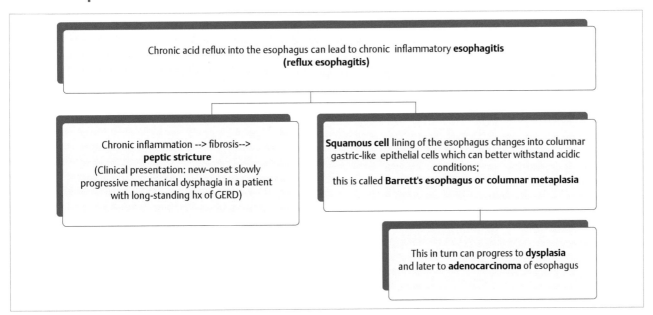

9.4.2 Management of GERD Complications Depend on EGD Findings

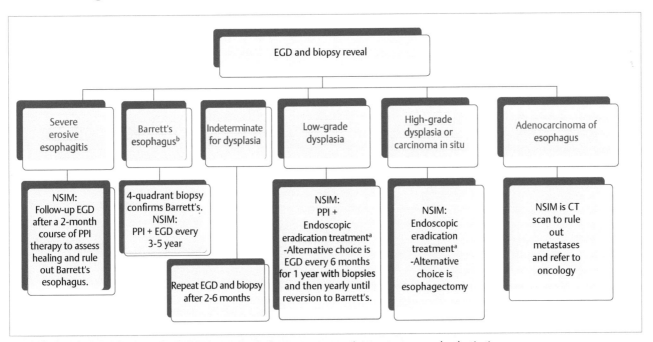

[a]Endoscopic eradication treatment involves using radiofrequency or cryotherapy to remove dysplastic tissue.

[b]When 1st EGD reveals gross findings suggestive of Barrett's esophagus, NSIM is to take 4-quadrant biopsies. Once biopsy confirms Barrett's, do EGD surveillance every 3–5 year. If biopsy reveals low-grade dysplasia or indeterminate for dysplasia manage as shown in the right.

Clinical Case Scenarios

1. A 28-year-old pregnant woman presents to emergency department with new-onset burning substernal chest pain. She does not have any risk factors for atherosclerotic disease. What is the NSIM?

   a) CXR

   b) EKG

   c) EGD

   d) Esophageal pH monitoring

9.5 Dyspepsia (Indigestion)

Definition: Presentation of vague epigastric pain, discomfort, or bloating is known as dyspepsia. Patient may have other symptoms of indigestion such as nausea, excessive flatulence, occasional exacerbation of pain or, in severe cases, diarrhea.

Etiology:

Helicobacter pylori infection	⇒	Helical gram-negative bacteria that is urease positive.
Significant alcohol, aspirin, and NSAIDs use	⇒	These can cause gastritis by inciting inflammation in mucosal lining of stomach.
Giardiasis: this can present with upper GI symptoms (dyspepsia)	⇒	Look for travel hx to high-risk areas for giardiasis. When suspected, NSIDx is to check for giardia stool antigen and do stool microscopy.

Other causes include severe stress, GI malignancy, chronic pancreatitis, infiltrative disease of stomach (e.g., eosinophilic gastritis), etc.

Abbreviations: GI, gastrointestinal; NSAIDs, nonsteroidal anti-inflammatory drugs.

9.5.1 Management Steps of Dyspepsia

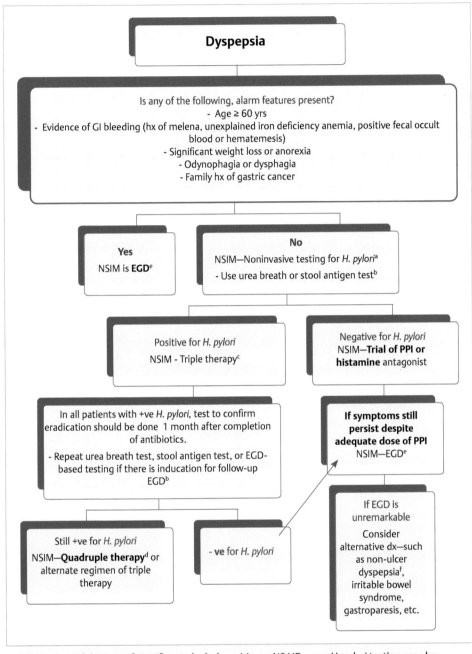

Dyspepsia

Is any of the following, alarm features present?
- Age ≥ 60 yrs
- Evidence of GI bleeding (hx of melena, unexplained iron deficiency anemia, positive fecal occult blood or hematemesis)
- Significant weight loss or anorexia
- Odynophagia or dysphagia
- Family hx of gastric cancer

Yes
NSIM is **EGD**[e]

No
NSIM—Noninvasive testing for *H. pylori*[a]
- Use urea breath or stool antigen test[b]

Positive for *H. pylori*
NSIM - Triple therapy[c]

Negative for *H. pylori*
NSIM—**Trial of PPI or histamine** antagonist

In all patients with +ve *H. pylori*, test to confirm eradication should be done 1 month after completion of antibiotics.
- Repeat urea breath test, stool antigen test, or EGD-based testing if there is induction for follow-up EGD[b]

If symptoms still persist despite adequate dose of PPI
NSIM—EGD[e]

Still +ve for *H. pylori*
NSIM—**Quadruple therapy**[d] or alternate regimen of triple therapy

- **ve** for *H. pylori*

If EGD is unremarkable
Consider alternative dx—such as non-ulcer dyspepsia[f], irritable bowel syndrome, gastroparesis, etc.

[a]In patients with history of significant alcohol, aspirin, or NSAIDs use, *H. pylori* testing may be deferred. Empiric antacid therapy and avoidance of precipitating factor can be tried first.

[b]Stop PPI therapy 1 to 2 weeks before *H. pylori* testing. PPI, antibiotics, and bismuth can lead to false negative result.

[c]Triple therapy for *H. pylori:* **P**PI + **A**moxicillin + **C**larithromycin. If patient is penicillin-allergic, use **M**etronidazole instead of amoxicillin;

[d]Quadruple therapy = **B**ismuth subsalicylate + **M**etronidazole + **T**etracycline (or doxycycline) + **P**PI. Alternative quadruple therapy is **P**PI + **A**moxicillin + **C**larithromycin + **M**etronidazole;

[e]During EGD, rapid urease testing can be done to detect *H. pylori*, which has urease activity.

[f]When no underlying pathology can be found for dyspeptic symptoms, dx of nonulcer (functional) dyspepsia can be made. As majority of dyspepsia are ultimately classified as nonulcer or functional; it is the **most common cause** of dyspeptic symptoms. NSIM is trial of PPI.

Serology (i.e., checking serum antibody against *H. pylori*) has low predictive value and is not recommended.

 MRS

CAP *H. pylori*
CMP (complete metabolic profile).

 MRS

MTBP (Master the boards points)
Quadruple CAMP.

9.6 Peptic Ulcer Disease (PUD)

Definition: Peptic ulcer disease (PUD) refers to gastric and/or duodenal ulcer.

Etiology: Major causes are *Helicobacter pylori* infection and nonsteroidal anti-inflammatory drugs (NSAIDs) use. Other causes of PUD include the following:

High-stress situations	– Severe burn injuries	Empiric PPI or H-2 blocker for ulcer prophylaxis is recommended in these situations.
	– Head trauma and increased intracranial pressure (traumatic brain injury)	
	– Intubation and mechanical ventilation > 48 hrs	
Stomach cancer	All gastric ulcers should be biopsied. By contrast, no need for routine biopsy of duodenal ulcer.	
Rare causes include MALToma, Zollinger–Ellison syndrome and Crohn's disease		

Abbreviation: PPI, proton pump inhibitor.

Presentation: PUD presents with dyspepsia +/– alarm features (as given before in algorithm).

Gastric ulcer	Classic presentation is epigastric pain worsened by eating food. Food stimulates production of gastric acid which irritates the ulcer.
Duodenal ulcer	Epigastric pain usually occurs within few hours after eating food, when gastric contents are being emptied into the duodenum. Eating food relieves pain, as this causes the pyloric sphincter to close, keeping the food and gastric acid in the stomach.

9.6.1 Diagnosis Is Based on Endoscopy Findings

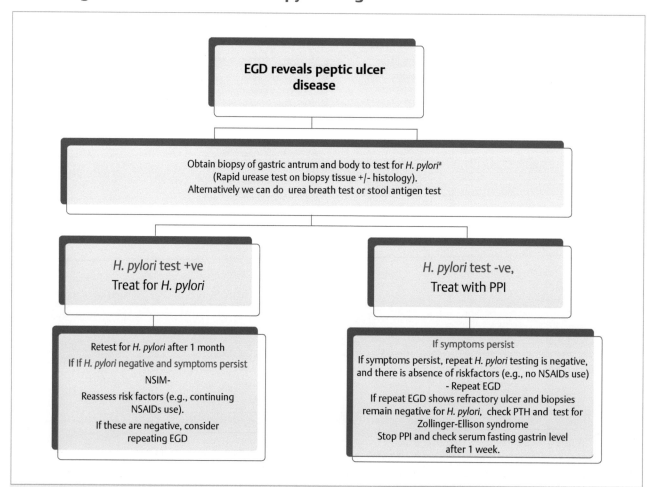

[a]Biopsy of the ulcer itself is not routinely recommended in patients with benign-appearing duodenal ulcer. For gastric ulcers, do biopsy.

9.7 Gastrinoma (Zollinger–Ellison Syndrome)

Background: Gastrinoma is a tumor that autonomously secretes a lot of gastrin. Common location of the tumor is in pancreatic or duodenal area. It can be associated with multiple endocrine neoplasia (MEN) I syndrome.

Pathophysiology:
- Hypergastrinemia stimulates gastric acid production, increases gastric pH and risk for subsequent ulcer formation (usually multiple).
- Hypergastrinemia stimulates gastric mucosal cells leading to mucosal hypertrophy and prominent gastric folds. There is an increased risk of gastric carcinoma.

Presentation:

Dyspeptic symptoms	Suspect gastrinoma if any of the following is present: • Multiple peptic ulcers • Ulcer in odd places like second or third part of duodenum or jejunum • Intractable ulcers or recurrent ulcers, particularly in patients with negative *H. pylori* testing and no hx of NSAIDs use
Malabsorption symptoms	Occur due to excessive gastric acid entering the duodenum, damaging small intestine mucosae, and inactivating pancreatic enzymes. Diarrhea is also present (mostly osmotic with some secretory component)

Abbreviation: NSAIDs, nonsteroidal anti-inflammatory drugs.

Workup:

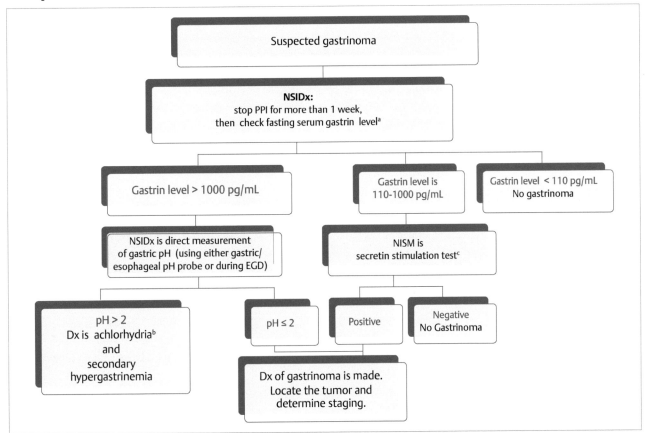

[a]PPIs decrease gastric acid production that leads to increase in compensatory gastrin secretion. So, PPI use can cause false positive hypergastrinemia.

[b]Achlorhydria is absence of gastric acid, that is, alkaline (elevated) pH. It leads to compensatory secondary hypergastrinemia. Causes of achlorhydria include atrophic gastritis (pernicious anemia), chronic renal failure, chronic *H. pylori* infection, surgical vagotomy, etc.

[c]**Mechanism:** Normal gastric acid production is inhibited by secretin. In contrast, gastrinoma cells secrete more gastrin in response to secretin hormone.

[d]1st step is to do an EGD (if not yet done), CT or MRI scan and somatostatin receptor scintigraphy (octreotide scan). If these tests are negative for primary tumor, NSIDx is endoscopic ultrasound. (This has greater sensitivity for diagnosing small tumors.)

Management:

- If gastrinoma is localized and/or with limited or isolated metastasis, NSIM is surgical resection. Do endoscopic ultrasound (US) prior to surgery to ensure proper staging.
- If widespread, do medical treatment with large doses of PPIs to block acid secretion.

[5]Para-pancreatic because these neuro-endocrine tumors can also be found in duodenum or jejunum.

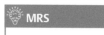

I HAD VIP guests today.

MAD glucagonoma

MEN I syndrome

Hereditary genetic syndrome associated with triad of pancreatic, parathyroid, and pituitary tumors (the board favorite): look for hypercalcemia (parathyroid adenoma), galactorrhoea-amenorrhea syndrome (pituitary adenoma), and features of gastrinoma or other pancreatic or parapancreatic[5] neuroendocrine tumors, as listed below:

	Features
VIPoma (hypersecretion of **v**asoactive **i**ntestinal **p**eptide)	**H**ypokalemia, **A**chlorhydria, **D**iarrhea (secretory type)
Glucagonoma	**M**igratory necrolytic erythema, **A**nemia, **D**iabetes or glucose intolerance
Insulinoma	Hypoglycemia, elevated blood C-peptide and insulin level

9.8 Stomach Cancer

Risk factors:

- Smoking and alcohol (they are synergistic).
- Diet rich in nitrosamines which are found in smoked, salted, or barbequed meat.
- Conditions that increase gastrin level: gastrinoma and chronic achlorhydria (due to pernicious anemia, chronic *H. pylori* infection, etc.).

[6]These are the alarm features for which EGD is recommended in patients with dyspepsia.

Presentation: early satiety, weight loss, dyspepsia, upper GI bleeding.[6]

Workup: NSIM is EGD and biopsy. If positive for malignancy, NSIM is CT scan. Depending on CT study results, positron emission tomography (PET)/CT, endoscopic US, or laparoscopy might be indicated for staging.

Rx: Localized disease is treated surgically. In advanced stages, chemotherapy +/− palliative surgery are indicated (e.g., patient has a bulky mass which is causing obstruction or inability to eat any solid food).

9.9 Gastric Muc`osa-Associated Lymphoid Tissue Tumor

Background: It is the MC type of extranodal marginal zone lymphoma and the only type associated with *H. Pylori* infection. Most MALTomas are of low grade and commonly remain localized.

Presentation: Symptoms or complication of PUD (e.g., upper GI bleeding or dyspepsia).

Workup:

- EGD will reveal ulcer or ulcerated mass. Biopsy will reveal non-Hodgkin's lymphoma. Testing for *H. pylori* should be done.
- NSIDx: CT scan of chest/abdomen/pelvis to look for metastasis.

Rx:

Localized disease	• If positive for *H. pylori*, start *H. pylori* eradication therapy; the tumor generally subsides after treatment. This is a unique treatment of this form of non-Hodgkin's lymphoma.
	• If negative for *H. pylori*, do radiotherapy for localized disease. Alternative regimen is rituximab.
Advanced disease	• If positive for *H. pylori*, start *H. pylori* eradication therapy.
	• When symptoms develop, treat with rituximab +/− chemotherapy.

Follow-up: Regular surveillance EGD.

9.10 Malabsorption Syndromes

There are various causes of malabsorption, but all usually share the following common features:

GI symptoms	**Chronic** diarrhea, bloating, flatulence (Note: **acute** diarrhea/bloating and flatulence is considered infectious until proven otherwise) Fatty greasy stools that float easily in the toilet (steatorrhea)
Features of malnutrition	
• Weight loss and fatigue • Children can present with failure to thrive	
Vitamin A deficiency	Follicular hyperkeratosis, squamous metaplasia of cornea (called Bitot's spot), night blindness, etc.
Vitamin K deficiency	Easy bruising and bleeding with elevated INR
Vitamin D deficiency	• Features of hypocalcemia • Bone loss/thinning in adults • Rickets in children
Other deficiencies	Vitamin B_{12}, folate, and/or iron deficiency can present with anemia
Hyperoxaluria	Normally free calcium in gut lumen binds with dietary oxalate; calcium oxalate, as a compound, cannot get absorbed through intestinal epithelial cells and gets excreted with stool. In malabsorption, increased fatty acids in stool bind with enteral luminal calcium, which in turn frees up oxalates to be absorbed into the circulation. This leads to hyperoxaluria and increased risk of calcium oxalate stones formation

9.10.1 Diagnostic Workup of Malabsorption

To diagnose malabsorption, do fecal fat quantification test. Spot test can be done for screening, but if negative and when suspicion is high, 72-hour fecal fat testing is recommended which has high sensitivity and specificity to diagnose steatorrhea (malabsorption). Generally, malabsorption should be confirmed before doing invasive procedures such as EGD with biopsy.

9.10.2 Different Etiologies of Malabsorption

In malabsorption, patient's history generally provides clues to etiology:

Malabsorption + history of the following	Think of	Workup	Management
Travel to developing countries	**Giardiasis**	Giardia stool antigen or nucleic acid testing.[a] Also, do stool microscopy for cysts, ova, parasites, and leukocytes. If these tests are negative consider serology to look for other infections such as Strongyloides, *Entamoeba histolytica*, etc. If all the above tests are negative, do fecal fat quantification to document malabsorption and celiac sprue testing (which is the major differential dx), prior to doing EGD with small bowel biopsy	If stool antigen or nucleic acid testing is positive for giardia, start treatment. **Rx:** depends on age • > 3 yrs of age- tinidazole (single dose) • 1-2 yrs of age-nitazoxanide • < 1 year of age -metronidazole • For pregnant patients in their 1st trimester,if treatment is deemed necessary, paromomycin is preferred. In 2nd or 3rd trimester, any of the medication mentioned here can be given.
	Tropical sprue (unknown microbiological cause)		If small bowel biopsy reveals blunting of villi/chronic inflammation, celiac sprue testing is negative, and there is positive travel history, preliminary dx is made. **Rx:** oral tetracycline for few months

(continued)

Malabsorption + history of the following	Think of	Workup	Management
– Bowel anatomical issues (e.g., strictures, fistula, anastomosis) – Risk factors for reduced peristalsis (e.g., diabetes, scleroderma, Crohn's disease) – Immunosuppression	**Small bowel intestinal bacterial overgrowth**	**Carbohydrate breath test:** after oral carbohydrate load, bacteria metabolize it to hydrogen and methane, which gets absorbed into circulation, excreted in breath and can be measured. Diagnostic test is EGD with jejunal aspirate culture growing > 1,000 CFU of bacteria, but this may not be needed.	**Rx:** (amoxicillin + clavulanate) or (rifaximin)
Migratory arthralgia, lymphadenopathy +/− skin hyperpigmentation[b] +/− central nervous system involvement (e.g., memory impairment)	**Whipple's disease** (caused by infection with *Tropheryma whipplei*)	EGD with small bowel biopsy with **PAS** (periodic acid–Schiff) staining	**Rx:** IV ceftriaxone or penicillin G, followed by oral trimethoprim-sulfamethoxazole (or doxycycline)

MRS

Whipple PASSes trophy

[a] Alternatively, patients with recent hx of travel and acute onset of symptoms suggestive of malabsorption can be empirically treated with metronidazole. If symptoms resolve, it is most likely giardiasis.

[b] Caution: Looks somewhat similar to hemochromatosis. Hemochromatosis can also present with malabsorption (due to pancreatic insufficiency), joint pain, and skin pigmentation. Presence of lymphadenopathy points toward Whipple's disease.

Malabsorption + History of the following	Think of	Workup	Management
Recurrent epigastric pain +/− diabetes mellitus (due to endocrine pancreas deficiency) Exam CCS may give hx of alcoholism or lab/clinical features suggestive of chronic alcohol use (e.g., macrocytosis, elevated GGT, AST > ALT)	Chronic pancreatitis	Document presence of the following: **Pancreatic calcification:** do either US, CT, or plain X-ray **Presence of ductal pathology:** do MRCP **Abnormal pancreatic exocrine function:** do either fecal elastase or 72-hr fecal fat test See chronic pancreatitis section for further details	**Rx:** oral pancreatic enzymes supplements
Epigastric pain: Endoscopy shows multiple ulcers in the stomach +/− duodenum or ulcers in unusual places like second or third part of duodenum or jejunum	Zollinger–Ellison Syndrome	Hold PPI and check serum fasting gastrin level after 1 week	Surgical resection if localized disease or with surgically resectable metastasis. If widespread, do medical treatment with large doses of PPIs to block acid secretion

Hx of anxiety or bulimia nervosa	Factitious diarrhea due to laxative abuse	Colonoscopy can reveal dark brown discoloration of colon (melanosis coli)	Rx: cognitive behavioral therapy + nutritional rehabilitation +/− SSRI or olanzapine
Intensely pruritic papulovesicular lesions on the extremities (dermatitis herpetiformis) Or Malabsorption without any other history suggestive of abovementioned conditions	Celiac sprue[a]	**See below for diagnostic algorithm**	Remove BReWed beer from diet (i.e., Barley, **R**ye, **W**heat, and beer, which is made from barley). These grains contain gluten protein, which when ingested, elicits an immune reaction in susceptible individuals

[a]Patients with celiac sprue may have increased risk of lymphoma and GI malignancy.

Abbreviations: ALT, alanine aminotransferase; AST, aspartate aminotransferase; CFU, colony forming unit; EGD, esophagogastroduodenoscopy; GGT, gamma-glutamyl transferase; MRCP, magnetic resonance cholangiopancreatography; PPI, proton pump inhibitor; SSRI, selective serotonin reuptake inhibitor.

9.10.3 Diagnostic algorithm of celiac disease

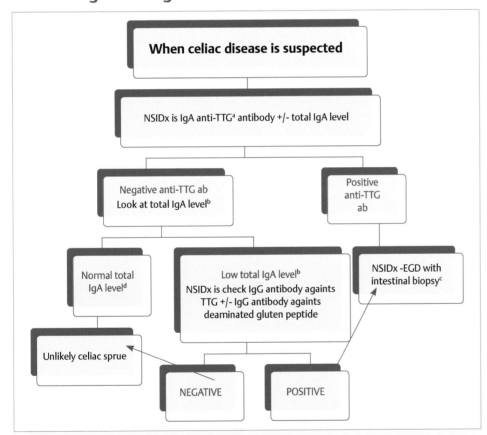

[a]IgA anti-tissue transglutaminase (TTG) antibody. Another antibody that can be checked is IgA antiendomysial antibodies.[7]

[b]Selective IgA deficiency is common in celiac sprue and can lead to false negative IgA anti-TTG.

[c]Best test is small bowel biopsy (biopsy of duodenal bulb + other duodenal areas +/− jejunum), which typically shows blunting or loss of villous architecture with increased inflammatory cells. Note: tropical sprue has the same picture. Absence of travel history to tropical countries points toward celiac. Note that in some patients with high probability of celiac (e.g., positive dermatitis herpetiformis or coexistent autoimmune disease such as type I DM, autoimmune hepatitis), we can go directly for EGD along with serology.

[d]If patient is already on gluten-free diet, antibody serology testing can be negative. In this instance, we can check HLA DQ2 and DQ8 genotypes. If positive, gluten challenge and repeat serology need to be done.

[7]Do not choose anti-gliadin antibodies, which has low specificity.

D-xylose test
Even if D-xylose test for malabsorption is not used anymore, the basic science behind it is interesting, hence questions on it are still asked on exam.
D-xylose is a simple sugar that does not need to be digested for absorption.
• If D-xylose is not absorbed into the circulation, then there is a problem with the absorptive surface (e.g., celiac sprue, tropical sprue).
• If D-xylose is absorbed into the circulation, then we can conclude that malabsorption is not due to problem with the absorptive surface; think of other causes such as chronic pancreatitis.

🔍 Clinical Case Scenarios

2. A 45-year-old female presents with long-standing history of symptoms of periodic diarrhea and weight loss. There is no history of travel. EGD with intestinal biopsy reveals blunting of villi. What is the best treatment? Antibiotics or dietary intervention?

9.11 Inflammatory Bowel Disease: Ulcerative Colitis and Crohn's Disease

	Ulcerative colitis	Crohn's disease
Idiopathic inflammatory process involves	**Only colon** • Ileitis might occur, but it is almost always in presence of right-sided colitis. (This is due to inflammation of colon spilling into ileum and is known as backwash ileitis.)	Can involve the **whole GI tract,** including mouth
MC location	• **Rectum:** inflammation can extend from there to involve the whole **colon.**	• Ileum
Common presentation	• Diarrhea, weight loss, fever, abdominal pain, etc. • Disease course is usually remitting-relapsing (periods of acute flare-ups followed by dormant phase).	
MC presentation scenarios	**Proctitis:** abdominal pain, tenesmus, stool urgency, and if severe, bloody diarrhea	• **Ileitis:** right lower quadrant abdominal pain and tenderness • **Malabsorption** (chronic diarrhea, weight loss, calcium oxalate stones, vitamin B_{12} deficiency, etc.) can result from: ○ Ileal involvement and bile salt malabsorption ○ Small intestinal bacterial overgrowth
Both can have extraintestinal manifestations[a]	• Erythema nodosum, pyoderma gangrenosum, uveitis/iritis, arthritis, etc. • They have increased risk for venous thromboembolism	
Laboratory workup	• Look for elevated ESR, leukocytosis, and/or reactive thrombocytosis. (These are important clues to diagnosis, but these can be normal in patients with mild disease or in remission.) • Both UC/CD can have positive fecal occult blood and stool leukocytes	

	Ulcerative colitis	Crohn's disease

Pathology
 	
Both UC/CD are diagnosed with endoscopy and biopsy
	Colonoscopy will show superficial inflammation with **continuous** GI mucosal involvement	• Granulomatous **transmural inflammation** which may lead to
		  – Perforation due to transmural involvement
		  – Fibrosis → stricture formation → intestinal obstruction → perforation
		  – Fistula formation → development of abscess
		• Granulomatous inflammation is a characteristic feature that differentiates CD from UC
		• Endoscopy will show **skip** lesions (lesions are not continuous)

MRS

COlitis is **CO**ntinous
Crohn's **DIS**ease is **DIS**continous

MRS

PAIR of B27 (bombers)
where
I = inflammatory bowel disease, the UC type

[a]UC is associated with HLA-B27 related disorders, which include **p**soriatic arthritis, **p**rimary sclerosing cholangitis, **a**nkylosing spondylitis, and **r**eactive arthritis.

Abbreviations: CD, Crohn's disease; ESR, erythrocyte sedimentation rate; GI, gastrointestinal; UC, ulcerative colitis.

Management:

	Ulcerative colitis	Crohn's disease
First treatment of choice: Both are treated with anti-inflammatory 5-ASA derivatives[a] and immunosuppressive agents such as steroids, 6-mercaptopurine, azathioprine, etc.	**Mild disease** • **Proctitis:** suppository Canasa • **Proctosigmoiditis:** suppository (Canasa) +enema (Rowasa) • **Left-sided or diffuse colitis:** oral 5-ASA derivatives and enema/suppository **If no response,** use oral glucocorticoid. (Budesonide is preferred, as it has high topical GI effect and low systemic effect due to extensive first pass metabolism by liver.)	**Mild flare-up** with no systemic symptoms: • Oral 5-ASA derivative may be tried first • **If not responding,** do a trial of oral antibiotics +/– oral steroids (e.g., budesonide). Transmural inflammation and gut bacterial infection more likely play a role in CD
	More Severe disease: For example, frequent bloody stools, frequent diarrhea, or signs of systemic toxicity such as fever, tachycardia. • Systemic steroids (e.g., prednisone or IV glucocorticoids) + oral and/or rectal ASA derivatives +/– antibiotics • If refractory to steroids, use any of the following: anti-TNF agents (infliximab, adalimumab) or vedolizumab (anti-integrin antibody). Cyclosporine is another option for UC and certolizumab for Crohn's disease	
Long-term treatment for prevention of flare-ups	If steroid dependent or frequent exacerbations, start steroid sparing agents such as 6-mercaptopurine or azathioprine. Other options are biologic agents (e.g., infliximab, adalimumab). Methotrexate is an additional option for CD	
Other additional management	After 8–10 years of dx of UC, colonoscopy with multiple blind biopsies should be done to screen for development of colon cancer, followed by serial colonoscopies at 1–3-year intervals. ! Any grade of dysplasia in biopsy warrants colectomy	• For active colonic disease or in patients with fistula, ciprofloxacin and metronidazole alone or in combination is commonly used • For CD with fistula, also use immunosuppressive agents. Systemic steroids and ASA derivatives have NOT been shown to induce closure of fistula

	Ulcerative colitis	Crohn's disease
Indications for surgery	• Toxic megacolon refractory to medical management • Severe flare-up refractory to medical management • Frequent exacerbation of disease despite medical management • After more than a decade of dx of UC prophylactic proctocolectomy might be offered to patients, instead of screening colonoscopy every 1–3 year	• Symptoms refractory to medical treatment (e.g., high dose of steroids required to control symptoms) or frequent exacerbation of disease despite adequate medical therapy • Severe fistulating disease • Bowel obstruction refractory to conservative management • Abscess formation • Bowel perforation

[a]5-ASA derivatives are olsalazine (oral), balsalazide (oral), sulfasalazine (oral), and mesalamine-derived compounds (oral or topical): discussed further in the below table.

Abbreviations: ASA, aminosalicylic acid; CD, Crohn's disease; GI, gastrointestinal; TNF, tumor necrosis factor; UC, ulcerative colitis.

Topical 5-ASA derivatives	Oral 5-ASA derivatives
Rowasa is a rectal enema[a] Canasa is suppository[a]	• Pentasa is released in both small and large bowel.[a] • Asacol is efficacious mostly in ileum and colon.[a] • Sulfasalazine[b] is only effective in colon. (Colonic bacteria are required to cleave this drug into 5-ASA which is the active form.)

[a] Mesalamine-derived ASA compounds are topical Can**asa**, Row**asa**, and oral **Asa**col, Pent**asa**.

[b] Sulfasalazine is usually not the first line as it has higher risk of side effects. It can cause GI disturbances, skin rash, hepatitis, pancreatitis, pneumonitis, agranulocytosis, and aplastic anemia.

MRS

• Asa**col** is for **Col**itis.
• PENTasa—Pan ENTeric ASA: is effective for both small and large bowel inflammation, so useful in Crohn's disease.
• **R**owa**S**a = **R**ectal enema for rectum + **S**igmoid colon involvement.

Clinical Case Scenarios

3. A man with hx of Crohn's disease presents with complain of fecal material in his urine. What is the likely dx?

Patient with prior long-standing history of nonspecific GI complaints presents with high fever and abdominal pain. Abdominal exam reveals diffuse tenderness and decreased bowel sounds. Lab tests reveals leukocytosis, thrombocytosis, and elevated lactate.

4. What is the best NSIDx?
5. Abdominal X-ray reveals the following. What is the likely dx?
6. What is the NSIM?
7. Patient with history of ulcerative colitis presents with few months' hx of progressive itching and fatigue. Liver function tests (LFTs) reveal ↑ gamma-glutamyl transferase (GGT) and ↑ alkaline phosphatase (AKP). What is the likely dx?

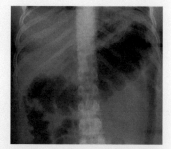

Source: In: Gunderman R, ed. Essential Radiology. Clinical Presentation, Pathophysiology, Imaging. 2nd ed. Thieme; 2000.

9.12 Lactose Intolerance

[8]It has higher incidence in people of Asian descent.

Background: Virtually everyone is born with **lactase**, an intestinal brush border enzyme that splits lactose into glucose and galactose and helps digesting milk. Later during life, people can lose this enzyme either spontaneously (genetically determined[8]) or due to villous pathology (e.g., giardiasis, celiac sprue).

Pathophysiology: When lactose-containing food is ingested, the undigested lactose remains in the GI lumen, which is then fermented by bacteria producing hydrogen gas (resulting in flatulence, bloating) and osmotically active compound (osmotic diarrhea so stool osmolar gap is typically increased).[9]

Presentation: Explosive diarrhea with flatulence and bloating any time one ingests dairy products. Exam question might not include hx of dairy ingestion. If weight loss is present, think of alternate dx.

Management: Avoid dairy products[10] and if symptoms resolve dx is made. If patient does not want to avoid lactose and wants to confirm the dx first, do hydrogen breath test after ingesting dairy products. In addition, lactase enzyme supplements can be used.

[9]Stool osmolar gap is increased in osmotic diarrhea. Osmotic diarrhea occurs due to presence of osmotically active particles in gut lumen.

Etiology:
- Lactose intolerance
- Osmotic laxative abuse (MgSO$_4$, magnesium citrate, lactulose or polyethylene glycol)
- MgOH$_2$ (antacid) ingestion
- Fat malabsorption

9.13 Diverticular Disease

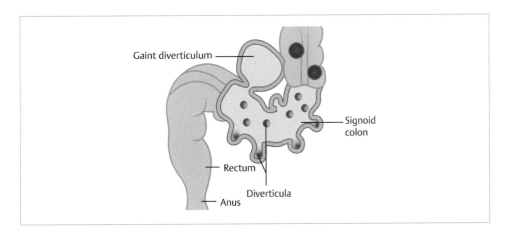

Gaint diverticulum

Signoid colon

Rectum

Diverticula

Anus

[10]Some types of yogurt (e.g., Greek yogurt) or aged cheese are better tolerated.

Background: It refers to the formation of multiple outpouchings in colon. This is common in older age population. MC location is in sigmoid colon. Risk factors include constipation, obesity, use of NSAIDs/opiates, etc.

Presentation:
- Hx of chronic constipation alternating with diarrhea.
- Sometimes patients have mild abdominal pain or bloating relieved by defecation.
- Chronic lower GI bleeding can lead to iron deficiency anemia.
- Acute painless lower GI bleeding.[11]

Management: High fiber diet and stool softeners as needed. Diet low in red meat and total fat can reduce likelihood of symptomatic diverticular disease.

[11]Typical hx is of bright red blood per rectum and passage of blood clots.

9.14 Acute Diverticulitis

Pathophysiology: Blockage of diverticula by colonic contents that results in peridiverticular inflammatory process.

Presentation: Acute abdominal pain and tenderness +/− signs of sepsis. MC location of abdominal tenderness is in left lower quadrant but it can occur anywhere (e.g., right lower quadrant tenderness due to pericecal diverticulitis).

Management:

Mild disease (low-grade fever, mild pain, and able to take PO intake)	Can be treated on an outpatient basis with clear liquid diet and oral antibiotics that cover gram negatives and anaerobes. For example, (amoxicillin-clavulanate) or (cefpodoxime + metronidazole). CT scan is not necessarily indicated but may be indicated in patients not responding to outpatient therapy.
Severe disease (severe pain, high fever, or high leukocyte count)	NSIM is hospitalization, bowel rest, IV fluids, and IV antibiotics (e.g., ceftriaxone + metronidazole). Then NSIM is **CT scan** to assess severity.
If patient hasn't had a recent colonoscopy, NSIM is to schedule colonoscopy after resolution of acute episode.	
For recurrent diverticulitis, elective diverticulectomy can be done on a case-by-case basis.	

9.14.1 Complication of diverticulitis

Clinical case scenarios

- Patient hospitalized for diverticulitis is not clinically improving. Repeat CT scan reveals large diverticular abscess. NSIM is radiologically guided percutaneous drainage. Abscess develops due to macro- or microperforation. Note: Small microabscesses can be managed conservatively.
- Patient with hx of recurrent diverticulitis presents with fecal material coming out of an opening in anterior abdominal wall. Dx is enterocutaneous fistula formation. NSIM is surgical fistulectomy. Fistula can also form in-between colon and bladder, vagina, uterus, etc.
- Other potential complications of diverticulitis include perforation, peritonitis, obstruction, etc.

9.15 Irritable Bowel Syndrome

Background: It is a chronic functional disorder of GI tract.

Criteria: Chronic recurrent abdominal pain with two or more of the following, in absence of organic GI pathology:

- **Pain related with defecation:** pain typically improves after bowel movement.
- **Change in stool frequency:** classic presentation is alternating diarrhea and constipation (constipation or diarrhea can be predominant).
- **Change in stool appearance:** mucous stools can be present, but is usually non-bloody.

These symptoms are usually not present at night. Alarming features such as presence of nocturnal symptoms, weight loss, iron deficiency anemia, or other features suggestive of celiac sprue or inflammatory bowel disease require further testing.[12]

[12]To make the dx of IBS, there should be no associated abnormal findings in colonoscopy +/– biopsy, blood tests or stool examination.

Management:

• First SIM: lifestyle and dietary modification, which includes avoiding diet that is high in FODMAPs (fermentable oligo, di- and monosaccharides and polyols) such as beans, lentils, etc. • In patients with constipation symptoms, add psyllium.	
If patients fail to respond to above measures or if they have severe symptoms, then treatment is targeted toward the problematic feature—pain, diarrhea, and/or constipation, as given below.	
Diarrhea-predominant IBS	Use antidiarrheals such as loperamide. Second-line agents are bile acid sequestrants (e.g., cholestyramine, colesevelam, colestipol).
Constipation-predominant IBS	Second-line agent is polyethylene glycol. Third-line treatment is lubiprostone or linaclotide.
For abdominal cramps	Several antispasmodics can be tried, e.g., hyoscyamine, dicyclomine, or the belladonna alkaloid derivatives. In patients with coexistent depression or as a second-line drug, a trial of amitriptyline can be done (amitriptyline also has M-antagonist effect that reduce spasms).

In a nutshell

Irritable Bowel Syndrome vs. Diverticulosis

- Both can have clinical features of alternating diarrhea with constipation and occasional abdominal pain relieved by defecation.

- But note that **diverticulosis** typically has other features as well, such as iron deficiency anemia, abnormal barium enema/colonoscopy; whereas all tests findings are normal in IBS.

9.16 Colon Cancer Screening[13]

9.16.1 At What Age Do We Start Screening?

In non-high-risk population	⟹	Begin screening at age 50
Hereditary colon cancer syndromes	⟹	See table below
In patients with family hx of colon cancer • In any first-degree relative before age 60 OR • In two or more first-degree relatives at any age	⟹	Begin screening at age 40, or 10 years before the youngest case in the family, whichever is earlier

What screening test to use? Preferred test is colonoscopy. In patients who decline colonoscopy, use any of the following:

– CT colonography every 5 years.
– Flexible sigmoidoscopy every 10 years + fecal immunochemistry stool testing (FIST) on a single sample every year, or fecal occult blood test on three samples.
– Annual FIST on single sample or fecal occult blood test on three samples.
– Annual fecal DNA + FIST testing. (Fecal DNA testing identifies abnormal DNA associated with colon cancer or polyps; FIST testing is a special test for occult blood in stool).
– If any of the above test is abnormal, do colonoscopy.[14]

9.16.2 Hereditary Colon Cancer Syndromes[15]

Hereditary colon cancer syndromes	Additional information

Familial adenomatous polyposis coli (FAP) syndrome	**Pathophysiology:** inherited autosomal dominant disorder due to mutation in tumor suppressor gene—APC (adenomatosis polyposis coli) gene
	– **FAP:** 100 or more colonic polyps are diagnostic of FAP. NSIM is total proctocolectomy
	– **Attenuated form of FAP** is when more than 10 but < 100 colonic polyps are found during life time. NSIM is polypectomy (if feasible) and yearly surveillance
	– **Colon cancer screening:** for at risk individuals **defined by genetic testing**
	  ○ **Individuals at risk of FAP** should start screening at **10–12** years of age with either proctosigmoidoscopy or colonoscopy. **Do annual** colonoscopy until indication for colectomy arises
	  ○ **Individuals at risk for attenuated form of FAP** should start screening at **25** years of age. Screening colonoscopy is recommended every 1–2 years. Sigmoidoscopy is not done for screening as these patients typically have distal polyps not seen by sigmoidoscopy.
	In addition, screen at regular intervals for gastric/duodenal tumors (with EGD) and thyroid tumors (with thyroid US). In patients with family hx of hepatoblastoma, do screening with AFP and liver US.

Gardner's syndrome is an FAP variant	– Associated with benign extracranial tumors such as **F**ibrosarcomas, **F**ibromas, **O**steomas, **LI**pomas, **E**pidermoid **C**ysts, etc. – Manage as above for FAP.

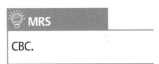 **MRS**

CBC.

---

[13]There are only few cancers in which regular screening in general population have been shown to decrease mortality and morbidity. They are **C**olon, **B**reast, and **C**ervical cancer.

[14]Example CCS: If found to have polyp in sigmoidoscopy, NSIM is full colonoscopy.

[15]If a patient has multiple relatives with colon cancer, then it can be one of hereditary colon cancer syndromes. NSIDx is genetic testing.

 MRS

GARDEN plants provide a lot of **FOLIC** acid)
F for folic: F for FAP variant

Hereditary colon cancer syndromes	Additional information
Turcot syndrome	– Brain tumor + polyposis colon cancer syndrome – Manage as above for FAP
Hereditary nonpolyposis Colorectal cancer syndrome (a.k.a. Lynch syndrome)	**Background:** Inherited autosomal dominant disorder due to mutation in DNA mismatch repair gene. In this disorder, there are no polyps in colon, hence called nonpolyposis **Colon cancer screening:** – Start **ANNUAL** screening colonoscopy at 20–25 years of age or 2–5 years before the youngest case in the family, whichever comes earlier – Also, screen at regular intervals for gastric cancer (with EGD), and in females, **E**ndometrial and **O**varian cancer (with TVUS, endometrial sampling and pelvic exam)

Abbreviations: EGD, esophagogastroduodenoscopy; TVUS, transvaginal ultrasound; US, ultrasound.

9.17 Polyps in Colonoscopy

When polyps are seen during colonoscopy, the whole polyp needs to be removed (polypectomy) and sent for pathology.

Type of polyp	Risks for colon cancer	Management
Hamartomatous polyps[a]	**Usually low risk**	Reassure patient
Hyperplastic or inflammatory polyps	**No risk**	Reassure patient
Adenomatous polyps	Can be premalignant[b]	Screening colonoscopy is done every 3–5 years, after this finding

[a]These polyps can occur in juvenile polyposis syndrome, Peutz–Jeghers syndrome, etc.

[b]Morphologically, sessile polyp has higher risk than pedunculated polyp and histologically; villous adenoma has higher risk than tubular. Size > 1 cm also has higher risk.

9.18 Colorectal Cancer

Risk factors:

– **Inherited genetic mutations:** hereditary nonpolyposis colorectal cancer (aka Lynch syndrome), familial adenomatous polyposis, etc.
– Alcohol, smoking, sedentary life style, poor diet (e.g., diet high in processed meat or red meat).
– Inflammatory bowel disease.
– Radiation.

Presentation:

Left-sided colon cancer	Right-sided colon cancer
– The left side of colon has a small diameter, so tumor typically grows in a circumferential growth pattern and obstructs the lumen. – On top of having a small diameter, the left side has presence of hard stool (as most of the water is already absorbed in the right side of the colon). This is likely to aggravate obstruction. – Clinical features are related to partial obstruction (constipation, pencil-shaped stool, tenesmus), and friable mass (blood-streaked stool).	– The right-sided colon is relatively larger in diameter and the tumor grows inside the lumen with typical polypoid growth pattern. – Typical presentation—chronic bleeding (e.g., melena) leading to iron deficiency anemia.[a]

[a]In patients > 50 years of age with iron deficiency anemia, do colorectal cancer screening. First SIDx is fecal occult blood test, followed by colonoscopy and biopsy. Even if occult blood test is negative, we should proceed for colonoscopy, as the occult blood test might be false negative.

Management steps:

– After dx of colon cancer is made with colonoscopy and biopsy, NSIDx is staging with CT scan of chest, abdomen, and pelvis with intravenous (IV) contrast.

Stage	Simplified definition	Treatment
I	Cancer hasn't grown into the outermost layer of the colon (serosa) and there is **no** lymph node spread	Curative-intent surgery
II	Cancer has grown into the outermost layer of colon and there is **no** lymph node spread	Curative-intent surgery +/– chemotherapy
III	Cancer has spread into lymph nodes	Surgery + chemotherapy
IV	Limited metastasis to liver[a] or lung	Curative-intent surgery can be done in the primary site as well as the site of metastasis with adjuvant chemotherapy
	Distant metastasis	Palliative chemotherapy

[a]For example, solitary metastasis to liver or few metastases limited to a one lobe of liver.[16]

Follow-up: Carcinoembryonic antigen (CEA) is used for follow-up. Increasing CEA levels point toward recurrence.

9.19 Carcinoid Syndrome

Definition: A neuroendocrine carcinoid tumor that secretes serotonin.

Clinical pathophysiology: Serotonin produced by a primary tumor in the small intestines gets rapidly metabolized by liver, and does not produce systemic symptoms of excessive serotonin (carcinoid syndrome), unless the disease is so advanced that it overwhelms liver's ability to metabolize serotonin. In contrast, primary carcinoid tumor in lung or ovary or metastatic disease can produce carcinoid syndrome as it bypasses portal liver pathway.

Presentation: Weight loss along with following:

– **F**acial **F**lushing.
– **E**xpiratory wheezing.
– **D**iarrhea (secretory type).
– **T**ricuspid **I**nsufficiency and **P**ulmonary **S**tenosis (TIPS).

Workup:

NSIDx is 24-hour urine hydroxy-indole-acetic acid (HIAA) which is a metabolite of serotonin. After biochemical confirmation, NSIM is to localize the tumor, which can be done with CT scan, MRI, PET/CT or octreotide scan (a.k.a. somatostatin receptor scintigraphy).

Treatment:

If tumor is resectable, then proceed with surgery. Note that a solitary liver metastasis with primary tumor in gut can be resectable.

If tumor is not amenable to resection (e.g., multiple metastases), then octreotide is the drug of choice (DOC), which is a somatostatin analogue that decreases serotonin secretion.

Complications:

Secondary niacin deficiency with features of pellagra[17] may develop in patients with carcinoid syndrome. This is because serotonin and niacin are both derived from tryptophan. If serotonin is overproduced, then there is less tryptophan remaining for production of niacin.

[16]Carcinomas usually metastasize via lymph nodes, but colorectal cancer frequently metastasizes to **liver** via **hematogenous** portal pathway.

MC primary location of carcinoid tumor is in gastroduodenal area (foregut) but tumor in this location is less likely to cause carcinoid syndrome.

MC primary location of carcinoid tumor that causes carcinoid syndrome is mid gut (distal small intestine and proximal colon).

 MRS

I was **FED TIPS** for diagnosing carcinoid syndrome.

⚠ **Caution**

Do not confuse carcinoid syndrome (due to chronic excessive serotonin) with serotonin syndrome (acute serotonin toxicity in the central nervous system due to combination of two serotonergic drugs).

[17]**Niacin** deficiency results in **PE**llagra: clinical features include **D**iarrhea, **D**ementia, **D**ermatitis (in sun-exposed areas) and may result in **D**eath.

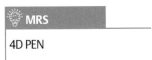 **MRS**

4D PEN

9.20 Gastrointestinal Bleeding

Initial stabilization: In any patient with ongoing moderate to severe GI bleeding, first SIM is to secure airway, check volume status of the patient, send for cross matching of blood, and insert two large gauge peripheral lines immediately.

Example scenarios	Best NSIM
A patient with altered mental status and active hematemesis	Intubation to protect airway
Hypotensive patient	IV fluid resuscitation +/− packed red blood cell (PRBC) transfusion
Severely anemic patient	PRBC transfusion

Specific management: depends on the type of GI bleeding (upper GI bleeding or lower GI bleeding).

9.20.1 Upper GI Bleeding

Presentation: Hematemesis (vomiting coffee ground material) or melena (black-colored stools) is suggestive of upper GI bleeding. Look for disproportionately elevated blood urea nitrogen (BUN) in respect to creatinine. Elevated BUN/Cr ratio means blood digested in gut becomes a source of urea.

Management:

- All patients with active upper GI bleeding should receive proton pump inhibitors (intravenous if severe) followed by endoscopy to find and treat the bleeding source. MCC is peptic ulcer disease.

- In patients with hx or stigmata of cirrhosis, suspect variceal bleeding. NSIM is adding IV octreotide (somatostatin analogue that decreases portal pressure) + antibiotics(e.g., ceftriaxone) for SBP (spontaneus bacterial peritonitis)prophylaxis while waiting for EGD.

9.20.2 Active Bleeding per Rectum (Hematochezia)

Maroon-colored stools, blood clots, or bright-red blood per rectum is suggestive of lower GI bleeding; however, this can also occur in cases of brisk upper GI bleeding, especially the ones that result in hemodynamic instability.

Management:

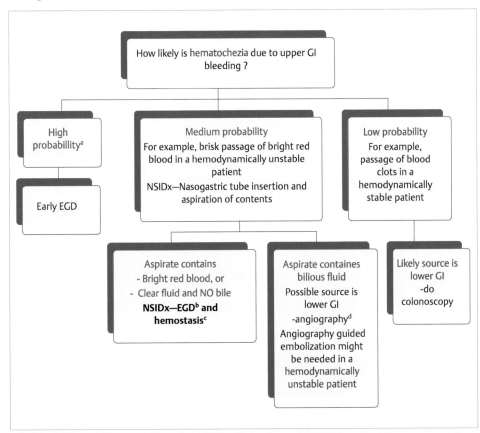

^a**Presence of the following suggest upper GI bleeding:** hemodynamic instability, elevated BUN/ Cr ratio > 30:1, **dark-maroon-colored stool** in a patient with hx of PUD or gastric cancer.

^bIf aspirate reveals bright red blood, then the dx of upper GI bleed is made comfortably. If aspirate reveals clear fluid which is not green, then bleeding up to the level of **pyloric antrum** is ruled out. Beyond the pyloric antrum, there is still the possibility of bleeding from a duodenal ulcer, so EGD is still done.

^cIn most situations, the initial treatment of choice is endoscopic methods of hemostasis (e.g., laser photo coagulation of the bleeding vessel).

^dCT arteriography or tagged RBC scan might help with localization prior to angiography.[18]

[18] **Duodenal** ulcer bleeding is from gastro-**duodenal** artery.
Gastric ulcer bleeding is from left-**gastric** artery.

Other diagnostic options include small bowel enteroscopy, Meckel's scan (in a young patient), laparoscopy or laparotomy.

Clinical Case Scenarios

8. A 60-year-old patient presents with hematemesis. EGD reveals old blood, no active bleeding and no obvious source of bleeding is identified. What is the most likely cause of bleeding?

a) Mallory–Weiss tear

b) Dieulafoy's lesion

c) Meckel's diverticulum

d) PUD

9.20.3 Etiology of lower GI bleeding

Hemorrhoids and fissure	Bleeding occurs in relation to defecation.[a] Bleeding is usually mild and not life threatening with minimal rectal bleeding. NSIDx is anoscopy.
AV malformation (aka angiodysplasia)	Can be associated with aortic stenosis, ESRD, Osler–Weber–Rendu[b] syndrome, CREST syndrome, etc. It is the second MCC of life-threatening painless bleeding.
Diverticulosis	MCC of life-threatening painless bleeding.[c]
Ischemic bowel disease	Bleeding + abdominal pain and tenderness
Polyps	Usually causes minor and non-life-threatening bleeds.

[a]One important diagnostic clue of hemorrhoidal bleeding is that it occurs in relation to passing regular stool. In nonhemorrhoidal bleeding, patients just pass bloody stool.

[b]Osler–Weber–Rendu syndrome (aka hereditary hemorrhagic telangiectasia) is a syndrome with formation of multiple telangiectasias in multiple locations which can bleed easily. Patients can present with GI bleeding, nose bleeding, facial telangiectasia, etc.

[c] Bleeding due to diverticulosis and AV malformation is painless. Bleeding due to ischemic bowel disease or ulcerative colitis occurs with abdominal pain.

Abbreviation: ESRD, end-stage renal disease.

9.21 Ischemic Bowel Disease

Definition: Small bowel ischemia is called mesenteric ischemia; large bowel ischemia is ischemic colitis.

Risk factors: Similar to cerebrovascular disease: cardioembolic (e.g., a-fib) or atherosclerotic disease of mesenteric blood vessels. In addition, it can occur after abdominal aortic aneurysmal repair (due to arterial occlusion by aortic graft).

Presentation:

Acute ischemia	Abdominal pain, diarrhea (may be bloody), and elevated lactic acid – Abdominal pain is the most prominent symptom (pain is very severe and out of proportion to exam findings)	Colonic ischemic bowel disease typically affects the watershed areas, which are the splenic flexure and the rectosigmoid junction.
Chronic ischemia	Postprandial pain and weight loss – Pain location depends on the site of atherosclerotic narrowing; e.g., celiac artery atherosclerotic narrowing might present with postprandial epigastric pain	

Superior mesenteric artery

Inferior mesenteric artery

Ileocolic artery

Management:

	Acute ischemia/infarct	Chronic disease
Small bowel mesenteric ischemia	If hemodynamic instability, or signs of peritonitis, NSIM resuscitation, and plain abdominal X-ray (also add antibiotics). If free air under-diaphragm or pneumatosis intestinalis, NSIM is explorative laparotomy. Surgical resection is needed for necrotic bowel. If viable, intraoperative angiogram and surgical embolectomy or bypass can be done.	Angioplasty +/− stenting for significant cases
	For all other cases, NSIDx is CT angiography. In patients with evidence of major vessel occlusion, start anticoagulation. In certain cases, percutaneous thrombectomy + angioplasty (for atherothrombotic disease) or pharmacologic/mechanical thrombolysis (for cardioembolic disease) might be done.	
Colonic ischemia	CT scan is commonly done first. Colonoscopy is done for equivocal cases	Mostly supportive
	Treatment is mostly supportive (IV antibiotics, IV fluids, GI rest). In severe cases, explorative laparotomy +/− resection might be needed.	

Differential diagnosis of abdominal pain after eating:

- Cholelithiasis: usually no weight loss
- Peptic ulcer disease
- Chronic pancreatitis: weight loss, hx of alcoholism
- Mesenteric angina: most patients avoid food as it precipitates severe pain, and this commonly results in weight loss.

🔍 Clinical Case Scenarios

A child presents with few months hx of painless melena.
  9. What is the NSIDx?
10. What is the treatment of choice?

An intubated patient in ICU develops acute hematemesis. EGD reveals multiple superficial ulcerations and hemorrhagic gastritis.
11. What prophylactic measure could have decreased the bleeding risk?
12. What are the other indications for stress-ulcer prophylaxis in ICU patient?

13. Patient presents with hx of several episodes of vomiting followed by hematemesis. What is the likely dx?
14. What cause of lower GI bleeding is associated with systolic murmur?
15. Patient presents with acute onset severe abdominal pain with bloody and mucous stools. Exam reveals irregularly irregular heart rhythm. What is the likely dx?
16. A 34 weeks pregnant patient complains of sore throat especially in the morning for the last few weeks. There are no other associated symptoms. What is the likely dx?
17. Patient on warfarin presents to your clinic with hx of intermittent melanotic bowel movements for 6 months. Lab reveals mild iron deficiency anemia and occult blood is positive for stool. EGD and colonoscopy reveals no source. What is the NSIDx?
18. A hypertensive patient started on calcium-channel blocker develops paroxysmal episodes of cough especially at night for the last few weeks. There are no other associated symptoms. What is the like dx?

9.22 Liver

Important liver function	Effect of liver failure or cirrhosis	Testing
Liver produces albumin,[a] which carries lipid-soluble substances in the plasma and is a major contributor of oncotic pressure that holds the plasma volume in the vascular compartment	Low albumin leads to low oncotic pressure that results in vascular fluid seeping out of blood vessels into the extracellular space leading to edema, ascites, and pleural effusion	Serum albumin
Synthesis of most proclotting factors	Increased bleeding tendencies	PT/INR[b]
Through phase 1 and phase 2 reactions, liver metabolizes toxic substances, drugs, hormones, etc.	– Decreased metabolism of drugs – Increased estrogen in blood leading to palmar erythema, spider angioma, etc. – Increased progesterone can cause respiratory alkalosis	
Liver conjugates lipid-soluble substances, making them water soluble, thus facilitating excretion through bile or urine	Decreased conjugation and excretion of bilirubin and lipid-soluble drugs	Conjugated and unconjugated bilirubin levels
With the help of hormones, such as glucagon and cortisol, liver maintains blood glucose during fasting state by glycogenolysis and later gluconeogenesis	Fasting hypoglycemia	
Blood detoxification: toxic ammonia (a byproduct of protein metabolism) is metabolized into urea (a less toxic substance) by urea cycle in liver.	Increased ammonia in blood enters the brain and produces false neurotransmitters causing changes in brain function. This can present as hepatic encephalopathy.	Serum ammonia

[a]Besides albumin, liver synthesizes all other kinds of necessary transporting proteins, such as transferrin, transcobalamin, transcortisol, ceruloplasmin, which carry and transfer iron, cobalamin (vitamin B_{12}), cortisol and copper, respectively.

[b]Production of functioning coagulation factors 2, 7, 9, 10 requires vitamin K-mediated gamma carboxylation in hepatocytes. Since factor 7 has shortest half-life of all the clotting factors, abnormal PT is the earliest seen abnormality in acute liver failure. Hence PT/INR is the most sensitive marker of hepatic function derangement and liver failure.

Abbreviations: INR, international normalized ratio; PT, prothrombin time.

9.22.1 Other Tests to Assess Status of Liver

Tests to assess necrosis of hepatocytes	Tests that signal obstruction in the biliary outflow
– Aspartate amino transferase (AST) – Alanine amino transferase (ALT) Death of hepatocytes leads to spill-over of these hepatic intracellular enzymes into blood	– Alkaline phosphatase (AKP) – Gamma-glutamyl transferase (GGT) – 5' nucleotidase

9.22.2 Liver Function Test Abnormalities and Underlying Pathology

ALT/AST	AKP	GGT[a] and 5' nucleotidase	Underlying pathology
↑	↑ ↑ ↑	↑ ↑ ↑	Obstruction of hepatobiliary outflow tract. Elevated bilirubin is commonly present.
Normal	↑ ↑	Normal	• Bone disorders such as Paget's disease, bone loss of immobility, etc. • AKP elevation of placental origin
↑ ↑ ↑	↑	↑	This combination signifies ongoing inflammation and death of hepatocytes AST/ALT ratio > 2 pattern is commonly seen in alcoholic hepatitis.[b] AST/ ALT ratio < 2 pattern is commonly seen in other causes of hepatitis (e.g., viruses, toxins)

[a]Chronic alcoholics typically have increased GGT and increased ferritin.

[b]Do not forget to order screening hepatitis panel to rule out coexistent Hep C or Hep B infection, and screen for other common liver toxins (e.g., tylenol intake), even if alcoholic patient and AST/ALT ratio is >2, because this pattern is commonly seen but is not exclusive to alcoholic hepatitis.

Abbreviations: AKP, alkaline phosphatase; ALT, alanine amino transferase; AST, aspartate amino transferase; GGT, gamma-glutamyl transferase.

9.22.3 Hepatitis and Acute Liver Failure

Presentation: Acute hepatitis typically presents with right upper quadrant (RUQ) pain and jaundice. Exam will likely reveal tender hepatomegaly. NSIDx is LFTs which typically reveal elevated ALT, AST and mixed bilirubinemia.

Most important step in dx is taking a thorough history, which should include:

- Exposure to other patients with jaundice.
- Risk factors, such as unprotected sex or intravenous drug abuse (IVDA).
- Alcohol and drug use, etc.

Etiology: Multiple diseases and chemicals can cause liver damage. Depending on degree of exposure and toxicity, liver damage can range from hepatitis to acute liver failure.

Acetaminophen (commonly called Tylenol)	Exam question will say that the patient took an over the counter medication (acetaminophen may be mentioned or not) **Clinical tip:** Check Tylenol level in all patients with significant hepatitis
Other drugs	Isoniazid, amiodarone, methotrexate, halothane, non-nucleoside reverse transcriptase inhibitors, etc.
Alcohol	Exam question might not give you a clear history of alcohol intake. For example, homeless person is found inebriated
Viruses	Hepatitis viruses (A, B, C, D, E), EBV, CMV, etc.
Autoimmune hepatitis	Can present similarly to chronic hepatitis B or C. Consider this as a differential diagnosis when hepatitis serology is negative, and no other obvious cause of hepatitis found (e.g., chronic Tylenol use)
Wilson disease	Liver abnormalities + movement disorder
Mushroom ingestion	*Amanita phalloides* species
Reye's syndrome	Occurs in children in the setting of acute viral infection and aspirin use. Exam question may say that the child was given some over-the-counter medication or living with grandmother.
Ischemic hepatitis	Acute significant increase in AST/ALT after a hypotensive event – Commonly seen in patients with shock (in ICU)
HELLP syndrome and acute fatty liver of pregnancy	– **HELLP = H**emolysis, **E**levated **L**iver enzymes (AST/ALT), **L**ow **P**latelets – Acute liver failure in pregnancy in absence of hemolysis suggests acute fatty liver of pregnancy
Budd–Chiari syndrome	**Pathophysiology:** Thrombosis of hepatic vein and/or inferior venacava leads to development of acute to subacute hepatitis and ascites/splenomegaly – Typically occurs in patients with myeloproliferative disorder and/or hypercoagulable disorder
Chronic exposure-to/infection-with any of the above can lead to cirrhosis	

Abbreviations: ALT, alanine amino transferase; AST, aspartate amino transferase; EBV, Epstein–Barr virus; CMV, cytomegalovirus; NNRTIs, nonnucleoside reverse transcriptase inhibitors.

Pathophysiology: Inflammation leads to necrosis of liver cells (↑ALT/ ↑AST). Severe inflammation may lead to extensive necrosis of liver cells and produce acute derangements of liver function. Development of elevated international normalized ratio (INR) or encephalopathy herald poor prognosis.

Terminology	Features	NSIM
Hepatitis	Only ALT/AST elevated; INR is < 1.5	Supportive and symptomatic treatment
Acute liver failure	PT prolongation (INR ≥ 1.5) with hepatic encephalopathy (elevated ammonia)	Patients with high grade encephalopathy and high PT/INR may be candidates for liver transplant.

Abbreviations: ALT, alanine amino transferase; AST, aspartate amino transferase; INR, international normalized ratio; PT, prothrombin time.

9.23 Specific Causes of Hepatitis

9.23.1 Alcoholic Liver Disease

Alcohol is the costliest health problem in the world and the third leading cause of death in the United States.

Different spectrums of alcoholic liver disease	Disease features	Pathological changes in liver	Reversibility after alcohol cessation
Fatty liver	Usually asymptomatic, but sometimes can present with tender hepatomegaly Slight elevation of AST and ALT	Macrovesicular steatosis	Reversible
Alcoholic hepatitis to acute liver failure	Marked elevation of AST > ALT Elevated INR and hyperammonemia signals development of liver failure	Balloon degeneration, neutrophilic infiltrate, and Mallory bodies (intracellular pink eosinophilic inclusion bodies)	Reversible Prednisolone[a] or pentoxifylline may be indicated in severe hepatitis
Fibrosis to cirrhosis	Low albumin, elevated INR, and other stigmata of cirrhosis	Cirrhosis is a form of advanced fibrosis, with disruption of normal liver architecture[b]	Fibrotic changes are usually irreversible

[a]Prednisolone is preferred over prednisone in patients with severe hepatitis, as prednisone requires conversion by liver into its active form of prednisolone.

[b]*FYI—only a small percentage (around 15%) of chronic alcoholics develop cirrhosis and it takes at least 10 years to develop cirrhosis. More rapid development of cirrhosis suggest co-existent liver pathology/toxin exposure (e.g., coexistent chronic Hep B or Hep C infection).*

9.23.2 Fatty Liver

Normally, liver cells are not supposed to store fat. If fat droplets are present in liver cells, the condition is called **fatty liver.** Fatty liver is histologically divided into two categories:

Microvesicular steatosis	**Etiology** – Sodium valproate-induced liver toxicity – Reye's syndrome – Acute fatty liver of pregnancy These are less common and more likely to present with severe hepatitis or liver failure.
Macrovesicular steatosis	This is more common. It is found in alcoholic liver disease, nonalcoholic fatty liver disease (NAFLD),[a] and other forms of liver damage. Depending on severity of underlying pathology and etiology, fatty liver may be asymptomatic, present as tender hepatomegaly and mild liver function test abnormalities, or as acute hepatitis, acute liver failure or cirrhosis in advanced stages.

[a]Develops due to constant unhealthy diet (e.g., high-fructose corn syrup, potato chips, high-glycemic-index foods), when body starts storing extra calories as fat in liver and other organs. NAFLD is closely associated with metabolic syndrome X, obesity, diabetes, etc. NASH (nonalcoholic steatohepatitis) is the more severe form of NAFLD. Chronically this can lead to cirrhosis.

9.23.3 Infectious Viral Hepatitis

- Viruses that cause hepatitis are **A, B, C, D,** and **E**. Other causes of viral hepatitis include Epstein–Barr virus, cytomegalovirus, herpes simplex virus, etc.
- Hep **A** and Hep **E** viruses are both transmitted by fecal–oral route and **never** cause chronic hepatitis.[19] Both are treated supportively. For Hep A, consider postexposure prophylaxis (PEP).
- Hep B and C can cause chronic hepatitis, cirrhosis, and increase risk of hepatocellular cancer. Both are transmitted by blood/blood products and are common in patients with IVDA (intravenous drug abuse).

[19]MCC of infectious hepatitis in USA is Hep **A**.
MCC of infectious hepatitis in developing countries is Hep E.

9.23.4 Postexposure Prophylaxis (PEP) for Hepatitis A

Consider PEP (within 2 weeks of exposure) for unvaccinated persons in the following situations:

All household and sex contacts of the case patient should receive PEP for Hep A			
In child-care centers[a]	Where children are wearing diapers		There is higher risk of transmission, so all staff and all other children in the center need to receive prophylaxis.
	Where children are not wearing diapers		Only the classroom contacts (the staff of that classroom and only the children in that classroom) are at risk and should be offered prophylaxis.
For a single case of food handler	For patrons of that place	Institutional cafeterias	Repeated exposure might have occurred (PEP is reasonable for patrons of that place).
		Noninstitutional cafeterias	Patrons do not need to be vaccinated in this setting, unless the case patient had poor hygienic practices or diarrhea and had handled foods following cooking.
	For other food handlers		All other food handlers in that establishment must receive PEP.

[a]PEP is not indicated in school, office, or hospital settings where a single case of Hep A is thought to be acquired outside of these settings.

What to use for prophylaxis?

For healthy patients 1 to 40 years of age	Hep A vaccine
Patients with chronic liver disease, immunosuppression, or age > 40 years	Hep A immunoglobulin + Hep A vaccine
<12 months of age	Hep A immunoglobulin only

Clinical Case Scenarios

A patient presents with acute hepatitis. He was in close contact with someone who was recently diagnosed with infectious hepatitis and was told by a doctor that it did not cause chronic infection.

19. What is the single test you would order?

20. If antibody is found to be positive, what is the NSIM regarding family members?

9.23.5 Hepatitis B
Hep B virus serology markers

HBs Ag = Hep B surface antigen	Presence of HBs Ag means that patient has an ongoing infection with Hep B virus; the virus is present in patient's body.
Anti-HBs antibody = anti-Hep B surface antibody	Presence of anti-HBs antibody indicates that patient is immune to Hep B virus and that he will never get Hep B infection again. The next question is how did he get this immunity? • Was patient infected with the virus and his immune system was able to get rid of it? (In this case, anti-HBc antibody will be positive.) • Patient got protective antibody after he was vaccinated. (In this case, anti-HBc will be negative, as the patient was only exposed to HBs Ag through vaccination.)
Anti-HBc = anti-Hep B core antibody	There are two different types: IgM anti-HBc denotes recent infection IgG anti-HBc denotes past infection
HBe Ag = Hep B envelope antigen	Presence of this antigen implies that the virus is actively replicating, patient has a high viral load and hence is contagious
Hep B viral DNA	Presence of viral DNA means that patient is infected with Hep B virus. Viral DNA quantification (viral load) gives an idea about how infectious patient is. Patients with high viral load are more infectious. It is also used to assess the need for antiviral therapy

Note that HBc **antigen** is not found in blood and we cannot test it.

 Caution

Do not choose Hep B viral DNA to diagnose Hep B.

Look at the following practice table, cover the last column with your hand and think what might be the diagnosis and why?

HBs Ag	Anti-HBs Ab	Anti-HBc Ab	HBe Ag	Dx
+	−	+ IgM type	+/−	Recently infected patient (point A in **Fig. 9.1** and **Fig. 9.2**) NSIM is repeat serology after 6 months
−	−	+ IgM type	−	This is called the window period and can only be diagnosed if anti-HBc serology is included in screening[a] (point B in **Fig. 9.1**)
−	+	+ IgG type	−	Cured of natural infection (point C in **Fig. 9.1**)
+	−	+ IgG type	+/−	Chronic infection (point D in **Fig. 9.2**)
−	+	−	−	MC serological profile in general population, because of the widespread use of vaccination

[a]That is why patients with acute hepatitis must be screened for Hep B by checking IgM anti-HBc antibody along with HBsAg and HBsAb.

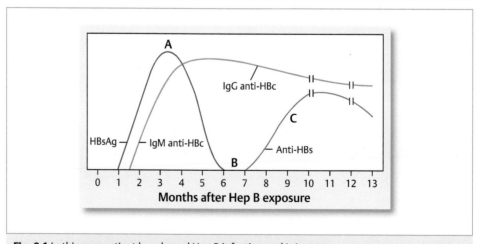

Fig. 9.1 In this case patient has cleared Hep B infection and is immune.

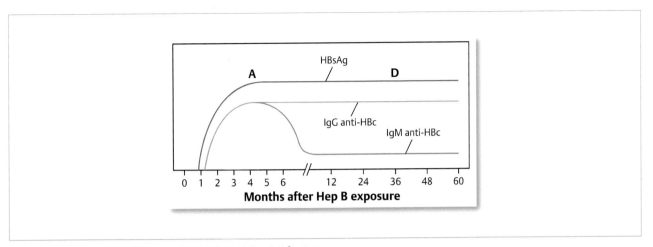

Fig. 9.2 In this case patient has developed chronic Hep B Infection

---

Clinical Case Scenarios

A patient presents with acute hepatitis. Hepatitis serology reveals positive anti-HBc IgM and HBsAg.

21. What is the NSIM?

22. HBs Ag after 6 months is still positive. NSIM?

9.24 Management of Chronic Hep B

9.24.1 Indication for treatment of chronic hepatitis B

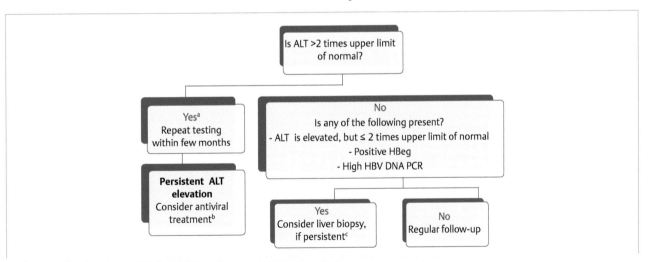

[a] Treat immediately if evidence of decompensated liver disease or jaundice.

[b] Usually before initiation of treatment, liver biopsy is considered.

[c] Consider treatment if it shows moderate to severe hepatitis or fibrosis. If biopsy is normal, no need for treatment.

[20]Interferon cannot be used in decompensated liver disease and is relatively contraindicated in patients with severe depression.

Choice of therapy:

- Anti-hepatitis B virus (HBV) treatment includes monotherapy with Entecavir, Tenofovir, or pegylated Interferon-α.[20] Other choices include lamivudine, adefovir, etc.
- Patients with decompensated liver disease should be referred to a transplant center.

Clinical Case Scenarios

ALT (FYI: normal range of ALT = 10–40)[a]	HBe Ag or HBV DNA PCR	NSIM
90, repeated after 2 months is 100 which is two times the upper limit of normal	Positive	Initiate treatment
50	Positive	Repeat test after few months Consider liver biopsy if persistent
20	Positive	Repeat test after few months Consider liver biopsy if persistent
20	Negative	No indication for treatment. Do regular follow-up

[a]FYI: no need to remember numerical values, just understand the concept.

9.24.2 Postexposure Prophylaxis for HBV

Scenario: A nurse had a needle-stick injury from a patient with hepatitis B. What is the NSIM? It depends upon vaccination status of the nurse.

Vaccination status	Post-vaccine anti-HBs titer	NSIM
Complete	Not checked	Check anti-HBs titer
Complete	> 10 mIU/mL	Reassure
Complete	< 10 mIU/mL (dx is vaccine nonresponder)	Anti-Hep B immunoglobulin + start Hep B vaccination
Not completed the vaccine series or never vaccinated		

Hepatitis D and B

Note, that Hep D is an "incomplete" virus and requires coinfection with Hep B to cause clinical disease.

In following situations of hep B, look for coinfection with Hep D:

– Patient with chronic Hep B infection suddenly develops new acute hepatitis.

– Hep B infection with fulminant course (i.e., severe disease).

Vaccination against Hep A and B

Following patients MUST receive routine hepatitis A and B vaccination:

- Patients with any form of chronic liver disease.
- HIV positive patients.
- Hemodialysis patients.
- IVDA.
- Men who have sex with men.
- Patients with clotting factor disorders.

[21]MCC of transfusion-associated hepatitis.

MC reason for liver transplantation in the United States.

9.25 Hepatitis C[21]

Presentation: Usually does not cause acute hepatitis and has more chronic, indolent course with majority of patients being asymptomatic. Commonly Hep C is diagnosed when screening test is positive or when patient is found to have abnormal LFTs and hepatitis panel is checked.

Diagnosis: Screening for hepatitis C virus (HCV) is done by HCV antibody. If HCV antibody is positive, NSIDx is HCV RNA polymerase chain reaction (PCR). **In patients with acute hepatitis or recent definite exposure to Hep C,** obtain antibody and PCR both at the same time. Testing for antibody alone might be falsely negative, as it takes some time to mount an immune response.

Management:
- If HCV PCR is positive, it needs to be repeated in 6 months. If PCR remains positive, consider treatment.
- Treatment choice depends on HCV genotype and presence of liver fibrosis.[22] Multiple antivirals are available nowadays, but unlike Hep B, Hep C is commonly treated with combination of two antiviral agents (e.g., ribavirin + sofosbuvir).
- Patients with decompensated liver disease are referred for transplant therapy.

Additional Notes on Hep B and C

Natural history:
- More than 50% of people who get infected with HCV develop chronic infection; whereas only about 20% of people with HBV develop chronic infection.
- Most common course of HBV is subclinical disease (asymptomatic) with complete recovery. Exception is primary HBV infection in an infant; most of these infants develop chronic infection.
- HCV acquired at a relatively young age is less likely to progress into chronic infection.

Contagiousness:
- Not wearing condoms is acceptable when HCV infected patient has a stable long-term monogamous relationship; no change in sexual practice is recommended. In contrast, in Hep B, which can have high viral load, a single sexual contact is considered high risk and PEP is recommended.
- All household contacts of chronic HBV carrier should be vaccinated with Hep B vaccine.

Specific conditions associated with Hep B and Hep C infection

	Think of
Hep B infection + kidney disease	Membranous glomerulopathy (nephrotic syndrome)
Hep B + kidney disease + skin rash	Polyarteritis nodosum
Hep C + kidney disease	Membranoproliferative glomerulonephritis
Hep C + kidney disease + skin rash	Cryoglobulinemic vasculitis
Hep C + skin rash only	Can be two different things:
	Porphyria cutanea tarda (photosensitive rash distributed in sun-exposed areas)
	Lichen planus

9.26 Autoimmune Hepatitis

Presentation: This can present with acute hepatitis, acute liver failure, or chronic progressive disease with flare-ups.

Diagnosis: It can be diagnosed with combination of serology and elevated total IgG, after excluding other causes of hepatitis. Best test is liver biopsy but may not be necessary to confirm diagnosis.

Treatment: Immunosuppressive agents (steroids +/− azathioprine).

Clinical Case Scenarios

A patient with history of IVDA comes to your clinic to establish care.

23. What is the NSIDx regarding hepatitis?

24. If hepatitis serology is negative, what is the NSIM?

A patient with history of IVDA presents with acute jaundice, urticarial rash, and joint pain.

25. What is the likely Dx?

26. What is the NSIDx?

[22]To detect liver fibrosis, liver biopsy may not be needed, as currently available noninvasive testing methods (e.g., ultrasound-based elastography) can detect stages of liver fibrosis and influence treatment decisions.

MRS

Antibodies found in autoimmune hepatitis are antibodies against "SNL LAMPS."
- S = smooth muscle = antismooth muscle antibody
- N = nuclear = antinuclear antibody
- L = liver/kidney microsomal-1 = anti-LKM1 antibodies
- L = liver cytosol-1 = anti-LC1 antibodies
- A = actin antibodies = antiactin antibodies
- M = mitochondrial antibodies = antimitochondrial antibodies
- P = p-perinuclear antineutrophil cytoplasmic antibodies
- S = soluble liver/liver pancreas antigen = anti-SL/LP antigen

9.27 Cirrhosis

Background: Cirrhosis develops due to chronic liver inflammation with underlying pathology severe and/or persistent enough to cause widespread damage and loss of hepatocytes, resulting in widespread liver fibrosis and disruption of liver architecture. Disruption of portal venous system leads to increased pressure and portal hypertension.

Causes of cirrhosis

Causes	Diagnostic clues	Additional points
Alcohol	Patient with hx of alcohol abuse	MCC of cirrhosis in the United States
Hep C	Features suggestive of IVDA are present	MCC of liver transplant in the United States[a]
Hep B	Patient with high risk sexual behavior or IVDA	Hep D coinfection can accelerate development of cirrhosis.
NAFLD/NASH	Obese patients with features of metabolic syndrome	Pathologically indistinguishable from alcoholic liver disease
Hemochromatosis	Liver abnormalities + skin hyperpigmentation +/− diabetes mellitus +/− arthritis +/− heart conduction defects or cardiomyopathy +/− hypogonadism	**NSIDx:** serum ferritin and iron saturation. Iron saturation of > 45% and elevated ferritin of >200 ng/mL in men or >150 ng/mL in women is consistent with iron overload. NSIDx is HFE genotyping (C282Y and H63D mutations). If ferritin> 1000 ng/ML, do MRI to quantify iron amount in liver and/or heart. Liver biopsy is only done in patients with suspected cirrhosis or fibrosis.[b] To screen first degree relatives of the patient, use genetic testing along with iron saturation and serum ferritin. Patients have very high risk of hepatocellular cancer.
Wilson disease (aka hepatolenticular degeneration)—an autosomal recessive disorder	Liver abnormalities + neurological disorder[c] +/− Coomb's negative hemolytic anemia (due to copper-mediated oxidative damage). Note: it can present as acute hepatitis and liver failure.	**NSIDx:** eye slit lamp exam (best initial test) + serum ceruloplasmin level and 24-hour urinary copper excretion. Presence of Kayser–Fleischer ring (a ring of brown discoloration in the periphery of cornea due to copper deposition), low ceruloplasmin, and high urinary copper levels confirm the diagnosis. If the above tests are equivocal, consider liver biopsy.[d] Source: Biousse V, Newman N, ed. Neuro-Ophthalmology Illustrated. 2nd ed. Thieme; 2015.
Alpha-1 antitrypsin deficiency	Lung + liver[e] abnormalities	**NSIDx:** serum antitrypsin level. **Treatment:** infusion of alpha-1 antitrypsin.[f] Patients should be counseled for complete smoking cessation.
Primary biliary cholangitis (aka primary biliary cirrhosis)	Present with generalized itching, fatigue, marked hypercholesterolemia (eye xanthelasma)	More common in females (discussed further after cirrhosis section)
Primary sclerosing cholangitis		More common in males (discussed further after cirrhosis section)

[a]Even though chronic alcoholism is the MCC of cirrhosis, this group of patients often continue to drink, which is an exclusion criterion for liver transplant.

[b]Iron overload/deposition can be detected with MRI of liver or heart, obviating the need for liver biopsy. Treatment of choice is regular interval phlebotomies which remove excess iron. Oral iron chelators such as deferasirox or deferoxamine are used only in patients who cannot tolerate phlebotomy. In contrast, for secondary hemochromatosis that occurs after multiple packed red blood cell transfusion for anemia, oral iron chelators are the treatment of choice. Note: Patients with hemochromatosis are more susceptible to *Listeria monocytogenes, Vibrio vulnificus,* and *Yersinia enterocolitica* as these bacteria thrive in iron-rich conditions.

[c]Patients can present with difficulty in speaking, excessive salivation, ataxia, mask-like facies, hands clumsiness, personality changes, etc. (Any neurological problem + liver issue, think of this.)

[d]**Rx:** Copper chelators—penicillamine and trientine. Liver transplant is curative because primary pathology is inability of the liver to excrete copper in bile.

[e]The hepatic cells produce alpha-1 antitrypsin but cannot secrete it into the circulation; hence it accumulates in hepatocytes causing liver damage.

[f]Alpha-1 antitrypsin infusion contains small amount of IgA, hence in IgA deficient individuals, infusion can lead to anaphylaxis.

Abbreviations: IVDA, intravenous drug abuse; NAFLD/NASH, nonalcoholic fatty liver disease/nonalcoholic steatohepatitis.

Presentation of cirrhosis

- Generalized edema due to low albumin levels and low oncotic pressure
- Ascites due to low oncotic pressure and portal hypertension
- Palmar erythema ⎫
- Spider angioma ⎪ due to decreased metabolism of estrogen leading to hyperestrogenemia
- Testicular atrophy ⎬
- Sparse hair ⎪
- Gynecomastia ⎭

Clinical features of portal hypertension:

- **Splenomegaly:** splenic congestion leads to hyperactivity of splenic macrophages (hypersplenism), which can eat up blood cells and cause reduction in any or all the blood cell types (anemia, thrombocytopenia, or pancytopenia)
- **Caput medusae** due to umbilical vein recanalization
- **Esophageal varices:** increased pressure in portal system results in venous engorgement of left gastric vein which anastomose to lower esophageal veins. These dilated and thinned out veins (varicose veins) can easily bleed and can present with life-threatening hematemesis

Patients with liver cirrhosis can also present acutely with the following:

- Hepatic encephalopathy
- Spontaneous bacterial peritonitis
- Acute variceal bleeding episode
- **Hepatorenal syndrome:** Prerenal kidney failure, which typically progresses despite adequate fluid/colloid resuscitation. This is thought to be due to renal vasoconstriction. The best treatment is liver transplantation.

Hepatopulmonary syndrome: Intrapulmonary arteriovenous connections can develop in decompensated cirrhosis. Combined with intrapulmonary vasodilation +/– pulmonary hypertension, it can lead to increased arteriovenous shunting. Shunting worsens in upright position, presenting as **platypnea** (shortness of breath when standing or sitting up and relieved by lying flat).

Preventive management of patients with compensated cirrhosis in clinic setting (commonly asked on exam):

- Periodic surveillance with LFTs and clinical visits.
- US liver to screen for hepatocellular cancer every 6 months.
- EGD surveillance for variceal disease.
- Vaccination against Hep A and B.

9.27.1 Ascites

Presentation: Abdominal distention. Exam may reveal fluid thrill and shifting dullness.

Workup: To confirm presence of ascites, US abdomen can be done. New-onset ascites generally requires diagnostic paracentesis. Calculate serum ascites albumin gradient (SAAG) = serum albumin concentration – (minus) albumin concentration in ascitic fluid.

SAAG ≥ 1.1	Ascites is due to portal hypertension and increased hydrostatic pressure
	Causes: right heart failure, Budd–Chiari syndrome and cirrhosis
	If there is no evidence of cirrhosis, NSIDx is echocardiography. If echocardiography unremarkable, consider US doppler of abdomen to look for hepatic vein or IVC vein thrombosis, to look for Budd-Chiari syndrome.
SAAG < 1.1	Means portal hypertension is not present and higher albumin content in ascitic fluid is signifying an exudative pathology: cancer or infection (except spontaneous bacterial peritonitis)

Management of ascites:

- First step is to limit daily Na⁺ intake. Water restriction is recommended only if serum Na⁺ is ≤ 125 mEq/L.
- If not controlled, NSIM is combination diuretics—**spironolactone** and **furosemide**.
- If ascites is still not controlled by maximum doses of furosemide and spironolactone, NSIM is regular **paracentesis**.
- As a last resort, **T**ransjugular-**I**ntrahepatic **P**orto-**S**ystemic **S**hunt (**TIPS**) can be placed.

 MRS

SAAG: "AA" = "1" and "1", as "A" is the first alphabet. So, important SAAG value is 1.1.
Elevated SAAG is elevated portal pressure.

MRS

Always start with most conservative and least invasive treatment: dietary Na+ restriction → maximize medicines (diuretics) → paracentesis procedure → surgical procedure.
However, if a patient presents with significant symptoms, such as shortness of breath due to abdominal distenstion and increased abdominal pressure, NSIM is large volume therapeutic paracentesis.

Clinical Case Scenarios

A patient with diagnosis of hemochromatosis and cirrhosis now presents with few months hx of unintentional weight loss and increased abdominal distension. Abdominal paracentesis reveals hemorrhagic ascites and elevated alpha-fetoprotein levels.

27. What is the most likely dx?

28. What is the NSIM?

A 75-year-old female presents with 6-month hx of slowly progressive abdominal distention. Exam reveals fluid thrill and shifting dullness. Paracentesis is done. Her serum albumin is 3.6 g/dL and ascitic albumin is 2.8 g/dL.

29. What is the SAAG gradient?

30. What is the likely dx?

9.27.2 Acute Variceal Bleeding

Definition: Varices are dilated submucosal veins in gastroesophageal junction that have increased risk of rupture and bleeding.[23]

Presentation: Acute hematemesis +/- melena.

[23]Endoscopic view of esophageal varices

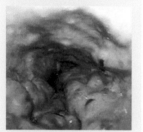

Source: Samir, Public domain, via Wikimedia Commons.

Management of Acute Variceal Bleeding

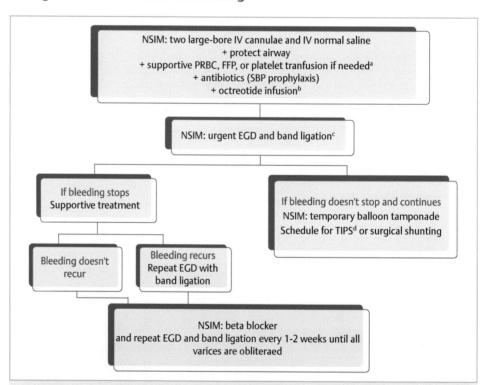

[a]Consider platelet transfusion if platelet count is <50,000/mm³.

[b]Octreotide is a somatostatin analogue which constricts splanchnic vessels and decreases portal pressure.

[c]Band ligation is preferred over sclerotherapy, because sclerotherapy is associated with increased risk of esophageal strictures and subsequent development of mechanical dysphagia.

[d]TIPS = **T**ransjugular-**i**ntrahepatic **p**orto**s**ystemic **s**hunting. A catheter, inserted through jugular vein, is used to create a shunt between portal (portal system) and hepatic veins (systemic circulation). This decreases the portal pressure, thus decreasing bleeding risk from varices. It also decreases ascitic fluid formation.

Note: The downside of TIPS procedure is that intestinal venous blood bypasses the natural detoxifying portal pathway, which leads to increased incidence of hepatic encephalopathy.

Abbreviations: EGD, esophagogastroduodenoscopy; FFP, fresh frozen plasma; PRBC, packed red blood cell transfusion; SBP, spontaneous bacterial peritonitis.

Prevention of variceal bleeding: All cirrhosis patients should be evaluated with EGD for detection of varices at regular interval. Use of nonselective beta blockers (e.g., nadolol or propranolol) is indicated if esophageal varices are found, as these medications reduce portal pressure and risk of bleeding. If beta blockers are contraindicated (e.g., refractory ascites or single episode of spontaneous bacterial peritonitis) or **patient has moderate to large varices, primary preventative endoscopic variceal ligation** can be done.

| Location of esophageal varices and the likely cause ||
Location of varices	**Likely cause**
Mid esophagus, with unaffected or mildly affected distal esophagus	Superior vena cava syndrome
Distal esophageal varices	Portal hypertension
Varices mostly in gastric antrum with unaffected esophagus	Splenic vein thrombosis

9.27.3 Spontaneous Bacterial Peritonitis (SBP)

Definition: Spontaneous infection of ascitic fluid with no clear extraneous source identified. MC bacteriological cause is *Escherichia coli*.[24]

Presentation: Fever, diffuse abdominal pain, hypotension, and/or sudden increase in abdominal distension.[25] Abdominal X-ray may reveal signs suggestive of paralytic ileus.

Diagnosis: Abdominal paracentesis and gram stain/culture. Absolute neutrophil count (polymorphonucleocyte count) ≥250/mm³ is diagnostic of spontaneous bacterial peritonitis (SBP).

Rx: Cefotaxime (preferred), ceftriaxone, or quinolones. Usual duration is 5 days.

Prophylaxis: A single episode of SBP warrants long-term antibiotic prophylaxis forever. Short-term prophylaxis **during hospitalization** is indicated in cirrhotic patients with either GI bleeding or ascitic protein of < 1 g/dL (long-term outpatient prophylaxis is not indicated in this situation). Use trimethoprim-sulfamethoxazole, oral quinolones, or IV cefotaxime or ceftriaxone.

9.27.4 Hepatic Encephalopathy

Pathophysiology: It occurs because of impaired liver detoxification of ammonia and increased ammonia (NH₃) load in blood which enters brain and stimulates production of false neurotransmitters (e.g., octopamine). These false neurotransmitters affect the synapses leading to changes in brain function (e.g., changes in sleep pattern, irritability, changes in personality, altered mental status, confusion, and coma when severe). Exam may reveal flapping tremor of extended hands (known as asterixis or hepatic flap).[26]

Management:
1. First SIM is to always address the precipitating cause.

Drugs	Eliminate use of sedatives and hypnotic drugs. Note, if sedatives are required in cirrhotic patients use oxazepam, temazepam or lorazepam, which are benzodiazepines not metabolized by the liver.
Uremia	
GI bleeding	Blood contents are metabolized by gut bacteria into urea and ammonia.
Hypokalemia	Promptly replace potassium in all patients with hypokalemia.
Excess dietary protein	Patients who develop recurrent encephalopathic episodes after high protein intake should be advised to restrict protein intake. However, most patients with cirrhosis are malnourished and it is more important to liberalize food intake.
PAracentesis	High volumes > 5 L. When > 5 L of ascitic fluid is removed with paracentesis, consider albumin replacement
Portosystemic shunts	TIPS or surgically created shunt
Trauma	Including surgery
Infection	For example, spontaneous bacterial peritonitis or urinary tract infection
Constipation	

[24] MCC of SBP in noncirrhotic ascites (e.g., ascites due to nephrotic syndrome in children) is *Streptococcus pneumoniae*.

[25]If a cirrhotic patient has any one of these features, think of SBP.

[26]*Google - video of hepatic flap*

MRS
Out The Liver

MRS
DUG HEPATIC

⚠ **Caution**
Both hepatic encephalopathy and SBP can present with altered mental status in a cirrhotic patient. Fever and enlarging ascites or tender abdomen points toward SBP. Also, SBP which is an infection may precipitate hepatic encephalopathy.

2. Second step is **lactulose** which has double effect:

Lactulose is fermented by gut bacteria into acid that supplies a lot of H⁺, changing NH_3 to NH_4^+. This ammonium ion isn't absorbed into the circulation and is subsequently trapped in the gut. It is also a laxative that flushes out gut NH_4^+ and protein (which is a substrate for conversion into ammonia). If there is no adequate response to lactulose, NSIM is broad-spectrum antibiotics, such as rifaximin, which kill bacteria that produces ammonia. Alternative antibiotic is neomycin.

9.27.5 Primary Biliary Cholangitis and Primary Sclerosing Cholangitis

	Primary biliary cholangitis (PBC) (formerly known as primary biliary cirrhosis)	Primary sclerosing cholangitis (PSC)
Pathophysiology	– Autoimmune inflammation and destruction of interlobular bile ducts inside liver parenchyma – Typically affects females, but can occur in males – It is associated with rheumatoid arthritis, Sjogren's syndrome, Raynaud's phenomenon, etc.	– Inflammation and destruction of large intra and extra hepatic bile ducts; hence liver biopsy might be normal. This is the **only** chronic liver disease in which liver biopsy is not the most specific test as primary pathology occurs in the ducts outside the liver parenchyma – Typical patient is a male, but it can occur in females. – It is closely associated with HLA-B27 related conditions (seronegative spondyloarthropathy)
Presentation	– Pruritus, fatigue, and evidence of cholestasis in liver function tests (↑AKP, ↑5′ nucleotidase, ↑GGT). Elevated bilirubin (jaundice) might present later in course and signals poor prognosis – Xanthelasma due to underlying hypercholesterolemia – When disease is advanced, bile salt deficiency can lead to fat malabsorption, steatorrhea, deficiency of fat-soluble vitamins (e.g., osteomalacia, vitamin A deficiency), etc.	
Workup	In patients with obstructive LFTs pattern, NSIDx is to rule out extrahepatic obstruction by doing abdominal US followed by MRCP	
	After ruling out obstructive lesions with MRCP, NSIDx is to check antimitochondrial antibody. Then do **liver biopsy**, which is the most accurate test. Liver biopsy might not be needed for dx in a classic case of PBC (a female patient, with elevated AKP and significant titers of antimitochondrial antibody)	– MRCP can show diagnostic beads (biliary duct dilatation) and strings (strictures) pattern in intrahepatic and/or extrahepatic ducts. ERCP (invasive but more sensitive than MRCP) can be done , if MRCP is negative , especially when PSC is suspected (e.g., male patient with coexistent ulcerative colitis). Also check serum antimitochondrial antibody (to exclude PBC) and IgG4 level (to rule out IgG4 associated cholangitis). – In rare cases, when small duct PSC is suspected and MRCP/ERCP is unremarkable, only then liver biopsy might be needed. Otherwise liver biopsy is rarely diagnostic and needed
Management	NSIM is ursodeoxycholic acid (slows the progression of disease). If no significant response, add obeticholic acid (increases synthesis of bile acid) or fibrates	Role of ursodeoxycholic acid is uncertain
	– For moderate to severe pruritus, bile acid binders, such as cholestyramine or colestipol, can be tried. Patients who cannot tolerate bile acid binders due to GI symptoms can try rifampin. – Liver transplant is recommended in advanced stages of both PBC and PSC.	

Abbreviations: AKP, alkaline phosphatase; ERCP, endoscopic retrograde cholangiopancreatography; GGT, gamma-glutamyl transferase; MRCP, magnetic resonance cholangiopancreatography; LFT, liver function test.

 MRS

PSC – Sclerosis = hard = men have harder muscles = occurs mostly in men; C = cholangitis = inflamed bile ducts → higher risk of cholangiocarcinoma. PSC is associated with a higher risk of cholangiocarcinoma and gallbladder cancer.

 MRS

Biliary MAMA - = Mothers Are Mitochondrial Antibody positive MAMA= mother = female

9.28 Jaundice

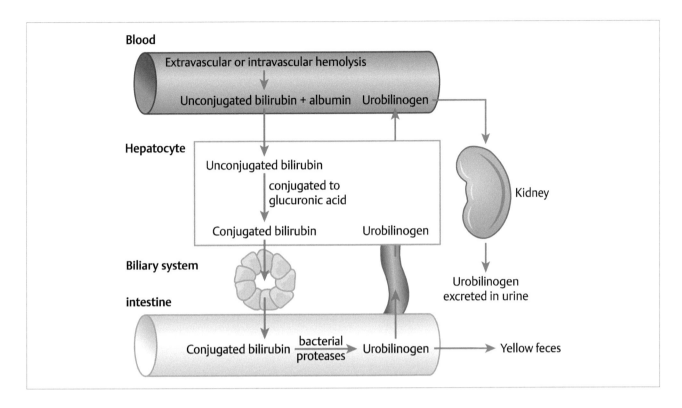

9.28.1 Background—The story of bilirubin:

When red blood cells (RBCs) die, either physiologically or pathologically, hemoglobin inside it is broken down. The heme part turns into bilirubin; this unconjugated bilirubin is lipid soluble and must be transported to liver through the blood highway, attached to albumin. Upon reaching the liver, the bilirubin is taken up by liver cells and then conjugated with a hydrophilic compound. This conjugated bilirubin is now water-soluble and can be excreted through the biliary/urinary system.

Unconjugated (indirect) hyperbilirubinemia	In this case the bilirubin is lipid soluble and is attached to albumin, hence it cannot be excreted in the urine. Pathology that results in increase in only unconjugated bilirubin does not result in yellow- or dark-colored urine and stool can be normal or pale.
Conjugated (direct) bilirubinemia	Bile flow obstruction and subsequent conjugated bilirubinemia has two bodily consequences:
	Pale stool: due to decreased passage of conjugated bilirubin to intestines. Normal stool color is a result of excretion of conjugated bilirubin through biliary system.
	Dark-colored urine: due to backflow of conjugated bilirubin into systemic circulation and henceforth kidney.

Definition: Jaundice is a clinical diagnosis of yellow discoloration of skin, sclera, conjunctiva, and nail beds. It can be due to rise in conjugated or unconjugated bilirubin or both.

9.28.2 Diagnostic approach to jaundice:

First SIDx is to look at LFTs	Second SIDx is to look at the following		Likely diagnosis
Normal LFTs	Direct/conjugated bilirubinemia		– Dubin–Johnson syndrome[a] – Rotor syndrome
	Indirect/ unconjugated bilirubinemia	No evidence of hemolysis or hematoma	– Gilbert syndrome (more common) or – Crigler–Najjar syndrome, type 2[b]
		Large hematoma	Due to increased breakdown of RBCs during reabsorption of hematoma
		Evidence of Hemolysis	Hemolytic anemia
Abnormal LFTs	Elevation of AST/ALT out of proportion to AKP		Look at Hepatitis Chapter (likely to have mixed bilirubinemia)
	Elevation of AKP and GGT out of proportion to ALT/AST		Obstructive jaundice (discussed below)

[a]For some reason if liver biopsy is done in Dubin–Johnson syndrome, it will reveal black pigment inside hepatocytes.

[b]Do not choose Crigler–Najjar type I in adults. Crigler–Najjar type I is the more severe form that occurs in infants and results in severe unconjugated hyperbilirubinemia. They end up requiring liver transplantation in early life.

Abbreviations: AKP, alkaline phosphatase; ALT, alanine amino transferase; AST, aspartate amino transferase; GGT, gamma-glutamyl transferase; LFT, liver function test.

All the above-mentioned "syndromes" are due to a hereditary defect either in bilirubin conjugation or transport. They are relatively benign except Crigler-Najjar type "I".

9.28.3 Obstructive Jaundice

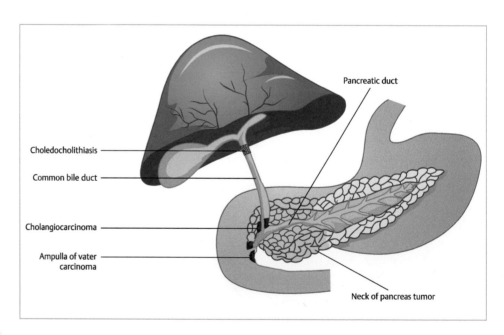

- In patients with obstructive jaundice and RUQ (right upper quadrant) pain, think of choledocholithiasis, and if there is fever then think of ascending cholangitis.[27]
- If patient presents with painless obstructive jaundice, look at the following algorithm:

[27]Jaundice + right upper quadrant pain along with mixed LFT pattern (significant elevation of ALT/AST) can be due to acute hepatitis too.

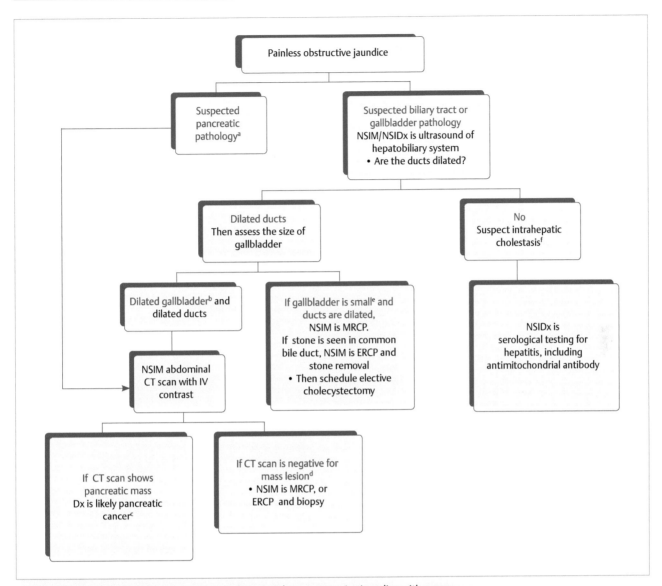

^aIf clinical vignette suggests pancreatic cancer (e.g., painless, progressive jaundice with vague epigastric pain and weight loss), NSIDx is abdominal CT scan with IV contrast.

^bDilated gallbladder means the obstruction is not due to stone and is likely due to malignant obstruction of biliary outflow.

^cIn pancreatic cancer, jaundice occurs due to obstruction of the **common bile duct**.(!) See algorithm below for further workup of pancreatic mass.

^dIf CT scan is negative for mass lesion, then extrinsic compression of biliary outflow is unlikely, but intrabiliary malignancy like cholangiocarcinoma is still possible which can cause early obstruction and can be hard to detect on CT scan, so ERCP and biopsy needs to be done (MRCP is an alternative). Risk factors for cholangiocarcinoma include chronic liver disease, primary sclerosing cholangitis, recurrent cholangitis, congenital biliary tree abnormalities, HIV or rare infection such as infection by *Clonorchis sinensis*.

^eIf gallbladder is small, then obstructive jaundice is likely due to biliary duct stone; it leads to reactionary inflammation and contracture of gallbladder.

^fCauses include primary biliary cholangitis, primary sclerosing cholangitis, infectious hepatitis, cholestasis of pregnancy, etc.

⚠ **Caution**

(!) Do not choose obstruction of **pancreatic duct** as a cause of jaundice in a patient with pancreatic mass.

9.28.4 Workup of Suspected Exocrine Pancreatic Cancer

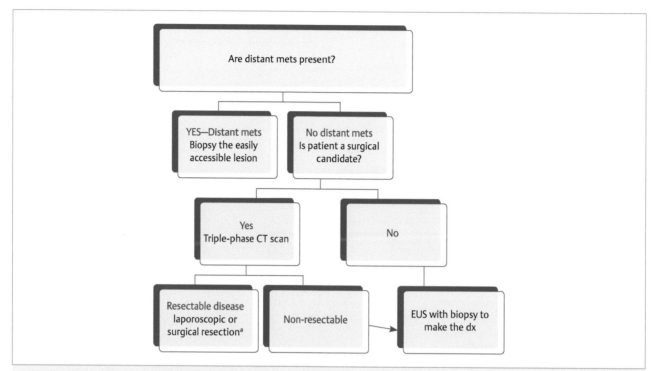

ᵃIf there is high probability of pancreatic cancer and patient is a surgical candidate, go directly for resection instead of doing biopsy. Rx of exocrine pancreatic cancer depends upon staging.

9.29 Cholelithiasis (Gallbladder Stone)

Background: There are two types of gallbladder stone.

Cholesterol gallstones (the most common one)	Calcium bilirubinate (black or brown pigment) stones
Risk factors:	**Risk factors:**
– The fat, female, fertile, and forties is the typical patient profile (four Fs). – Estrogen and progesterone predispose to formation of gall bladder stones. Estrogen increases the cholesterol content in bile and progesterone decreases gall bladder motility, leading to stasis. Use of oral contraceptive pills and pregnancy increases risk. – Fat cells due to their aromatase activity increase estrogen level in blood and hence obesity is also a risk factor. – Other causes of increased gall bladder stasis are low gallbladder function (e.g., in patients on total parenteral nutrition).	– **Chronic hemolysis:** sickle cell disease, hereditary spherocytosis, etc. – **Ileal disease:** Crohn's disease, ileectomy, ileal bypass, etc. This is due to increased enterohepatic circulation of bilirubin. – **Rare biliary tract infections** such as *Clonorchis sinensis*, *Ascaris lumbricoides*, etc.
They are typically radiolucent and not seen in plain X-ray films.	They are radiopaque and seen in plain X-ray films.

9.29.1 Clinical Pathophysiology

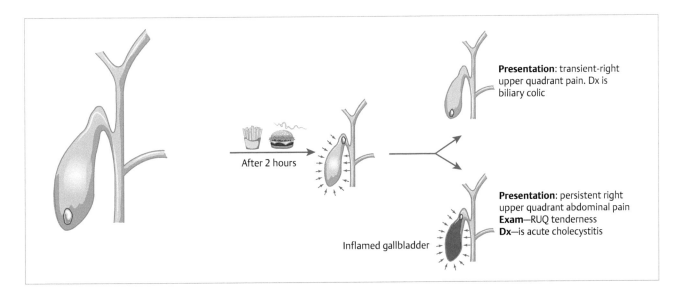

Presentation: transient-right upper quadrant pain. Dx is biliary colic

Presentation: persistent right upper quadrant abdominal pain
Exam—RUQ tenderness
Dx—is acute cholecystitis

After 2 hours

Inflamed gallbladder

9.30 Biliary Colic

Presentation: Transient band-like upper abdominal or RUQ (right upper quadrant) pain after eating. If the stone dislodges from the gallbladder neck, it no longer causes pain.

Management steps:

– NSIDx is US of the hepatobiliary system.
– After dx, NSIM is to schedule elective cholecystectomy. If patient does not want surgery, a trial of ursodeoxycholic acid can be done (it reduces cholesterol content in bile and may dissolve cholesterol gallstones).

9.31 Acute Cholecystitis

Presentation: Constant RUQ pain +/– fever. Complete blood count may reveal leukocytosis.
Physical exam: Palpation of the RUQ while patient takes a deep breath in causes acute tenderness, as inspiration causes the inflamed gallbladder to ascend onto the palpating fingers (Murphy's sign).
Diagnosis: US of the hepatobiliary system (best initial test). If it is unremarkable and if there is still high suspicion, NSIDx is hepatobiliary iminodiacetic acid (**HIDA) scan** aka cholescintigraphy (most accurate test).
Management: Full GI rest, i.e., nil per os (NPO), IV fluids and pain management.

– If symptoms subside, NSIM is schedule elective cholecystectomy in next 24 to 48 hours.
– If patient continues to have pain, fever or increasing leukocytosis, then do an emergent cholecystectomy.
– If patient is a poor surgical candidate, a percutaneous biliary drain may be placed.

9.31.1 Complications of Acute Cholecystitis

Gallbladder perforation and biliary peritonitis	**Typical CCS:** Look for acute clinical deterioration in a patient with acute cholecystitis (development of generalized abdominal pain, guarding, and rigidity).
Gallbladder abscess	**Typical CCS:** Persistent fever in a patient diagnosed with acute cholecystitis. Exam may reveal RUQ fluctuant mass. NSIDx is US of gallbladder. NSIM is IV broad-spectrum antibiotics + urgent gallbladder resection or percutaneous drainage in a hemodynamically unstable patient.
Fistula formation between gallbladder and intestine (cholecystointestinal fistula)	Sometimes gallbladder stones can pass into intestine through this fistula. If stones are big enough to get stuck in the narrow portion of ileocecal valve, it can cause intestinal obstruction (gallstone ileus).
Emphysematous cholecystitis	This occurs as result of gallbladder superinfection with gas-forming bacteria. Risk factors are immunosuppression, advanced age, and diabetes. US typically reveals increased echogenicity of gallbladder wall (due to gas formation). NSIM is urgent cholecystectomy and antibiotics (e.g., ceftriaxone + metronidazole).
Chronic cholecystitis	This can lead to **porcelain gallbladder** (intramural calcification of gallbladder due to chronic inflammation). For porcelain gallbladder, consider cholecystectomy, as it may be associated with increased risk of gallbladder cancer. Source: Herzog C. Differential diagnosis of diseases of the biliary system (CT). In: Burgener F, Zaunbauer W, Meyers S, et al., ed. Differential Diagnosis in Computed Tomography. 2nd ed. Stuttgart: 2011.

9.31.2 Complications of Gallbladder Stones which Are Small Enough to Pass into Biliary Ductal System

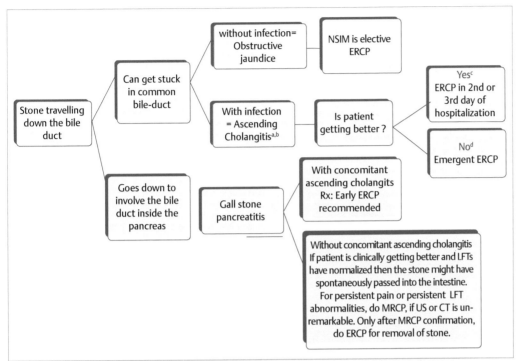

Clinical Tip: Even after cholecystectomy, common bile duct stone or sludge can form in the duct itself.

[a]**Presentation of ascending cholangitis:** fever, abdominal pain, and obstructive pattern in LFT. This can progress to severe sepsis or septic shock (with hypotension and mental status change). NSIM is IV fluids, antibiotics directed against GI pathogens, and ERCP, to extract the stone and/or sludge.

[b]Other causes of ascending cholangitis are Mirizzi's syndrome,[28] recurrent pyogenic cholangitis, etc.

[c]Improvement in clinical status (e.g., patient has less pain) and liver function tests are getting better.

[d]If patient does not improve within first day of hospitalization or becomes more septic, emergent ERCP and stone extraction is indicated.

[28]**Mirizzi's syndrome**

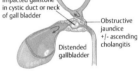

Impacted cystic duct stone can cause obstructive jaundice +/- ascending cholangitis

---

After treating the complication of biliary stone, elective cholecystectomy is scheduled.

9.32 Differential dx of Postcholecystectomy Biliary Colic Type Pain

Presentation: Patient continues to have RUQ or band-like upper abdominal pain after cholecystectomy.

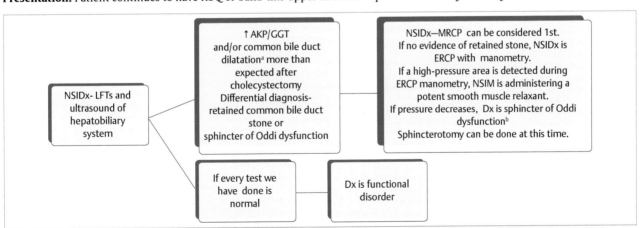

[a]In patients who present with postcholecystectomy obstructive jaundice and have biliary duct dilatation without involvement of common bile duct, think of the following: cystic duct stump stone (retained or recurrent) causing Mirizzi's syndrome or iatrogenic biliary stricture.

[b]Sphincter of Oddi dysfunction can also present with postprandial pain without hx of cholecystectomy. An attack can be precipitated by opioid analgesics as they cause sphincter contraction. US may reveal normal gallbladder with unexplained dilatation of common bile duct. LFTs may reveal obstructive pattern that normalize in between attacks.

9.33 Acute Acalculous Cholecystitis

Background: Inflammation (+/– necrosis of gallbladder) which most commonly occurs in patients who are very sick, or who have absent oral intake for a relatively long period.

Risk factors: Total parenteral nutrition, severe burns, severe trauma, ICU patients, etc.

Presentation: Its presentation is similar to acute cholecystitis. Consider this in critically ill patients with unexplained sepsis, leukocytosis, jaundice, or vague abdominal pain.

Workup: NSIDx is US of hepatobiliary system which will reveal features of cholecystitis but no evidence of cholelithiasis and no biliary ductal dilatation. If dx remains uncertain, do CT abdomen (to look for other causes of sepsis) and if needed go for HIDA scan.

Rx: Keep patient NPO, give broad-spectrum IV antibiotics directed against GI pathogens, and do cholecystectomy or, if patient is not a surgical candidate, cholecystostomy (surgical or interventional radiology guided drainage of gallbladder).

9.34 Pancreatitis

Background: Normally pancreatic enzymes are activated only when they reach intestinal lumen. Pancreatitis is caused by factors that lead to **activation** of pancreatic enzymes **within** the pancreas, which leads to autodigestion and inflammation of the pancreas.

Etiology:
- Gallstones.
- Ethanol, endoscopic retrograde cholangiopancreatography (ERCP).
- Trauma (blunt or penetrating trauma).
- Steroids, anti-seizure medications (sodium valproate).
- Scorpion venom.
- Mumps, 6-mercaptopurine.
- Azathioprine, autoimmune (elevated IgG4).
- Sulfa drugs (e.g., sulfamethoxazole-trimethoprim, sulfasalazine).
- Hypertriglyceridemia (triglyceride level > 1000 can lead to pancreatitis).[29]
- Hypercalcemia.[30]
- Embryological problems like pancreatic divisum and accessory pancreatic duct.
- Didanosine, zalcitabine (e.g., HIV patient with pancreatitis).
- Pentamidine (e.g., patient undergoing treatment for PCP develops pancreatitis).

Presentation: Epigastric pain/tenderness, +/– nausea and vomiting +/– fever. The pain can radiate to the back, since pancreas is mostly an extraperitoneal organ. Drug-induced pancreatitis can be very mild, and patient can even walk into your office with complaint of 1-week history of epigastric pain and mild fever.

Workup: NSIDx is serum lipase and/or amylase.

Presence of two out of the following three is diagnostic:
1. Lipase/amylase ≥ three times the upper limit of normal.
2. Acute onset persistent epigastric pain and/or tenderness.
3. Characteristic finding on imaging: CT scan (inflammatory stranding in peripancreatic area),[31] or US (hypoechoic and/or diffusely enlarged pancreas)

Rectal NSAIDs (e.g., indomethacin, diclofenac), immediately before or after ERCP, has been shown to reduce incidence of post-ECRP pancreatitis.

Gallstones, ethanol and trauma are the most common causes

 MRS

Pancreas GETS SMASHED

[29]For treatment of hypertriglyceridemia-induced pancreatitis, plasmapheresis or (insulin + glucose) infusion may be needed.

[30]Remember to send lipid profile and serum calcium in all patients admitted with acute pancreatitis

[31]If patient does not have either diagnostic lipase/amylase elevation or characteristic pain, then CT scan should be done to confirm diagnosis and to exclude other causes of abdominal pain.

Laboratory findings:

Hypo- or hyperglycemia	
Hypocalcemia	Multifactorial, due to • Fat saponification: spilled pancreatic lipase digests triglycerides, which leads to release of fatty acids that binds with free calcium • Hormonal imbalances, etc.
Acute renal failure	Can occur because of intravascular volume depletion due to third spacing of fluids and acute tubular necrosis

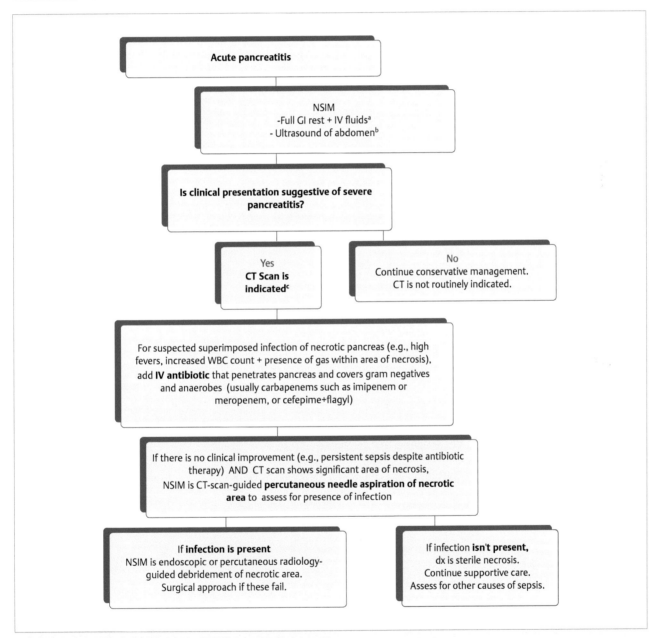

[a] IV fluid resuscitation is very important in early stages of pancreatitis.

[b] Ultrasound should be done in all patients with pancreatitis. US is more sensitive than CT scan in detecting gallbladder stone/sludge pathology. If presence of gallbladder stone/sludge is confirmed, cholecystectomy is indicated.

[c] CT scan is the most accurate method to determine **severity of pancreatitis**.

9.34.1 Complications of Pancreatitis

Systemic inflammatory response syndrome, which when severe can progress to acute respiratory distress syndrome, disseminated intravascular coagulation, septic or distributive shock, and multiorgan dysfunction syndrome	
Pancreatic abscess	Postpancreatitis mass in the epigastrium + features of sepsis point toward abscess
	For suspected abscess, NSIDx is CT scan of abdomen with IV contrast
	Rx: radiologically guided or surgical drainage
Splenic venous thrombosis	May present as hematemesis. EGD may reveal isolated gastric varices
– Ascites – Pleural effusion	fluid will have increased amylase content
Pancreatic pseudocyst-discussed below	

9.34.2 Pancreatic Pseudocysts and Walled-off Pancreatic Necrosis

Background: with pancreatitis or pancreatic trauma, cystic collections can form with maturation of wall after few weeks. If the collection is of pancreatic and/or peripancreatic necrosis, it is known as walled-off pancreatic necrosis.

If it is just walled-off fluid collection outside the pancreas, it is known as Pseudocysts; "pseudo" because cyst is usually lined by epithelial membrane while this one is not. Both have similar management and is discussed here.

Presentation: Can vary from vague epigastric fullness to obstructive jaundice and/or abdominal pain, usually after 5–6 weeks of acute pancreatitis episode.

Workup: NSIDx is ultrasound or CT scan. If both choices are given, it is wiser to choose US as next step, but CT scan is more accurate test and is usually done to confirm diagnosis and rule out cystic neoplasms or pseudoaneurysm.

Management:

- In asymptomatic patients, manage conservatively (in 40% of cases resolve on their own).
- In presence of symptoms and/or complications (e.g., compression of surrounding structures, pseudoaneurysm formation, hemorrhage, infection, rupture) surgical, radiologic, or endoscopic drainage is indicated.

9.34.3 Chronic Pancreatitis

Etiology: Recurrent and/or persistent pancreatitis can lead to chronic pancreatitis.

Causes of recurrent and/or persistent pancreatitis

CCS	Likely cause
Homeless person (exam question may not say chronic alcoholic)	Alcoholism (It is the MCC of recurrent or chronic pancreatitis)
Exam reveals xanthelasma. Patient has a family hx of early-onset heart attacks.	Familial hypertriglyceridemia
Recurrent pancreatitis in childhood or adolescence with family hx of similar kind of issues	Hereditary pancreatitis or cystic fibrosis
Recurrent pancreatitis in children or adolescents with no associated family history and no associated exam findings like xanthelasma	Think about congenital pancreatic abnormalities like pancreatic divisum and choledochal cyst. NSIM/NSIDx is MRCP (magnetic resonance cholangiopancreatography) or ERCP (endoscopic retrograde cholangiopancreatography)
An adult patient with recurrent idiopathic pancreatitis	Consider IgG4-mediated recurrent autoimmune pancreatitis or sphincter-of-Oddi dysfunction

Recurrent gallstones are less common as cholecystectomy is commonly done

Presentation: Chronic epigastric pain with episodic flare-ups, malabsorption +/− diabetes mellitus.

Diagnosis:

Requires all of the following:	Use the following test
Pancreatic calcification	Plain abdominal X-ray, CT scan, or abdominal US.
Ductal pathology	Magnetic resonance cholangiopancreatography is a very good test to assess pancreatic duct
Abnormal pancreatic exocrine function	Fecal elastase (test of choice), or 72-hour fecal fat

If above tests are unremarkable and chronic pancreatitis is still suspected, do the following test:

Secretin stimulation test: this test involves insertion of nasogastric tube followed by stimulation of pancreas by injecting secretin and checking duodenal secretion for pancreatic enzymes

+/−

Endoscopic ultrasound

Rx: Pancreatic enzymes and analgesics. In patients with intractable pain, MRCP or ERCP is done to assess for ductal or parenchymal pathology that might be amenable to surgical or endoscopic treatment.

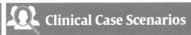
Clinical Case Scenarios

31. Patient with chronic pancreatitis now develops slowly progressive obstructive jaundice and increasing abdominal pain. What is the NSIM?

9.35 Liver Tumors

Condition	Additional points		Management	
Hepatocellular cancer (HCC)	Major risk factor is cirrhosis; these patients should undergo regular surveillance with abdominal US every 6 months to a year (+/- AFP: AFP is optional) Dx is mostly made with multiphase CT scan or MRI (liver tumor protocol). Also, look for elevated AFP		If resectable, and if patient is a surgical candidate then NSIM is resection. If not a candidate for resection (commonly due to advanced liver disease), NSIM is to evaluate for liver transplant.	
Solitary solid liver nodule	In patients with chronic Hep B infection or cirrhosis	< 1 cm nodule	Do follow-up US after 3 months or do MRI liver protocol.	
		≥ 1 cm	MRI or CT liver tumor protocol	If atypical for HCC, do the other test (e.g., if MRI was done, do CT liver protocol).
	In patients without chronic Hep B infection or	Elevated AFP, or size ≥ 1cm		
	cirrhosis, decision can be based upon AFP level	Normal AFP and size < 1 cm	Do follow-up US after 3 months or do MRI liver protocol.	
Imaging is suggestive of metastases to the liver	Most likely primary source is GI tract, lung, or breast		If mammogram and CT chest/abdomen/pelvis is negative for primary lesion, NSIDx is colonoscopy.	

Abbreviation: AFP, Alpha-fetoprotein.

9.35.1 Benign Liver Tumors

Hepatic adenoma Strongly associated with anabolic steroids and OCPs. So, first SIM is to stop these medications	– Most often found incidentally, but patients may present with acute abdominal pain due to bleeding. Hemorrhagic shock might also develop – **Imaging findings:** For dx, CT or MRI with contrast is the test of choice. Heterogenous mass with heterogenous arterial enhancement is seen	– **Indication for resection:** symptomatic, enlarging after stopping steroids/OCPs, and/or size > 5 cm. Note that percutaneous biopsy is not recommended due to increased risk of bleeding. With resection, histological picture will reveal adenomatous cells containing glycogen and lipid deposits. – **If > 2 cm and patient is contemplating pregnancy,** radiofrequency ablation can be done.
Hepatic hemangioma	– Most often found incidentally, but patients may present with acute complication of thrombosis (pain) or bleeding. Compression of surrounding structures may cause early satiety, anorexia, weight loss, etc. – **Imaging findings:** Highly echogenic on US. Contrast imaging shows peripheral enhancement + centripetal flow in late phase. In tagged-RBC scan, there is undetectable or decreased intensity compared to liver in flow images, but increased intensity in delayed images.	– Surgical resection for compressive symptoms – Observation for asymptomatic ones
Focal nodular hyperplasia Most often found incidentally	– **Pathology:** Reactive hyperplastic response to hyperperfusion by anomalous arteries. Histologically there is normal appearing liver cellular architecture, and presence of central scar with radiating fibrous septa. – **Imaging findings:** Dx is mostly through multiple imaging modalities, i.e., doppler ultrasound, CT or MRI with contrast. Look for well-demarcated central scar on imaging.	Usually **expectant management** is recommended as natural history is favorable without much complications.

Abbreviations: AFP, alpha fetoprotein; OCPs, oral contraceptive pills.

Answers

1. EKG. As with any patient who presents with chest pain, even if the pain is atypical for angina, we need to do an EKG. If EKG is unremarkable, then a preliminary diagnosis of GERD can be made.

2. Avoidance of Beer BReW diet. (Do not choose antibiotics in a patient with no history of travel).

3. Rectovesical or colovesical fistula.

4. Abdominal X-ray.

5. X-rays shows distended colon filled with gas. Dx is toxic megacolon.

6. Medical therapy with IV steroids, supportive fluid resuscitation, antibiotics, and bowel decompression (NG tube). Refractory cases may need emergent surgery.

7. Primary sclerosing cholangitis associated with ulcerative colitis.

8. Dieulafoy's lesion (aberrant arteriole in the submucosa). If the lesion is not actively bleeding at the time of EGD, it might be difficult to identify it.

9. NSIDx is Meckel scan (this identifies ectopic gastric in the small intestine). Likely dx is Meckel's diverticulum.

10. Surgical resection.

11. Prophylaxis with PPI or H_2 blockers is recommended in patients with mechanical ventilation for > 48 hours.

12. **Presence of any one of the following:** coagulopathy (platelet count < 50,000 or INR > 1.5), traumatic brain or spine injury, severe burns and hx of GI ulceration or bleeding in the last year.

13. Dx is Mallory–Weiss tears due to mechanical force causing tear and rupture of submucosal arteries in distal esophagus.

14. Think of angiodysplasia associated with aortic stenosis.

15. A-fib with cardioembolic bowel ischemia.

16. GERD.

17. Video capsule endoscopy. Patient ingests a tiny wireless camera pill and it takes pictures as it passes through the gut.

18. GERD.

19. IgM anti-Hep A antibody. History appears to be an acute infectious hepatitis. Unlike Hep E with no specific management, Hep A diagnosis has further clinical implications—consideration of PEP.

20. All household contacts of the patient should receive PEP.

21. F/U HBsAg after 6 months. Acute hepatitis requires symptomatic management only.

22. Dx is chronic hepatitis B.

23. Screen for both Hep B and Hep C.

24. Vaccinate against Hep A and Hep B.

25. Acute Hep B infection. Hep B overproduces HBsAg, so there is increased formation of HBsAg–HBsAb complexes. These immune complexes can deposit anywhere and present with serum sickness reaction.

26. Check HBsAg, anti-HBs, and anti-HBc antibody.

27. The patient most likely has developed hepatocellular carcinoma.

28. NSIM is CT scan of liver with IV contrast.

29. SAAG gradient = 3.6 − 2.8 = 0.8 (< 1.1). It is exudative as ascitic albumin is high.

30. Possible dx includes ovarian cancer.

31. Abdominal CT scan. Note that chronic pancreatitis with pancreatic calcifications is associated with higher risk of pancreatic cancer. Other major risk factor for pancreatic cancer is smoking.

10. Neurology

> *"In the grip of a neurological disorder, **I am fast losing control of words even as my relationship with the world has been reduced to them.**" -Tony Judt in the grip of ALS.*

10.1 Basics of Clinical Neurology

10.1.1 Cranial Nerves

MRS

Oh Oh Oh to try and feel very good vibes—Ah heaven

MRS	Name of cranial nerve	Numbering of cranial nerve	Function	Features of cranial nerve lesion
Oh	**Olfactory**	1	Sense of smell	Anosmia
Oh	**Optic**	2	Vision	Vision loss
Oh	**Oculomotor**	3	Supplies all muscles of eye, except superior-oblique and lateral rectus Also supplies parasympathetic innervation of eye (pupillary constriction and lens accommodation)	Double vision + ptosis+ eye is down and out. (This is due to unopposed actions of fourth and sixth CN)[b]
To	**Trochlear**	4	Supplies superior-oblique muscle of eye (which moves eye down and out)	Double vision + eye is "up and in" *(opposite of 3rd cranial nerve palsy)*
Try	**Trigeminal**	5	Sensation of face (including cornea)	Loss of sensation in face, and increased risk of corneal injury
And	**Abducens**	6	Lateral rectus muscle of eye	Double vision + eye is deviated inward[a]
Feel	**Facial**	7	Controls motor function of facial muscles	Ptosis, facial droop, and hyperacusis (facial nerve controls middle ear bones that help dampen loud sounds)
Very	**Vestibulocochlear nerve**	8	Hearing and balance	Tinnitus, hearing loss, and vertigo
Good	**Glossopharyngeal**	9	– Swallowing, speaking – Afferent-sensory arm of gag reflex	Dysphagia, dysarthria, and absent gag reflex
Vibes	**Vagus**	10	– Efferent-motor arm of gag reflex – Also controls swallowing and upper GI function	
Ah	**Accessory**	11	Movement of shoulder and neck	Weakness of shoulder and neck muscles
Heaven	**Hypoglossal**	12	Tongue movement	Tongue deviates to affected side

[a]Isolated cranial nerve VI palsy (abducens nerve) can be due to increased intracranial pressure, Wernicke's encephalopathy, etc.

[b]See table on next page.

Third CN palsy + ...		
+ diabetes or syphilis	**Pathophysiology:** microvascular infarct that usually affects only somatic nerves; parasympathetic nerves are usually not involved	
	Physical exam finding: ptosis with "down and out eye." As parasympathetic innervation is intact, pupils will constrict to light	
+ fever + headache + protruding eye	Cavernous sinus thrombosis	Both autonomic and somatic nerves are involved
+ severe thunderclap headache	Could represent subarachnoid hemorrhage and growing or budding of posterior communicating artery aneurysm compressing on the third cranial nerve	

In a nutshell

Cranial nerve (CN) innervation of eye

CN 2—optic	– Vision – The afferent (sensory) limb of the pupillary light reflex
CN 3—oculomotor	Most functions of eyes are mediated by CN 3 – For example, efferent arm of pupillary reaction, convergence, medial rectus
CN 4—trochlear	Superior oblique muscle
CN 6—abducens	Lateral rectus muscle (eye abduction)
CN 5—trigeminal	Sensory innervation of cornea

10.1.2 Eponymous Pupillary Abnormalities

Condition	Clinical findings	Anisocoria (unequal pupil sizes)	Underlying lesion
Hutchinson pupil	One pupil is dilated and nonreactive to light or accommodation	Yes	Compression of third cranial nerve (e.g., intracranial mass or tumor, aneurysm) – Parasympathetic fibers of the third cranial nerve are located peripherally and thus, in compressive pathologies, they are affected earlier than motor fibers
Adie's tonic pupil in Holmes–Adie syndrome	One pupil is **di**lated and does not react to light but has a slow tonic constriction in reaction to accommodation	Yes	Lesion in parasympathetic neurons of ciliary ganglion – It can occur due to viral or bacterial infection, or inflammation of other causes
Argy**ll** Robertson pupil	Both pupils are constricted (sma**ll**), and do not react to light, but react to accommodation (i.e., pupils become small when seeing near objects)	No (bilateral)	Bilateral damage of pretectal nuclei in midbrain – Cause: neurosyphilis, diabetes
Marcus–Gunn pupil	No reaction with direct light but constricts when light is shone in the other eye (consensual light reflex is present)	No (consensual eye is maintaining tone of both eyes)	Problem with eye, retina, or optic nerve in that eye (e.g., optic neuritis in multiple sclerosis)
Horner's syndrome	One side of face has small pupils, drooped eyelid, and absence of sweating	Yes	Lesion in sympathetic tract of eye (e.g., in brainstem, neck, upper chest, or in ganglion)

10.1.3 Upper Motor Neuron versus Lower Motor Neuron Lesion

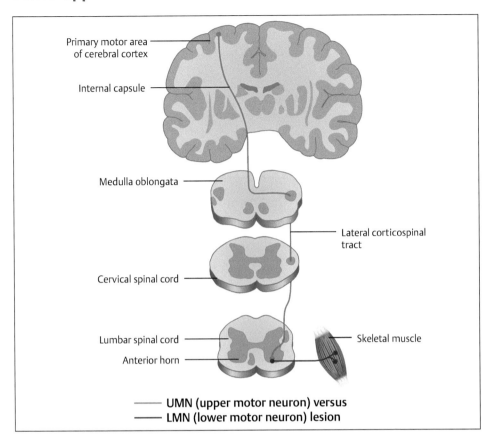

UMN (upper motor neuron) versus
LMN (lower motor neuron) lesion

	UMN lesion	LMN lesion
Etiology	Lesion occurring anywhere in the pathway of blue line in the picture above (e.g., stroke in internal capsule)	Lesion occurring anywhere in the pathway of red line in the picture above (e.g., lesion in the anterior horn of spinal cord)
Muscle tone	Initially muscle tone is flaccid, then spasticity develops slowly (may take weeks)	Flaccid
Deep tendon reflex	Just like muscle tone, it can be hypoactive in initial stages. In later stages, they are **increased**	Decreased (!)
Strength	↓ [1]	↓
Atrophy	Present (due to disuse atrophy)	Present (due to combination of disuse atrophy and loss of neurotrophic stimulation (denervation))
Associated signs	Babinski reflex Clonus	Babinski reflex is negative **Fibrillation:** these are small amplitudes of contraction which can be detected by EMG. The only place where fibrillation can be seen with naked eye is tongue **Fasciculation:** larger amplitudes of contractions seen by naked eye

⚠ **Caution**

(!) Elderly patients can have decreased or absent ankle and knee reflex. This is a normal aging phenomenon; so be very careful in interpreting such findings in elderly.

[1] Pronator drift test is a sensitive test for UMN lesion. Patients are asked to extend their hands with their palm up and close their eyes. If one hand slowly pronates (turns inside), then pronator drift is positive.

NSIDx	CNS imaging (CT or MRI of brain or spine)	EMG and NCS
Facial nerve	Only lower half of the face is affected. Frowning, raising eyebrow, and eye closing remain intact	The whole half of the face is affected (LMN facial nerve palsy is known as Bell's palsy. This diagnosis is made by physical exam only[a]

[a]**Bell's palsy**

Etiology: Lyme disease, sarcoidosis, viral infection (herpes virus), etc.

Management: In idiopathic cases or when viral infection is suspected, NSIM is oral glucocorticoids, preferably initiated within 3 days of onset. If patient has severe involvement, empiric oral valacyclovir should also be given in conjunction with steroids (disfiguring asymmetry of face, with no forehead motion and incomplete closure of eye are severe features). Most common (MC) complication is corneal ulceration due to difficulty closing the eye. Taping the eye shut and using ocular lubricants can prevent this.

Abbreviations: CNS, central nervous system; CT, computed tomography; EMG, electromyography; LMN, lower motor neuron; MRI, magnetic resonance imaging; NCS, nerve conduction study; UMN, upper motor neuron.

Clinical Tip: One of the easiest ways to approach a patient presenting with weakness is to look for UMN or LMN signs. If LMN/UMN signs are not present, think about disorders related to neuromuscular junction, myopathy or electrolyte imbalance.

Cerebellar Signs:

Cerebellum controls fine movement of our body. Cerebellar pathology may have the following clinical features:

- Dysdiadochokinesia = inability to perform a series of rapidly alternating movements. Ask the patient to keep one hand over the other and rapidly move the upper hand in alternating supination/pronation.
- Dysmetria = the patient overshoots when attempting to reach something.
- Ataxia = tendency to fall to the side of the lesion and broad based ataxic gait.
- Nystagmus +/- double vision.
- Intention tremor (because of dysmetria).
- Slurred speech (dysarthria).
- Hypotonia.
- Pendular knee reflex = persistent back and forth swinging of leg.

MRS

Danish pendulum

Patients who present with cerebellar signs, NSIDx is CNS imaging with CT or MRI scan.

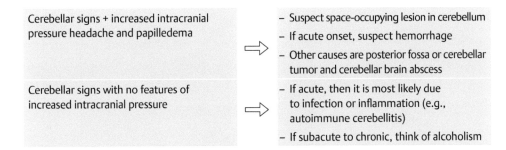

| Cerebellar signs + increased intracranial pressure headache and papilledema | ⇒ | – Suspect space-occupying lesion in cerebellum
– If acute onset, suspect hemorrhage
– Other causes are posterior fossa or cerebellar tumor and cerebellar brain abscess |
| Cerebellar signs with no features of increased intracranial pressure | ⇒ | – If acute, then it is most likely due to infection or inflammation (e.g., autoimmune cerebellitis)
– If subacute to chronic, think of alcoholism |

10.2 Cerebrovascular Disease

Definition: It is an umbrella term for conditions caused by abnormalities in cerebral blood vessels, such as transient ischemic attack (TIA), stroke (hemorrhagic or ischemic), subarachnoid hemorrhage (SAH), vascular dementia, and others.

TIA	Sudden onset **FND (focal neurological deficit)** that lasts **less** than 24 hours, and there is no evidence of infarction on MRI
Stroke (aka cerebrovascular accident) subtypes are hemorrhagic and ischemic	Sudden onset FND that lasts for more than 24 hours and/or CT/MRI is positive for hemorrhage and/or infarction In most cases, FND is permanent

Abbreviations: CT/MRI, computed tomography/magnetic resonance imaging; FND, focal neurological deficit; TIA, transient ischemic attack.

Etiology:

- **Atherosclerotic cardiovascular disease (ASCVD):** Formation of atheromatous plaque which can ulcerate and lead to acute thrombus formation (+/− further embolization) causing ischemia/infarction.
- **Lipohyalinosis of small vessels:** This may lead to small lacunar infarcts. This typically occurs in patients with uncontrolled hypertension (HTN), diabetes or active smoking.
- **Cardioembolic stroke:** Emboli from left heart mural thrombus.[2]
- **Paradoxical emboli:** In a patient with right to left shunt (e.g., due to Eisenmenger's syndrome) deep vein thrombosis (DVT) can embolize into arterial circulation.
- **Hemorrhage:** Rupture of blood vessel/aneurysms can lead to acute reduction in blood supply and can also cause mass effect.
- **Generalized decrease in blood pressure (hypotension)** can lead to anoxic brain injury (e.g., after cardiac arrest, or in a patient with severe persistent hypotension).

[2]**The following conditions increases risk of intra-cardiac thrombus:** a-fib, large anterior myocardial infarction, dilated cardiomyopathy, valvular heart disease, infective endocarditis, etc.

10.2.1 Presentations of Transient Ischemic Attack

- **CCS:** patient woke up with symptoms of difficulty speaking and weakness in his right leg that lasted for 3 hours. Patient is currently asymptomatic.
- **CCS:** sudden painless loss of vision (like a "dark curtain" over one eye) followed by spontaneous recovery. Dx is amaurosis fugax, which is a form of TIA involving the **retinal artery** (branch of internal carotid artery).

In a patient with stroke and hx of drug abuse, think of the following:
– Cocaine-induced vasospasm
– Cocaine-induced intracranial hemorrhage
– Embolization from infective endocarditis (in IV drug users)

10.2.2 Territorial Stroke, Involved Arteries and Corresponding Focal Neurological Deficit/s

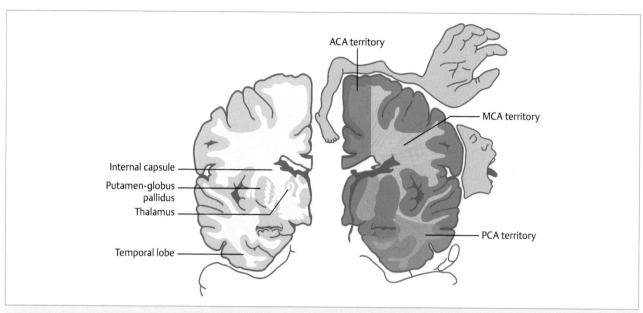

Abbreviations: ACA, anterior cerebral artery; MCA, middle cerebral artery; PCA, posterior cerebral artery

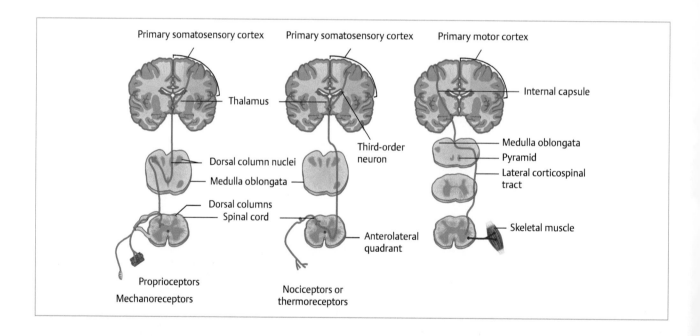

Artery/area involved	Motor weakness	Sensory deficits	Associated cranial nerve involvement	Associated neurological deficit/s	
Left MCA territory or **left** ICA territory	**Right** arm > right leg	**Right** arm > right leg	**Right** upper motor neuron facial palsy	• **Right** homonymous hemianopia (it is contralateral) • Dominant right lobe involvement = Broca's and Wernicke's aphasia	+/− Conjugate eye deviation to the side of the lesion For example, **left**-sided stroke has left deviation of eye
Right MCA territory or right ICA territory	**Left** arm > left leg	**Left** arm > left leg	**Left** upper motor neuron facial palsy	**Left** homonymous hemianopia (it is contralateral) Nondominant left lobe involvement = **left** hemi-neglect syndrome (one is neglecting the weaker side of the body)[a] Constructional apraxia[a]	
Left ACA territory	**Right** leg > right arm	**Right** leg > right arm	–	Incontinence (bladder involvement)	
Right PCA territory stroke	–	–	–	Visual field Left Right **Left** homonymous hemianopia **Note:** PCA area infarct causes contralateral homonymous hemianopia without motor or sensory deficits	
Pure motor stroke due to lacunar infarct in **left** penetrating thalamic branches in posterior limb (or sometimes genu) of left internal capsule[b]	**Right** arm, leg	–	+ Right UMN facial palsy +/− dysarthria/dysphagia	**No** visual loss and speech/praxis is normal (no involvement of other higher cortical functions)	
Pure sensory stroke due to lacunar infarct in penetrating thalamic branches usually in the **left** thalamus[b]	–	**Right** arm, leg	–		
Brain stem strokes[c]					
Left paramedian branches of PCA **Medial mid brain** infarction (Weber's syndrome)	**Right** arm, leg	–	**Left** CN III (3)	Right UMN facial palsy	
Left paramedian branches of basilar artery **Medial pons** infarction			**Left** CN VI (lateral gaze paralysis) with diplopia	–	
Left vertebral artery or spinal artery **medial medulla** infarction			**Left** CN XII (tongue deviates to left; to the side of the lesion)	–	

Artery/area involved	Motor weakness	Sensory deficits	Associated cranial nerve involvement	Associated neurological deficit/s
Left AICA or left (superior cerebellar artery) infarction of **lateral pons**	–	**Right** spinothalamic tract involvement (pain and temperature sensation loss)	**Left** CN VII (lower motor neuron facial palsy)	Lateral brainstem lesions may have the following common features: Ipsilateral Horner's syndrome (ptosis, miosis) Ipsilateral Vth nerve (trigeminal) nucleus involvement
Left PICA **lateral medullary infarction** (Wallenberg syndrome)			**Left** CN IX, X (dysphagia, hoarseness, absent gag reflex)	Ipsilateral VIII nerve involvement (vertigo, nystagmus, and vomiting) Ipsilateral limb cerebellar ataxia
Left thalamus (thalamic pain syndrome)	–	**Right**-sided pain aggravated by light touch (allodynia or dysesthesia) and hemi-sensory loss. Thalamic pain syndrome can be very problematic		+/– Athetosis, hemiballismus

[a]**Constructional apraxia and hemineglect syndrome:** when patient is asked to draw shapes or clock, this is what he will draw:

[b]**Lacunar strokes in internal capsule**

Stroke syndrome	Presentation	What part of internal capsule is involved?
Clumsy hand dysarthria syndrome	sudden-onset hand weakness and mild dysarthria	Anterior limb or genu
Pure motor stroke	Weakness of face, arm, and/or leg	Posterior limb
Ataxia hemiparesis	Leg > arm weakness + limb ataxia	Posterior limb

[c]To better understand brain-stem strokes, please refer to "In a nutshell" box in next page before proceeding further down the table. Abbreviations: ACA, anterior cerebral artery; AICA, anterior inferior cerebellar artery; ICA, internal carotid artery; MCA, middle cerebral artery; PCA, posterior cerebral artery; PICA, posterior-inferior cerebellar artery; UMN, upper motor neuron.

In a nutshell

Cortical versus brainstem lesions	Cortical lesions have unilateral defects Also look for defects in higher cortical functions (creating and understanding words, vision, reasoning, etc.)	Brainstem lesions have crossed deficits; i.e., contralateral motor or sensory deficit with ipsilateral cranial nerve involvement Absence of defects in higher cortical functions
Lateral versus medial brainstem lesions	Lesions in medial brainstem involve contralateral corticospinal tract (motor weakness)	Lesions in lateral brainstem involve contralateral spinothalamic tract (sensory loss)
To determine location of the brainstem lesion, look at the cranial nerve involved	Midbrain	3, 4
	Pons	6, 7
	Medulla	9, 10, 11, 12

Note: both CN 5 and 8 can be involved in *lateral lesion of pons and medulla*

 MRS

Medial = Motor weakness; M=M

 MRS

Lateral = Loss of sensation

 MRS

For medial brainstem lesions; from top to bottom, that is, from midbrain-pons to medulla, CN 3, 6, and 12 are involved respectively.

 Clinical Case Scenarios

1. Acute-onset right-sided hemiparesis with left-sided lateral rectus muscle weakness. Where is the lesion?

10.2.3 Aphasia

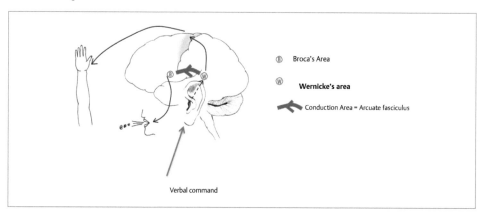

Aphasia type	Comprehension[a]	Fluency	Area involved
Broca's	Normal	Impaired	Dominant[b] frontal lobe (look for associated contralateral hemiparesis)
Conduction	Normal	Patient is fluent, but has garbled, paraphasic speech that does not make sense	Dominant[b] parietal lobe
Wernicke's	Impaired		Dominant[b] temporal lobe
Global	Impaired	Impaired	All of the above areas are affected

[a]**Comprehension:** Does the patient understand what you are saying. For example, does the patient follow commands such as "Raise your hand"?

[b]FYI, > 90% of right-handed and > 50 % of left-handed people have language area on the left side of the brain. If a left-handed person has Broca's aphasia, statistically, the lesion is more likely to be in the left frontal lobe.

 MRS

Broca is **bro**ken speech.
Wernicke is **w**ordy.

In all types of aphasia sentence repetition is impaired.

10.2.4 Management of TIA and Stroke

Emergency management of patients with suspected stroke (sudden onset persistent focal neurological deficit)

Legend: *NSIDx, next step in diagnosis; NSIM, next step in management; FND, focal neurological deficit; BP, blood pressure*

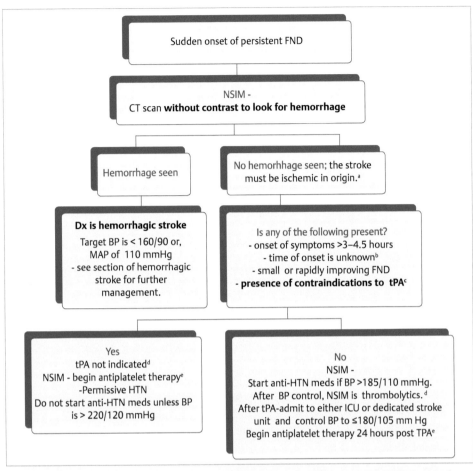

For TIA patient
- Check computed tomography (CT) to rule out hemorrhage.
- After bleeding is ruled out, start antiplatelet therapy (e.g., aspirin).
- Consider hospital admission for patients with new TIA, as TIA is a sign of impending stroke.

[3]MC side effect of ASA/ dipyridamole combination is headache).

Flowchart content:

Sudden onset of persistent FND

NSIM - CT scan **without contrast to look for hemorrhage**

Hemorrhage seen

No hemorrhage seen; the stroke must be ischemic in origin.[a]

Dx is hemorrhagic stroke
Target BP is < 160/90 or, MAP of 110 mmHg
- see section of hemorrhagic stroke for further management.

Is any of the following present?
- onset of symptoms >3–4.5 hours
- time of onset is unknown[b]
- small or rapidly improving FND
- **presence of contraindications to tPA**[c]

Yes
tPA not indicated[d]
NSIM - begin antiplatelet therapy[e]
-Permissive HTN
Do not start anti-HTN meds unless BP is > 220/120 mmHg

No
NSIM -
Start anti-HTN meds if BP >185/110 mmHg.
After BP control, NSIM is thrombolytics.[d]
After tPA-admit to either ICU or dedicated stroke unit and control BP to ≤180/105 mm Hg
Begin antiplatelet therapy 24 hours post TPA[e]

---

[a]In patients with significant FND who may be thrombectomy candidates, get CT angiography of head and neck as a part of stroke workup, after the initial CT head is negative for hemorrhage.

[b]If a patient cannot report the time of onset of symptoms, consider onset to be the last time when patient was seen normal. For example, patient presents with right arm weakness since waking up at 8 AM. At around 4 AM, he woke up and went to the bathroom at which time he did not have any weakness. In this case, the time of onset is considered to be at 4 AM.

[c]Presence of any of the following is considered contraindication to thrombolytics:
  – Ischemic stroke, intracranial or intraspinal surgery, or serious head injury within 3 months.
  – Major surgery (nonintracranial) or trauma within 2 weeks: this is a relative contraindication—physician judgment needed.
  – Prior history of hemorrhagic stroke at any time.
  – BP > 185/110 mmHg. In this case, NSIM is IV labetalol or nicardipine to lower BP before administering tPA.
  – Current use of anticoagulants or coagulopathy with international normalized ratio of >1.7.
  – Platelets < 100,000/mm³
  – Glucose < 50 mg/dL or > 400 mg/dL: correct glucose before administering tPA.
  – Arterial puncture in a noncompressible site within 7 days.
  – Hx of gastrointestinal or genitourinary bleeding within 3 weeks.

[d]For patients with major arterial occlusion on vascular imaging, intra-arterial catheter-directed procedure (thrombolysis or removal) can be done up to 24 hours after onset of symptoms. This is commonly known as embolectomy for stroke with emergent large vessel occlusion (ELVO) protocol. Patients who are candidates for ELVO and have received thrombolytic should not be observed until clinical improvement, but rather transferred to the center where thrombectomy can be performed.

[e]Start antiplatelet therapy in all cases of ischemic TIA or stroke within 48 hours. Use any one of them
- Clopidogrel alone
- Aspirin + extended-release dipyridamole³, or
- aspirin

All patients with TIA/stroke are considered to have atherosclerotic cardiovascular disease (ASCVD) and high intensity statin therapy is recommended.

If workup reveals cardioembolic source (e.g., EKG shows new-onset a-fib), start long-term anticoagulation such as warfarin, apixaban. This can be started 48 hours after symptom onset, if area of stroke is small. In patients with large stroke, wait 1 to 2 weeks before starting anticoagulation.

10.2.5 Diagnostic Evaluation of TIA/Ischemic Stroke

Purpose	Which test to choose?		
To look for infarct	Brain MRI[a]		
To look for cardioembolic source	EKG and cardiac telemetry to detect paroxysmal atrial fibrillation – Echocardiography is commonly done		
To look for atheroembolic source in arteries of the neck	CT angiography of head and neck (if CT ELVO protocol not done)	MRA of neck	carotid ultrasound
To look for atheroembolic source in arteries of the head		MRA of head	transcranial Doppler

[a]MRI may also show silent infarcts (i.e., infarcts with no obvious corresponding focal neurological deficit). Note that routine use of MRI has not been shown to improve outcome and is not recommended in low risk ischemic strokes.

Abbreviations: CT, computed tomography; EKG, electrocardiography; ELVO, embolectomy for stroke with emergent large vessel occlusion; MRA, magnetic resonance angiography; MRI, magnetic resonance imaging.

10.2.6 Cardioembolic TIA/Ischemic Stroke

TIA/ischemic stroke in a young person usually warrants an active search for cardioembolic source. Consider transesophageal echocardiography to look for cardiac source.

Suspect cardioembolic source in the following situations:
– Bilateral stroke.
– Stroke involving multiple vascular territories.
– Large middle cerebral artery stroke.

If transthoracic echocardiography (TTE), electrocardiography (EKG), and cardiac telemetry fail to reveal the source and cardioembolic mechanism is highly suspected, NSIM is transesophageal echocardiography (TEE). If intracardiac clot is discovered, start anticoagulation.

If no obvious source of stroke is identified, the following pathophysiology might account for the TIA/ischemic stroke

Small vessel atherothrombotic disease	Typically have small focal neurological deficit and/or infarct
Lipohyalinosis	They typically have hx of uncontrolled HTN (MCC) or diabetes mellitus, and present with pure motor or sensory stroke. MRI may show lacunar infarct/s
Cryptogenic TIA/stroke	Consider home cardiac monitoring to detect paroxysmal a-fib episodes (e.g. for 1 month)

10.2.7 Carotid Artery Stenosis

Background: Atherosclerotic narrowing of carotid artery is known as carotid artery stenosis. It typically occurs in patients with multiple risk factors for ASCVD.

Presentation: It may be detected incidentally on clinical exam when carotid bruit is heard. It can also present with stroke or TIA. Some patients may have hx of pulsatile tinnitus.

Diagnosis: Imaging of neck arteries will show the atherosclerotic narrowing and the degree of stenosis.

Management

Is the stenosis symptomatic or asymptomatic?	Patient group		Management
Symptomatic lesion (i.e., patient has hx of ipsilateral TIA or stroke)	≥70% stenosis and life expectancy of at least 5 years		Carotid endarterectomy (CEA)[a]
	50–69% stenosis	In men with life expectancy of at least 5 years	CEA[a]
		Women	Medical management
	< 50% stenosis		Medical management
Asymptomatic lesion (i.e., patient has **no** hx of ipsilateral stroke or TIA)	≥ **80%** stenosis with life expectancy of at least 5 years		CEA[a]
	< 80%		Medical management
100% occlusion	No intervention is recommended (blood supply occurs from collateral circulation and risk of stroke with procedure is very high in this case.)		

[a]A nonsurgical alternative for CEA is carotid artery angioplasty and stenting (CAS).[4] This may be preferred over CEA in the following situations:

- Radiation-induced stenosis.

- Surgically inaccessible lesion.

- Patients with significant cardiopulmonary disease who have increased risk of anesthesia-related complications.

[4]CAS is associated with higher risk of perioperative stroke.

Remember the cut-off numbers for CEA
- Symptomatic: 50 and 70%
- Asymptomatic-:80%

10.2.8 Long-Term Antiplatelet Therapy in Ischemic Stroke or TIA patients

Situation	Subcategory	Antiplatelet therapy
Intracranial large artery atherosclerosis (70 to 99 % stenosis) as the cause of TIA or minor ischemic stroke	NIHSS[a] ≤ 3	Dual antiplatelet therapy (DAPT)[b] for 3 months, followed by long term monotherapy[c]
	NIHSS > 3	Start ASA, then add clopidogrel when the risk of a hemorrhagic transformation is acceptable; continue DAPT[b] for 3 months, followed by long term monotherapy[c]
Symptomatic extracranial carotid artery stenosis with an indication for a vascular procedure	CEA (Carotid endarterectomy)	Aspirin monotherapy before and after CEA
	CAS (carotid artery stenting)	DAPT prior to CAS and continue DAPT for 1 month after CAS, followed by single-agent monotherapy[c]
-TIA without significant vascular disease -ischemic stroke due to small vessel disease -cryptogenic stroke	-TIA with ABCD2[e] score ≥4 -Lower severity ischemic stroke (NIHSS ≤ 3)	DAPT for 3 weeks, then monotherapy[c]
	-TIA with ABCD2 score <4 -Higher severity ischemic stroke (NIHSS >3)[d]	Long term monotherapy[b]

[a]The NIH Stroke Scale (NIHSS) is a clinical score to assess the severity of a stroke. Board exam will not ask you to compute it and the score will likely be given in the exam question.

[b]DAPT=Aspirin + Plavix (both need loading dose followed by maintenance dose).

[c]Anyone of them—clopidogrel, or aspirin-extended-release dipyridamole, or aspirin alone.

[d]Increased risk of hemorrhagic transformation in early stages so only monotherapy.

[e]How to calculate ABCD2 score to determine risk in TIA patients.

Risk factor	Points
Age >= 60 years	1
Blood pressure elevation (systolic > 140mmHg and/or diastolic >= 90mmHg)	1
Clinical features	
Unilateral weakness	2
Speech disturbance without weakness	1
Duration of symptoms	
>= 60 mins	2
10–59 mins	2
Diabetes mellitus	2

Additional points:

- For patients already on anticoagulation prior to stroke/TIA, determine the risk of hemorrhagic transformation. If small stroke, continue anticoagulation (no need for addition of antiplatelet agent). If large stroke, hold anticoagulation until deemed safe to start (usually 1–2 weeks later), and in the meantime bridge with aspirin.
- Long-term DAPT isn't recommended for stroke beyond 1–3 mos, even if the patient was on an antiplatelet agent prior to the current stroke.

[5]HTN is the **most important risk** factor for stroke and cerebrovascular disease (more than diabetes).

[6]Charcot–Bouchard aneurysms are tiny aneurysms in small penetrating blood vessels. They are a common cause of intracranial hemorrhage. Berry aneurysms occur in larger arteries.

Hypertension and Stroke[5]

HTN can predispose to the following pathologies that can lead to stroke:
- Generalized atherosclerotic disease leading to atheroembolic stroke.
- Lipohyalinosis of small arterioles which predisposes to lacunar stroke. MCC of lacunar stroke is HTN.
- Formation of Charcot–Bouchard aneurysm[6] and its subsequent rupture leading to hemorrhagic stroke.
- Formation of berry (saccular) aneurysms with subsequent rupture leading to subarachnoid hemorrhage.

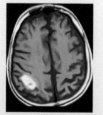

[7]

MRI scan of lobar hemorrhage: causes include amyloid angiopathy (particularly in elderly), HTN, cerebral aneurysm, etc.
Source: Amyloid Angiopathy. In: Sartor K, Hähnel S, Kress B. 1st ed. Thieme; 2007.

10.2.9 Intracranial Bleeding (Hemorrhagic Cerebrovascular Accident)

Etiology:
- MCC is HTN
- Amyloid angiopathy[7]
- Vascular malformation
- Coagulopathy and head trauma
- Cocaine and alcohol abuse

Presentation: Sudden-onset focal neurological deficit (FND) along with the following features that point toward hemorrhagic stroke[8]:
- Features of increased intracranial pressure (ICP): bradycardia, abducens nerve palsy (lateral rectus palsy), papilledema, etc.
- Severe headache
- Vomiting
- Altered mental status
- Loss of consciousness

[8]These features are not usually present in ischemic stroke.

10.2.10 Hypertension and Intracranial Bleeding

MC sites of hypertensive bleeding (given in order of frequency) and their clinical presentation:

1. Basal ganglia (putamen) and adjacent internal capsule	Contralateral sensory and motor FND – It may have UMN facial palsy and oculomotor nerve gaze palsy	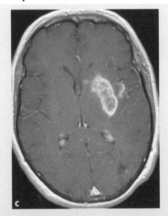 MRI scan showing left basal ganglia hemorrhage. Source: Nontraumatic Intracranial Hemorrhage. In: Mattle H, Mumenthaler M, Taub E. Fundamentals of Neurology: An Illustrated Guide. 2nd ed. Thieme; 2017.
2. Cerebellum	Patient can present with features of increased ICP[a] (e.g., sudden onset of headache, nausea/vomiting, vertigo, papilledema), along with cerebellar signs such as ataxia NSIM is immediate neurosurgical evaluation	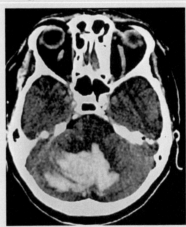 CT scan shows cerebellar hemorrhage. Source: Nonhypertensive Intracerebral Hemorrhage. In: Bähr M, Frotscher M, ed. Duus' Topical Diagnosis in Neurology: Anatomy, Physiology, Signs, Symptoms. 4th ed. Thieme; 2005.
3. Pons	May present initially with deep coma due to involvement of reticular activating system May present with locked-in syndrome: quadriplegic patient with intact eye movement (cranial nerve III in midbrain is not affected) [b]	

[a] There is not much room in posterior fossa, so even small cerebellar bleeds can increase ICP.

[b] Other causes of locked-in syndrome include:
– Central pontine myelinolysis: due to rapid correction of hyponatremia.
– Cardioembolic occlusion of paramedian branches of basilar artery which supply the central pons.
– Brainstem tumor or infection.

Abbreviations: FND, focal neurological deficit; ICP, intracranial pressure; UMN, upper motor neuron.

General management of intracranial hemorrhage:
– Reverse anticoagulation, if present.
– If there is extension of blood into the ventricles with hydrocephalus, emergent neurosurgical evaluation for shunting is recommended.
– For hemorrhagic stroke with elevated ICP leading to midline shift and worsening mental status, NSIM is stabilization with intubation, short-term hyperventilation and mannitol, followed by surgical evacuation.
– IV nicardipine or labetalol is used to target blood pressure < 160/90 or mean arterial pressure (MAP) of 110 mmHg.

10.2.11 Complications of Stroke (Ischemic/Hemorrhagic)

- Ischemic stroke can have hemorrhagic transformation: patient with large ischemic stroke is at higher risk.
- Seizure (caution: new-onset seizure is a contraindication for tPA).
- Aspiration pneumonia: all patients who present with stroke should have a bedside or formal swallow evaluation.
- Immobility that increases risk of urinary tract infection (UTI) and venous thromboembolism.

10.2.12 Differential Diagnosis of Stroke[9]

[9]Most of these conditions occur in young patients (< 50 years of age) with no risk factors for ASCVD or HTN.

Hemiplegic migraine	– Development of any form of new FND + coexistent pulsatile headache in a patient with prior hx of recurrent headaches points toward this dx
	– Some forms of hemiplegic migraine are due to familial autosomal dominant disorder; hence, family hx may be positive
	– In patients with hx of hemiplegic migraines triptans are contraindicated
Internal carotid artery dissection	**Background:** Patients usually have predisposing arteriopathic conditions, such as Marfan's syndrome, fibromuscular dysplasia, significant atherosclerotic disease, or vasculitis. This may be brought upon by excessive exertion, minor/or major trauma
	Presentation: Acute-onset headache **or** neck pain, +/- ipsilateral Horner's syndrome (sympathetic ganglion is very near to carotid artery), +/- FND due to embolic stroke from the dissection
	Management steps: Imaging test of choice is MRI of the soft tissues of the neck which will show the hematoma within internal carotid artery. NSIM is surgical evaluation
Multiple sclerosis	Discussed later in this chapter
Todd's palsy	Postseizure transient weakness (look for elevated lactic acid)
Subarachnoid hemorrhage and dural/cerebral venous thrombosis *(see below)*	
Abbreviations: FND, focal neurological deficit; MRI, magnetic resonance imaging.	

Clinical Case Scenarios

2. A 57-year-old male with hx of a-fib on warfarin presents with sudden onset severe headache + altered mental status. His INR is > 10. CT scan shows hyperdense white shadow. What is the best NSIM?

10.2.13 Subarachnoid Hemorrhage (SAH)

Etiology:
- MCC is rupture of berry (saccular) aneurysm. Risk factors for formation of berry aneurysm are HTN, smoking, adult polycystic kidney disease, and collagen disorders such as Marfan's and Ehlers–Danlos syndromes.
- Other rare causes of SAH are arteriovenous malformation (AVM) and mycotic aneurysms.

Presentation:
- Sudden onset of **severe headache** ("worst headache of my life," "thunderclap headache").
- Patients can also present with loss of consciousness and other features of increased ICP (e.g., abducens nerve palsy).
- Fundoscopy may reveal subhyaloid hemorrhage +/– papilledema.
- Exam reveals signs of meningeal irritation, for example, stiff neck (nuchal rigidity). Blood in cerebrospinal fluid (CSF) irritates the meningeal membranes.

- Most likely electrolyte abnormality in SAH is hyponatremia, due to increased secretion of atrial and brain natriuretic peptide (ANP and BNP).
- Most likely EKG finding is nonspecific ST-T changes or big/inverted T-waves.

- Other focal neurological findings may include the following:
  - ○ **Cranial nerve deficits:** oculomotor palsy is common (posterior communicating artery aneurysm is anatomically near to oculomotor nerve). Eye will be down and out.
  - ○ SAH can also present with any form of FND related to anterior, middle, or posterior cerebral artery territory. This might be due to arterial spasms, hypoperfusion, or intracerebral clot.

Diagnostic evaluation:

- Best initial test/NSIDx is CT scan without IV contrast. Earliest place where blood is typically seen is in the Sylvian fissure.[10]
- If CT scan is negative and if there is a high degree of suspicion for SAH, NSIDx is lumbar puncture which may show xanthochromia and increased RBCs. Lumber puncture is the most sensitive test for SAH.[11]
- NSIM after dx, is magnetic resonance angiography (MRA) to locate aneurysms.

Management:

- Most appropriate treatment is interventional coiling. It involves placing a platinum wire under radiological guidance to clog-up the aneurysm. This is preferred over neurosurgical clipping (which requires craniotomy).
- To prevent vasospasm, give **nimodipine** or verapamil (vasoactive calcium channel blockers) in all SAH patients. The major cause of morbidity and mortality in SAH is vasospasm of major arteries. The blood in the subarachnoid space may cause irritation of the smooth muscles of the major arteries causing vasospasms. This can cause infarction/ischemia in the corresponding arterial territories, causing TIA or stroke. This is called **delayed ischemic neurological deficit** as it can occur 3 days to 1 week after SAH.

Complications:

- **Hydrocephalus:** CSF outflows are not designed to drain out viscous and cellular blood. Therefore, blood components may clog up CSF outflow drains. If hydrocephalus develops, NSIM is ventriculoperitoneal shunting.
- **Seizures:** patient will generally require antiepileptic drug prophylaxis.

Prevention of SAH: Consider surgery for incidentally discovered aneurysms >7–10 mm in size.

Major differential diagnosis of SAH:

Dural or cerebral venous thrombosis

Risk factors: same as venous *thromboembolism (see Chapter 3, for further information)*

Presentation: symptoms of severe headache, altered mental status, seizures, and/or FND. Fundoscopy may reveal papilledema.

Workup: magnetic resonance venography (MRV) will confirm dx.

Rx: anticoagulation.

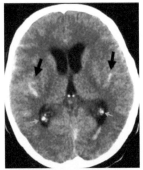

[10]The fine, dense lines in the Sylvain fissure (black arrows) correspond to blood in the subarachnoid space. A small amount of blood is also seen in the posterior horn of the left lateral ventricle(red arrow).The green arrows are choroid plexus calcifications commonly seen in adults.
Source: Perfusion Disturbances of the Brain. In: Eastman G, Wald C, Crossin J. Getting Started in Clinical Radiology. From Image to Diagnosis. 1st ed. Thieme; 2005.

[11]With every 500 to 1000 RBC that enters CSF, 1 WBC will enter CSF.
For example,
1. CSF reveals 100,000 RBCs and only 50–100 WBCs: This WBC count is related to hemorrhage itself and isn't a sign of meningitis.
2. CSF reveals 100,000 RBCs and 8,000 WBCs: There are more than expected WBCs for the number of RBCs. In this case, hemorrhage alone does not account for increased WBCs. The likely dx is infection with hemorrhage (e.g., herpes meningoencephalitis with hemorrhage).
Note: Major differential dx for SAH is meningitis.

10.3 Motor Neuron Diseases

The following are various degenerative motor neuron diseases. Their etiology is not clear, but some occur due to genetic mutation (familial forms) whereas others occur sporadically (due to various factors).

Types	Motor neuron involvement
Primary lateral sclerosis	Selective involvement of first order motor neuron cell in frontal lobe motor cortex Only UMN signs are present
Progressive muscular atrophy	Selective involvement of second order motor neuron cell in anterior horn of spinal cord Only LMN signs are present
Amyotrophic lateral sclerosis	Involvement of both first and second order motor neuron cell Both UMN and LMN signs are present

Legend:
- *UMN = upper motor neuron*
- *LMN = lower motor neuron*

10.3.1 Amyotrophic Lateral Sclerosis

Pathophysiology: Amyotrophic sclerosis (ALS) is a motor neuron disease with both upper motor neuron (UMN) and lower motor neuron (LMN) involvement. There is no cognitive, sensory, or autonomic involvement. This leads to a slow development of progressive paralysis in a patient who is mentally alert and fully competent.

Management: NSIDx is to do electromyography (EMG) and nerve conduction study (NCS) (for LMN lesion work up) and magnetic resonance imaging (MRI of brain and spinal cord; for UMN lesion work up). These will help to rule out other causes of reversible neurological disorder, or anatomic lesions. Riluzole (glutamate inhibitor), which is neuroprotective, may slow progression. Patients are legally competent, and they can refuse any medical treatment or procedures (such as feeding tube and intubation), even though it might be lifesaving at that time.

Complications: Respiratory failure and death, within 3 to 5 years, is common due to involvement of diaphragmatic nerve or due to aspiration.[12]

10.4 Multiple Sclerosis (MS)

Suspect MS when there are nerve deficits that cannot be explained by one CNS lesion alone and is separated by time and space.

Background: It is due to autoimmune central nervous system (CNS) inflammation and subsequent demyelination. This can occur anywhere in the white matter of CNS (brain, brainstem, and spinal cord).

Clinical pathophysiology:

Autoimmune inflammation and demyelination can involve the following systems	Clinical presentation
Optic nerve (optic neuritis)	Visual disturbances (blurry vision and loss of visual acuity) +/− pain behind the eyes (retrobulbar pain)
	Fundoscopy is commonly normal as the lesion is more commonly in retrobulbar region.
Motor nerve system	Weakness and spasticity (mostly UMN findings)
Sensory nerve system	Numbness and paraesthesias (tingling or pins and needle sensation)
	Unsteady limbs (sensory ataxia)
Spinal cord	Transverse myelitis
Cerebellum	Cerebellar ataxia and gait problems
Autonomic system	Urinary retention, gastroparesis, etc.
Cranial nerves	Any cranial nerve can be involved
	Bilateral trigeminal neuralgia is usually pathognomonic of MS
Medial longitudinal fasciculus lesion causing internuclear ophthalmoplegia (INO)	Failure to adduct affected eye

MRS

I NO ADD: i.e. In INO I cannot adduct my affected eye.

Other features:

– **Lhermitte's phenomenon:** flexion of the neck precipitates electric shock-like sensation travelling down the center of the back and into the limbs.

– **Heat sensitivity:** exposure to heat causes worsening of fatigue or neurological symptoms.

Different types of MS depending upon the progression of deficits

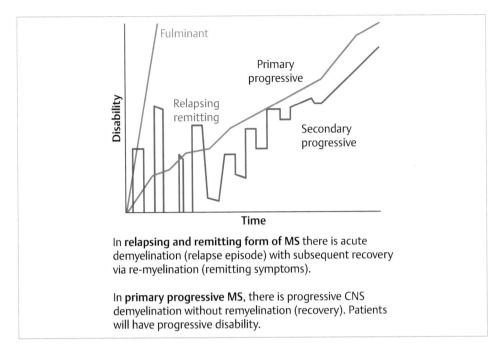

In **relapsing and remitting form of MS** there is acute demyelination (relapse episode) with subsequent recovery via re-myelination (remitting symptoms).

In **primary progressive MS**, there is progressive CNS demyelination without remyelination (recovery). Patients will have progressive disability.

Diagnostic evaluation:

– NSIDx/best SIDx is MRI with gadolinium contrast, which is the most sensitive and specific test. T2-weighted MRI images will show multiple well-demarcated increased-intensity lesions in periventricular areas. This signifies increased water content in the plaques.[13] T1-weighted images will show decreased intensities.

– When MRI is nonconfirmatory and clinical suspicion is high, NSIDx is lumbar puncture. Look for oligoclonal IgG bands and/or elevated IgG index in CSF.

Management of MS

– Treatment of acute exacerbation.
– Slowing the progression of disease.
– Symptomatic/supportive treatment.

10.4.1 Treatment of Acute Exacerbation

• Infections and trauma can trigger neurological worsening of underlying deficit (aka pseudorelapse). Always look for UTI and other sources of infection.

• Acute exacerbation of MS resulting in functional impairment (impaired vision, balance, strength, and coordination) should be treated with short course of **high-dose steroids**. It shortens the duration of episode. In severe case, where patient is unresponsive to steroids, use **plasma exchange**.

10.4.2 Slowing the Progression of MS

Choice of treatment depends on the type of MS.

– Is it on-and-off type with no residual or minimal residual symptoms? Or,
– Is it primarily progressive with increasing severity of symptoms with no remitting features?

** The following history is suggestive of relapsing/remitting form of MS.

– Three months ago, patient had transient left lower extremity weakness that lasted for days. One month ago, patient had transient right upper extremity numbness and paraesthesias for 1 week. Patient now presents with eye pain and blurry vision. Presentation of relapsing and remitting form of MS, particularly during the earlier course of disease, with no resultant disability or FND, can often sound like TIA. **To differentiate know the following:** MS is characterized by on and off neurological symptoms that persist for several days to weeks. TIA usually lasts < 24 hours.

A rare form of MS is neuromyelitis optica (NMO). As the name implies, it only affects spinal cord and the optic nerve. Also, NMO will not have the characteristic MRI brain lesions seen in MS. NMO-IgG antibody may be present.

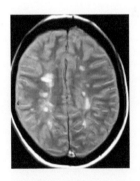

[13]T2 image showing focal hyperintensities in the periventricular white matter.
Source: Multiple Sclerosis (MS). In: Sartor K, Hähnel S, Kress B, ed. Direct Diagnosis in Radiology. Brain Imaging. 1st ed. Thieme; 2007.

Steroids have effect on acute exacerbation, but **no** effect on progression of disease or prevention of MS relapses.

MRS

BIG dx of MS

Cigarette smoking is associated with worsening symptoms; hence, all patients should stop smoking.

Relapsing and remitting	CCS: First attack of MS with no residual FND. MRI findings are highly suggestive of MS. NSIM: start one of the following first-line disease-modifying agents for relapsing forms of MS. – Recombinant INF β1a and IFN β1b: side effects are liver failure (monitor LFTs) and depression – Glatiramer acetate aka copolymer 1 Other options of immunosuppressive therapy for relapsing-remitting MS include the following: – **Natalizumab:** it is a monoclonal antibody to cell-adhesion molecule in T cells. Dreaded side effect is progressive multifocal leukoencephalopathy (see Chapter 8, for further details) – **Oral dimethyl fumarate:** side effects include lymphocytopenia and liver injury – Oral **teriflunomide:** side effects include liver injury – **Fingolimod** is a sphingosine 1- phosphate modulator: side effects include serious herpes virus infection, lymphopenia, heart blocks, and abnormal LFTs
Secondary progressive	– In patients that have progressed from relapsing-remitting to secondary progressive forms and who have evidence of active disease and lesions, try switching immunosuppressives and adding **pulse steroids, cyclophosphamide, or methotrexate** – **Mitoxantrone** is cardiotoxic and associated with increased risk of leukemia. Its use is limited by side effects
Primary progressive	– Ocrelizumab (anti-CD20 monoclonal antibody). Screen for Hep B prior to initiating treatment (active Hep B is a contraindication). – In patients who have evidence of active disease and lesions try immunosuppressives such as pulse steroids, cyclophosphamide, cladribine, methotrexate, etc.

Abbreviations: IFN, interferon; MS, multiple sclerosis; LFTs, liver function tests.

Supportive management of neurological symptoms in MS and of any other neurological disorder (e.g., stroke patient with spasticity)

Neurological symptom	Treatment
Spasticity	– Baclofen (muscle relaxant which opens up K⁺ channel), or – M-blockers such as tizanidine, cyclobenzaprine, or – Botulin toxin injection
Fatigue	– Amantadine, or – Modafinil
Urinary incontinence due to bladder hyperactivity	Bladder antispasmodics such as oxybutynin or tolterodine (M-blockers)
Urinary retention due to bladder weakness	Bethanechol (M-agonist)
Painful neuropathy such as trigeminal neuralgia or dysesthesia	This responds well to agents that decrease electric potential propagation in nerves—carbamazepine, oxcarbazepine, gabapentin, phenytoin, tricyclic antidepressants, etc.
Erectile dysfunction	Sildenafil citrate

Pregnancy and MS
- There are generally fewer attacks during pregnancy.
- General recommendation is to discontinue disease-modifying drugs during pregnancy.
- Steroids or plasmapheresis can be used for acute exacerbation.

Differential diagnosis of MS

Acute disseminated encephalomyelitis (ADEM): This is similar to Guillain–Barre syndrome (GBS) in that it is a postinfectious autoimmune demyelination syndrome; but unlike GBS it affects CNS. It is similar to MS in this regard. Just like MS, ADEM can involve any part of CNS, that is, cerebrum, cerebellum, brainstem, and spinal cord. Now what differentiates MS from ADEM is that ADEM generally consists of a single attack, while MS has multiple attacks. The presence of older well-healed lesions and new lesions in MRI, denoting various periods of attacks of demyelination, point toward MS.

Clinical Case Scenarios

Patient presents with double vision for 1 week. Two months ago, patient had transient right arm weakness and numbness for 1 week. Current exam findings include the following: When patient is asked to look right, the right eye will look right but the left eye will not move. When asked to look left, the left eye will look left but the right eye won't move. When asked to converge, both eyes can converge.

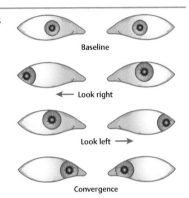

Baseline

⟵ Look right

Look left ⟶

Convergence

3. What is the eye finding called?

4. What is the likely dx?

10.5 Myasthenia Gravis (MG)

Pathophysiology: It is due to autoimmune antibody production to acetylcholine (Ach) receptors in neuromuscular junction. This results in depletion of Ach receptors in neuromuscular junction, leading to muscular weakness as the primary symptom.

Presentation: Earlier in the course, weakness mostly involves small muscles such as face (facial droop), eyes (ptosis, diplopia),[14] and throat (dysphagia and difficulty speaking). Later on, it involves arms and legs. Weakness gets worse with repetitive actions and is more pronounced during later in the day. Sensory system is not involved, and autonomic system involvement is rare.

Weakness can be worsened by concurrent illness (infection) or medications such as beta-blockers, antiarrhythmics, and antibiotics (e.g., aminoglycosides, tetracycline).

Management steps:

Legend: *NSIM, next step in management; NSIDx, next step in diagnosis; DOC, drug of choice; MG, myasthenia gravis*

Tip: One of the easiest ways to approach a patient with weakness is to look for UMN or LMN signs. If no UMN/LMN signs are there, think about disorders related to neuromuscular junction, myopathy, or electrolyte imbalances.
- Look for chronic or recurrent ptosis or diplopia to suspect myasthenia gravis.

[14]A certain subset of patients may have ocular symptoms only. This is called ocular MG.

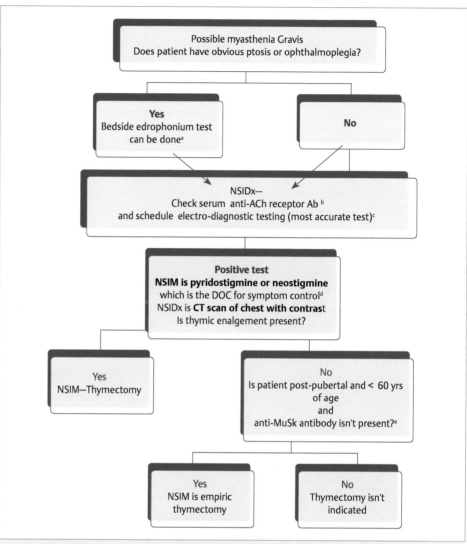

[a]Injectable edrophonium is a fast-acting acetylcholinesterase inhibitor. It is used in patients in whom improvement can be easily observed; as in patients with obvious ptosis, or ophthalmoplegia. In certain subset of patients with obvious ptosis, in whom edrophonium testing is contraindicated (e.g., severe heart disease), bedside ice pack test can also be done. Ice pack decreases temperature and improves neuromuscular conduction, which will improve ptosis in patients with MG.

[b]If anti-ACh receptor antibody is negative, NSIDx is to test for anti**mu**scle **s**pecific tyrosine **k**inase antibody (anti-**MuSK** ab).

[c]Electrodiagnostic testing for MG includes repeated nerve stimulation and single-fiber EMG. Progressive decrease in strength of muscle contraction on repeated stimulation is diagnostic of MG.

Thymectomy is the best treatment to induce remission and provide symptomatic relief.

[d]If patient still has significant symptoms despite initial therapy, consider immunomodulatory agent. They have variable onset of clinical response. Steroids *(onset of effect around 2–3 weeks)* are preferred in most patients (especially if patient remains asymptomatic on low-dose steroids). Steroids are also used as bridge therapy when using steroid-sparing agents (azathioprine, mycophenolate mofetil, cyclosporine, etc.), as these have slow onset of action (e.g., azathioprine *starts working in a year*).

[e]Patients who have not yet reached puberty have increased chances of spontaneous remission. Older patients, > 60 years of age, generally have increased negative outcome from surgery and they also have natural thymic involution, so thymectomy is not found to be beneficial in this group. Thymectomy is also beneficial in patients with positive anti-MuSK antibody.

Abbreviation: DOC, drug of choice.

 MRS

Ach-receptor antibody is pro-thymectomy and anti-MUSK is anti-thymectomy.

Acute Myasthenic Crisis

Background: Precipitating factors include infection, surgery, tapering of immunosuppression, or can be spontaneous.

Presentation: Profound weakness +/− respiratory distress.

Management:

- Intravenous immunoglobulin or plasmapheresis and steroids. Steroid, as a standalone treatment is reserved for milder flares.
- Monitor bedside pulmonary function test (spirometry). Especially important is the serial measurement of vital capacity and negative inspiratory force or maximal inspiratory pressure.
- If there is a serial decline in spirometry values (usually accompanied by weak respiratory effort), NSIM is intubation. Hold acetylcholinesterase inhibitor to reduce secretions in intubated patients.

Clinical Case Scenarios

A 45-year-old female presents to your clinic complaining of diplopia that worsens near the end of the day. She also has problem keeping her eyes open, especially in the evening. She also complains of arm and leg muscle weakness mostly at the end of an activity. During evaluation, when patient is asked to look up, her eyelid falls down within a few minutes. This issue is significantly impacting her life.

5. What is the likely dx?

6. What is the NSIDx?

7. If anti-ACh receptor antibody is negative, what additional antibody test should you order?

8. If electrodiagnostic test is diagnostic for MG, what imaging test should you order?

9. If CT chest is negative for thymic enlargement, and patient is positive for anti-MUSK-antibody, is thymectomy indicated?

10. What if the patient was negative for both anti-Ach receptor antibody and anti-MUSK-antibody; is thymectomy indicated?

10.6 Guillain–Barre Syndrome (GBS)

Background: GBS is an autoimmune inflammatory demyelination of peripheral nerves. It can involve motor, sensory, and autonomic peripheral nerves. This autoimmunity can be incited by any infection such as gastrointestinal infection (*Campylobacter jejuni* is the MCC in the United States), upper respiratory tract infection (influenza virus and *Haemophilus influenzae*), HIV, Zika infection, etc. Other inciting factors are surgery, trauma, or immunization.

Clinical presentation:

- Progressive ascending paralysis with distal to proximal progression (weakness starts from feet, then to knees, thighs, and so on).[15]
- Areflexia (absent reflex).
- Disease course is < 4 weeks.
- It can also involve cranial nerves and cause facial nerve palsy, blurred vision, dysphagia, etc.
- Associated symptoms of autonomic neuropathy (e.g., orthostatic hypertension alternating with hypotension).
- Fever, constitutional symptoms, and bladder dysfunction are rare in GBS; if present consider another dx.

Workup:

- Best initial test is lumbar puncture; look for albumin cytological dissociation (cell count is normal, but protein is high).

Management steps:

When GBS is suspected, treatment should be initiated immediately; before confirmatory test such as EMG/NCS (electromyography and nerve conduction study).[16]

[15]A rare variant of GBS can present with cranial nerve involvement.

[16]EMG/NCS is usually hard to get inpatient, even in resource rich countries. Dx of GBS is often made clinically with supportive CSF findings.

- Intravenous immunoglobulin treatment (IVIG) or plasmapheresis is indicated in patients with significant disease (patients who are nonambulatory) or who are not improving within 4 weeks of onset of symptoms.
- Monitor bedside pulmonary function test (spirometry). Especially important is the serial measurement of vital capacity and negative inspiratory force or maximal inspiratory pressure.
- If there is a serial decline in spirometry values (usually accompanied by weak respiratory effort), NSIM is intubation.

 In a nutshell

	Myasthenic crisis	GBS	MS flare-up
Best SIM	Intravenous immunoglobulin or plasmapheresis + steroids	Intravenous immunoglobulin or plasmapheresis Steroids not indicated	Steroids Patients who have significant disease and not improving on steroids, NSIM is plasmapheresis
	Monitoring: Bedside pulmonary function test (spirometry). If there is a serial decline in spirometry values (usually accompanied by weak respiratory effort), NSIM is intubation		

 In a nutshell

Differential diagnosis of muscle weakness

Clinical features	Likely Dx		Additional differentiating feature
Weakness that primarily involve small muscles – Face, – Eyes (ptosis, diplopia) and – Throat (dysphagia and difficulty speaking)	**Myasthenia gravis.** It has a chronic course. Exam: diminished tendon reflexes		Never affects pupils
	Botulism Course is acute. Look for descending paralysis. Associated with coexistent gastrointestinal symptoms (nausea, vomiting, abdominal pain, etc.).		Affects pupil (they are dilated)
Weakness that primarily involve proximal muscles of arms/legs: the ones used for climbing upstairs, combing hair, and standing up	Normal deep tendon reflexes suggest myositis/ myopathy syndromes	**Dermatomyositis**	ESR and CK elevated Presence of dermal signs such as heliotrope rash or Gottron's plaques
		Polymyositis	ESR and CK elevated Rash not present
		Autoimmune myositis in cancer	ESR and CK elevated Associated with malignancy, for example, small cell cancer of lung
		Steroid-induced myopathy	ESR and CK normal ! In a rare form of steroid-induced acute myopathy CK can be elevated
		Hypothyroid myopathy	CK elevated; ESR normal Other features of hypothyroidism are usually present
	Abnormal/slow deep tendon reflex suggest nerve pathology	**Eaton–Lambert syndrome**	Associated with malignancy, for example, small cell cancer of lung

Clinical features	Likely Dx	Additional differentiating feature
< 4 weeks' duration of weakness that's ascending in nature (begins in feet and spreads to thighs). Sensory system is also involved	Guillain–Barre syndrome	Hx of precedent infection, surgery, trauma, or immunization. It may also involve autonomic nervous system
Weakness that's ascending in nature and patient quickly deteriorates (one extremity is worse than the other)	Tick paralysis (neurotoxin secreted by the attached tick causes paralysis) NSIDx is meticulous search for the tick on patient's body	Sensory or autonomic nervous system is not involved (however mild paraesthesias might be present)
Subacute to acute generalized weakness and hyporeflexia (generalized flaccid paralysis)	NSIDx is check electrolytes. Severe electrolyte abnormalities can do this.	

Statin-induced myopathy usually presents with muscle pain and tenderness and less likely with weakness. CK is typically elevated and ESR is normal.

10.7 Spinal Cord Pathology = Myelopathy

Background: It helps to think of myelopathies in two different categories: compressive versus noncompressive and acute versus chronic.

Etiologies

Compressive myelopathy	Noncompressive myelopathy
• Spondylotic myelopathy • Traumatic (e.g., burst fracture, hematoma) • Infectious (e.g., abscess) • Tumors • Syringomyelia	• Transverse myelitis due to infectious or inflammatory etiology (e.g., multiple sclerosis, acute disseminated encephalomyelitis) • Vascular (e.g., anterior spinal artery thrombosis) • Familial degenerative neuron disease (e.g., primary lateral sclerosis) • Metabolic (e.g., vitamin B12 or copper deficiency) • Toxins

Acute myelopathy	Chronic myelopathy
Trauma, infection, tumors, spinal infarcts, transverse myelitis, etc.	Spondylotic myelopathy, HIV-associated vacuolar myelopathy, syringomyelia, subacute combined degeneration of cord, multiple sclerosis, tabes dorsalis[a]

[a]Tabes dorsalis is associated with syphilis and mostly involves **dorsal** column-medial lemniscal system.

Presentation of myelopathies:

Myelopathy can present with various combination of neurological abnormalities, depending on the following:

– **Level of lesion**: cervical, thoracic, lumbar, or sacral
– **Location of lesion**: anterior, central or posterior cord, and
– **The extent of the pathology:** compression of spinal cord from one side by a tumor versus complete cross-sectional involvement of spinal cord.

A classic presentation of complete cross-sectional involvement would include the following:

– Paraplegia (UMN signs below the level of lesion and LMN signs at the level of lesion).[17]
– Bladder/fecal incontinence.
– Sensory level +/– Back pain.

It is very important to differentiate acute compressive from acute noncompressive myelopathy, as the management strategy is different.

Terminology:
- *Spondylopathy = vertebral bone pathology.*
- *Spondylotic myelopathy = vertebral bone/disc disease leading to spinal cord dysfunction.*
- *Myelitis = spinal cord inflammation/infection*

[17]Initially flaccid paresis that later evolves into spastic paresis over days to weeks.

10.7.1 Acute Compressive Myelopathy

Suspect this in patients with acute myelopathic symptoms and any one of the following:
- Fever
- Saddle anesthesia
- Hx of malignancy, trauma, or IVDA
- Acute urinary/fecal incontinence[18]

Management: First step is high-dose dexamethasone. Then only, MRI of spine with contrast is done. Urgent surgical evaluation is indicated.

10.7.2 Acute Noncompressive Myelopathies (aka Acute Transverse Myelopathies)

Causes:
- Spinal cord infarction (see below)
- Transverse myelitis due to:
    - Systemic disorders such as systemic lupus erythematosus[19] and sarcoidosis
    - Infectious especially viral (herpes family is the MCC of acute transverse myelopathy due to infection)
    - Demyelinating disease such as multiple sclerosis or acute demyelinating encephalomyelitis

Presentation: Typically, present with signs of cross-sectional involvement of spinal cord, with bilateral involvement of sensory and motor system. There are clearly defined sensory level.[20]

Management steps:

NSIM/NSIDx is MRI of spine with IV contrast to rule out compressive pathology. If MRI is negative for compressive lesion, NSIDx is lumbar puncture.[21]

After dx, treat the underlying cause. All of the abovementioned causes (except for spinal cord infarction) are treated with high-dose steroids. Addition of plasmapheresis is recommended in patients with motor impairment.

Anterior, posterior, and central cord syndrome + Brown–Sequard syndrome

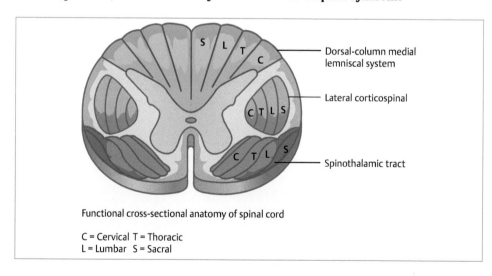

Functional cross-sectional anatomy of spinal cord

C = Cervical   T = Thoracic
L = Lumbar   S = Sacral

[18]See acute back pain section in Chapter 11 for further information

[19]FYI, in approximately 25% of cases where underlying cause of transverse myelitis is not found, patients later develop MS or SLE.

[20]Back pain can develop at the level of acute transverse myelopathy but is usually not severe, and it is not associated with radiculopathic features (e.g., pain shooting down from back to knee).

[21]Other tests that are done to look for cause of transverse myelitis are:
MRI of brain (look for brain lesions), serum NMO-IgG antibodies, serum level for vit B_{12}, methylmalonic acid, HIV, syphilis serology, and autoimmune workup (e.g., ANA).

Anterior cord syndrome	**Etiology**: MCC is spinal cord infarction, with anterior spinal artery involvement due to the following: – Aortic pathology (e.g., aortic dissection or aneurysm, direct trauma to aorta, neurosurgery) – Any condition that can cause of arterial thrombus (e.g., sickle cell crisis, polycythemia) – Vasculitis Anterior spinal cord syndrome can also occur due to burst vertebral fracture **Presentation**: acute sudden-onset bilateral flaccid paresis accompanied with bilateral loss of pain and temperature sensation. There is sparing of vibration and proprioception modalities
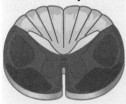	
Posterior cord syndrome (very rare)	Posterior column is exclusively supplied by posterior spinal artery. Posterior spinal artery infarction causes bilateral loss of proprioception and vibratory sense below the level of the injury (it will only involve distal medial-lemniscal system)
Brown–Sequard syndrome 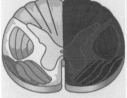	**Etiology:** occurs due to hemisection of spinal cord (e.g., patient with knife injury to one side of spinal cord or spinal cord compression from tumor) **Presentation:** – Ipsilateral loss of corticospinal tract (motor weakness) and dorsal column-medial lemniscal system (loss of joint position and vibration sense) – Contralateral loss of spinothalamic tract (loss of pain and temperature sensation)

Treatment: There is no specific treatment for these cord syndromes. Treatment should be directed towards to the primary cause.

10.7.3 Central Cord Syndrome

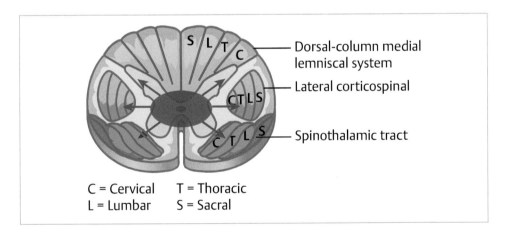

C = Cervical   T = Thoracic
L = Lumbar   S = Sacral

Etiology:
MCC is syringomyelia. Other causes include intramedullary tumor and the result of hyperextension injury in individuals with long-standing cervical spondylosis.
Syringomyelia: It is a term that refers to cystic cavity formation within the spinal cord.
● Acquired syringomyelia can be caused by trauma, inflammation/infection, or tumor in spinal cord.
● Congenital syringomyelia is associated with downward (caudal) displacement of cerebellar tonsils through foramen magnum. This syndrome is called Arnold–Chiari malformation.[22]

[22]**Arnold–Chiari malformation:** Depending on the degree of the herniation and pathology, it is divided into four categories, out of which type I is the mildest (may or may not have syringomyelia) and type IV is the most severe and rarest form.

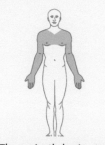

[23]The spinothalamic tract from both sides cross the spinal cord in close proximity to center of the spinal canal. In central cord syndrome, spinothalamic system is typically affected first, in bilateral fashion. Hence, the cape-like distribution of sensory loss.

[24]Onset of clinical disease is generally after the age of 50 years.
Spondylopathy = osteoarthritis of the vertebral joints.

Clinical presentation:

- First presenting sign might be loss of spinothalamic pain and temperature sensation in bilateral upper extremities. MC location of syringomyelia is cervical spinal cord region.[23]
- As the syrinx or intramedullary tumor expands it will involve cervical, thoracic, lumbar, and sacral in a progressive serial fashion. Weakness in arm is more pronounced than in legs.
- Further extension into the anterior horn of spinal cord will result in LMN involvement at the level of lesion (typically in upper extremities) and UMN below the level of lesion (hyperreflexia in lower extremities).

Management steps: NSIDx is MRI of spine with contrast. Surgical treatment may be needed.

10.7.4 Cervical Spondylotic Myelopathy

Background: These are degenerative and hypertrophic changes in vertebra, ligaments, and discs (spondylopathy) which can result in cervical nerve root impingement (radiculopathy), disc herniation, narrowing of spinal arteries and may also narrow the spinal cord causing spinal cord compression from outside (myelopathy).[24]

Clinical pathophysiology:

Compression of cervical nerve roots or injury to the anterior horn cells of cervical spinal cord	Clumsy-weak-atrophic hands (i.e., LMN signs in upper extremities)
Compression of cervical nerve roots	Radiculopathic pain in upper extremities
Spinal cord compression from the lateral side causes early involvement of descending sacral and lumbar corticospinal tract. (*To get a better picture see spinal cross-sectional image in central cord syndrome section.*)	Asymmetric UMN signs in lower extremities—lower extremity spastic leg weakness, leg stiffness, unsteady gait, and hyperreflexia
Compression of dorsal column-medial lemniscal system	
Loss of joint and vibration sense in lower extremities	

- Similar to multiple sclerosis patients may have Lhermitte's sign—neck flexion precipitates electric shock-like sensation travelling down the center of the back and into the limbs. This sign is nonspecific, as it can occur in any form of myelopathy that involves cervical spinal cord
- Neck pain

Workup: Vertebral X-ray shows the presence of vertebral bony spurs, sclerotic facet joints, and narrowing of disk spaces. Dx is usually made by correlating clinical exam with MRI findings.

Rx: Surgical decompression is recommended for acute severe myelopathy or progressive symptoms. Similar pathophysiology in lumbar spine can present with back pain, sciatica symptoms, and neurogenic claudication. For further info on neurogenic claudication, see rheumatology chapter.

10.7.5 Subacute Combined Degeneration

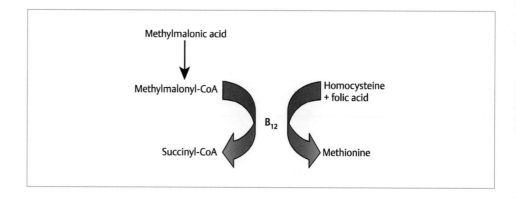

Pathophysiology: Vitamin B_{12} deficiency leads to increased methylmalonyl-CoA (which is toxic to myelin sheaths) with subsequent development of demyelination of neurons in brain, spine, and periphery. This can involve any nervous system, but the ones that are affected earlier are the heavily myelinated dorsal column medial lemniscal system and corticospinal tract.

Etiology: Pernicious anemia, strict vegetarian diet for years, small bowel disease, etc.[25]

Clinical pathophysiology:

Demyelination of	Clinical presentation
Dorsal column medial lemniscal sensory system	– Loss of joint position and vibration sense – Paraesthesia (pins and needle sensation)
Corticospinal tract	– Spastic paresis (UMN signs) – Paresis can be symmetric, involving both legs
Brain nerves	– Dementia
Hematologic abnormalities may or may not be present, hence absence of hematologic abnormality does not rule out this condition.	

Abbreviation: UMN, upper motorneurons.

Diagnostic evaluation: NSIDx is serum vitamin B_{12} level. If vitamin B_{12} level is low, it is diagnostic. If vitamin B_{12} level is in indeterminate range, NSIDx: check serum methylmalonic acid level.

Treatment: Intramuscular vitamin B_{12} is recommended with neurological symptoms.

10.8 Headache

The single most important tool for diagnosis of headache is patient's history. In all patients presenting with headache, ask the following questions:

- Is this the first time you have had this kind of headache?
- Is this a new type of headache in a person > 40 to 50 year of age? (*In a patient with a history of chronic headaches, ask if this headache is similar to previous ones.*)
- Is this a sudden onset "thunderclap" headache, classically described as the worst headache of life? (suggests *subarachnoid hemorrhage*)
- Do you have fever?
- Is it a progressively worsening headache?
- Is the headache aggravated by sexual activity, exertion, bending, coughing, Valsalva maneuver? Is it most severe early in the morning? (*suggests increased intracranial pressure*)
- Is there associated FND, change in mental status, change in personality, or papilledema? (*suggests space-occupying lesion such as brain abscess or brain tumor*)

If any of the above is present, then NSIM is brain imaging. However, note that brain imaging is not the initial test of choice in the following situations:

Fever + headache + stiff neck	Possible meningitis. Consider lumbar puncture first if there are no contraindications
Headache + eye pain, red eye + photophobia + mildly dilated pupils	Likely dx is acute angle closure glaucoma. NSIDx is tonometry, which detects increased intraocular pressure

Primary Headache Disorders (Migraine, Tension, and Cluster Headache) Migraine

10.8.1 Primary Headache Disorders (Migraine, Tension, and Cluster Headache)

Migraine

Background: Exact etiology is unknown; a mix of environmental and genetic factors is thought to be the cause. It is related to abnormal neurovascular reactivity.

Presentation: Migraine usually presents as a pulsating (pounding) headache of unilateral location with multiple attacks each lasting 48 to 72 hours (on average lasting one day), associated with nausea +/– vomiting, photophobia, and phonophobia. If severe enough, it can be disabling.

[25]See Chapter 7, vitamin B_{12} deficiency section for further information.

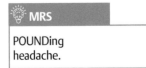

MRS

POUNDing headache.

Forms of migraine:

Classic migraine	Migraine with aura.
	Aura = characteristic sensory or visual symptoms before the onset on headache, such as visual scotomas (dark spots or zig zag lines in the visual field before the onset of headache)
Common migraine	Migraine without aura
Hemiplegic migraine	Coexistent pulsatile headache and development of any form of focal neurological deficit points toward this dx
	Some forms of hemiplegic migraine are due to familial autosomal dominant disorder; hence, family hx may be positive
Basilar migraine	Pathology starts from the brainstem; therefore, patients might have aura of dizziness, dysarthria, double vision or lack of coordination before the onset of headache

Management (Treatment of acute migraine attack and preventive management)

In all patients, identify and avoid triggers. Known migraine triggers are certain foods (e.g., chocolate, cheese, monosodium glutamate, and artificial sweeteners), alcohol, hunger, irregular meals, caffeine, and lack of sleep.

Treatment of acute migraine attack

Mild to moderate symptoms	**Initial treatment:** NSAIDs or acetaminophen, or their combination
	Use triptans[a] in patients with hx of not responding to simple analgesic
	Add antiemetics in patients with nausea
Moderate to severe symptoms, or migraine upon **waking up** (in absence of vomiting or significant nausea)	Initial treatment is with oral triptans[a] +/− NSAIDs
Severe symptoms with vomiting or significant nausea, or when patient is not responding to oral therapy	First-line treatment: subcutaneous or nasal triptans[a]
	IV prochlorperazine, chlorpromazine, or metoclopramide are second-line agent. As they are dopamine blockers, consider adding diphenhydramine to prevent dystonic reaction or akathisia
	Consider adjunctive treatment with parenteral dexamethasone
For patients who continue to have **debilitating migraine,** despite treatment	Sodium valproate, or
	Parenteral dihydroergotamine

[a]Triptans (sumatriptan, zolmitriptan, rizatriptan, almotriptan, naratriptan, eletriptan) are serotonin receptor agonists. Pathogenesis of migraine is thought to be vasodilation in cerebral vessels. Triptans by causing vasoconstriction, relieve acute migraine headache. The side effects of triptans are also related to vasoconstriction in other sites such as limb heaviness, paraesthesias, chest/neck/throat tightness and flushing; however, these are mostly benign side effects. Triptans are contraindicated in the following situations:

- Pregnancy: if there is a chance that patient might be pregnant, pregnancy test should be done prior to giving a following situations[26]:

- Known coronary artery disease: because vasoconstriction in already narrowed vessels coronary vessels may exacerbate angina or even cause infarction.

- Uncontrolled HTN: generalized vasoconstriction can precipitate acute hypertensive crisis.

- Hemiplegic or basilar migraine.

Abbreviation: NSAIDs, nonsteroidal anti-inflammatory drugs.

[26]Vasoconstrictors such as triptans or prostaglandin analogues may induce abortion.

Migraine prevention

Indications for initiation of prophylactic pharmacotherapy include presence of any one of the following:
- Migraine attacks > four times a month or headaches that last > 12 hours.
- Headaches that are prolonged and debilitating despite abortive treatment.
- Hemiplegic/basilar migraine.
- Migraine with aura that lasts for more than hour.

Choose any one of the following prophylactic treatment:
- β-blockers: metoprolol, propranolol, timolol
- Antidepressants: amitriptyline, venlafaxine
- Anticonvulsants: valproic acid, topiramate

Specific scenarios with migraine

- **Pregnancy**
- Migraine control usually improves in the last 6 months of pregnancy.
- Since most prophylactic migraine drugs are associated with fetal risks, their use should be reserved for patients with severe or frequent migraine attacks.
- Migraine has been associated with low birth weight, preterm delivery, abruption of placenta, and eclampsia.
- **Menstruation:** migraine can be worse during perimenstrual period. In selected patients, with predictable perimenstrual episodes, oral triptans can be given prophylactically.
- **Oral contraceptive pills** are avoided in patients with hx of migraine with aura, as there might be increased risk of stroke in these patients.

Cluster Headache

Background: It is an idiopathic primary headache disorder.

Presentation:
- Severe pain behind the eyes (retro-orbital pain) that can later become generalized. Pain can be pulsating in character. Usual hx is headache upon waking up.
- Look for signs of ipsilateral autonomic dysregulation such as runny nose, teary red eyes, ipsilateral Horner's syndrome (ptosis, miosis).
- Another important clue for diagnosis is the timing of headache; as name gives all, it occurs in clusters (1–8 times a day for few weeks to months) and then disappears for some time; and then comes again in clusters.
- As opposed to migraine, which can last for many hours to days, cluster headache usually lasts for less than 3 to 4 hours.

Treatment:

For acute headache	Acute abortive treatment is indicated. Best initial treatment is 100% oxygen. Adjunctive triptans can be given
For ongoing episode of clusters of headache	Steroids can be used for breaking a new cluster cycle
For prophylaxis	Verapamil is the drug of choice

Tension Headaches

Background: Tension headaches are typically due to a lot of stress in patient's life. It is the MC of primary headache disorder. Social issues are an important causative factor. It is associated with depression and anxiety.

Presentation: Headache is typically continuous, band like, crushing in character and especially severe in the evenings. It can be associated with neck pain and neck muscle stiffness. Absence of features suggestive of migraine points toward this diagnosis. It rarely awakes patient from sleep.

Management: First of all address patient's source of stress. In addition, the following medical therapy can be offered to the patients:
- Simple analgesia such as nonsteroidal anti-inflammatory drugs (NSAIDs) or aspirin. Acetaminophen is preferred in pregnancy.
- Addition of caffeine with NSAIDs or aspirin increases efficacy and can be used if monotherapy is not effective.

For prevention:

- Relaxation, biofeedback, and cognitive behavioral therapy is likely beneficial.
- Prophylactic low-dose amitriptyline can be used.

10.9 Pseudotumor Cerebri (aka Benign or Idiopathic Intracranial HTN)

Pathophysiology: Pathogenesis is unknown. It can occur in any age group, even in children. Drugs associated with this disorder include oral contraceptive pills, growth hormone, anabolic steroids, isotretinoin and tetracyclines. It is also associated with steroid withdrawal and hypervitaminosis A.

Presentation: Headache (MC symptom) with features of increased ICP.[27]

Additional findings:

- Papilledema: an early sign of disease is transient vision loss precipitated by maneuvers that increase ICP (e.g., hx of visual blurring when patient bends over).[28]
- Most commonly involved cranial nerve is CN VI (abducens nerve palsy).

Diagnostic evaluation:

- NSIM/NSIDx is CNS imaging: CT or MRI scan of brain, to rule out intracranial pathology and space-occupying lesions +/– magentic resonance venography (to rule out cerebral venous sinus thombosis). Imaging may show incidental empty sella syndrome (high ICP pushes CSF and the meningeal layer membrane into the sella turcica displacing the functional pituitary gland).
- NSIM/NSIDx, after ruling out space-occupying lesion, is lumbar puncture which will show increased CSF pressure. It is also for therapeutic purposes, which will lead to transient decrease in ICP and improvement of symptoms. The CSF cell counts are unremarkable.

Treatment:

- Best SIM is weight loss if obese and avoiding offending agents. For example, if the patient is on oral contraceptive, advise patient to discontinue it and provide alternative method of contraception.
- The first drug of choice (DOC) is acetazolamide which decreases the production of CSF and decreases ICP. Lasix can be added. In pregnant patients, serial lumber puncture is the treatment of choice.
- If the symptoms are refractory to medical management, then NSIM is either shunting or optic nerve sheath decompression (these are the two forms of definitive treatment). While waiting for surgery, some patients may need bridging options such as repeated lumbar punctures or oral steroids, for significant symptoms.

10.10 Trigeminal Neuralgia (aka Tic Douloureux)

Pathophysiology: Abnormal blood vessel (most commonly superior cerebellar artery and anterior inferior cerebellar artery) has been implicated in vascular compression of the trigeminal nerve root microvasculature leading to demyelination of trigeminal nerve roots.[29] This leads to abnormal firing and neuropathic pain in trigeminal nerve root distribution.

Presentation: Multiple episodes of sudden-onset lightning-like sharp pain in the face region[30] which is typically aggravated by touch or movement stimuli (e.g., pain is aggravated while brushing teeth or even while talking or eating).

Management: MRI of the brain should be done first to rule out compressive lesions. MRA can be done to look for vascular compression.

- **First-line drugs:** Carbamazepine (dreaded side effect is aplastic anemia, so complete blood count (CBC) should be checked at regular intervals). Oxcarbazepine is a good alternative.
- **Second-line drugs** are gabapentin, baclofen, lamotrigine, and clonazepam.
- **If refractory to medical management** then surgical option is considered. Microvascular decompressive surgery separates the compressing vessel from the nerve. Rhizotomy (selective nerve fiber destruction) is also an option.

[27]Features of headache related to intracranial HTN
- Hx of headache that worsens when leaning forward, coughing, with Valsalva maneuver, and in the mornings.
- Papilledema may develop causing vision loss. MC intracranial nerve involvement is abducens nerve palsy (with associated double vision). Tinnitus may also be present.
- Physical exam may reveal HTN and bradycardia.
- Causes: intracranial hemorrhage, primary or metastatic intracranial tumors, brain abscess, idiopathic intracranial hypertension, etc.

[28]The most likely complication, if not treated, is permanent visual loss due to optic nerve atrophy.

[29]Patients with multiple sclerosis can have **bilateral** trigeminal neuralgia, due to noncompressive autoimmune demyelination.

[30]Fleeting, lightning-like, sharp pain points toward neuropathic pain.

Clinical Case Scenarios

A 25-year-old female presents to emergency department with complaint of severe pulsating headache and visual field defects prior to the onset of headache. She has severe nausea. Upon further questioning, she reveals this is the first time she had such headache. She has family hx of migraine disorder.

11. What is the NSIDx?

12. What is the best abortive treatment in this case?

    a) Oral triptan + NSAID,

    b) NSAIDs + tylenol,

    c) Subcutaneous triptan

13. A 55-year-old female patient presents with few months' history of dull, vice-like, crushing type of headache especially severe in the evenings. She also gives hx of neck stiffness and neck pain. What is the likely Dx?

A 45-year-old male patient presents with severe headache that started from behind the eyes and later got generalized. He also complains of runny eyes and runny nose. Exam reveals left eye erythema, lid lag, and small pupil. He gives hx of five similar episodes in the last 1 week. Few months ago, he had 15 episodes like these that lasted for 20 days.

    14. What is the likely dx?

    15. What is best NSIM for this headache episode?

    16. What can you give to terminate this episode of cluster headaches?

17. A 35-year-old obese female, on oral retinoic acid treatment for acne, presents with pulsatile headache and tinnitus that typically wakes her from sleep. Exam reveals lateral gaze palsy. What is the likely dx?

18. A 24-year-old female on prophylactic migraine therapy started 2 to 3 weeks ago, comes to emergency department with another headache episode. Abortive therapy at this time was successful. What is the NSIM regarding preventative migraine treatment?

10.11 Dizziness (Presyncope versus Vertigo)

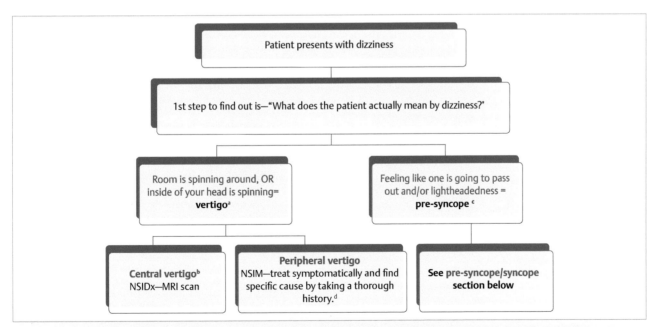

[a]After establishing that patient has vertigo, next step is to find out whether it is **central vertigo** (usually caused by cerebellum or brainstem problem) or **peripheral vertigo** (caused by CN VIII and inner ear problems). *Look at table on next page.*

	Peripheral	Central
Symptoms related to inner ear (tinnitus and/or hearing loss)	Usually present	No
Other neurological symptoms (e.g., diplopia, cortical blindness, dysarthria)	No	Usually present
Persistence of dizziness	Transient (on and off), but can be continuous	Usually continuous

[b]Causes of central vertigo: vertebrobasilar or cerebellar TIA/stroke, tumor, infection, etc.

[c]Coexistent **palpitations** and/or **dyspnea** point toward underlying cardiac disease (severe aortic stenosis, silent MI in diabetics, HOCM, etc.).

[d]Peripheral causes of vertigo and distinguishing features are discussed below.

Condition	Presentation – Note that vertigo is usually associated with nausea/vomiting		Management [a]
Meniere's disease (Proposed pathogenesis is increase in endolymphatic pressure)	**Intermittent** vertigo + hearing loss + tinnitus		NSIDx is to rule out syphilis by doing VDRL or RPR. **Rx:** salt restriction and diuretics. If no improvement with medical treatment, then surgical decompression is offered
Vestibular neuronitis/ neuritis	It is often caused by viral infection, or less commonly bacterial infection	Sudden acute-onset vertigo lasting up to several days	**No** tinnitus and **no** hearing loss: preserved auditory function	Supportive treatment May use short course of steroids
Vestibular labyrinthitis		Rarely can have recurrence	Hearing loss and/ or tinnitus is present	
Benign positional paroxysmal vertigo (BPPV) (It is due otoliths in inner ear and is associated with aging)	Episodes of transient vertigo (+/- nausea) exacerbated by head movements, rolling over, or getting out of bed		NSIDx is Dix–Hallpike maneuver (positional head maneuvering re-elicits transient vertigo/ nystagmus). Treatment is often supportive. If symptoms persist, certain maneuvers can be tried to dislodge the otolith from the semicircular canals (e.g., Epley maneuver)
Perilymphatic fistula	Vertigo that started after a blunt trauma to the ear or while scuba diving or after a vigorous Valsalva maneuver		Supportive
Vestibular schwannoma aka acoustic neuroma (It is a Schwann cell derived tumor, most commonly from vestibular portion of 8th cranial nerve.)	Progressive symptoms of nonspecific vertigo (disequilibrium), tinnitus and asymmetric hearing loss		An audiogram is important in documenting sensorineural hearing loss. MRI is preferred imaging modality. **Rx:** surgical or radiation therapy
Motion sickness	Vertigo + nausea/vomiting induced by motion		Scopolamine (parasympathetic M-blockers), ephedrine, or promethazine (anti-histamine) can be used

[a]**Supportive Rx:** alleviate vertigo symptoms with drugs, such as meclizine (anti-histamine) or diazepam, if severe.

⚠ Caution

Vertigo with hearing loss

- In **Meniere's disease,** there are recurrent relapsing-remitting episodes.
- In **acoustic neuroma,** patients have progressive symptoms.
- In **vestibular labyrinthitis,** the symptoms are acute, and there is no hx of prior episodes.

10.12 Presyncope and Syncope

Any pathology that leads to acute decrease in blood supply to the brain can cause presyncope/syncope.

Definition:

- **Presyncope:** Decrease in brain blood supply is low enough to cause symptoms of dizziness (+/– confusion), but not severe enough to cause loss of consciousness.
- **Syncope:** Decreased brain blood supply results in loss of consciousness.

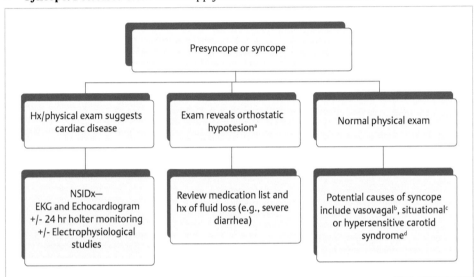

[a]Orthostatic or postural presyncope/syncope	Attacks are precipitated by sudden standing, or in severe cases, even sitting up and dangling their legs at the side of the bed can precipitate an attack. NSIDx is to check orthostatic vital signs.	
	If acute, it is commonly caused by volume depletion related to diarrhea/diuretic use or use of new medications that can cause postural hypotension (e.g., α_1-blockers, tricyclic antidepressants). Elderly patients can be very vulnerable to dehydration and medication side effects, as they poorly tolerate even seemingly minimal fluid loss or small dose of medication.	
	If chronic, it can be related to chronic autonomic neuropathy (due to diabetes, alcoholism, Parkinsonism, Vitamin B_{12} deficiency, etc.).	Orthostatic syncope is a common cause of falls in elderly.
	Medications to treat persistent orthostatic hypotension include fludrocortisone, midodrine (α_1- agonist), pyridostigmine.	
[b]Vasovagal syncope (aka neurocardiogenic syncope)	Vagal mediated response to situations such as intense emotion or prolonged standing in heat. Patients might have nausea and intense feeling prior to fainting. Increased vagal activity may lead to marked bradycardia in some patients. Recurrent attacks might be present in a young patient.	
	– If hx of such kind of recurrent episodes, NSIDx is tilt-table test	
[c]Situational syncope	Occurs in specific situation	
	– **Micturition Syncope:** - typically occurs in patients with hx of bladder outlet obstruction, who have to strain to pass urine (e.g., benign prostatic hyperplasia)	
	– Syncope related to coughing spells	
[d]Hypersensitive carotid sinus syndrome	As name gives all, this is due to exaggerated vagal response to carotid sinus stimulation which leads to decreased cardiac output. Attacks can be precipitated by seemingly mundane stimuli such as moving the neck or wearing garments with tight neck collars	

10.13 Seizures

Definition: Seizures are repetitive, abnormal firing of a group of nerve cell in the brain.

How to differentiate syncope from a seizure? Sometimes seizures (particularly unwitnessed) are difficult to differentiate from a syncopal attack. Also note that sometimes syncope can be followed by movements that mimic seizures (e.g., transient generalized movement, focal myoclonic jerks, tonic stiffening).

MRS

How to differentiate syncope from a seizure? that's **A CATCH**!!!

	Seizures (fits)	Syncope (faints)
Aura (pre-ictal)	May be present	Usually absent
Confusion (post-ictal)		
Amnesia (retrograde or anterograde)		
Tongue biting (ictal)		
Continence loss (ictal)		
Headache (postictal)		

Etiology of seizures:

MRS

VITAMINS

- **V**ascular: stroke, intracranial hemorrhage, AV malformation.
- **I**nfection: meningitis, encephalitis, brain abscess.
- **T**rauma/**T**oxins: motor vehicle accident, neurosurgery, cocaine, methamphetamines, etc.
- **A**utoimmune: encephalitis, vasculitis (e.g., SLE).
- **A**lcohol or other sedative withdrawal (benzodiazepine, barbiturates, etc.).
- **M**etabolic: severe electrolyte/metabolic/oxygen imbalances can cause seizures (e.g., hypo/hypernatremia, hypo/hypercalcemia, hypoglycemia, hypomagnesemia/hypophosphatemia, hypoxemia).
- **I**diopathic epilepsy syndrome.
- **N**eoplastic: primary or metastatic brain tumors.
- p**S**ychiatric or p**S**eudoseizure: patient is faking an episode of seizure (look for to and fro head movement, pelvic thrusting, and generalized body involvement without loss of consciousness in patient with hx of psychiatric disorder).

Presentation: Seizures can manifest clinically as different types, depending on the initial location and subsequent propagation of the abnormal firings of electrical activity. Differentiating seizure type (partial, focal or generalized) is important because treatment varies.

Seizure classification	Type	Clinical features
Partial seizures, aka focal seizures occur due to abnormal firing from a discrete portion of brain	**Simple partial seizure**	No loss of consciousness (LOC) and patient is responsive during the episode Usually involves single neurological function (motor, sensory, olfactory, visual, etc.)
	Complex partial seizure	No LOC (loss of consciousness) but patient is not responsive to external stimuli during the episode (unaware of environment—might be seen staring blankly into space) Usually arises from the temporal lobe which affects awareness
	Partial seizure with secondary generalization	If the abnormal firing spreads throughout the brain, it can now lead to LOC, which may be followed by tonic/clonic phase
Generalized seizures (usually have no aura)	**Generalized tonic-clonic seizure**	With tonic (muscle rigidity) and clonic (muscle contractions) phase LOC is typically present
	Absence seizure	Looks like the patient is day-dreaming (see below for further info) Brief LOC may be present
	Atonic seizure	Drop attacks, i.e., sudden loss of muscle tone Typically lasts for < 15 seconds May or may not have postictal confusion or LOC
	Myoclonic seizure	Sudden or brief muscle contraction involving one part of the body or the entire body patient typically remains conscious (no LOC)

Progression of a seizure:

> **Pre-ictal i.e., before seizure**
> Aura which can be visual, olfactory or auditory hallucinations (This is mostly seen in partial seizures)

> **Ictal (during seizure)**
> **Any of the following can occur**
> - Cyanosis
> -Tongue biting
> -Loss of bladder control—incontinence
> -Loss of consciousness (LOC)
> -Abnormal repetitive movemements like lip-smacking, frequent blinking and picking on clothes
> -Increased tonicity of limbs (tonic), and/or violent contraction of limbs (clonic) can be present

> **Post-ictal (after-seizure)**
> -Headache
> -Confusion
> -If seizure involved repeated muscle contractions, patients may have elevated lactate (anion gap acidosis), and transient muscle weakness (Todd's palsy).

10.13.1 Additional Information on Different Types of Seizures

Generalized tonic–clonic seizures (GTCS)

- Abrupt onset with loss of consciousness (LOC). In primary GTCS, there is usually no aura.
- Tonic phase = abrupt onset generalized stiffness of the limb (muscle tone is increased in most of the muscles groups).
- Clonic phase = tonic phase is followed by phase of generalized repeated contraction of the limbs.
- Tonic–clonic phase is accompanied with ictal incontinence, tongue biting, and postictal confusion. Preictal/postictal amnesia usually occurs.

Absence Seizure

Background: It usually occurs in school-age children.[31]

Presentation:
- Each episode lasts around 10 seconds and can occur multiple times in a day.[32]
- Presents as frequent staring and blinking episodes (looks like the child is day-dreaming a lot).
- Children may have deteriorating school performance because of the frequency of seizures during school time.
- This seizure is different from other seizures: "ACATCH" is absent.

Workup: Best step for dx is EEG (which may reveal 3 Hz spike-and-wave discharge pattern). As absence seizures occur very frequently, EEG is most likely to detect abnormal firing. If there is no spontaneous detection, patient is asked to hyperventilate (seizures can be precipitated by hyperventilation).

Rx: DOC is ethosuximide (most important side effect is gastrointestinal disturbance). If gastrointestinal side effects are not tolerable, other options are lamotrigine or valproic acid.

Complex partial seizure

- These typically arise from temporal lobe.[33] So, it is often preceded by preictal aura such as hallucinations, déjà vu, jamais vu,[34] depersonalization, tunnel vision, etc.
- These typically last for few minutes (in contrast to absence seizures which last 10 seconds or so).
- Automatisms (e.g., lip smacking, swallowing, hand picking movements) are present. "A CATCH" may be present.

[31]Caution: *Do not make this dx in an adult.*

[32]To give you the magnitude, children may have 10–100 episodes/day.

 MRS

ELVes are absent from children books.

[33]Some patients with temporal lobe epilepsy disorder may have evidence of mesial temporal sclerosis (hippocampal atrophy).

[34]**Déjà vu** = feeling that a completely new experience has already happened in the past.
Jamais vu = feeling of a familiar experience being unfamiliar.

Other seizure syndromes

Lenox–Gastaut syndrome	⇒	Childhood onset epilepsy with multiple types of seizures in the same patient. For example, patient presents with hx of GTCS, myoclonic and atonic seizures
Juvenile myoclonic epilepsy	⇒	Hx of multiple episodes of morning myoclonus or jitteriness. Despite the name, it can be seen in adults too
Frontal lobe epilepsy (aka recurrent Jacksonian seizure)	⇒	This is a form of simple partial seizure involving the motor cortex. It starts with repeated contractions of a specific muscle followed by involvement of other muscle groups. For example, patient presents with jerking of leg that progresses to arm and then head

Management of first seizure episode in adults

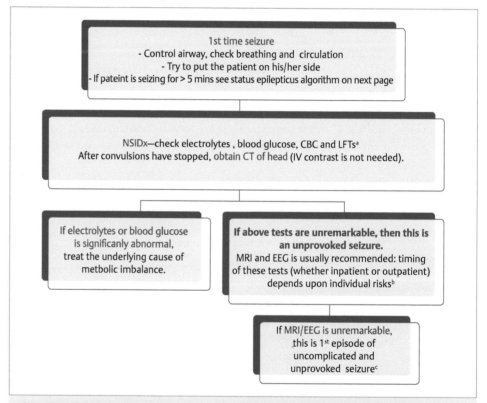

[a] If a patient with hx of seizure disorder on antiepileptic drug (AED) presents with seizure, check AED level (check for noncompliance or inadequate dosage)

[b] Do stat EEG in patients whose level of consciousness is not improving after 10 minutes of seizures, or who continue to have abnormal mental status 30 minutes after seizures, or who have waxing and waning mental status or persistent FND. In this case, subclinical nonconvulsive status epilepticus needs to be ruled out. Patients can have mild confusion or twitching that can be overlooked by clinicians.

[c] In patients with first episode of unprovoked seizure, consider AED only if one of the following is present: status epilepticus, strong family hx of seizures, hx of significant head trauma, focal seizure, abnormal neurological exam, and/or focal findings on EEG or CNS imaging.

If none of the above present, AED is indicated only if patient has second episode of unprovoked seizure.

EEG for diagnosis of seizures/epilepsy
- EEG is specific (can confirm diagnosis) but not sensitive (can't exclude dx) for seizures.
- Inpatient EEG monitoring is considered when patient is not responding to 2 or more AED.

10.14 Status Epilepticus

Definition: When a patient is continuously seizing for ≥5 minutes[35] or when the patient has multiple seizures without regaining consciousness in between.

Management:

MCC of status epilepticus is low AED level.

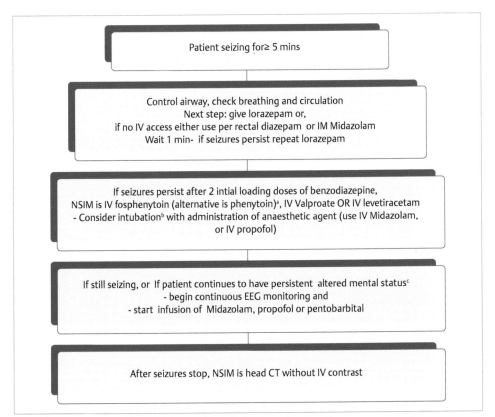

Patient seizing for≥ 5 mins

Control airway, check breathing and circulation
Next step: give lorazepam or,
if no IV access either use per rectal diazepam or IM Midazolam
Wait 1 min- if seizures persist repeat lorazepam

If seizures persist after 2 intial loading doses of benzodiazepine,
NSIM is IV fosphenytoin (alternative is phenytoin)[a], IV Valproate OR IV levetiracetam
- Consider intubation[b] with administration of anaesthetic agent (use IV Midazolam, or IV propofol)

If still seizing, or If patient continues to have persistent altered mental status[c]
- begin continuous EEG monitoring and
- start infusion of Midazolam, propofol or pentobarbital

After seizures stop, NSIM is head CT without IV contrast

[a]Fosphenytoin is preferred over phenytoin whenever available, as it is can be infused faster and does not cause skin necrosis (extravasation of phenytoin can cause skin necrosis). Both drugs can cause hypotension.

[b]Intubation might be indicated earlier if patient is hemodynamically unstable.

[c]Nonconvulsive status epilepticus needs to be ruled out in patients with persistent altered mental status. Continuing seizure activity signals poorer prognosis.

Patients with epilepsy disorder have higher risk of:
- Mood disorder
- Cognitive issues
- Osteoporosis

Complications of seizure:
- Rhabdomyolysis
- Anion gap metabolic acidosis, due to elevated lactic acid
- Pulmonary edema
- Neuroexcitotoxicity can result in cortical laminar ischemia/necrosis leading to transient or persistent focal or global neurological deficit. MRI may show increased intensity in affected areas.
- Aspiration pneumonitis/ pneumonia

10.14.1 Antiepileptic Drugs (AED)

The choice of seizure medication depends on the type of seizure, availability, side effects, and cost. Differentiating seizure type (partial or focal vs generalized) is important.

Gabazepines treat Partial focal only; - GABA = GABAergic meds - Zepines = AEDs with suffix "azepine" - P = AED that start with letter "P" - "ocal" of Focal in reverse is "Laco"samide	**Narrow-spectrum AED** These work mostly for specific type of seizure (such as partial, focal, absence, or myoclonic seizures) GABAergic AEDs: Ezogabine, gabapentin, pregabalin, tiagabine, vigabatrin AEDs with suffix "azepine": carbamazepine, eslicarbazepine, oxcarbazepine, AED that start with letter "P": perampanel, phenobarbital, phenytoin, primidone, Lacosamide Out of all these medications, carbamazepine and oxcarbazepine are preferred first-line agents for partial seizures	**Broad-spectrum AED** These can be used for all seizure types (generalized and partial seizures) Valproate (valproic acid), lamotrigine, levetiracetam, zonisamide, Clobazam, felbamate, rufinamide, topiramate

As a side note, narrow-spectrum drugs are also often used for neuropathic pain syndromes (e.g., for trigeminal neuralgia, herpetic neuralgia, diabetic neuropathy).

AED can be stopped if patient is seizure free for more than 2 years. Sleep deprivation test can be done before stopping AED. If seizures are not precipitated by sleep deprivation, then it's relatively safe to discontinue AED. Normal EEG, MRI, and neurologic exam also can indicate that AEDs may probably be discontinued.

Common side effects of AED

Carbamazepine	Aplastic anemia, hepatic failure, rash, Stevens–Johnson syndrome, severe hyponatremia, agranulocytosis (neutropenia)	– Most AEDs can cause diplopia, ataxia, CNS depression, especially when serum AED levels are high – AEDs may also inhibit cytochrome P450 enzyme system resulting in multiple drug interactions – Most AEDs require routine CBC and LFTs follow up
Phenytoin	Rash, Stevens–Johnson syndrome, hepatic failure, gingival hyperplasia Cardiac arrhythmias and hypotension if administered too rapidly IV	
Ethosuximide	Gastrointestinal distress	
Valproic acid	Thrombocytopenia, aplastic anemia, hirsutism, and hepatotoxicity (MC)	
Lamotrigine	Stevens–Johnson syndrome, hepatic failure, rash	
Felbamate	Aplastic anemia, hepatic failure	
Topiramate	Kidney stones, renal tubular acidosis	
Zonisamide	Kidney stones, rash	

Abbreviations: AED, antiepileptic drug; CBC, complete blood count; CNS, central nervous system; LFTs, liver function tests.

10.14.2 Pregnancy and Antiepileptic Drugs

- The general rule is to continue the current AED in lowest possible dosage and to use a single AED.
- Avoid valproate in patients who are planning to conceive. However, in patients with established pregnancy, AED should not be changed (even if patient is on valproate), as typically this change will require overlapping of AEDs, exposing the fetus to multiple medications (which can be more harmful than continuation of original AED).
- Neural tube defects are commonly associated with the use of AED; hence, patients should be on folate supplement. Early detection of neural tube defects with serum AFP, amniocentesis or ultrasound **can be offered** to pregnant patients on AEDs.
- There is no specific contraindication to breastfeeding; however, lamotrigine (a sedating medication) may be an exception.

10.15 Dementia

Definition:

Mild cognitive impairment = age-related memory loss only	Important differentiating feature from dementia is that patient is able to perform activities of daily living, such as paying bills, driving, shopping, and cooking. They are able to use common appliances and are not lost in familiar environment in which they have lived for years
Dementia = memory loss + impairment of ability to perform activities of daily living	For example, inability to use common appliances, or are lost in familiar environment in which they have lived for years

Diagnostic evaluation:

The best way to diagnose dementia is **M**ini **M**ental **S**tatus **E**xamination (MMSE). It is a series of questions designed to test memory and other cognitive functions.[36]

After dx of dementia is made, first SIM is to rule out reversible causes of dementia.

Rule out vitamin B$_{12}$ deficiency	Check serum vitamin B$_{12}$ level
	Patients may or may not have associated features of macrocytosis, anemia, and/or subacute combined degeneration of spinal cord
Rule out hypothyroidism	Check TSH
	Look for constipation, weight gain despite poor appetite and slow reflexes
Rule out syphilis and HIV, in patient with risk factor/s for STD	Check RPR or TPHA and HIV antigen/antibody

– Brain imaging should always be done to rule out other pathologies.

Abbreviations: HIV, human immunodeficiency virus; RPR, rapid plasma reagin; STD, sexually transmitted disease; TSH, thyroid-stimulating hormone.

After reversible causes have been ruled out, we have to consider primary dementia-related disorders. See the table below for this. Important associations and diagnostic clues will point towards the underlying cause:

Dementia +.......	Most likely dx is
Urinary incontinence + broad-based gait	Normal pressure hydrocephalus[a]
Dementia with fluctuating course + visual hallucination +/-Parkinsonism (rigidity and bradykinesia)	Lewy body dementia[b]
EEG abnormalities + sudden jerky movements of limb Any age group	Spongiform encephalopathy[c]
Slow-writhing movements of limb (chorea) +/- myoclonus + family hx Onset < 50 yrs of age (can also occur in children /adolescents)	Huntington's disease[d]
Personality change → onset of dementia (Personality change precedes onset of dementia)	Frontotemporal dementia[e]
Dementia → personality change → psychotic features (Dementia precedes onset of personality change)	Alzheimer's dementia[g]
Features suggestive of depression[f]; here patient does not care about memory loss, so patient is frequently brought to clinic by a relative	
Features suggestive of depression[f] + patient is very distressed about cognitive impairment	Pseudodementia[h]
Features suggestive of depression[f]+ patient has features of parkinsonism (see 10.17 Parkinson's Disease)	Parkinson disease
Patient with multiple risk factors for atherosclerotic disease presents with **stepwise progression of cognitive decline,** or gait instability (falls)	Vascular dementia (a.k.a. multi-infarct dementia)
Dementia + focal neurological deficit	
Hx of HTN + slowly progressive dementia + CT scan reveals diffuse involvement of subcortical white matter	Binswanger disease aka subcortical dementia

[a]**Normal pressure hydrocephalus (NPH)**

Pathology: It occurs due to decreased CSF absorption, mostly in older adults.

Management steps:

– NSIDx is CNS imaging (CT or MRI). It will show dilated ventricles (hydrocephalus) disproportionate to cortical atrophy.[37]

[36]If you want to see what MMSE looks like, Google it.

Management of chronic progressive dementia should involve education of family members, optimization of dementia-oriented structural/functional housing and provision of optimal psychosocial support.

 MRS

triad of DUG for NPH
– Dementia, Urinary incontinence and Gait disturbance
("wacky, wet , wobbly")

[37] CT scan picture of NPH.

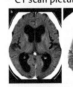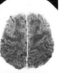

Source: Idiopathic Normal-Pressure Hydrocephalus.
In: Sartor K, Hähnel S, Kress B. Direct Diagnosis in Radiology. Brain Imaging. 1st ed. Thieme; 2007.

– After CNS imaging, NSIDx is lumbar puncture which will reveal normal pressure and normal cell counts. Usually large volume of CSF is removed for therapeutic purpose.

– If patient's gait and cognitive function improves after lumber puncture, then patient will likely benefit from ventriculoperitoneal shunt, which is the definitive surgical treatment.

[b]Lewy body dementia

Pathology: It is an idiopathic neurodegenerative disease due to deposition of abnormal protein called alpha-synuclein in the brain.

Presentation: fluctuating memory loss and confusion (hx may sound like recurrent episodes of delirium). Patients usually have associated visual hallucination (e.g., talking to people when no one is there, or seeing tigers) +/– features of Parkinsonism.

Rx: Supportive.

[c]Spongiform encephalopathy (of which Creutzfeldt–Jakob a.k.a. mad cow disease is the MC type)

Pathology: It is a neurodegenerative prion disease acquired by contact with infected tissues, or through rare spontaneous mutation.

Presentation: rapidly progressive dementia (progressive memory loss within a few weeks/months) and sudden jerky movements of limb or muscle twitching (myoclonus).

Workup: EEG will reveal periodic sharp waves. Get MRI brain and lumber puncture to check for 14-3-3 protein in CSF.

There is no treatment; disease is universally fatal within 1 year of dx.

[d]Huntington's disease

Pathology: It is a neurodegenerative disease occurring due to trinucleotide repeats mutation, inherited in autosomal dominant fashion.

Presentation: patients usually present with irritability, mood disturbance, and movement abnormalities such as slow-writhing movement of limbs (chorea) or sudden, involuntary jerky movements (myoclonus). Dementia also occurs.

Diagnostic evaluation: Brain imaging will reveal prominent atrophy of caudate nucleus.

Rx: For chorea, dopamine blockers such as haloperidol or risperidone may help. It is a progressive fatal condition.

[e]Frontotemporal dementia

Pathology: It is an idiopathic neurodegenerative disease with predilection for frontal and temporal cortex. Pick's disease is a subtype due to deposition of abnormal protein called tau.

Presentation: Onset is usually around the age of 40 to 50 years. Patients present with new-onset personality changes such as disinhibition (using dirty language and unprovoked shouting at friends or family). Exam reveals grasp reflex and snout reflex (primitive reflexes). (!)

[f]Old patients with depression can have memory loss (called pseudodementia) and patients with dementia (due to Alzheimer's, Parkinson's disease) can have features of depression; therefore, it can be hard to differentiate them in exam question. Look at the table below for differentiating features

MRS

Dementia in Lewy sounds like recurrent episodes of delirium.

Most forms of dementia occur in patients > 50 years of age. In younger patients with dementia, think of spongiform encephalopathy, frontotemporal dementia (in 40s), neurosyphilis, and Huntington's disease.

MRS

CC = chorea and caudate nucleus: atrophy of Caudate nucleus in Huntington chorea

⚠ **Caution**

(!) As frontotemporal dementia can occur in younger patients (in their 40s), it should be differentiated from neurosyphilis, since it can also present with social disinhibition and personality changes. Check TPHA/VDRL/RPR and look for risk factors for sexually transmitted diseases.

	[g]Alzheimer's disease Pathophysiology: neurodegenerative disease due to idiopathic deposition of amyloid protein. Genetics is implicated only in certain subset of cases.	[h]Pseudodementia due to depression		
Features	They usually are not concerned about their cognitive impairment, hence most of the time they are brought in by their family member. *These patients may have "SPACE" features but usually not the "DIGS feature" (see table on the next column.)* If you ask them MMSE questions they frequently confabulate, or they start telling you something that is really off topic	Patient is distressed about memory loss. They also have most of the SPACEDIGS features of depression.		
				Symptoms
			S	Sleep loss or gain
			P	Psychomotor retardation or agitation
			A	Appetite loss or gain
			C	Concentration loss or cognitive function loss
			E	Energy loss, or Easy fatigability
			D	Depressed mood
			I	Interest loss or pleasure loss (anhedonia)
			G	Guilt or feeling of worthlessness
			S	Suicide thoughts, ideations or preoccupation
CNS imaging	CNS imaging may show diffuse cortical and subcortical atrophy, particular in temporal and parietal region. The most affected area is hippocampus within the temporal lobe Do not choose imaging to confirm the dx of Alzheimer's because it is a clinical dx. However, neuroimaging is recommended in all cases of dementia to rule out reversible causes	Normal		
Hx of progression	From mild memory loss in initial stage to severe impairment of functioning	Usually nonprogressive		
NSIM	See below	SSRI's and psychotherapy		

Pharmacological treatment of Alzheimer's disease

- **Acetylcholine-esterase inhibitors (donepezil, rivastigmine, or galantamine)** may show small improvement in cognitive function. They are used in patients with mild to moderate dementia. If there is no improvement in cognitive function after 6 months of treatment, then these drugs should be discontinued.
  - Remember the cholinergic side effects, which are high yield; gastrointestinal stimulation (nausea, vomiting), cardioinhibition (bradycardia, heart blocks), etc.
- **Memantine** (a glutamate receptor antagonist) may be used in moderate to advanced disease.
- **Vitamin E** supplementation may be used in patients with mild to moderate dementia.

Acetylcholine-esterase inhibitors (donepezil, rivastigmine, or galantamine) may show small improvement in cognitive function in all forms of dementia.

10.16 Acute Delirium

Definition: Acute deterioration of cognitive function and/or mental status due to underlying sickness.

Background: Most common underling risk factors for delirium are dementia (any type) and advanced age. But note that it can occur even in relatively young patients, without underlying dementia, if underlying sickness is severe (e.g., intubated patient in ICU with severe pneumonia).

Precipitating factors: Infection (UTI is a common scenario), myocardial infarction, medications (e.g., benzodiazepines, opiates, anticholinergics, opiates, antipsychotics, anti-Parkinsonism drugs), etc.

Presentation:
- Hyperactive delirium: acute confusion and/or agitation +/- hallucinations +/- delusion
- Hypoactive delirium: lethargic patient (sleeps throughout the day and is not responsive)

In earlier/milder phase, symptoms can be waxing/waning. When severe, it can be persistent for days or weeks.

Management steps:

- First SIDx (step in dx): CBC, serum electrolytes, and consider urinalysis (to look for UTI). Find and treat underlying cause.
- Supportive treatment: Behavioral interventions (e.g., minimize staff changes, providing a quiet room, reorientation). If patient has severe agitation that interferes with treatment or patient is at harm to self or others, antipsychotics such as haloperidol, quetiapine or risperidone can be used with caution.

10.17 Parkinson's Disease

Background: It is an idiopathic disorder with progressive neurodegenerative loss of dopaminergic neurons in substantia nigra.

Clinical features:

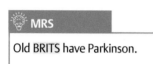

MRS

Old BRITS have Parkinson.

(!) If similar presentation occurs in children, think of Wilson's disease (due to copper deposition in basal ganglia)

Bradykinesia	Slow and stiff movement
Rigidity	In upper extremities, patients usually have cogwheel rigidity (due to resting tremor + increased tone of muscles)
	In lower extremities, patients usually have only rigidity (as resting tremor is usually absent in lower limbs)
Instability of posture	Leads to imbalance and falls
Tremor (resting)	It is present at rest and improves/resolves with intentional activity
	Tremor initially might involve only one finger resulting in the classic pill-rolling tremor
Shuffling gait	A succession of short small steps or slow hypokinetic gait
Other features that may be present are expressionless face (mask facies), stooped posture, and small handwriting (micrographia)	

Diagnosis: Clinical dx is made if exam finding includes bradykinesia + one or more of RITS. It does not require any specific diagnostic test.

Next step is to look for underlying secondary causes of Parkinsonism:

Medications	Chronic use of the following medications can cause Parkinsonism:
	Dopamine blockers such as antipsychotics (fluphenazine, haloperidol) and antiemetics (metoclopramide, prochlorperazine)
	Dopamine-depleting agents such as methyldopa or reserpine
Illegal drug use	MPTP: a synthetic analogue of meperidine has been shown to cause Parkinsonism
Any form of pathology (stroke, infection, tumor or trauma) involving **midbrain** can produce Parkinsonian features. Brain MRI can be done to rule out these conditions	
If no underlying cause is identified dx is **Parkinson's disease** (a primary disorder).	

Management:

The most disabling of all symptoms is bradykinesia. The slowness of movement makes patients' normal daily activities impossible. Therefore, management primarily depends upon the presence of bradykinesia.

Legend: DOC, drug of choice

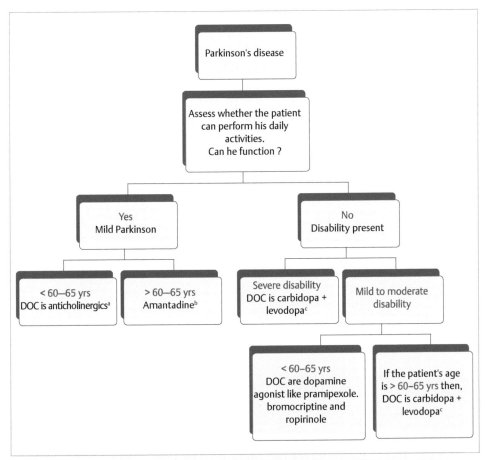

38 **On-off phenomenon**
After about 30 minutes of taking the medication patient may develop dopaminergic side effects such as dyskinesia (e.g., choreic twisting writhing movements) which is the "on effect." As the drug level drops down, patient may develop bradykinesia, rigidity, and tremors which is the "off effect."
For managing the "on-off" effect, we can add medications such as tolcapone and entacapone (they inhibit COMT enzyme, which degrades dopamine). Additionally, all patients should be advised to restrict protein intake at night.

ᵃAnticholinergics (benztropine and trihexyphenidyl) are particularly useful for patients with significant tremor. They are relatively contraindicated in old patients because they are more vulnerable to anticholinergic side effects such as dry mouth, urinary retention, and confusion.

ᵇAmantadine is an antiviral drug with anti-Parkinsonian effect. It probably works by increasing release of dopamine and decreasing its reuptake. It also blocks M-receptors.

ᶜThe combination of carbidopa and levodopa is the most effective medication for Parkinson's disease. Carbidopa inhibits extracerebral dopa-decarboxylase, which allows more levodopa to enter CNS to be converted into dopamine, where it has the most therapeutic benefit. Major disadvantages of this combination drug are dyskinesias, on-off phenomenon[38] and, sometimes, gradual loss of effect of this drug. So, it is usually not started unless required, and also not preferred as the initial agent in younger patients with mild to moderate disability.

Other therapies:

– Monoamine oxidase (MAO) inhibitors such as rasagiline and selegiline can be used in patients with early disease. Some studies report that these medications may delay disease progression, however it is controversial.

– Deep brain stimulation can be considered in some carefully selected patients with advanced disease. It has been shown to improve symptoms. Target areas for stimulation include subthalamic nucleus, globus pallidus, and thalamus.

Notable side-effects of Parkinson medications

Medication	Side effect	
Carbidopa–levodopa, dopamine agonist or COMT inhibitors (These medications increase dopamine transmission)	Dopaminergic side effects: **Early:** Psychosis, nausea and vomiting, anxiety, agitation, somnolence, confusion, and hallucination. **Late:** Dyskinesias, dystonia, akathisia, and on-off effect	The dopaminergic side effects are seen more commonly with levodopa–carbidopa combination

In patients with Parkinson's presenting with features of confusion, agitation, nausea, vomiting, it may be confusing to differentiate between dopaminergic and anticholinergic side effects. Look for other associated anticholinergic features (mydriasis for example).

Medication	Side effect
Trihexyphenidyl/ benztropine	Anticholinergic (atropine-like) side effects: confusion, constipation, urinary retention, tachycardia, angle closure glaucoma (headache, eye pain), dry skin or mouth, and GI stimulation (nausea, vomiting, diarrhea)
Selegiline	Coadministration with other serotonergic agents can lead to serotonin syndrome
Amantadine	Ankle edema, livedo reticularis (purplish meshwork-like rash), CNS excitation (hallucination and agitation), etc.

Dopamine related clinical effects

Too less dopamine = Parkinsonism	Too much dopamine = psychosis and impulsive behavior
Treatment of Parkinson is dopamine precursors or agonists	Treatment of psychosis = block dopamine
One possible side effect of dopaminergic treatment of Parkinson is psychosis and impulsive behavior	One possible side effect of psychosis treatment by blocking dopamine is Parkinsonism. They also have other extrapyramidal side effects such as dystonia, akathisia, etc.

Disease entities that have features of Parkinson's disease

BRITS + relative lack of response to carbidopa-levodopa +/- dementia + the following....	Diagnosis
Autonomic disturbance (impotence, orthostatic hypotension, dry mouth, dry skin) + ataxia	Multiple systems atrophy (aka Shy–Dragger syndrome)
Visual hallucinations + fluctuating cognition	Lewy body dementia
Prominent ataxia	Olivopontocerebellar atrophy
Vertical gaze palsy	Supranuclear palsy

10.18 Tremors

Cause of tremor	At rest	Goal-directed activity (e.g., finger to nose testing)	Additional pointers to dx	Management
Essential tremor	Usually absent, but can be present in severe cases	Tremor worsens	– May have positive family hx (familial tremor) – Is usually bilateral – Sedatives like alcohol make it better – Head bobbing might be present	Pharmacotherapy is initiated when symptoms are problematic DOC for intermittent disability is propranolol as needed. For more severe/persistent disease, use continuous therapy propranolol or primidone. If not significantly controlled, NSIM is combination therapy with propranolol + primidone[a]
Cerebellar tremor aka intention tremor[b]	Usually absent	Tremor is seen and worsens on activity	Other cerebellar features such as ataxia or nystagmus are present	Brain imaging: CT scan or MRI

Cause of tremor	At rest	Goal-directed activity (e.g., finger to nose testing)	Additional pointers to dx	Management
Parkinson's disease	Present	Better with movement	• Usually unilateral at onset • Look for other features of BRITS	For patients < 60 to 65 years DOC is anticholinergics such as benztropine or trihexyphenidyl For patients > 60 to 65 years, DOC is amantidine[c]

[a]Topiramate, atenolol, metoprolol, and alprazolam can also be used.

[b]Intentional tremors are tremors that worsen with goal-directed activities such as finger-to-nose testing or when reaching for a cup of coffee. Both cerebellar and essential tremor may fall into this category, but traditionally intention tremor is a name given for cerebellar tremor.

[c]Old patients > 60 to 65 years of age can develop significant side effects with anticholinergics. Amantadine is given instead of anticholinergic in this age group.

10.19 Peripheral Nerve Disorders

Presentation	Diagnosis and etiology	Management[a]
Atrophy of thenar eminence Loss of thumb adduction and opposition Sensory loss/paraesthesias in palmar surface of first to third fingers Cutaneous innervation of the ulner ulnar nerve — Cutaneous innervation of the median nerve	**Carpal tunnel syndrome** (Median nerve compression commonly in carpal tunnel) Etiology: hypothyroidism, diabetes mellitus, amyloidosis, pregnancy, occupational (typist, carpenters, etc.)	For moderate to severe case, especially with motor impairment, NSIDx is EMG and NCS. If it shows axonal loss or denervation, NSIM is surgical decompression. If no evidence of neuronal injury in EMG and NCS, and for mild to moderate cases, first SIM is nocturnal splinting. If still problematic, NSIM is glucocorticoid injection, or short course of oral glucocorticoids, along with continuation of splinting. Other conservative measures include carpal bone mobilization and yoga. For patients who continue to have moderate to severe symptoms despite conservative measures, surgical decompression can be done.
Sensory loss or paraesthesias in palmar and dorsal surface of fourth and fifth fingers Weakness in interosseous muscles (weakness in spreading out fingers) Atrophy of hypothenar area Clawing occurs late in the disease	**Ulnar nerve compression:** Occurs commonly in the elbow (in cubital tunnel) due to repeated elbow flexion or trauma/fracture Can occur in the wrist in the Guyon's canal (particularly in avid cyclist)	First SIM is elbow splinting and/or pads. In cyclists, use wrist splinting. For patients who have moderate to severe features despite conservative measures, NSIM is surgery
Sensory loss/paraesthesias in great toe and along medial foot Pain and numbness	**Tarsal tunnel syndrome** due to compression of posterior tibial nerve Etiology: flat feet, local swelling, arthritis, etc.	First SIM is conservative (orthotics, NSAIDs, shoe modification). If still problematic, NSIM is local corticosteroids injection. For patients that have moderate to severe features despite conservative measures, NSIM is surgery
Sensory loss/paraesthesias in lateral abdomen and thigh (usually unilateral)	**Meralgia paresthetica** due to compression of lateral cutaneous nerve of thigh Etiology: tight clothing, obesity, pregnancy, significant abdominal distention (e.g., large ascites)	Treat underlying cause

Foot drop (weakness of dorsiflexion of foot, which results in the whole foot touching the ground while walking), and Sensory loss/paraesthesias over dorsum of the foot and lateral shin	**Common peroneal nerve palsy:** commonly injured just below the knee, near the fibular neck. This can occur due to prolonged lying, leg crossing, squatting, leg cast or fibular neck fracture	Supportive management (extra-cushioning in affected knee while sleeping and avoidance of crossing legs), ankle foot orthotics, splint and physical therapy
Multiple, peripheral nerves are involved and may be separated in time and space. (Think of it as the multiple sclerosis of peripheral nerves.)	**Mononeuritis multiplex** Etiology: vasculitis, sarcoidosis, HIV, paraneoplastic, diabetes mellitus, etc.	Treat underlying disorder
Symmetric distal to proximal progression of paraesthesias and sensory loss (glove–stocking distribution)	**Axonal polyneuropathies** Etiology: systemic, endocrinal, autoimmune, medication related Diabetes mellitus (MCC), alcohol, uremia, hypothyroidism, certain heavy metal exposures, vitamin B_{12} deficiency, myeloma, paraneoplastic syndrome, chemotherapy (cisplatin, vincristine)	Treat underlying disorder
Unilateral lower extremity motor and sensory nerve involvement For example, severe unilateral leg pain and leg muscle weakness/atrophy	**Proximal diabetic neuropathy** (aka diabetic amyotrophy or diabetic lumbosacral radioplexus neuropathy)	Treat diabetes

[a]For most neuropathies, clinical dx is usually supported with EMG and NCS. EMG/NCS studies are mandatory prior to any surgical intervention. For persistent and/or problematic pain gabapentin, pregabalin, tricyclics, or duloxetine can be given.

Abbreviations: EMG, electromyography; NCS, nerve conduction study; NSAIDs, nonsteroidal anti-inflammatory drugs.

10.20 Neuro-oncology

10.20.1 Brain Tumors

Presentation: Patients may present with features of increased ICP such as slow-onset headache that is worsened by coughing or bending over. Depending on the location of the tumor, it can manifest with various types of FNDs (e.g., astrocytoma in the frontal lobe tumor can present with personality changes). They can also cause seizures by directly irritating the nerves.

Meningioma (Primary brain tumor)	MC intracranial tumor usually of benign histology. It is typically discovered incidentally. CNS imaging will typically show a partially calcified mass attached to or arising from the dura Management: surgery for enlarging or symptomatic lesion and observation for a small mass	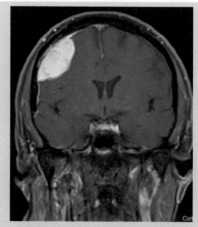 Source: Pathology. In: Gunderman R. Essential Radiology. Clinical Presentation, Pathophysiology, Imaging. 3rd ed. Thieme; 2014.

Astrocytoma (Primary brain tumor)	Astrocytomas are tumors arising from glial astrocytes. Low-grade astrocytomas are more often found in children, while high-grade types are more often found in adults. Best noninvasive test is MRI with IV contrast. Most accurate test is brain biopsy. Treatment options are surgery (debulking), chemotherapy, and radiation therapy Prognosis mostly depends upon histological grading, with grade IV astrocytoma (aka glioblastoma multiforme) having the worst prognosis. (Unfortunately, this is the MC primary malignant brain tumor.)	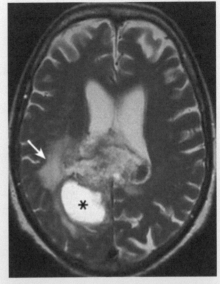 Glioblastoma multiforme: This T2-weighted image reveals a butterfly-shaped tumor in the splenium of the corpus callosum and adjacent regions of the two cerebral hemispheres. A cyst (*) in the right occipital lobe is part of the tumor; like the rest of the tumor, the cyst wall displays contrast enhancement. Source: Brain Tumors. In: Mattle H, Mumenthaler M, Taub E. Fundamentals of Neurology: An Illustrated Guide. 2nd ed. Thieme; 2017.
Metastatic	– Imaging can reveal multiple lesions located in grey–white matter junction. – Most common primary cancers are lung, breast, and melanoma. **Rx:** – For multiple metastasis of solid tumor, NSIM is palliative whole brain radiation. – For a solitary metastasis, with limited systemic solid tumor, NSIM is surgical resection, followed by whole brain radiation.	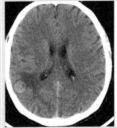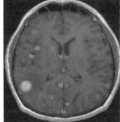 (Left image) CT demonstrates a round, hyperdense mass in the right hemisphere. (Right image) MRI of the same patient demonstrates numerous hyperintense lesions throughout both hemispheres, which are consistent with metastatic disease.

10.21 Additional Ancillary Topics

10.21.1 Restless Leg syndrome

Background: This is a common disorder. This condition is associated with sleep deprivation, caffeine, pregnancy, uremia, iron deficiency anemia, and peripheral neuropathy.

Presentation: Patients complain of creeping or crawling dysesthesias in the calves or feet or sometimes even in upper extremity, which is associated with irresistible urge to move one's leg or hands. As opposed to dysesthesias of peripheral neuropathy, which persists with activity, this condition is exacerbated/precipitated by rest and temporarily relieved by movement. Sometimes patient's sleep partner may report of patient having frequent involuntary flinging movements of the legs during sleep and the sleep partner may show multiple bruises sustained during the nights.

Management steps:

NSIDx is rule out easily treatable condition such as iron deficiency by doing iron panel.

If patient has evidence of iron deficiency, first SIM is iron replacement. In patients with end-stage renal disease, short-term intensification of hemodialysis can be tried.

Specific therapy:

- In patients with troubling symptoms and who are requesting therapy, dopamine agonists such as pramipexole and ropinirole are generally used as first-line therapy. If patient is having intermittent but troubling symptoms that are not frequent enough to get daily therapy, PRN dopamine agonist can be tried.
- If patient has comorbid insomnia, anxiety, fibromyalgia, or neuropathic pain gabapentin or pregabalin are generally tried first instead of dopamine agonist.
- If severe and unresponsive, other treatment options are benzodiazepine, opiates, or levodopa/carbidopa.

10.21.2 Brain Death

Background: Diagnosis of brain death is important in critical care medicine. This is of paramount importance in counseling patient's family member and for organ transplantation. An example of a scenario where brain death is considered would be in a patient after a prolonged cardiac arrest who has no obvious brain activity for 6 to 7 days.

How to make the diagnosis: First step is to exclude medical conditions that can confound clinical exam and/or cause coma (e.g., severe hypothermia, shock, severe electrolyte/acid-base/endocrine disturbances, drug intoxication and poisoning).

After excluding these conditions, do testing for brainstem and cortical functions.

There should be no cranial nerve reflexes[39] (pupillary, vestibulo-ocular, corneal reflexes, etc.) and no spontaneous respiration after hypercapnia challenge. Hypercapnia challenge is done by preoxygenating patient and pausing ventilator support.

[39]Deep tendon reflexes are preserved in brain death because it is purely a spinal cord reflex and not related to brain function.

10.21.3 Acute Intermittent Porphyria

Background: This is a rare autosomal dominant disorder related to deficiency of an enzyme in hemoglobin synthesis pathway.

Presentation: The following are the features of this disorder:

- **P**ain: patients usually present with recurrent episodes of acute abdominal pain. They may have multiples surgical scars in the abdomen for suspected acute abdomen.
- **P**eripubertal onset
- **P**henobarbital/primidone or other cytochrome inducers (e.g., alcohol) can precipitate an episode.
- **P**sychosis: acute hallucination/delusion and confusion
- **P**eripheral neuropathy with sensory and motor nerve involvement. Acute **p**aralysis with areflexia may occur.

Diagnostic workup:

First SIDx is to measure urine porphyrins and porphobilinogen.

Management of acute attack: IV hemin or carbohydrate load, which decrease porphyrin synthesis.

Prevention of attacks: avoidance of medications, smoking, alcohol, diet that can precipitate attacks. In more severe cases, other preventive treatment options include scheduled IV hemin infusions, gonadotropin-releasing hormone (GnRH) analogue , Givosiran (small interfering RNA directed against hepatic *enzyme*), and liver transplantation.

MRS

The 5 P's of AIP

MRS

Think Guillain-Barre syndrome with Psychosis.

10.21.4 CSF Leak

Etiology: spontaneous CSF leak, trauma, osteomyelitis, etc.

Presentation:

- Tinnitus
- Low ICP headache: headache is better when supine, or when tying shoes but worse while standing (orthostatic headache which is opposite of increased ICP headache).
- Patients usually have hx of clear nasal or ear discharge.

Diagnostic work up:

NSIDx is to check ear/nasal discharge for beta-2 transferrin (this is a protein found uniquely in CSF). MRI or radionucleotide cisternography is done for further dx.

Management: For new onset mild leak and mild headaches, do conservative treatment.If severe disabling low ICPheadaches, consider epidural blood patch (injecting patients blood into the epidural space). If the CSF leak doesn't heal on its own or a large leak, surgical repair is indicated.

Complication: Meningitis is the MC complication; MC bacteriological cause being streptococcus pneumonia.[40]

[40]MC bacterial cause is similar to the ones seen in otitis media, bronchitis and sinusitis.

Answers

1. These following points describe the location of lesion:

   - "Is it cortical versus brainstem lesion?" Crossed deficits mean it is brainstem.
   - "Is this lateral or medial brainstem lesion?" In this case motor weakness means medial brainstem lesion.
   - "Is the lesion in midbrain, pons, or medulla?" 6th nerve arises from pons, so this is medial pontine lesion. Do you remember which artery supplies this area?

2. Reverse anticoagulation (give fresh frozen plasma or prothrombin complex concentrate + vitamin K).

3. Bilateral internuclear ophthalmoplegia (INO). Remember the MRS: INO ADD. The affected eye has "NO ADDuction." In this case both eyes cannot adduct.

4. Bilateral INO is suggestive of multiple sclerosis.

5. Myasthenia gravis.

6. Check serum anti-Ach receptor Ab and schedule electrodiagnostic testing.

7. Anti-MUSK antibody.

8. CT chest with IV contrast.

9. No.

10. Yes (patient is < 60 years old and is postpubertal).

11. CNS imaging, as this is the first time presentation. If CT scan is normal, then the likely dx is migraine. If the same patient presents later with similar recurrent headaches, then dx of migraine can be comfortably made.

12. c: subcutaneous triptan, as patient has significant nausea.

13. Tension headache.

14. Cluster headache with associated Horner's syndrome (lid-lag + miosis).

15. 100% oxygen.

16. Steroids (e.g., prednisone).

17. Idiopathic intracranial HTN.

18. Continue the same drug because it can take weeks for the preventative medication to take a full effect. See below:

    - Delay for therapy to take effect for various conditions

Prophylaxis of migraine	Wait at least 4 weeks
Treatment of myasthenia gravis	*For steroids, the onset of effect is around 2–3 weeks and for azathioprine—onset of effect is around 1 yr*
Treatment of depression	Wait at least few weeks

11. Rheumatology and Musculoskeletal System Disorders

The Army Within

Our immune system fights against bacteria, viruses, fungi, protozoa, and rogue cancer cells. When the "army-within" fails to recognize our own cells and starts attacking them, it results in autoimmunity. Medications needed to treat autoimmune diseases, sadly, also weaken our own "army," increasing risk of infections and malignancies.

11.1 Autoimmune Conditions: General Points

Sometimes it is helpful to think of autoimmune conditions in two broad categories:

Primary mediator of autoimmunity	Humoral B-cell autoimmunity	T-cell-mediated autoimmunity
Gender	Female predominant	Male predominant
Conditions[a]	• Rheumatoid arthritis (RA) • Scleroderma • SLE (systemic lupus erythematosus) • Primary biliary cirrhosis • Autoimmune hepatitis • Sjögren's syndrome • Myositis syndrome • Autoimmune thyroiditis	• **P**rimary sclerosing cholangitis • **P**soriasis • **A**nkylosing spondylitis • **I**nflammatory bowel disease—ulcerative colitis • **R**eiter's syndrome or **R**eactive arthritis
Serological tests	Mostly seropositive, e.g., antinuclear antibody (ANA), rheumatoid factor (RF)[b] antimitochondrial antibody, anti-SSA, anti-SSB	Mostly seronegative, but may be p-ANCA positive • Associated with HLA-**B27**
Associated condition	• Increased risk of non-Hodgkin lymphoma and Raynaud phenomenon	
General treatment strategy	• Flare-ups usually can be treated with steroids. • In moderate–severe persistent disease, use steroid-sparing agents, such as methotrexate, azathioprine, mycophenolate, etc. As it takes some time for these to work, steroids are used as a "bridging" treatment.	

MRS

PAIR of B27

[a]Patients with one condition have increased risk of other conditions in the same group. For example, patients with RA have increased risk of Sjogren: patients with psoriasis have increased risk of ankylosing spondylitis.

[b]Note: ANA and RF are not only found in SLE and rheumatoid arthritis, but also in other autoimmune conditions and also in females and old patients with no connective tissue disease. Hence, presence of ANA and RF in serum is very nonspecific.

CCS	Dx
An old patient with positive RF and ANA, but no other features suggestive of inflammatory disorder	Normal
Positive ANA, RF, and symmetrical arthritis of hand–joints with deformity	RA

When asked about the most common cause (MCC) of death in a specific condition (e.g., what is the MCC of death in SLE, RA, ankylosing spondylitis, peripheral vascular disease?), the safest bet is to answer cardiovascular cause (it is the MCC of death in general population too). Also note that chronic inflammatory conditions such as SLE and RA are associated with accelerated atherogenesis.

It is easier to remember only the exceptions to this rule, e.g., for scleroderma, the MCC of death is lung disease, and for primary biliary cirrhosis-liver failure, etc.

11.2 Joint Pathology

Inflammatory versus noninflammatory: Presence of any of the following suggests an inflammatory arthritis:

- Morning stiffness >1 hour[1]
- Red, hot joint
- Elevated ESR (erythrocyte sedimentation rate) and/or CRP (C-reactive protein)

Acute versus chronic:

Acute (< 6 weeks)	Chronic (> 6 weeks)
Gout, pseudogout, and septic arthritis	RA, psoriatic arthritis, osteoarthritis, etc.

11.3 Rheumatoid Arthritis

Pathophysiology: In a patient with genetic susceptibility, an inciting factor (e.g., infection, smoking) leads to activation of autoimmune T-helper cells, causing joint inflammation.

Diagnosis: Made on clinical and lab findings, which include the following:

- Inflammatory erosive arthritis involving three or more joints: arthritis is typically symmetric and commonly involves metacarpophalangeal and proximal interphalangeal joints.
- Elevated ESR/CRP.
- Positive serum RF (rheumatoid factor)[2] or anticyclic citrullinated peptide.
- Extra-articular features are rheumatoid nodules, anemia of chronic inflammation, splenomegaly, amyloidosis, interstitial lung disease, etc.
- Duration of symptoms for > 6 weeks
- Debilitating joint deformities are common.[3]

[2]Rheumatoid factor is autoimmune antibody against our own Immunoglobulin G (IgG). Immunoglobulin M (IgM) rheumatoid factor is commonly tested and is specifically helpful in assessing the course and prognosis. But note that negative serum rheumatoid factor does not rule out rheumatoid arthritis.

[3]Typical hand deformities in rheumatoid arthritis.

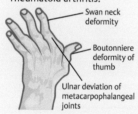

Swan neck deformity

Boutonniere deformity of thumb

Ulnar deviation of metacarpophalangeal joints

Management: Initiate DMARD (disease-modifying antirheumatic drug) as soon as diagnosis is made. DMARDs slow the progression of disease.

Severity	Choice of DMARDs
Mild disease	Hydroxychloroquine or sulfasalazine
Moderate to severe disease	Methotrexate

As DMARDs take some time to work, we can use nonsteroidal anti-inflammatory drugs (NSAIDs) or steroids for immediate symptomatic relief (bridging therapy).

Side effects of common DMARDs

DMARD	Side effect	
Methotrexate	• Hepatotoxicity and liver cirrhosis (with long-term use) • Megaloblastic anemia: use leucovorin or folic acid to prevent this.	In patients taking methotrexate, follow CBC (complete blood count) and LFTs (liver function tests) regularly.
	• Pulmonary fibrosis • Stomatitis (mouth ulcers and pain)	
Azathioprine	• Pancreatitis • Hepatotoxicity • Bone marrow suppression	
TNF antagonist (etanercept, infliximab, adalimumab)	Can cause reactivation of tuberculosis, so do PPD (purified protein derivative) test before starting treatment	
Hydroxychloroquine	Cinchonism (gastrointestinal and visual disturbances) • In patients taking this for long-term, perform regular eye exam	
Sulfasalazine	Side effects are similar to sulfonamides and penicillin (rash, hemolysis, Stevens–Johnson syndrome, etc.) Additionally, can cause drug-induced lupus	

Anti-**TNF** agents are **INFl**iximab (MAB = monoclonal antibody to **TNF**), eTaNeRCept (**TNF** Receptor antagonist), etc.

Disease associations

Rheumatoid arthritis	Dx
+ Lung problem (pneumoconiosis)	Caplan's syndrome
+ Neutropenia + splenomegaly	Felty's syndrome
+ Heart problem or kidney problem	Secondary amyloidosis

Complications:

Atlanto-axial subluxation	Patients with hx of RA who need to undergo anesthesia and intubation should get a cervical spine X-ray. If found to have rheumatoid cervical spine involvement, patients need measures to stabilize spine before intubation, as they are at increased risk of Atlanto-axial subluxation. This can lead to anterior displacement of vertebral bone into the spinal canal causing acute spinal cord damage.
Increased risk of Baker's cyst	This can form when inflamed synovium extends into the popliteal space. If it ruptures, it can present with swollen and tender calf (similar in presentation to deep venous thrombosis of calf).
Increased risk of osteoporosis	Screen with DEXA (dual-energy X-ray absorptiometry) scan regularly

11.3.1 Differential Diagnosis of Rheumatoid Arthritis

Parvovirus Infection in Adults

Risk factor: Frequent exposure to children (e.g., school teacher or day-care center worker).

Presentation: Recent-onset symmetrical polyarthralgia/arthritis with or without hx of classical rash (slapped cheek rash, or lacy rash that looks a like a fish net). It may be confused with RA due to symmetric inflammatory arthritis. Look for acute onset and history of contact with children.

Diagnosis: Check antiparvovirus IgM in immunocompetent patients. In immunosuppressed individuals, check viral polymerized chain reaction (PCR), as they are less likely to mount an antibody response.

Treatment: NSAIDs. It is usually a self-limiting condition.

Complication: Aplastic crisis or chronic pure red cell aplasia can occur in patients with hematologic disorder or who are immunosuppressed. Primary infection during pregnancy can lead to intrauterine fetal death and/or hydrops fetalis (due to severe fetal anemia).

Juvenile Rheumatoid or Idiopathic Arthritis (JRA aka JIA)

Pathology: Autoimmune joint inflammation. The difference between JRA and RA is that many people with JRA outgrow their disease, whereas RA is usually a lifelong disease.

Presentation: Can initially present with indolent isolated hip pain and progress on to polyarticular symmetric arthritis. Joint disease can progress rapidly.

Dx: Made clinically with the help of inflammatory markers such as elevated ESR, ferritin, and autoimmune markers.

Serology in JRA	
Positive ANA	May not be related with disease severity, but does signal increased risk of uveitis
Positive RF	May signal poor prognosis and increased chances of having disease into their adulthood

Management: NSAIDs + DMARDs (except in patients with low-disease activity). All patients are recommended to have periodic slit lamp examination, as coexistent asymptomatic iridocyclitis can lead to blindness, if left untreated.

[4]Even though rare, adult-onset Still's disease can occur.

Systemic-Onset Juvenile Idiopathic Arthritis (Formerly Known as Systemic JRA or Juvenile-Onset Form of Still's Disease[4])

Background: Idiopathic inflammatory condition that rarely occurs in patients older than 35 years. It is a subtype of JRA with prominent extra-articular manifestations.

Clinical dx:

- History of fever (intermittent high-spiking fevers for at least 2 weeks)
- Arthritis
- Salmon-pink maculopapular skin rash
- Increased inflammatory markers such as leukocytosis, elevated ESR, ferritin, etc.
- Patients may also have reticuloendothelial system involvement (tender cervical lymph nodes, splenomegaly, sore throat, etc.), and
- Serositis (e.g., pericardial effusion, pleuritis).

 MRS

Still too FAST
- Still = Still's disease
- Too = 2 weeks of fever spikes
- F = Fever
- A = arthritis
- S = Skin rash (salmon-red/pink colored), Splenomegaly, Serositis
- T = Tender lymphadenopathy

Rx: (low yield)

Severity	
Mild disease	NSAIDs
Severe disease, or not responding to NSAIDs	Anakinra OR canakinumab (these are IL-1 antagonists)

11.4 Sjögren's Syndrome

Pathophysiology: Autoimmune destruction of salivary and lacrimal glands.

Presentation:

Lacrimal gland involvement (known as keratoconjunctivitis sicca)	Burning and foreign-body sensation in eyes. Severe eye dryness can lead to corneal ulceration and scarring.
Salivary gland involvement	Results in difficulty in swallowing food (loss of salivary lubrication effect), dental caries (loss of protective effect of salivary secretions), and fissures in mucosa. Patients may have parotid gland enlargement.

Work-up: NSIDx is bedside Schirmer's test (a filter paper is placed in the eye and the extent of wetness is measured). Check anti-Ro(SSA) and anti-La(SSB), which are specific serologic findings. Most specific test is salivary gland biopsy of lower lip, but may not be necessary.

Treatment: Maintain oral hygiene (avoid sugary drinks and drink water frequently to keep the mouth wet), and use artificial tears and/or saliva. Second-line agents are pilocarpine or cevimeline (these are procholinergic agents that promote glandular secretion).

Disease association: Other female-predominant autoimmune syndromes (e.g., RA, primary biliary cirrhosis).

Complication: Predisposes to malignant lymphomas. MC type is mucosa-associated lymphoid tissue (MALT) lymphoma, which commonly arises from salivary glands but can occur anywhere.

11.5 Systemic Lupus Erythematosus (SLE)

Description: SLE is an autoimmune disorder that can affect multiple systems.

Patients can present with any of the following:

MRS		Additional info
SOAP BRAIN MD	Serositis	Inflammation of serosal membranes (e.g., pleurisy, pericarditis)
	Oral ulcers	They are painless.
	Arthritis	Migratory, symmetrical arthritis that is nonerosive.[a] X-ray of joints is normal. (This is in contrast to RA, which is erosive, and X-ray is abnormal).
	Photosensitivity	Sun exposure can cause flare-ups of malar or discoid rash.
	Blood disorder	Anemia, leukopenia, and/or thrombocytopenia
	Renal problems	Discussed in next page
	ANA positive	Sensitive but not specific test
	Immunological tests	Antiphospholipid, anti-Smith, and anti-dsDNA antibody may be positive.
	Neurological disorder	Psychosis, seizures, cerebral vasculitis, etc.
	Malar rash	Butterfly-shaped rash in the face
	Discoid rash[b]	This can cause scarring and atrophy

(a) Early lesion. **(b)** Late lesion with scarring. Source: Chronic Cutaneous Lupus Erythematosus. In: Sterry W, Paus R, Burgdorf W, eds. Thieme Clinical Companions - Dermatology. 1st ed. Thieme; 2006.

[a]Additional MRS ☺ I'M SANE even though I have SLE arthritis. SLE has Migratory, Symmetrical Arthritis that is Non-Erosive.

[b]Presence of only discoid rash is called discoid lupus. Patients with discoid lupus can have positive ANA, but anti-dsDNA or anti-Smith antibody is usually negative.

Work-up: If patient has any of the features of "SOAP BRAIN MD," NSIDx is serum ANA (which is the screening test). If ANA is positive, NSIDx is anti-Smith and anti-dsDNA antibodies (these antibodies are specific to SLE, but not sensitive).

11.5.1 Renal Involvement in SLE

SLE can cause nephrotic or nephritic syndrome.

Pathophysiology: Immune complexes (anti-dsDNA antibody and antigen complex) are deposited in the glomerulus with subsequent activation of complement pathway, hence anti-dsDNA titers usually correlate with the severity of renal disease. Patients with high anti-dsDNA titer and low complement levels most likely have severe renal disease.[5]

Work-up: In patients with SLE, always check urinalysis and serum creatinine to screen for renal involvement. UA may show RBC casts and/or proteinuria. If significant renal involvement is suspected, NSIM is renal biopsy.

[5]Also, anti-dsDNA titer and C3 levels are used to assess treatment response.

11.5.2 Management of SLE

Mild disease	Antimalarials (hydroxychloroquine, chloroquine)
Moderate disease (nonorgan threatening)	Short-term prednisone + antimalarials
Severe disease (organ threatening, e.g., diffuse proliferative glomerulonephritis)	High-dose IV steroids + mycophenolate or cyclophosphamide[a]
Skin disease	Topical steroids. Oral antimalarials if refractory or generalized disease

[a]**Side effects of cyclophosphamide**
- Like any other antineoplastic agents, it can cause mucositis with gastrointestinal tract involvement (nausea, vomiting, diarrhea, stomatitis, etc.).
- Acute hemorrhagic cystitis: Mesna is co-administered to reduce risk. (Mesna inactivates the toxic component of cyclophosphamide in urine.)
- Increased risk of bladder cancer with chronic use.

11.5.3 Obstetric/Gynecological Issues Related with SLE

- Combined oral-contraceptive pills are absolutely contraindicated in active SLE (can worsen disease) and in antiphospholipid syndrome (double trouble for the thrombotic state).
- Screen all pregnant patients with SLE for SSA antibody (anti-Ro antibodies). These autoantibodies can cross the placenta causing neonatal lupus and congenital heart block.[6]
- In SLE patients with positive antiphospholipid antibody and history of prior fetal loss, use low-molecular-weight heparin and low-dose aspirin during pregnancy.

[6]Anti-La (SSB antibody) cannot cross placenta.

MRS

cROSS A placenta:
Ro = anti-Ro antibodies;
SSA = SSA antibody.

11.5.4 Drug-Induced Lupus

Etiology: It has been associated with the following drugs: **C**hlorpromazine (antipsychotic), **Car**bamazepine, Captopril, **H**ydralazine, **I**soniazid, **M**ethyldopa, Minocycline, **P**rocainamide, Penicillamine, Phenytoin, **S**ulfasalazine, Sodium valproate, **Quin**idine, **TNF** inhibitors (e.g., infliximab, etanercept), **Di**ltiazem, etc.

Presentation: Fever, arthralgia/arthritis, serositis, rash, pulmonary infiltrates, hepatosplenomegaly, etc.

Diagnosis: Specific test for drug-induced lupus is antihistone antibody. Presence of anti-dsDNA can occur with minocycline or TNF-inhibitor-induced disease. Low complement levels and kidney or CNS involvement are rare.

Management: Discontinue offending agent. Use NSAIDs for mild disease and steroids for severe disease. For persistent disease, start hydroxychloroquine.

MRS

CHIMP'S Queen Tonight Died of drug-induced SLE.

11.5.5 Other Causes of Migratory Arthralgia or Arthritis Besides SLE

Presentation: Joint pain (arthralgia) ± swelling and redness (arthritis) in different joints at different times. For example, CCS: patient presents with pain in the right knee joint. He also gives history of pain, swelling in the right wrist 3 days ago and left knee involvement 7 days ago.

Migratory arthralgia or arthritis + following findings	Likely Dx
Painless pustules (dermatitis) Pain and inflammation in tendons (tenosynovitis) ± signs of septicemia	Disseminated gonococcal infection. Complication is gonococcal septic arthritis.
+ Fat malabsorption + Skin pigmentation + Generalized lymphadenopathy	Whipple disease
+ Hiking trip + Hx of target-like rash + Living in areas endemic for Lyme disease	Lyme disease
Recent hx of infection (diarrhea or urethritis)	Reactive arthritis due to *Campylobacter jejuni* or *Chlamydia trachomatis* infection
+ Hx of strep infection + Carditis, chorea, subcutaneous nodules, or erythema marginatum	Rheumatic fever

11.6 Sclerosis (Scleroderma[7])

11.6.1 Systemic Sclerosis (aka Systemic Scleroderma)

[7]
- Localized to specific organs = **CREST syndrome**.
- Systemic involvement = **systemic sclerosis**.

Background: An autoimmune disorder involving multiple organs in which normal tissues are replaced by fibrous tissues.

Organ affected by fibrosis	Clinical effect
Lung	• Acute interstitial lung inflammation (indistinguishable from usual interstitial pneumonia) can be seen in earlier stages. Recurrent or persistent inflammation can lead to interstitial fibrosis (restrictive lung disease). • The combination of pulmonary artery smooth muscle fibrosis and interstitial lung disease can lead to pulmonary hypertension (HTN) and cor pulmonale (MCC of death in scleroderma). NSIDx is high-resolution computed tomography (CT) scan.
Heart	Myocardial fibrosis, heart blocks
Subcutaneous tissue of skin	Skin thickening in face, trunk, hands, and fingers • Some patients with systemic sclerosis may not have the skin findings (this is called systemic sclerosis sine scleroderma). *This is why I think systemic sclerosis is a better name than scleroderma.*
Esophagus and lower esophageal sphincter (LES)	Normal contracting smooth muscles are replaced by fibrous tissue, resulting in • Acid reflux and peptic stricture (mechanical dysphagia), and/or • Failure of LES to relax causing pseudoachalasia (nonmechanical dysphagia)
Small intestine	Fibrosis replaces intestinal smooth muscles causing stasis, which can lead to bacterial overgrowth and malabsorption.
Large intestine	Constipation and diverticulosis
Smooth muscles of renal vasculature	**Scleroderma renal crisis:** Abrupt-onset malignant HTN + acute renal failure ± microangiopathic hemolytic anemia. **Rx:** ACE (angiotensin-converting enzyme) inhibitor (drug of choice).

Patient also commonly have Raynaud phenomenon. Nail fold microscopy to look for underlying vascular changes helps in making the dx of systemic sclerosis.

Diagnosis: Made on clinical grounds and serology, as following:

Anti-Scl-70 antibody (anti-DNA topoisomerase antibody)

Anti-RNA polymerase III antibody

ANA with nucleolar pattern

Rx: Treatment is nonspecific and organ based. It also depends upon presence of ongoing inflammation. Commonly used drugs are immunosuppressants, such as methotrexate, steroids, hydroxychloroquine, etc.

11.6.2 CREST (Localized Form of Scleroderma)

Crest	Features
Calcinosis	Nodular swelling in the skin which can be painful or painless. X-ray will show subcutaneous calcification.
Raynaud phenomenon	See box below.
Esophageal involvement	Acid reflux and peptic stricture (mechanical dysphagia), and/or Failure of lower esophageal sphincter to relax causing pseudoachalasia (nonmechanical dysphagia)
Sclerodactyly	Thickening of skin folds in fingers or hands (sausage-shaped digits with very few wrinkles) 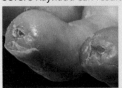Source: Fever in autoimmune diseases. In: Siegenthaler W, ed. Siegenthaler's Differential Diagnosis in Internal Medicine: From Symptom to Diagnosis. 1st ed. Thieme; 2007.
Telangiectasia	Dilated blood vessels on the face and neck

Diagnosis: Made with clinical picture and presence of serum anti-centromere antibody.

Raynaud phenomenon

Background: Can be primary (isolated disorder) or secondary (associated with underlying autoimmune condition such as scleroderma, SLE, RA, dermato/poly-myositis, etc.).

Presentation: Triggers such as cold exposure or emotional upset may incite an episode which typically occurs in the following sequence:

- **P**allor and **P**ain (due to vasoconstriction) → **C**yanosis (deoxygenation) → **R**edness (reactive vasodilation after ischemia).

Severe Raynaud can result in prolonged cyanosis, finger-tip necrosis, and ulcer.

Ulcers on the fingertips in severe Raynaud.
Source: Fever in autoimmune diseases. In: Siegenthaler W, ed. Siegenthaler's Differential Diagnosis in Internal Medicine: From Symptom to Diagnosis. 1st ed. Thieme; 2007

Diagnosis: Nailfold microscopy is most commonly used for aiding in diagnosis (underlying vascular changes point toward underlying autoimmune disorder). NSIDx: check ANA.

Treatment: Try conservative measures first—avoid smoking and cold exposure (use gloves and wool stockings). If not responding, use nifedipine or amlodipine (decreases vasoconstriction).

MRS

Scl-70 = **scl**erosis in **70** organs = systemic diffuse sclerosis.
Anti-**DNA** (topoisomerase) and **RNA** (polymerase) antibodies occur in sclero**DeRMA**.
Both DNA and RNA are located chiefly in the **nucleolus** of nucleus. So, ANA is chiefly of nucleolar pattern.

MRS

CREST = **C**entro**mere** antibody.

MRS

PCR of Raynaud

11.6.3 Differentiating CREST and Scleroderma

- In CREST syndrome, skin involvement is localized to the face, hands, and forearm (i.e., acral distribution only). In systemic sclerosis, the skin involvement can involve the whole body including trunk and arms.
- Any feature of CREST with additional involvement of any other organ, except isolated pulmonary HTN, is systemic sclerosis. **Note:** CREST can also be associated with pulmonary HTN (loud P2 sound on heart auscultation), but is usually not accompanied by pulmonary parenchymal fibrosis.

Nephrogenic systemic fibrosis
Gadolinium contrast (given with magnetic resonance imaging [MRI]) is almost exclusively excreted by kidney. If given to patients with advanced kidney disease, it can remain in tissues causing reactive fibrosis. Skin findings include patches, plaques, and peau d'orange appearance, along with sclerodactyly and other features similar to systemic scleroderma.

11.7 Dermatomyositis and Polymyositis

	Dermatomyositis		Polymyositis
Pathophysiology	Autoimmune inflammation of muscles		
Presentation	• Symmetrical proximal muscle weakness (e.g., difficulty climbing stairs, getting up from the chair, combing, carrying grocery bags) • Patients can also have swallowing problems (oropharyngeal dysphagia, nasal regurgitation, and/or aspiration)		
Differentiating features	**Rash present**		**No rash**
	Scaly, red or violaceous, papule or plaques on the dorsal surface of small hand joints (Gottron's plaques) Source: Clinical features. In: Sterry W, Paus R, Burgdorf W, eds. Thieme Clinical Companions — Dermatology. 1st ed. Thieme; 2006.	Red or violaceous rash around eyes (aka heliotrope rash) and nose Source: Dermatomyositis. In: Laskaris G, ed. Color Atlas of Oral Diseases: Diagnosis and Treatment. 4th ed. Thieme; 2017.	
	Could be paraneoplastic (associated with underlying malignancy)[a]		Not associated with malignancy
Steps in Dx	**First step:** Muscle creatine kinase (CK) and enolase (both will be high). Additionally, check myositis-specific antibodies (e.g., anti-Jo-1 antibody[MRS-1]). **Second step:** Electromyography (shows spontaneous fibrillation and decreased muscle potential). **Third step:** Muscle biopsy (most specific test).		
Initial treatment to achieve remission	Oral corticosteroids as a bridging therapy with initiation of azathioprine, methotrexate, or mycophenolate at the same time when steroid is started.		
After achieving disease remission	If patient remains stable, try to taper off steroids. If no flare-up after a slow steroid taper, can attempt to taper off immunosuppressant.		

[a]Think of the following conditions when muscle weakness is associated with malignancy:
- **M**yasthenia **g**ravis: typically associated with thymoma which can be benign or malignant.
- **D**ermato**m**yositis: various malignancies.
- **L**ambert–**E**aton: small-cell cancer.

MRS

Think **MG, DM, LE**.

MRS

MRS-1 **M**O**J**O—**M**y**O**sitis **J**o-1 antibody. This antibody is directed against histidyl-tRNA synthetase. Presence of this antibody is associated with higher incidence of lung fibrosis.

11.8 Mixed Connective Tissue Disorder

Presentation: Overlapping symptoms of SLE, scleroderma, and/or myositis.

Various presentation scenarios:

- 35 y/o F presents with complain of food getting stuck in the chest while swallowing and skin thickening (sounds like systemic scleroderma). She also gives hx of difficulty to climb stairs (sounds like myositis).
- 45 y/o F presents with symmetrical skin thickening of hands (scleroderma). She also gives hx of photosensitive facial rash and has hx of pericarditis (sounds like SLE now).
- Patients can have positive RF and ANA.

Serology: Serum antiribonucleoprotein antibody (specific test).

Rx: Depending upon severity, can be treated with antimalarials, steroids, or immunosuppressants.

Prognosis: Patients with features of systemic sclerosis or polymyositis have poorer prognosis.

11.9 Polymyalgia Rheumatica (PMR)

Presentation: Poly = multiple, myalgia = muscle pain, rheumatica = joint pain. Patients have chronic malaise, muscle pains, joint pains, and/or stiffness which is typically proximal and bilateral (e.g., neck, shoulder, hips, and thighs).

It can be associated with giant-cell arteritis, so patients presenting with PMR should be asked about presence of temporal headache or tenderness, recent-onset visual problems, and jaw claudication.

Work-up: NSIDx is ESR (it is usually ≥40 mm/h). Check muscle enzymes to rule out myositis. If both ESR and CRP are low, diagnosis is very less likely.

Rx: Low-dose prednisone. If patients have symptoms suggestive of giant-cell arteritis, NSIM is high-dose prednisone and temporal artery biopsy.

11.10 Fibromyalgia

Background: Thought to be related to underlying psychological stress affecting nerve fibers, causing their hyperactivity and increased sensitivity.

Presentation: Chronic pain in multiple areas (including myalgia, muscle stiffness, and/or arthralgias), which typically coexists depression–anxiety disorder (e.g., presence of sleep disturbances, chronic fatigue).

Clinical findings: Physical exam may elicit pain in tender points (shoulder, knee, buttocks, etc.). Usually there are no objective findings of inflammation such as erythema or edema. ESR and CK are normal.

Management:

- First SIM is exercise program, yoga ± trial of low-dose tricyclic antidepressants (e.g., amitriptyline).
- Second line:

| Fatigue-dominant disease | Use duloxetine or milnacipran |
| Insomnia-dominant disease | Pregabalin (night time) or gabapentin |

- Third-line treatments: Combination drug therapy, monitored physical therapy, cognitive behavioral therapy, etc.

Differential Dx: chronic fatigue syndrome: Patients present with extreme fatigue of more than 6 months' duration in absence of muscle pain and/or tenderness. Dx is made only after all other conditions are ruled out (including hypothyroidism).

In a nutshell

Differential dx of muscle weakness/stiffness and/or pain[8]

Dx	ESR	CK	TSH
Poly- or dermatomyositis	↑ ↑	↑ ↑	N
PMR	↑ ↑	N	N
Hypothyroidism	N	↑ or N	↑ ↑
Fibromyalgia	N	N	N

 Clinical Case Scenarios

1. A 65 y/o female patient presents with 6 months hx of generalized muscle pain, malaise, and low-grade fever. ESR is elevated and CK is normal. What is the like dx?

2. A 35 y/o female patient presents with 6 months hx of generalized muscle pain, malaise, and low-grade fever. Exam reveals extreme tenderness in shoulder girdle and medial knee area. ESR, CRP, thyroid stimulating hormone (TSH), and CK are normal. Patient is not on any statin or steroid therapy. What is the likely dx?

3. A 45 y/o female patients present with extreme fatigue of more than 8 months' duration. There is no history of muscle pain and/or tenderness. Physical exam is unremarkable. What is the NSIDx?

11.11 Seronegative Spondyloarthropathy

- **R**eactive arthritis
- **E**nteropathic arthritis
- **A**nkylosing spondylitis
- **P**soriatic arthritis

As the name implies, seronegative spondyloarthropathy is a group of inflammatory joint conditions in which rheumatoid factor is negative. They have the following features in common (let's name them *REAP features*):

- They are male-predominant autoimmune conditions associated with HLA-B27.[9]
- The REAP conditions, unlike rheumatoid arthritis, are likely to involve lower back and sacroiliac joint (sacroiliitis). Back pain is usually associated with morning stiffness that improves with activity.
- Most of the time when patients present with back pain and if one of REAP condition is suspected, the best initial test is lumbosacral spine X-ray (not HLA-B27 testing).
- They may also involve other joints (knee, hands, etc.).
- Enthesopathy (inflammation of tendons and/or ligaments) is common. Patients may present with heel pain (Achilles tendonitis), pain in iliac crest, or tibial tuberosity.
- Dactylitis is common in psoriatic arthritis, but can occur in any of the REAP. Look for asymmetric involvement of fingers, with diffuse finger edema (sausage-shaped digits) and pain.
- Any of the REAP can be associated with anterior uveitis. NSIM in this case is steroids and urgent referral to an ophthalmologist.
- ESR/CRP may be elevated.

11.11.1 Reactive Arthritis

Presentation: Acute joint pain with preceding hx of infection. Look for history of nongonococcal urethritis or infectious diarrhea (*Campylobacter, Shigella, Salmonella, Yersinia,* etc.).

Besides the common *REAP features,* reactive arthritis can the following unique features:

Keratoderma blennorrhagica	The name may sound complex, but when broken down, keratoderma = keratinized skin (typically in palms and soles); blenno = mucousy or slimy; rrhagia = rupture or discharge. The rash in mild or early stages can have vesicles on a clean base, in later stages can look severe with a red surface and ulcers.	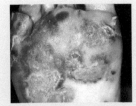 Source: Reactive arthritis. In: Laskaris G, ed. Color Atlas of Oral Diseases: Diagnosis and Treatment. 4th ed. Thieme; 2017.
Circinate balanitis	Circular painless shallow ulcers around the glans penis (balanitis)	

Reiter's syndrome is a subset of reactive arthritis that presents with the triad of reactive arthritis, conjunctivitis, and urethritis. It is commonly caused by *C. trachomatis*.

Work-up: Do X-ray of involved joints. In patients with joint effusion, arthrocentesis is recommended. Do HLA-B27 testing in equivocal cases. If patient history is suggestive of infection, do stool culture or nucleic acid testing for STD.

Rx: NSAIDs provide symptomatic relief. Treat underlying cause (e.g., in patient with chlamydial urethritis treat with doxycycline).

11.11.2 Enteropathic Arthropathy (Arthritis Associated with Inflammatory Bowel Disease)

Presentation: REAP features in a patient with symptoms of bowel disease. Arthritis can occur with intestinal disease flare-up or independently of it. This presents a diagnostic challenge when it occurs independent of intestinal disease.

Diagnosis: Made with clinical history and X-ray of involved joints. In patients with chronic vertebral joint arthritis, X-ray of spine may show findings typical of ankylosing spondylitis.

Rx: Treat underlying inflammatory bowel disease. In severe cases, a short course of steroids is used. NSAIDs are avoided as they may cause increase leukotriene production, aggravating bowel inflammation.

Differential dx: Reactive arthritis caused by gastrointestinal infection. When a patient presents with abdominal pain and bloody diarrhea with arthritis, look for prior hx of bowel disease or signs of chronic inflammation (anemia of chronic disease, thrombocytosis) which point toward enteropathic arthritis.

11.11.3 Ankylosing Spondylitis

Background: A chronic inflammatory disease of the spine and sacroiliac joint leading to joint rigidity and fusion.

Presentation: Look for chronic back pain in a male with onset in the late teens or 20s. In addition to the common REAP features, it can also involve heart causing atrioventricular block or aortic regurgitation.

Work-up:
- *Schöber's* test is a physical exam test to measure flexion of the back. It will reveal reduced flexion of spine.
- X-ray of the **sacroiliac joint** is the best initial test. Earliest changes are sacroiliac joint inflammation and squaring of vertebra may be visible. Later "bamboo spine" develops.[10]
- If X-ray is negative and there is still a strong suspicion, then MRI (which is the best test to diagnose sacroiliac joint inflammation) or CT scan can be done.[10]

Rx:
- NSAIDs are the mainstay of therapy for symptomatic control.
- Regular exercise and physiotherapy may decrease disease progression.
- If unresponsive to NSAIDs and symptoms are affecting life, NSIM is anti-TNF agents (infliximab, etanercept, or adalimumab). They slow disease progression.

[10]These changes are not specific to ankylosing spondylitis, as it can also be seen in chronic reactive, enteropathic, and psoriatic arthritis involving the lower spine.

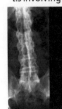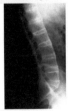

Bamboo spine.
Source: Imaging signs. In: Reiser M, Baur-Melnyk A, Glaser C, ed. Direct Diagnosis in Radiology. Musculoskeletal Imaging. 1st ed. Thieme; 2008.

11.11.4 Psoriatic Arthritis

Presentation: Arthritis may precede skin disease, so absence of skin lesions does not rule out psoriatic arthritis. Look for hx of asymmetric, distal hand-joint involvement, and sausage-shaped fingers. In physical exam, look for pitting of nails and rash (scaly plaques).

Work-up: X-ray of the involved joint typically reveals bony erosion and irregular bone destruction.

Treatment: NSAIDs as initial treatment for mild disease. Methotrexate for patients with more severe disease (e.g., presence of joint erosion or deformity) or when not responding to NSAIDs.

11.12 Gout and Pseudogout

	Gout	Pseudogout
Pathophysiology: Neutrophilic inflammation of joint incited by deposition of crystals	Uric acid crystals	Calcium pyrophosphate (CPP) crystals
Risk factors	Alcohol abuse, myeloproliferative disorders, diet high in purines, congenital enzyme deficiency (Lesch–Nyhan syndrome, glycogen storage disease, etc.)	Trauma or surgery[a]
Classic presentation: Fever, elevated ESR, and leukocytosis are common during an acute attack	• Most commonly involves the first metatarsophalangeal joint (podagra), but any other joint can be involved. • Diffuse erythema that looks like cellulitis may also be present and usually occurs with oligo- or monoarthritis.	Mostly involve big joints (MC is knee)
X-ray findings (not always present, but supports diagnosis if seen)	**Chronic gouty arthritis:** Well-defined punched-out erosion with a thin rim of calcification. Gouty tophi might be present.	Chondrocalcinosis (calcification seen in cartilages and/or ligaments)
NSIDx is joint fluid aspiration and polarized light microscopy	Presence of negatively birefringent needle-shaped crystals in joint fluid is highly specific for gout.(Elevated serum uric acid alone is neither sensitive to be reliable nor specific to be accurate.)	**Rhomboid**-shaped **positively** birefringent crystals[MRS-2]
Treatment of acute attack	**First line:** Oral glucocorticoids or NSAIDs if no contraindication (e.g., no creatinine elevation and no active peptic ulcer disease. NSAIDs are most effective if started within 48 hours of onset of symptoms. If one or two joints are involved, intra-articular steroids can be given. **Second line:** Colchicine (usually not effective if pain started >24 hours ago).	
Preventive treatment	Allopurinol[b] is indicated in the following situations: • Gouty tophi[c] • Two or more attacks per year, despite adequate life style modification[d] • Estimated glomerular filtration rate (GFR) < 60 • Hx of uric acid stone • Urinary uric acid excretion > 800 mg/day	Use colchicine[e] for prevention when three or more attacks per year. Manage underlying metabolic disease if present.

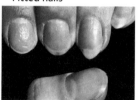

[a]In patients aged <50 years look for the secondary metabolic causes of pseudogout.

- Hyperparathyroidism
- Hemosiderosis or hemochromatosis[11]
- Hypothyroidism
- Wilson's disease

[b]Uric acid is insoluble and can easily precipitate. Allopurinol decreases uric acid production by competitively inhibiting xanthine oxidase, thereby decreasing conversion of soluble xanthine and hypoxanthine into uric acid. Allopurinol's side effect profile is similar to penicillin and sulfonamides (e.g., rash, hemolysis, allergic interstitial nephritis).

[c]Other urate-lowering options are Febuxostat and Pegloticase (a new agent that dissolves uric acid).

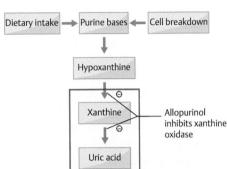

[11]If hemochromatosis is suspected, What is the NSIDx?

Answer: Iron panel and serum ferritin.

[d]**Examples of gouty tophi:**

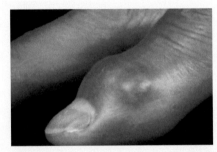

Source: Inflammatory rheumatic joint disorders. In: Siegenthaler W, ed. Siegenthaler's Differential Diagnosis in Internal Medicine: From Symptom to Diagnosis. 1st ed. Thieme; 2007.

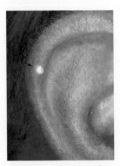

Source: Earrings. In: Bull T, Almeyda J, eds. Color Atlas of ENT Diagnosis. 5th ed. Thieme; 2009.

[e]**Lifestyle modification:**

- Avoid alcohol.
- Avoid high purine diets like organ meats (e.g., liver, kidney), certain seafood, etc.
- Avoid drugs which can cause hyperuricemia—diuretics (hydrochlorothiazide), pyrazinamide (antituberculosis drugs), etc.

[f]Side effects of colchicine include diarrhea and GI upset. Chronic therapy may cause bone marrow suppression.

Clinical Case Scenarios

Patient with no prior hx of gout presents with acute-onset severe knee pain, swelling, and erythema that started 4 days ago. He is found have few episodes of fever. He has baseline eGFR of 40. Serum uric acid is 9.

4. What is the NSIM?

5. Arthrocentesis reveals 20,000 WBCs/μL, negatively birefringent crystals, and bacterial Gram stain is negative. What is the dx?

6. What is the NSIM?

7. Patient's pain is relieved. Would you start him on allopurinol, or colchicine, or both?

11.13 Noninflammatory Joint Conditions

11.13.1 Osteoarthritis

Background: This is an age-related disorder due to wear and tear of the joint cartilage. It commonly involves weight-bearing joints like ankle, knee, hip, and vertebra. It is more common in patients who are obese or inactive (who have poor muscle strength to support joints). Hand-joint involvement is typical for people who perform manual labor (e.g., farmers).

Examples of presentation:
- Bilateral or asymmetric knee or hip pain that is progressively worsening, and pain gets worse on weight bearing and walking. Exam reveals decreased range of motion, crepitus, and joint deformity in the involved joints. Morning stiffness can occur, but there are no other signs of inflammation.
- Patient has hx of years of manual labor with hands. His hands show deformity and enlargement of proximal interphalangeal joint (which is called *Bouchard's nodes*) and distal interphalangeal joint *(Heberden's nodes).*
- In later stages joint effusion, tenderness, and instability can be present.

Work-up: Do X-ray of the affected joints. Typical changes seen are narrowing of joint space, marginal osteophyte formation (*blue arrows*), and subchondral sclerosis (increased radiodensity below the articular cartilage) (*red arrows*).

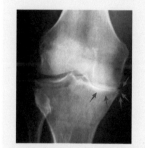

Note that lateral half of knee joint is not involved.

Management:
- If the patient is obese (i.e., BMI > 30), the single best SIM is **weight reduction**. Weight reduction reduces the stress in the joints and hence can decrease the progression.
- NSIM: **Acetaminophen (first line) along with** muscle-strengthening exercises. Second-line agents include NSAIDs (oral or topical forms) or topical capsaicin cream. Third line: intra-articular glucocorticoids or intra-articular hyaluronate.
- If no response to the above measures and symptoms are bothersome, surgery can be done (e.g., total knee replacement for knee joint involvement).

11.13.2 Charcot Joint

Etiology: Sensory neuropathy due to diabetes mellitus (most common), vit B12 deficiency, spinal cord injury, hereditary conditions, etc.

Pathophysiology: It is an extreme form of degenerative joint disease, in which absence of sensory nerve feedback (which normally prevents joint damage) leads to repetitive joint trauma. Repetitive trauma leads to stress fractures and bony deformities. Furthermore, skeletal deformities may result in pressure necrosis of skin, ulceration, and increased risk of infection. Weight-bearing joints such as knees, ankles, or feet are typically affected.

Presentation: Severe acute disease can present with swelling, erythema, and increased warmth which can be mistaken for inflammatory arthritis or cellulitis.[12] Recurrent attacks can occur. Patients can also present with slowly progressive arthropathy.

Diagnosis: X-ray is suggestive of very severe osteoarthritis with large osteophytes, bony fragments, and significant deformity.

Management: Acute presentation requires immobilization (casting) and off-loading. Long-term management includes decreasing further damage by using braces and customized footwear. Orthopedic/podiatric procedures might be necessary. There is a lower threshold for surgery in patients without diabetes (lesser risk of vascular nonhealing). If underlying disease is severe and complicated, amputation might be needed.

[12]In patients with joint effusion, arthrocentesis may be needed to rule out infection.

In a nutshell

Typical X-ray findings in various conditions:

Condition	X-ray findings	Insert picture	Pattern of hand involvement
Psoriatic arthritis	Marginal bony erosions *(white arrow)* with irregular fuzzy-appearing bone *(red arrow)* • Note the heterogeneity (different stages and sparing of other joints)	Source: Mc Ardle A, Flatley B, Pennington SR, FitzGerald O. Early biomarkers of joint damage in rheumatoid and psoriatic arthritis. Arthritis Res Ther. 2015; 17(1): 141.	DIP = distal interphalangeal joint PIP = proximal interphalangeal joint MCP = metacarpophalangeal joint OA= Osteoarthritis RA= Rheumatoid arthritis
Osteoarthritis	Joint space narrowing, osteophyte formation and subchondral sclerosis	Source: Diseases of the joints. In: Eastman G, Wald C, Crossin J, eds. Getting Started in Clinical Radiology: From Image to Diagnosis. 1st ed. Thieme; 2005.	
RA	Joint space narrowing with bony erosions and joint fusion[a] in later stages.	Source: Pathology. In: Gunderman R, ed. Essential Radiology. Clinical Presentation, Pathophysiology, Imaging. 3rd ed. Thieme; 2014.	
Gout	Well-defined punched-out erosion with a thin rim of calcification	Source: Inflammatory rheumatic joint disorders. In: Siegenthaler W, ed. Siegenthaler's Differential Diagnosis in Internal Medicine: From Symptom to Diagnosis. 1st ed. Thieme; 2007.	Can occur in any hand joint

[a]Joint fusion suggests inflammatory arthritis. Not present in osteoarthritis.

In a nutshell: Types of arthritis

Disease[a]	Distribution	Duration	Additional points
Rheumatic arthritis	Polyarticular and symmetric	Chronic	– Subcutaneous nodules on extensor surfaces – Cardiac, pulmonary and/or renal involvement
REAP	Can be oligo- or polyarticular, symmetric or asymmetric	Chronic[b]	Low back pain, anterior uveitis, dactylitis, enthesopathy, etc.
SLE	Migratory symmetric polyarticular arthritis that is nonerosive	Chronic	Multisystem involvement-skin, kidney, lung, blood, etc. (SOAP BRAIN MD)
Viral (MCC Parvo B19)	Polyarticular and symmetric	Acute	– May have hx of coexistent slapped cheek rash, or lacy rash that looks a like a fish net – Look for history of contact with children
Osteoarthritis	Mono- or oligoarticular, asymmetric or symmetric	Chronic	– Joint crepitus, decreased range of motion – Absence of inflammatory markers
Septic	Monoarticular	Acute	– Acute hot, red, painful swollen joint – Dx confirmed by arthrocentesis fluid showing gram stain organism or when culture positive
Gout/pseudogout	Mono- or oligoarticular	Acute	Gout—MC involved joint is first metatarsophalangeal Pseudogout—commonly involves knee or ankle joints

[a]All the following are inflammatory joint conditions, except osteoarthritis.

[b]Reactive arthritis can be acute or chronic.

11.13.3 Osteoporosis

Description: Diffuse thinning of bone due to defective mineralization mostly related to aging. This can lead to pathologic fractures. Diagnosis is most often made with screening DEXA scan (dual-energy x-ray absorptiometry or bone densitometry) test.

Indications for osteoporosis screening:

- All women aged > 65 years.
- Postmenopausal women < 65 years of age, and men with the following risk factors:
    - Active smoking
    - Excessive alcohol consumption
    - Chronic steroid use
    - Parental history of hip fracture
    - Rheumatoid arthritis
    - Estrogen-deficiency states: anorexia nervosa, low body weight, hypogonadism (e.g., Turner syndrome), etc.

Protective factors for osteoporosis:

- Obesity: adipose cells convert testosterone to estrogen
- High calcium diet
- African-American race
- Weight-bearing exercises[13]

[13]Swimming is not a weight-bearing exercise, so it is not protective of osteoporosis.

Other presentation scenarios of osteoporosis:

- **Vertebral compression fracture:** Sudden-onset acute back pain without hx of trauma. Back exam reveals point vertebral tenderness.
- **Colles' fracture:** Fall on an outstretched hand leading to distal radius fracture with dinner fork deformity.

Diagnosis: Made with DEXA scan which gives a T-score number. T-score compares patient's bone density to mean bone density of young adults.

T-score	Dx	NSIM (along with lifestyle and risk-factor modification)
Between −1 and −2.5[a]	Osteopenia (low bone mass)	Calcium/vitamin D supplementation In high-risk cases, consider oral bisphosphonates[c]
−2.5 or less[b]	Osteoporosis	Calcium/vitamin D supplementation + oral bisphosphonates[c]

[a]This means patient's bone density is 1 to 2.5 standard deviation below normal.

[b]This means patient's bone density is >2.5 standard deviation below normal.

[c]Bisphosphonates are drugs that have the suffix "+ dronate or dronic acid" in their name (e.g., alendronate, zoledronic acid, and risedronate). They work by inhibiting osteoclasts. Their notable side effects include esophagitis, bone pain, and osteonecrosis of jaw. In patients with gastric disorders, parenteral bisphosphonates can be given. In patients who cannot tolerate bisphosphonates, options include teriparatide[14], denosumab[15], and selective estrogen receptor modulators.

11.13.4 Avascular Necrosis (Aseptic Necrosis) of Femoral Head

Pathophysiology: Compromised vascular supply to femoral head leading to femoral head infarction and joint changes.

Risk factors: **C**hronic steroid therapy, **H**IV, **A**lcoholism, **O**rgan transplantation, **S**ickle cell disease, and **S**LE.

Presentation: Progressive unilateral hip pain which gets worse with ambulation.

Diagnosis: X-ray of hip may be normal (particularly in mild or early cases). If X-ray is normal and diagnosis is still suspected, NSIDx is MRI of hip (most sensitive and best test).

Treatment: Conservative management or surgical treatment depending upon severity and effect on lifestyle.

11.13.5 Paget's Disease of Bone (aka Osteitis Deformans)

Pathophysiology: Idiopathic increase in bone turnover, with rapid cycles of osteoclastic destruction of bone and osteoblastic bone reformation.

Presentation: Majority of patients are asymptomatic and have isolated rise in alkaline phosphatase. Symptomatic presentation is usually due to bony deformities causing nerve impingement (e.g., hearing loss, radiculopathic symptoms), morphological changes (increased hat size) or due to pathological fractures. Sometimes, high cardiac output failure can occur due to development of extensive arteriovenous shunting in hypervascularized bone marrow.

Diagnosis: X-ray usually reveals islands of bone thinning, sclerosis, and bony deformities. Serum calcium and phosphorus are normal. AKP and markers of bone destruction are increased (e.g., hydroxyproline, telopeptide).

Treatment: Bisphosphonates.

Complication: Most dreadful is **osteosarcoma:** look out for marked bone pain, new lytic changes in X-ray and sudden increase in AKP in a patient with preexisting Paget's disease.

11.14 Bone Cancers

Background: Bone cancers are more common in young adults and adolescents, as there's rapid bone growth and development in this age group.[16] However, certain bone cancers are more common in **older age** (e.g., chondrosarcomas, secondary osteosarcoma).[17]

Presentation: Bone pain, pathological fracture, weight loss, etc.

[14]Teriparatide is a synthetic parathyroid hormone. It is associated with an increased risk of osteosarcoma.

[15]Denosumab binds to RANK-ligand receptor and decreases osteoclast function and numbers.

CHAOS caused by decreased blood supply to hip.

POD

[16]Some cancers occur more often in young, e.g., **bone cancers and testicular cancers**.

[17]Conditions of high bone turnover, like **Paget's disease of bone**, increase **risk of secondary osteosarcoma**.

Type of bone cancer	Typically arises from	X-ray findings	
Giant cell tumor	Epiphysis	Soap-bubble appearance

Giant cell tumor of the distal metaphysis and epiphysis of the femur.
Source: Localized bone changes. In: Siegenthaler W, ed. Siegenthaler's Differential Diagnosis in Internal Medicine: From Symptom to Diagnosis. 1st ed. Thieme; 2007. |
| Osteosarcoma | Metaphysis | Periosteal elevation (Codman's triangle—*red arrow*) and sun-burst appearance |

Source: Pathology. In: Gunderman R, ed. Essential Radiology: Clinical Presentation, Pathophysiology, Imaging. 2nd ed. Thieme; 2000. |
| Ewing's sarcoma | Diaphysis | Onion skinning |

Note the marked lamellar periosteal reaction.
Source: Clinical aspects. In: Reiser M, Baur-Melnyk A, Glaser C, eds. Direct Diagnosis in Radiology: Musculoskeletal Imaging. 1st ed. Thieme; 2008. |

Management: Refer to orthopedic oncology.

MRS

E.G. MODE from top to bottom, starting with epiphysis.

11.15 Musculoskeletal Issues[18]

11.15.1 Musculoskeletal Disorders of Elbow and Hands

Pattern of injury and presentation	Physical exam findings	Dx
Hx of repetitive wrist extension movements (e.g., hitting backhand stroke while playing tennis). • Presents with lateral elbow pain	Tenderness in the lateral[MRSIII] epicondyle of elbow (origin of tendon of extensors of wrist). Pain is classically reproduced by forced wrist extension.	**Lateral epicondylitis of elbow**[b]
Hx of repetitive wrist flexion movements (e.g., playing golf or hitting forehand stroke of tennis) • Presents with medial elbow pain	Tenderness in medial[MRS-3] epicondyle (origin of tendon of flexors of wrist). Pain is reproduced by forced wrist flexion	**Medial epicondylitis of elbow**[a]
Hx of repetitive extension of thumb (e.g., repetitive lifting of infants) • Presents with pain in the lateral aspect of wrist (area around the anatomic-snuff box).	Tenderness in anatomic snuff box area. Passive flexion of thumb may exacerbate pain 	**De Quervain's tenosynovitis**[a]
Hx of too much use of fingers in a flexed position (e.g., barbers). It results in thickening of flexor tendon. **Presentation:** Finger stiffness, followed by finger getting locked in a flexed position. A popping or clicking sound is heard as one extends the finger.	Trigger finger (aka stenosing flexor tenosynovitis)	**Trigger finger (aka stenosing flexor tenosynovitis)**[a]
Presentation: Superficial cystic nodules that can be tender. MC location is the extensor surface of wrist and hand joints.	Compressible, mobile, cystic swelling that transilluminates.	**Ganglion cysts** **Rx:** For symptomatic or bothersome cysts, do aspiration, and if aspiration fails, do surgery.
Presentation: Progressive tightness in palmar aspect of hand **Risk factors:** Alcoholism, HIV, diabetics, etc.	Tight waxy skin in the palmar area with nodularities. Extension of fingers is limited due to subcutaneous fibrosis and contracture of palmar fascia. Fourth and fifth fingers are most commonly involved.	**Dupuytren's contracture.** **Rx:** Steroid or collagenase injections may help.

[a]**General management of inflammation in tendons, ligaments, and bursa.**

• First-line treatment is conservative management: avoidance of aggravating factors, joint protection (e.g., braces or splints), and NSAIDs as needed. Physical therapy is also helpful.
• Second-line treatment options include injection of corticosteroids, local anesthetics, or both in affected area.

[18]Most of the tables in this section is formulated in such a way that presentation and physical exam is given in the first two columns, and diagnosis is given in the last column. This type of arrangement helps students think about the diagnosis.

> **MRS**
>
> [MRS-3]**ELF M**an has elbow pain: **E**xtensor = **L**ateral Epicondyle: **F**lexor = **M**edial epicondyle.

11.15.2 Shoulder Pain (Rotator Cuff Dysfunction)

Mechanism of injury: Repetitive overhead movements (like swimming, playing tennis, or using a hammer) can stress the shoulder joint, causing frequent friction between tendons, muscles, bursa, and bone in shoulder. It can also occur in older patients as a part of degenerative wear and tear process, or due to intrinsic joint pathology.

The process starts with inflammation of rotator cuff tendons (rotator cuff tendinitis); this commonly occurs in supraspinatus tendon. Irritation of adjacent bursa can occur (e.g., subacromial bursitis). Calcification in the tendons can result (supracalcific tendinitis).	This presentation is known as **impingement syndrome**	Both presents with pain with overhead movements and inability to raise arm above a certain level. Pain of bursitis or tendinitis improves with lidocaine injection, whereas pain of rotator cuff tear does not improve.
With continued overuse this can lead to partial or complete tear of the tendon.	**Rotator cuff tear** This can also occur with sudden forceful movement of shoulder.	

Chronic/recurrent damage can lead to **frozen shoulder (a.k.a. adhesive capsulitis)**. This primarily presents with stiffness of the shoulder joint with or without pain. On exam both active and passive ranges of motion are decreased in all directions.

Work-up: Best initial test is shoulder X-ray. MRI is the most accurate test.

Treatment: Follow general management of inflammation in tendons, ligaments, and bursa (e.g., NSAIDs and physical therapy, steroid injection may help). Surgery, if significant disability or no response to conservative measures.

Thoracic Outlet Syndrome

Pathophysiology: Obstruction of thoracic outlet can occur due to cervical rib (congenital abnormality with an extra rib above the first rib), abnormal scalene muscles (e.g., hypertrophy due to excessive weightlifting), or congenital fibromuscular bands. This can put pressure on the neurovascular bundle.

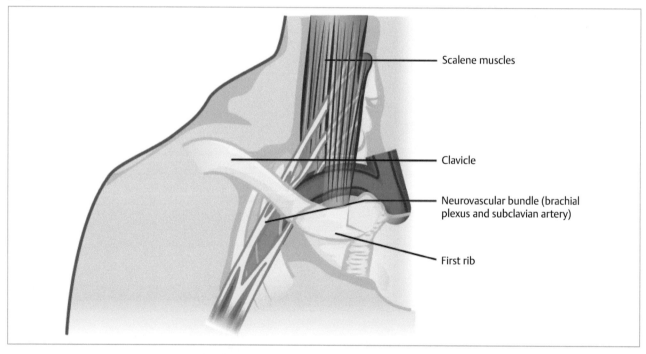

Presentation: Pain along the inner aspect of hand and/or arm, especially at night. The affected arm may be colder. On physical exam, the pulse disappears on deep inspiration when the affected arm is elevated, as the obstruction typically worsens when arm is elevated.

NSIDx: Doppler vascular studies.

Treatment: Mostly conservative, but in severe cases surgical decompression can be done.

11.15.3 Acute Back Pain

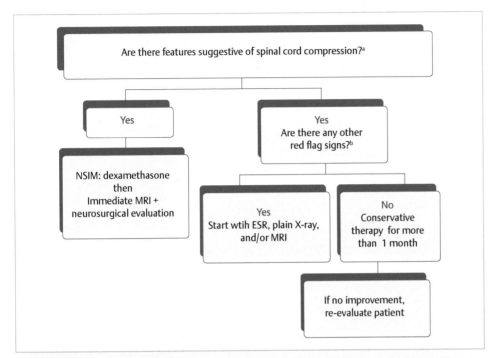

[a]Signs of spinal cord compression

Compression of the spinal cord	Loss of motor and/or sensory nerve function not localized to a single nerve root. Look for combination of *upper motor sign* (e.g., hyperreflexia) and lower motor neuron signs (e.g., absent reflex).[19]
Compression at the level of cauda equina	• Urinary incontinence/retention • Fecal incontinence • Saddle anesthesia: loss of sensation in the perianal area (the area upon which one sits on while riding a horse). • Absent anal and bulbocavernosus reflex[20] • Lower extremity sensory loss or motor weakness

[b]Similar to danger signs in headache. Look for the following:

• Fever or unexplained weight loss.

• Hx of intravenous drug abuse (IVDA).

• Exam shows exquisite vertebral tenderness.

• Back pain duration of >1 month.

• Nighttime symptoms interfering with sleep.

• Sudden back pain with spinal tenderness (especially with history of osteoporosis, cancer, steroid use) suggests vertebral compression fracture.

• New-onset back pain in age >50 years.

• Hx of trauma.

• Serious underlying medical condition (e.g., cancer, severe immunosuppression)

[19]Lower motor neuron symptoms (absent reflex, muscle weakness) in one nerve group alone do not point to compressive myelopathy, as this might be due to radiculopathy.

[20]Anal reflex: reflexive contraction of the external anal sphincter upon stroking of the skin around the anus Bulbocavernous reflex: reflexive contraction of internal/external anal sphincter in response to squeezing the glans penis or clitoris, or tugging on an indwelling Foley catheter.

In patients with acute low back pain with severe motor weakness , even though limited to 1 single nerve root, should be considered for an early MRI (e.g., acute severe foot drop).

CCS	Additional points	Possible dx and additional info
Sudden-onset severe back pain after lifting a light object in a patient with multiple risk factors for osteoporosis	Exam reveals point vertebral tenderness	**Vertebral compression fracture** • NSIDx is X-ray of spine
Low back pain in a patient with risk factors for bacteremia (e.g., IVDA)	Exam reveals paravertebral spasm and point vertebral tenderness. Fever is present.	**Vertebral osteomyelitis and/or abscess.** NSIM: blood culture, antibiotics, and MRI with IV contrast. If abscess is present and large enough, do drainage.
Back pain after lifting or carrying a heavy object	Pain may radiate to foot or knee. Straight leg raising test is positive. Radiculopathic signs might be present.[a]	**Prolapsed intervertebral disc causing back pain.**[b]
	Pain may radiate to buttocks, thigh, or groin (but usually not lower than these areas). Paravertebral spasm or tenderness is usually present.	**Lumbago a.k.a. lumbosacral muscle strain** It has good response to conservative measures[c]
Continuous lower back pain (that interferes with sleep) + hx suggestive of malignancy	Point tenderness might be present. Cord compression might develop.	**Malignancy is the likely dx** NSIDx: MRI with contrast.
A young adult presents with low back pain with stiffness in the morning that gets better after exercise	Look for other extra-articular findings	Ankylosing spondylitis
Low back pain in pregnancy	X-ray reveals increased lumbar lordosis	**Lumbar hyperlordosis**
Low back pain worsened by extension and relieved by flexion. It is worse with exertion, particularly when walking uphill.	Radiculopathic signs might be present.	**Lumbar spinal stenosis** (neurogenic claudication)

[a]Please see the image on the right to get an idea of what nerve root is likely affected when specific joint reflex is absent. For example, in a patient with acute left-arm radiculopathic pain and absent left elbow reflex, C (5,6) nerve root is likely involved.

[b]Management: early mobilization and adjunctive NSAIDs for pain. Second line for pain management is steroid injection. Imaging is indicated if pain persists after 1 month.

[c]Most helpful in preventing such episodes are keeping the waist straight and knees bend while lifting objects (i.e., bend at knee not at waist). Appropriate sleeping posture such as avoiding sleeping on stomach will also help.

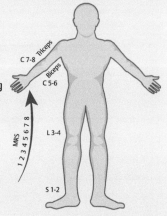

Clinical Case Scenarios

8. A patient presents with acute back pain after lifting or carrying a heavy object. The pain radiates to right knee. The patient has absent knee reflex in the right side. What nerve root is involved?

9. A patient presents with acute back pain after lifting a heavy object.
   Straight leg raising test elicits pain and radiation into the right buttock. There is right paravertebral area tightness. What is the likely dx?

   a) Prolapsed intervertebral disc disease

   b) Acute lumbago

   c) Lumbar lordosis

11.15.4 Hip Pain

CCS	Clinical findings	Dx
Recent-onset hip pain after running on a hard ground	Tenderness in the lateral hip area (cannot sleep on that side)	Subtrochanteric bursitis[b]
Pain in posterior thigh or buttock area brought upon by bicycle riding, running, or sitting for a long period of time	Sciatica nerve compression by hypertrophied piriformis muscle causes sciatic type of pain that radiates into the leg.	Piriformis syndrome
Chronic insidious-onset hip pain relieved by rest and worsened by weight bearing	Reduced range of motion, crepitus,[a] and tenderness in the hip joint area. Bland effusion might be present.	Osteoarthritis of hip joint, or in younger patients with risk factors, suspect avascular necrosis of the femoral head

[a]Crepitus is not a specific sign for osteoarthritis and can be present in other conditions.

[b]Manage as per inflammation of ligaments, tendons, and bursa.

11.15.5 Knee Pain

CCS	Clinical findings	Dx
Chronic insidious-onset knee pain relieved by rest and worsened by weight bearing	Reduced range of motion, joint crepitus, and knee tenderness. Bland effusion might be present.	Osteoarthritis of knee
Pain in the medial side of the knee that can result from acute trauma or due to repetitive side-to-side movements (such as in playing basketball or soccer)	Tenderness, swelling, and/or erythema in the medial side of the knee	Anserine bursitis[a]
Pain and swelling in the anterior aspect of the knee just in front of the patella. This can be due to acute trauma or excessive kneeling at work.	Erythema, tenderness, and/or edema over the patella	Prepatellar bursitis
Anterior knee pain specifically aggravated by knee flexion movements (e.g., pain aggravated by using stairs, squatting)	Elicitation of pain with pressure on patella	Patellofemoral syndrome

[a]Differential dx is proximal tibial stress fracture. Think of stress fracture when there is extreme pain or tenderness, and there is absence of inflammation overlying the bursa.

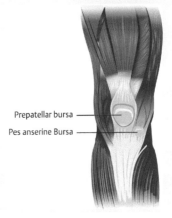

Prepatellar bursa

Pes anserine Bursa

Differential diagnosis of "leg pain when walking, but goes away with rest"

	Neurogenic claudication	Vascular claudication
Pathophysiology	Lumbar spinal stenosis can present as neurogenic claudication. Spinal stenosis occurs due to a combination of *vertebral osteoarthritis* and degenerative disc disease. The osteophytes from the vertebral joints along with prolapsed intervertebral disc can lead to compressed nerve roots and cause pressure on the spinal cord.	This is due to atherosclerotic narrowing of arteries supplying the leg. Increased metabolic demands, brought upon by exertion, can precipitate relative ischemia and leg pain.
Presentation	There is a relationship of pain with posture: buttock, thigh, leg, and/or calf pain *occurs or worsens* while standing straight and walking. Pain is relieved by resting, sitting, and bending forward. Similarly, pain is aggravated by walking uphill and goes away when walking downhill.	Depending on the severity of vascular disease, exertional leg pain can occur at various distances. If the vascular obstruction is severe, it can occur at rest. There is no relationship of pain to posture.
Associated features	• Preservation of pedal pulses • Coexistent low back pain • Can have radicular signs and straight leg raising test might be positive	• Diminished or absent pulses • Decreased warmth in the affected extremity • If hx of impotence is present, think of aortoiliac disease (Leriche syndrome).

Spinal X-ray	Changes of osteoarthritis can be seen	Normal X-ray
Best SIDx	MRI scan	Ankle: brachial index ≤ 0.9 is diagnostic.
Management	The mainstay of treatment is physiotherapy, along with NSAIDs as needed. Steroid injections may improve pain. Surgery is recommended when there is significant radiculopathy and/or myelopathy.	Aspirin, statin, and exercise treatment program ± cilostazol If patients have functional impairment, then bypass surgery or stenting can be done.

11.15.6 Foot Pain

Condition	Features	Management
Plantar fasciitis	Pain and point tenderness in plantar surface—commonly in the heel area. Pain is worse with the first step of the day or when initiating running/walking.	• NSAIDs, stretching exercises and shoe inserts. • Steroid injection is second line.
Stress fracture	• Focal point tenderness in foot • Commonly involved bones are the navicular bone and metatarsals. • **Risk factors:** Increased intensity of running and low BMI	See Chapter 25, General surgery for management.
Motor neuroma	• Pain or numbness at the base of 2nd, 3rd or 4th toe • When metatarsals are squeezed, there is a clicking sensation with elicitation of pain. • **Risk factor:** Runners, tight shoes	• Metatarsal support or padded shoe inserts • Surgery might be needed if refractory
Achilles tendinopathy (tear or rupture)	• **Risk factor:** Sports, avid running, or quinolone use • **Exam:** Pain in the posterior ankle area	• For tear, do conservative management (NSAIDs and avoidance of inciting factors). • For rupture, do surgical repair.

Acute Painful Leg or Toes with Signs of Decreased Perfusion

Signs of vascular compromise (pain, decreased warmth, and cyanosis) are usually present in the following disorders:

Single or multiple microvessel emboli	**Etiology:** Cholesterol emboli that can occur after manipulation of atherosclerotic arteries[a] Microvascular disease **Clinical involvement:** Only one or few toes (blue toe syndrome) are involved. In this case, pulses can be normal.
Acute macrovascular occlusion	**Etiology:** Acute cardioemboli or atheroembolism from proximal atherosclerotic vascular disease **Clinical involvement:** All the digits of one extremity can be involved and there is diminished pulse in that extremity.
Severe peripheral vasoconstriction	**Etiology:** Use of vasopressors (e.g., norepinephrine or phenylephrine) in ICU patients. **Clinical involvement:** Can have acrocyanosis of all digits (hands + toes). Significant pain is typically absent.

[a]Patients can have eosinophilia and renal failure.

11.15.7 Complex Regional Pain Syndrome (aka Reflex Sympathetic Dystrophy)

Pathogenesis: Possibly related to neurogenic inflammation due to excessive sympathetic nerve hyperactivity.

Inciting factors: Trauma/injuries (e.g., after orthopedic surgery or fracture), poststroke, etc.

Presentation: Intermittent or persistent neuropathic pain, sweating, and redness of involved extremity. Livedo reticularis (vague purplish net-like rash) can be seen in affected extremities. In chronic cases, X-ray can reveal osteopenia of bones in the involved area.

Dx is often made on clinical grounds.

Management: Analgesics, physical therapy, and for neuropathic pain, use amitriptyline, nortriptyline, or gabapentin. In patients with increased uptake in bone scan, use bisphosphonates. In severe cases, sympathetic nerve excision can be done.

11.16 Vasculitis

Behcet's syndrome	**Presentation:** Recurrent painful ulcers in the oral cavity or genital area, anterior uveitis, erythema nodosum. **Pathergy phenomenon:** Development of nonhealing skin lesions even after a minor trauma. **Rx:** Depending upon severity, colchicine, oral steroids, or immunosuppressants are used.
Relapsing polychondritis	**Presentation:** As the name giveth all, it presents as recurrent episodes of inflammation of cartilaginous structures. • Ear involvement: Pain in external ear + signs of inflammation. This condition does not involve the lowest part of the ear (ear lobule), as this area lacks cartilage, which helps to differentiate it from ear cellulitis. • Eye involvement: Scleritis, episcleritis, and/or conjunctivitis • Others: Larynx (hoarse voice), nasal septum, joints, etc. Source: Earrings. In: Bull T, Almeyda J, eds. Color Atlas of ENT Diagnosis. 5th ed. Thieme; 2009. **Rx:** Depending upon severity, NSAIDs, dapsone, oral steroids, or immunosuppressants are used.

Common features that could be seen in all types of vasculitis are fever, myalgia, arthralgia/arthritis, and weight loss. Also depending on the severity, vasculitis can be treated with NSAIDS, steroids, and other immunosuppressive agents.

11.16.1 Temporal Arteritis (aka Giant Cell Arteritis)

Pathophysiology: Autoimmune granulomatous large artery vasculitis. Its more commonly recognized symptoms, however, are due to involvement of smaller arteries in the head.

Presentation: Typical age of onset > 50 years of age. Patients with headache and temporal tenderness. Visual field defect, jaw pain, jaw claudication, and coexistent PMR (polymyalgia rheumatica) might be present.

Workup: First SIDx is ESR and CRP (ESR is usually ≥ 40 mm/hour). In patients with unilateral vision loss, urgent ophthalmic evaluation is recommended. In centers where cranial doppler ultrasound and expertise is available, it should be done to look for changes suggestive of temporal arteritis. Temporal artery biopsy is the gold standard, but diagnosis is often made of clinical grounds supported by ESR/CRP and ophthalmologic findings. It can however be done in equivocal cases, along with CT or MRI angiography of aorta and subclavian artery.

Management: High-dose corticosteroid (to prevent blindness) and patients might need long-term steroid therapy, on a lower dose.

Complication: MC is thoracic aortic aneurysm.

11.16.2 Other Types of Vasculitis

Condition	Arteries involved	Disease features
Takayasu's arteritis	Large vessel vasculitis—involving aortic arch and its branches	• Involvement of subclavian artery results in arm claudication and diminished or absent upper extremity pulses (therefore it is also known as pulseless arteritis) • Involvement of carotid artery can result in stroke • Aortoiliac involvement can result in Leriche syndrome (Dx is usually made on clinical grounds supplemented by MRI or CT angiography.)
Buerger disease (thromboangiitis obliterans)	Small- and medium-sized vessels (can also involve veins)	Major risk factor is smoking. Clinical features include the following: • Digit ischemia (e.g., ischemic toe or hands) • Vascular claudication with diminished leg pulses • Migratory thrombophlebitis: exam may reveal presence of red, tender, palpable cords in multiple areas. • Raynaud's phenomenon in legs or arms (Dx is usually made on clinical grounds supplemented by angiography. Immediate smoking cessation is recommended.)

Condition	Arteries involved	Disease features
Polyarteritis nodosa	Medium-vessel vasculitis	• Associated with chronic hepatitis B virus (HBV) and hepatitis C virus (HCV) infection (Hep B is more likely than Hep C) • Has multisystem involvement. It can involve nerves (neuritis), skin (palpable purpura[a]), renal (glomerulonephritis), gastrointestinal (abdominal pain after eating), and brain (stroke). Does not usually involve lung. • Arterial aneurysms can develop anywhere. (Dx is made by biopsy.)
Kawasaki disease		See the Pediatric chapter (Chapter 22).
Microscopic polyangiitis (MPA) Granulomatosis with polyangiitis (GPA)—used to be known as Wegener granulomatosis	ANCA-associated small-vessel vasculitis	• GPA is primarily associated with PR-3 ANCA (a.k.a. c-ANCA) and granulomatous inflammation. • **MP**A is primarily associated with **MP**O-ANCA (**p**-ANCA) and nongranulomatous inflammation. Except the above differences, GPA and MPA have very similar features and treatment: • They cause ANCA-positive necrotizing vasculitis, predominantly affecting vessels in lung, kidney, and ear–nose–throat. • Hemoptysis and nodular cavities in the lung • Nephritic syndrome and rapidly proliferative glomerulonephritis • Rhinosinusitis and otitis media • May also have uveitis • Can also involve skin causing palpable purpura[a] Treatment in severe renal involvement is with cyclophosphamide and prednisone.
Eosinophilic granulomatosis with polyangiitis (a.k.a. Churg–Strauss syndrome)		Triad of: • **A**sthma • **R**hinosinusitis • **E**osinophilia
Cryoglobulinemic vasculitis	Immune-complex-mediated small-vessel vasculitis	• Cryoglobulins are IgM antibodies that precipitate in cold temperatures[b] • Associated with Hep **C**, HIV, endocarditis, plasma cell disorders (e.g., multiple myeloma), chronic rheumatologic disease, etc. • Typically affects kidney (glomerulonephritis), skin (palpable purpura[a]), and nerves (neuritis)
Henoch–Schonlein purpura		Most often occurs in children **Presentation:** Abdominal pain, palpable purpura,[a] and renal involvement (hematuria).

[a]Palpable purpura = vasculitis. Biopsy typically reveals leukocytoclastic vasculitis.[21]

Nonpalpable purpura is either due to platelet issues or due to poor connective tissue support (senile purpura, long-term steroid use, etc.).

[b]They are different from cold agglutinins, which cause hemolysis in cold temperature.

MRS

Churg and Strauss **ARE** **E**asy **G**oing (**E**osinophilic **G**ranulomatosis)

[21]Leukocytoclastic vasculitis

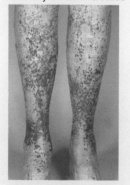

Source: Skin. In: Siegenthaler W, ed. Siegenthaler's Differential Diagnosis in Internal Medicine: From Symptom to Diagnosis. 1st ed. Thieme; 2007.

Clinical Case Scenarios

A patient with hx of SLE presents with *few months* of progressive left hip pain. X-ray of left hip is negative.

10. What is the likely Dx?

11. How would you confirm the dx?

12. A 75 y/o male is found to have elevated AKP and normal GGT. Differential AKP reveals increased bone isoform of AKP. He also has few months' history of hearing loss. What is the likely Dx?

    a) Osteitis imperfecta

    b) Osteitis deformans

    c) Osteodystrophy

    d) Osteomalacia

    e) Adynamic bone disease

Answers:

1. Polymyalgia rheumatica.

2. Fibromyalgia. This condition is common in outpatient setting.

3. TSH. Hypothyroidism should be ruled out in this case.

4. Arthrocentesis.

5. Gout.

6. Intra-articular steroid injection. Here NSAIDs are contraindicated because of kidney disease, and colchicine is likely to be ineffective as the onset started >24 hours ago.

7. Both. Start daily colchicine and wait for 2 weeks before starting allopurinol. Allopurinol is indicated to prevent gout flare-ups, because even if this attack was the first one, it was severe, and the patient has a GFR of <60. Also, starting or changing dose of urate-lowering therapy leads to acute changes in uric acid concentration. This increases risk of precipitating a gout attack , so concomitant colchicine prophylaxis is given to prevent acute flare-up, and continued for at least 3 to 6 months after achieving goal urate level.

8. L3–4 nerve root.

9. (b) Acute lumbago. Note that straight leg raising test is not a specific test for herniated discs. Also, the pain is radiating only to buttocks.

10. Avascular necrosis of left femur with a history of SLE.

11. MRI of left hip.

12. (b) Osteitis deformans (a.k.a. Paget's disease). Remember ☺ MRS. POD.

12. Allergy and Clinical Immunology

A tick bite from the Lone Star tick can trigger a severe allergy to red meat.

This specific allergy is related to a carbohydrate called alpha-gal found in red meat. So do patients become allergic to themselves? No! Interestingly, the alpha-gal molecule is found in all mammals except apes, humans, and Old World monkeys.

12.1 Hypersensitivity Reactions

Types of hypersensitivity reactions	Timing of presentation after allergen exposure	Major mediators	Presentation	Treatment (first step is to remove offending agents)
Type I—immediate	Occurs fast (*within minutes* to hours of exposure)	• Initial exposure leads to antigen-specific immunoglobulin E (IgE) formation.[a] • Subsequent exposure leads to formation of antigen–IgE complexes that crosslink → *mast cell* degranulation → release of *histamine* and other mediators.	**Urticaria:** edema of epidermis and dermis **Angioedema:** • *Edema of deep dermis*, e.g., lip or eyelid swelling. Overlying skin may or may not have urticaria. • *Edema of submucosal tissue* may involve respiratory mucosa causing respiratory compromise[b] **Anaphylaxis:** involvement of respiratory (respiratory compromise[b]) *and/or* circulatory system (vasodilatory shock) • Can present with or without urticaria or angioedema	• Mild to moderate urticaria: antihistamines • Severe urticaria or uncomplicated angioedema: antihistamines + oral steroids. • Severe angioedema or anaphylaxis (e.g., with respiratory distress): immediate *parenteral epinephrine* + oral steroids and antihistamines.
Type II	Occurs 1 or more weeks after allergen exposure, but can also manifest much later	Antibody mediated	Presentation depends on the target of autoantibody: • Autoimmune thrombocytopenia • Autoimmune hemolytic anemia, • Pemphigus/pemphigoid disorders, etc.	For severe, persistent disease, treatment options include steroids and other immunosuppressants. In acute severe cases, use plasmapheresis or IVIG. Splenectomy can be done if chronic and refractory.
Type III		Primary damage is from *immune complexes* (antigen–antibody complexes). Complement levels are typically low.	• Serum sickness reaction • Various forms of vasculitis • Immune-complex glomerulonephritis	For severe persistent disease, can use steroids, azathioprine, methotrexate, mycophenolate mofetil, etc.
Type IV cell mediated	Delayed (>48 hours after allergen exposure; sometimes may take days or weeks to develop)	T-cell mediated	Poison ivy, Crohn's disease, multiple sclerosis, morbilliform drug eruption, Stevens–Johnson syndrome, toxic epidermal necrolysis, DRESS syndrome, etc.	Varies

[a]Can be caused by anything: drugs, infection, foods, latex, bee sting, etc. Note that in a lot of cases history of sensitization might not be present.

[b]Severe angioedema and can overlap with early anaphylaxis.

Abbreviations: DRESS, drug reaction with eosinophilia and systemic symptoms; IVIG, intravenous immunoglobulin.

12.1.1 Highly Allergenic Drugs

Theoretically, almost *any drug* can cause hypersensitivity reaction, but the most notorious ones are the following:

- Sulfa drugs[1]
- Penicillins and cephalosporins
- Antiseizure medication (phenytoin, lamotrigine, valproic acid, carbamazepine, phenobarbital)
- NSAIDs (nonsteroidal anti-inflammatory drugs)

These drugs can cause all four types of hypersensitivity (urticaria, anaphylaxis, autoimmune hemolytic anemia, serum sickness, allergic interstitial nephritis, maculopapular rash, toxic epidermal necrolysis, Stevens–Johnson syndrome, etc.). They will be called "highly allergenic drugs" for the purpose of this book.

These drugs are commonly implicated but any medication has the potential to cause allergic reaction in a genetically susceptible individual

- Example: Allopurinol, various ACE inhibitors and proton-pump inhibitors are implicated in inciting all types of allergic reaction , but is less common than the highly allergenic drugs.

🔍 Clinical Case Scenarios

1. With diagnosis of otitis media, patient was started on amoxicillin more than a week ago. Patient now presents with new onset fever, rash, joint pain, and lymphadenopathy. ANA is negative. What is the likely dx?

An adult patient has hypotension and shortness of breath after a bee sting. Patient reports <u>no hx</u> of bee sting in the past. Exam reveals diffuse swelling of eyelids, lips, and bilateral extensive wheezing. He then develops hypotension.

2. Is this anaphylaxis?

3. What is the treatment?

12.1.2 Urticaria (Hives)

Pathophysiology: Edema of epidermis[2] and dermis due to mast-cell degranulation, most commonly as a result of type I hypersensitivity. Antibody (type II), immune-complex, or T-cell-mediated urticaria can also occur.

Classification	Acute urticaria	Chronic urticaria
Definition	Urticaria of <6 weeks duration	Urticaria for >6 weeks
Pathology	Most commonly due to allergic triggers	Mostly nonallergic
Likely etiology	Food (e.g., peanuts, shellfish, eggs), medications, insect bites, latex, infection, etc.	Physical urticaria[a], or underlying systemic disorder (autoimmune, vasculitis, malignancy, etc.)
Rx	Antihistamines (H$_1$- blockers)[b] For moderate to severe disease, also add H$_2$-blockers (e.g., ranitidine, famotidine)	
	Steroids can be used in significant cases not responding to above regimen.	In severe cases not responding to above regimen, use omalizumab (anti-IgE antibody). If not responding, use anti-inflammatory agents such as dapsone, sulfasalazine, hydroxychloroquine, or in more severe cases, immunosuppressives such as tacrolimus.

[a]**Physical urticaria:** Mast-cell degranulation due to physical factors such as exercise, sunlight, hot or cold temperatures, etc.

[b]Few notes on antihistamines (H$_1$- blockers).

---

[1]**Sulfa drugs**
Most of the drugs that fall into this category have the word "sulf" in them:

- **Sulf**amethoxazole (antibiotic)
- **Sulf**asalazine (anti-inflammatory drug)
- **Sulf**inpyrazone (uricosuric drug)

Additionally, drugs *which have the suffix "ide"* (e.g., chlorpropam**ide**—antidiabetic drug, *diuretics—furosem**ide**, acetazolam**ide**, hydrochlorothiaz**ide**, bumetan**ide***) have some sulfa component, but most are well tolerated and have very low cross-reactivity with other sulfonamides.

[2]**Classic rash description:** red or flesh-colored itchy bumps, with blanching erythema.

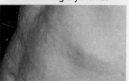

Source: Hyper84 at English Wikipedia, Public domain, via Wikimedia Commons.

Antihistamines (H$_1$- blockers)	Side effects
Promethazine, diphenhydramine	Sedation Also blocks alpha-receptors[a] and M-receptors[b]
Hydroxyzine	Less sedating (less blocking effect on alpha-receptors and M-receptors)
Newer generation antihistamines like loratadine, fexofenadine, cetirizine, etc.	Least sedating of antihistamines with minimal side effects, hence drug of choice for initial treatment of urticaria

[a]Can lead to orthostatic hypotension.

[b]Due to significant M-blocking effect, these can also be used for muscle spasms (e.g., for dystonia).

12.1.3 Angioedema

Definition: Edema of deep dermis, subcutaneous and/or submucosal tissue due to increased vascular permeability.[3]

Edema of	Clinical effect
Deep dermis and subcutaneous tissue	Puffy eyes, lips, face, genitals, etc.
Respiratory submucosa	Respiratory distress and arrest[a]
Intestinal submucosa	Colicky abdominal pain CT imaging may show bowel-wall thickening.

[a]In a patient presenting with angioedema, the first step is to assess airway. If there is impending airway compromise, NSIM is intubation.

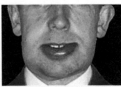

[3]Angioedema of lower lip
Source: Localized Edema. In: Siegenthaler W, ed. Siegenthaler's Differential Diagnosis in Internal Medicine: From Symptom to Diagnosis. 1st ed. Thieme; 2007.

Types:

Histamine-mediated angioedema or mast-cell-mediated angioedema (allergic reaction)	Bradykinin-mediated angioedema
Etiology: Most commonly due to allergic triggers such as foods (e.g., peanuts, shellfish, eggs), pollen, medications (highly allergenic drugs), insect bites, rubber latex, contrast media, etc. This can also be due to physical factors such as exercise, sunlight, hot or cold temperatures, etc. **Presentation:** Can present with urticaria or anaphylaxis (as this is an IgE-mediated reaction)[a] **Another rare cause** is mast cell hyperactivity due to systemic mastocytosis (a mast cell malignancy).	There are two major types: 1. **Bradykinin-mediated angioedema due to ACE-i:** this is the most common form of bradykinin-mediated angioedema (it can occur any time after initiation)[b] 2. **Bradykinin-mediated angioedema not related to ACE-i:** This can be hereditary or acquired • **Hereditary:** Genetic mutation resulting in decreased production or loss of function of *C1 inhibitor* (normal levels of C1 inhibitor is seen in the latter). • **Acquired:** Autoimmune antibody against C1-inhibitor due to autoimmune conditions like SLE or underlying myeloproliferative disorder that increases risks for autoimmunity (e.g., CLL) **Pathophysiology:** Decreased activity of C1 inhibitor → *increased C1 activity* → increased activation and consumption of complement proteins (low C3, C4) → increased production of *bradykinin* and other edema mediators.
Urticaria is mostly present	Urticaria is absent, and usually not itchy.

Histamine-mediated angioedema or mast-cell-mediated angioedema (allergic reaction)	Bradykinin-mediated angioedema
Rx[c]: • Antihistamines (H$_1$ and H$_2$ blockers) and glucocorticoids • Add epinephrine, if having breathing issue or hypotension. • After one episode of anaphylaxis, patients must always carry epinephrine injection. • Desensitization can be done when the trigger cannot be avoided[d]	Rx: • Supportive • For significant bradykinin-mediated angioedema not related to ACE-i, C1 inhibitor concentrate or bradykinin inhibitor (icatibant or ecallantide) is given. Second-line treatment includes solvent-detergent treated plasma or fresh-frozen plasma (they contain multiple enzymes which degrade bradykinin) • For significant bradykinin-mediated angioedema due to ACE-i, icatibant, ecallantide, or FFP can be tried, but is not of proven benefit.

[a]After an anaphylaxis episode, the serum tryptase level increases (tryptase is a unique mast cell protein). This is useful for diagnosis in atypical cases, but the level needs to be drawn within few hours of symptom onset, as it rapidly falls to normal levels within few hours of the episode.

[b]*Angiotensin-receptor blockers (ARBs), unlike ACE-i, do not decrease bradykinin metabolism. They act only by blocking angiotensin receptors. Hence ARBs can be given to patient with ACE-i-related angioedema.*

[c]If angioedema is idiopathic and does not fit into the above classification, treat as histamine-mediated angioedema.

[d]For example, patient has anaphylaxis due to bee sting, but he is a bee farmer and would like to continue to work. Prior to desensitization any adrenergic blocking agents (such as B-blockers) must be stopped, because epinephrine might be required if the patient develops an anaphylactic reaction during the procedure.

Abbreviations: ACE-i, angiotensin-converting enzyme inhibitor; CLL, chronic lymphocytic leukemia; SLE, systemic lupus erythematosus.

Clinical Case Scenarios

4. Patient started on lisinopril 6 months ago, now presents with lip swelling and respiratory distress. What is the likely dx?

5. A 24-year-old female with abdominal pain for the last few days. She has hx of intermittent abdominal pain and occasional lip, eyelid swelling for the last 3 years. Her father's two sisters have "some kind of recurrent swelling problem." Exam reveals nonspecific abdominal tenderness. CT scan reveals nonspecific small bowel-wall thickening and small amount of ascites. What is the likely dx?

12.1.4 Erythema Multiforme, Stevens–Johnson Syndrome, and Toxic Epidermal Necrolysis

Background: All of these are type IV cell-mediated hypersensitivity reactions that can occur with various drugs (especially "highly allergenic drugs") or infections (viral or bacterial). All can start with prodromal syndrome of fever, malaise, myalgia, etc.

	Erythema multiforme	Stevens–Johnson syndrome (SJS)	Toxic epidermal necrolysis (TEN)
Target lesions or bull's-eye rash	Usually present (*left picture below*)	Usually present	Might be absent
Extent of skin involvement	• Only a small area is involved (can occur in palms and soles) • *Can have* minimal mucous membrane involvement[a]	• < 10% of body-surface area is involved[b] • Mucous membranes are classically involved[a]	• > 30% of body surface area is involved[b] • Mucous membranes are usually involved[a]
	Source: Skin. In: Siegenthaler W, ed. Siegenthaler's Differential Diagnosis in Internal Medicine: From Symptom to Diagnosis. 1st ed. Thieme; 2007.	Severe lesions on the lips Source: Stevens–Johnson Syndrome. In: Laskaris G, ed. Color Atlas of Oral Diseases. Diagnosis and Treatment. 4th ed. Thieme; 2017.	Source: Qadir SN, Raza N, Qadir F. Drug induced toxic epidermal necrolysis: two case reports. Cases J. 2009; 2: 7765.
Management	• For symptomatic treatment, use topical antihistamines or topical steroids. • For severe mucosal involvement, oral steroids can be used. • Treat the underlying condition[c]	• Skin biopsy is useful in confirming the dx.[d] • Supportive treatment • In patients with extensive skin denudation, admit patient to a burn unit. Treat similar to burn patients. • Complications are also similar to severe burn—septic shock, ARDS, acute pancreatitis, acalculous cholecystitis, etc. • Respiratory mucosal involvement may require intubation.	

[a]For example, patients can have oral, ocular, or genital membrane involvement. Oral cavity involvement can present with odynophagia. Ocular involvement can lead to keratitis and scarring.

[b]Note: 10–30% is considered as overlap disease.

Description of skin involvement in SJS/TEN: Erythematous macules, papules, or target lesions which may later coalesce to form a diffuse erythema pattern. Look for multiple bulla formation and/or denuded skin (as bullae rupture). Nikolsky's sign is positive (gentle rubbing of the area near to bullae results in skin peeling off easily).

[c]For example, treat concurrent herpes simplex virus infection or mycoplasma pneumonia.

[d]Differential dx is staphylococcal scalded skin syndrome (discussed in next table).

FYI: Approximate mortality of TEN is around 40%, vs. SJS 5%. The larger the area of denuded skin, the higher the risk of mortality.

In a nutshell

	Clinical situation	How to differentiate	Skin biopsy findings
TEN/SJS	Look for highly allergenic drugs	Blisters/bulla + denuded skin Nikolsky's sign is present. It typically has mucous membrane involvement.	Involves subepidermal splitting of skin (at dermoepidermal junction)
Staphylococcal scalded skin syndrome[a] due to infection with *Staph. aureus* that produces an exotoxin called exfoliatin, which cleaves a desmosome protein.	It typically occurs in children or in immunosuppressed patents. May present with symptoms of primary infection that was the original source of exfoliatin (e.g., bullous impetigo, conjunctivitis, pharyngitis), followed by → diffuse red rash → fluid-filled blister formation → denuded skin.	Blisters/bulla + denuded skin Nikolsky's sign is present. *No* mucous membrane involvement	Desquamation of superficial layer of epidermis (intraepidermal separation)
Toxic shock syndrome[b] (another complication of staphylococcal infection, this time with production of a superantigen that nonspecifically activates T-cells)	Look for risk factors (use of tampons, nasal packing, surgical wound infection, postpartum patient, etc.)	Diffuse red rash Nikolsky's sign *is absent*. Hemodynamic instability and shock Superficial ulcerations in mucous membranes can occur. Desquamation, especially in extremities (including palms and soles) occurs 1–2 weeks after illness.	It is a clinical dx and biopsy is usually not done.

[a]**Rx:** IV antibiotics against *S (IV nafcillin or cefazolin). aureus*. If significant area is involved, may need to admit to a burn unit.

[b]**Rx:** Removal of foreign body and broad-spectrum antibiotics (e.g., Vancomycin + Piperacillin - tazobactam + clindamycin)

Abbreviations: SJS, Stevens–Johnson syndrome; TEN, toxic epidermal necrolysis.

In a nutshell

Target Lesion Aka Bull's-Eye Rash

Description: Erythematous rash with a central spot

Classic rash can occur in the following conditions	The following rash might also look like bull's-eye or target lesions
Lyme disease (erythema migrans)	Tinea corporis
Erythema multiforme	Granuloma annulare
Stevens–Johnson syndrome (SJS)	
Toxic epidermal necrolysis (TEN)	

[4] Fixed drug eruption

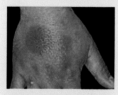

Source: Fixed Drug Eruption. In: Sterry W, Paus R, Burgdorf W, ed. Thieme Clinical Companions - Dermatology. 1st ed. Thieme; 2006.

12.1.5 Fixed Drug Eruption or Reaction

Description: The rash occurs in the same location every time after exposure to offending drugs.

Etiology: Typically caused by one of the "highly allergenic drugs."

Physical exam: Round rash with demarcated borders[4] that may leave behind a hyper/hypopigmented spot.

Rx: Topical steroids can be tried with withdrawal of the offending drug.

12.1.6 DRESS Syndrome (Drug Reaction with Eosinophilia and Systemic Symptoms)

Etiology: Type IV hypersensitivity reaction to drugs (typically "highly allergenic drugs").

Presentation: Morbilliform skin rash[5] + fever and generalized lymphadenopathy. Liver or kidneys might also be involved. Eosinophilia is usually present.

Rx: Withdrawal of offending agent, and systemic steroids in severe cases.

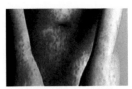

[5]Morbilliform drug exanthem Source: Skin. In: Siegenthaler W, ed. Siegenthaler's Differential Diagnosis in Internal Medicine: From Symptom to Diagnosis. 1st ed. Thieme; 2007

Differential diagnosis	
DRESS—type IV reaction	Serum sickness—type III reaction
Both can be due to one of the highly allergenic drugs (e.g., penicillin)	
Both can have fever, lymphadenopathy, morbilliform rash, and splenomegaly	
Look for end organ dysfunction (e.g., creatinine elevation, hepatitis) and eosinophilia	Look for arthralgias

12.2 Clinical Immunology

How to recognize immunodeficiency disorders with history of recurrent infections:

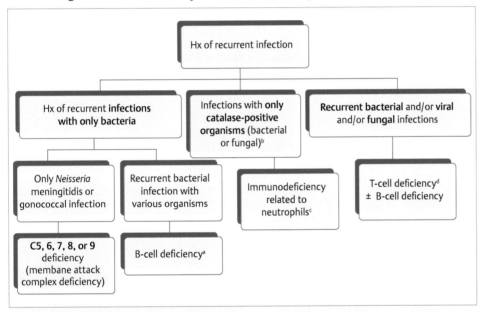

[a]For example, Bruton's agammaglobulinemia, common-variable immunodeficiency syndrome, hyper IgM syndrome, etc.

[b]Catalase-positive organisms are **E**. *coli*, **S**erratia, **P**seudomonas, **N**ocardia, **L**isteria, **A**spergillus, **C**andida, **K**lebsiella, **S**. *aureus*, etc.

[c]Neutropenia, leukocyte-adhesion deficiency, chronic granulomatous disease, Chediak–Higashi syndrome, etc.

[d]Adenosine deaminase deficiency, HIV, DiGeorge syndrome, Wiskott–Aldrich syndrome, etc.

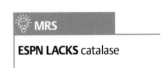

MRS

ESPN LACKS catalase

12.2.1 Complement Pathway Deficiency

A good screening test for **C**omplement pathway deficiency is CH50.

*It is a test that measures hemolytic activity of patient's serum against test antigen–antibody–RBC complexes. One **CH50** is defined as the volume dilution of serum that **h**ydrolyzes **50**% of RBCs.*

Complement proteins	Deficiency leads to the following issues
1, 2, or 4	Predisposes to autoimmune disorders such as SLE
3	Recurrent infections with encapsulated organisms (especially with pneumococcus and *H. influenzae*)
5, 6, 7, 8, 9, (or properdin)	Recurrent *Neisseria* infection (gonococcus or meningitis)

Abbreviation: SLE, systemic lupus erythematosus.

12.2.2 Humoral Issues

These typically present with recurrent **bacterial** infection (sinopulmonary and gastrointestinal infection).

Condition[a]	B cell numbers	Immunoglobulin affected
X-linked Bruton's agammaglobulinemia (defective tyrosine kinase in B-cells)	Low	All low[b]
Hyper-IgM syndrome		All low[b] (with exception of high IgM)
Hyper-IgE syndrome[c]		• Elevated IgE and eosinophilia • IgG, IgA, and IgM are typically normal
IgA deficiency	Normal	Low IgA
CVID (common-variable immunodeficiency syndrome)[d]		IgG should be low. IgM and IgA may also be low.
IgG subclass deficiency[d]		Typically affects a specific IgG subclass. Total IgG might also be low.

[a]Patients with these conditions and low IgG levels need regular infusion of intravenous immunoglobulin.

[b]In congenital disorders with low IgG levels, maternal transfer of IgG can prevent early infections up until 6 months.

[c]Additional feature includes dermatitis (similar to atopic dermatitis).

[d]Age of onset is variable; can present in adults.

12.2.3 Immune Deficiency Related to Neutrophils[6]

[6]Significant periodontal infection is a common feature of these disorders.

Recurrent infections due to catalase-positive organisms (e.g., *E. coli, Serratia, Pseudomonas, Nocardia, Listeria, Aspergillus, Candida, Klebsiella, S. aureus*) point towards neutrophil dysfunction. Think of the following conditions:

Condition[a]	Inheritance	Pathophysiology	Additional info
Chronic granulomatous disease	Most cases are X-linked, but can also be autosomal recessive	Genetic defect in NADPH oxidase results in inability of neutrophils to digest the bacteria/fungal elements in the lysosomes. Microscopy will show neutrophils filled with bacteria that are not digested.	Neutrophil function test and nitroblue tetrazolium test are abnormal
Chediak–Higashi syndrome[b]	Autosomal recessive	Altered function of lysosomes and granules in neutrophils with abnormal degranulation. Melanosomes are also involved leading to albinism	Test reveals neutropenia and *giant lysosomes*

Condition[a]	Inheritance	Pathophysiology	Additional info
Leukocyte-adhesion deficiency[b]	Autosomal recessive	Genetic defect with neutrophils not being able to adhere to and get out from blood vessels to infected tissues. (Neutrophils are forever stuck in blood vessels).	**Presentation:** delayed separation of umbilical cord and neutrophilia. In infected tissue samples, no neutrophils are seen and hence there is no pus.

Inherited Myeloperoxidase Deficiency
It results in a mild neutrophil defect, which commonly presents with recurrent *Candida* infection.

[a]For all these conditions, treatment is bone-marrow stem-cell transplant.

[b]Both Chediak–Higashi syndrome and leukocyte adhesion deficiency can also have recurrent *Streptococcus* infections. *Strep.* is less common in chronic granulomatous disease.

12.2.4 Primary T-cell Issue

Look for recurrent bacterial, viral, and/or fungal infections.

Condition[a]	Pathophysiology	Clinical presentation[b]
Adenosine deaminase deficiency	Autosomal recessive disorder that leads to intracellular accumulation of adenosine, which is toxic to lymphocytes (leading to deficiency of both T-cell and B-cell)	It is a form of severe combined immunodeficiency and presents in first few months of life.
DiGeorge syndrome	Autosomal dominant disorder due to deletion of a small segment in chromosome 22 that leads to defective development of pharyngeal arch, resulting in thymic and parathyroid gland hypoplasia.	**C**ardiac abnormality (especially tetralogy of Fallot) **A**bnormal facies **T**hymic aplasia **C**left palate **H**ypocalcemia/**H**ypoparathyroidism Severity can range from recurrent sinopulmonary infections only to severe combined immunodeficiency.
Wiskott–Aldrich syndrome	**X**-linked genetic disorder (occurs in men) that results in abnormal cellular signaling pathways involving cytoskeletons. Severity of immunosuppression depends upon underlying mutation.	Thrombocytopenia Eczema (may resemble atopic dermatitis) Autoimmune conditions (e.g., hemolytic anemia) Malignancy (lymphoma/leukemia) risk is increased

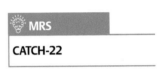

MRS
CATCH-22

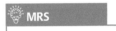

MRS
TEAM Wiskott: Wiskott is a guy's name, so it is X-linked.

[a]In all these conditions, treatment is hematopoietic stem-cell transplant. In patients with low IgG levels, consider regular infusions of intravenous immunoglobulin.

[b]Lymphopenia and absent or very small thymus can occur in all three disorders. Do not automatically choose DiGeorge syndrome when an exam vignette says absent thymic shadow.

Clinical Case Scenarios

6. A 4-year-old male baby is brought in by his mother because the child bruises easily. He also has had 4–5 episodes of infection (pneumonia, sinusitis, etc.). Upon examination of his neck, you note an area of dry scaly skin. CBC reveals thrombocytopenia. What is the likely diagnosis?

    a) Ataxia-telangiectasia
    b) Wiskott–Aldrich
    c) Severe combined immunodeficiency disease
    d) DiGeorge syndrome

Answers:

1. Serum sickness reaction. Drug-induced lupus can have similar presentation, but ANA is usually positive, and serositis might be present. Also, amoxicillin is not associated with drug-induced lupus.

2. Yes. Absence of prior hx of exposure does not rule out anaphylaxis because one might not be able to remember bee stings during childhood. He has evidence of angioedema too.

3. Immediate epinephrine injection, IV steroids and antihistamine.

4. ACE-i mediated angioedema. It can occur any time after initiation of the drug.

5. Hereditary angioedema.

6. The correct answer is b. The patient has all three criteria of Wiskott–Aldrich syndrome: thrombocytopenia, evidence of infection, and eczema found on the neck.
   Regarding option (a), ataxia-telangiectasia also affects the immune system (T-cells and B-cells). It commonly manifests as a recurrent bacterial sinopulmonary infection. Opportunistic infections and infections outside of sinopulmonary location are rare.

13. Dermatology

Few snippets

Extensor versus flexor skin surfaces: skin over the extensor surface is thicker and darker in color. This is designed to withstand trauma which is more likely to occur with extension movements than with flexion movements.

- *Skin in the back of your arm and upper body (extensor surface) is thicker and darker than skin in the front of your upper body or arm.*
- *Skin in the front part of your leg is thicker and darker than in the back of your leg.*

Intertriginous area (skin fold) is where skin touches skin frequently (e.g., groin and axilla). These areas are more likely to get infection with Candida, scabies, hidradenitis suppurativa, etc.

Rash variations: we included few classic pictures of various rashes, but in your free time try to look for other variations online. This can help you on exam. Just as humans, of the same Homo sapiens species, look different from one another, rashes of the same condition can look different too. If you Google search for atopic dermatitis or lichen planus, you will be amazed at how many variations you can find.

Terminology to describe skin lesions

Skin lesion type	Small (< ½ cm)	Big (> ½ cm)
Flat (non-elevated)	Macule	Patch[a]
Elevated	Papule	Nodule
Fluid-filled blisters[b]	Vesicle	Bulla
Red lesions	Petechiae	Purpura
	Source: James Heilman, MD, CC BY-SA 4.0, via Wikimedia Commons.	Source: Coagulopathic Forms. In:Riede U, Werner M, ed.Color Atlas of Pathology: Pathologic Principles, Associated Diseases, Sequela. 1st ed. Thieme; 2004.[a]
Loss of skin integrity	Ulcer — Epidermis[c] equivalent to mucosa — Dermis (submucosa) — Fissure — Erosion	

[a]Patches that are palpable, or with corrugated, elevated surface are called plaques.[1]
[b]If the fluid inside blister/bullae is yellow, then it is called a pustule.
[c]Similar to this principle, gastric erosion affects only mucosa, if there is involvement of submucosa, it is called an ulcer.

[1]

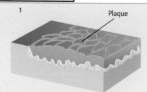

Plaque

13.1 Skin Infections (Folliculitis, Furuncles, Carbuncles, Skin Abscess, Paronychia, and Hidradenitis Suppurativa)[2]

13.1.1 Folliculitis

Definition: Superficial infection around a hair follicle, most commonly due to *Staphylococcus aureus*.

Exam: Pinpoint erythema or pustules around follicles. It can be tender.[3]

Rx: Depends on the area of involvement and severity.

Mild, with involvement of limited areas	Topical mupirocin or topical clindamycin
Extensive area involvement	Oral Staph drugs such as cephalexin or dicloxacillin. If methicillin-resistant S. aureus (MRSA) risk factor is present, use doxycycline or trimethoprim-sulfamethoxazole.

Differential dx: Bathtub folliculitis due to Pseudomonas. The lesions typically start below the neck (bathtub water submersion pattern). **Treatment** is avoidance or chlorination of hot tub. In severe cases use ciprofloxacin.

13.1.2 Furuncles, Carbuncles, Skin Abscess, and Paronychia

Definition:

Furuncles, carbuncles, skin abscess	Folliculitis can progress to small collection of infected material known as **furuncle**. When several furuncles come together to form a larger pus collection, it becomes a **carbuncle**, and a skin abscess forms.	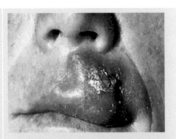 Furuncle on upper lip with edema. Source: Furuncle. In: Sterry W, Paus R, Burgdorf W, eds. Thieme Clinical Companions—Dermatology. 1st ed. Thieme; 2006.
Paronychia	Localized redness, swelling, ± abscess in skin surrounding a nail area	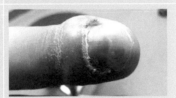 Source: Cgfalco, CC BY 4.0, via Wikimedia Commons.

Microbiology: Most common (MC) organism is *S. aureus*.

Physical Exam: As opposed to folliculitis which might not be tender, these are usually tender. A small collection or fluctuant mass is felt, with surrounding erythema and swelling.

[2] Common risk factors of skin infections: diabetes, immunosuppression, obesity, infancy.

[3]

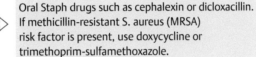

Source: In: Sterry W, Paus R, Burgdorf W, eds. Thieme Clinical Companions - Dermatology. 1st ed. Thieme; 2006.

Management:

Small furuncles and mild case of paronychia	⇒	Warm compress to promote drainage
Larger furuncles, carbuncles, or paronychia with abscess	⇒	Incision and drainage
In patients with any of the following: – multiple lesions or severe infection – significant surrounding area cellulitis – systemic symptoms – immunosuppression	⇒	Incision and drainage + oral Staph drugs such as cephalexin or dicloxacillin. If MRSA risk factor is present, use doxycycline, or trimethoprim-sulfamethoxazole.

13.1.3 Hidradenitis Suppurativa

Predisposing factors: Obesity, smoking, genetic susceptibility, and postpuberty. Occurs in intertriginous areas (arm pits, inguinal, genital, and perianal area).

Pathophysiology	Presentation
Follicular occlusion → inflamed nodules	Recurrent painful inflammatory nodules in inner folds. As opposed to folliculitis, it is a recurrent chronic process that is potentially disfiguring and debilitating.
→ abscess → drainage	Purulent or serosanguinous discharge that might be foul-smelling
→ sinus tract and fibrous bands. Multiple recurrences can lead to scarring and severe deformity.	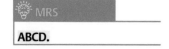 **Right inguinal area.** Source: Alharbi Z, Kauczok J, Pallua N. A review of wide surgical excision of hidradenitis suppurativa. BMC Dermatol. 2012; 12: 9.

Dx: Made clinically.

Rx: Lifestyle modification (e.g., maintaining hygiene) and, depending on severity, topical or systemic antibiotics and/or surgery (punch debridement or unroofing).

13.2 Other Bacterial Infections Involving Skin

	Causative organism	Presentation	Management	Additional info
Leprosy	Mycobacterium leprae	Hypopigmented patch with anesthesia (i.e., loss of sensation in the lesion).	**NSIDx:** skin biopsy to demonstrate acid-fast bacilli. **Rx:** dapsone	Disseminated leprosy infection can result in permanent damage to skin, nerves, limbs, eyes, etc.
Anthrax	Bacillus anthracis (cutaneous infection acquired from direct contact with infected livestock, e.g., in wool sorters).	A papule that progresses to ulcer with development of central necrosis and black eschar.	**NSIDx:** Gram stain and culture of ulcer. **Rx:** ciprofloxacin or doxycycline[a]	Bacillus can cause severe pulmonary disease with spore inhalation. As spores are very resistant (even to drying), powdered forms can be used as biological agents for terrorism.

MRS

ABCD.

13.3 Viral Skin Infections-HSV-1, HSV-2 and Herpes Zoster[4]

13.3.1 Herpes Simplex Virus (HSV) Infection

	HSV-1	HSV-2
Presentation	A single or multiple cluster of small vesicles, pustules, and/or multiple superficial ulcerations	
Typical location	Oral area; rash most commonly occurs in vermilion borders of lip (known as herpes labialis or cold sores)	Genital area
Transmission	Infected oral secretions	Exposure to infected genital secretions during sex or child birth
Potential complication	• Gingivostomatitis ± pharyngitis • Eczema herpeticum • Recurrent aseptic meningitis • Primary HSV-1 infection can cause meningoencephalitis (typically with temporal lobe involvement)	• *Usually* does not cause encephalitis • Can cause recurrent aseptic meningitis
Rx	• Consider antiviral valacyclovir, famciclovir, or acyclovir (+ clovir) during an episode. • In patients with frequent infections (4–6 episodes/year), consider chronic suppressive therapy with antivirals.	

• Dx is usually made clinically, but when in doubt we can do viral culture, viral polymerase chain reaction (PCR), direct fluorescent testing on sample, or Tzanck smear (to look for multinucleated giant cells).
• Both can have dormant stage with recurrent reactivation and infection.

[4]The herpes group of viruses can remain dormant in a nerve ganglion for a long period of time. Certain precipitating factors such as stress (surgery, trauma, burn, etc.), or immunosuppression (e.g., advanced age or use of immunosuppressive medication) can lead to reactivation of the dormant virus.

13.3.2 Herpetic Whitlow

Background: Cutaneous herpes simplex virus (HSV-1 or -2) can be acquired through contact with infected herpes genitalia or cold sores (e.g., dentist gets exposed to patient's oral lesions). It can occur as a result of self-infection, too.

Presentation: Clear fluid-filled vesicles or pustules in fingers or hands. It is usually tender and can be recurrent.

Dx: Clinical, but when in doubt, we can do viral culture, viral PCR, direct fluorescent testing on sample, or Tzanck smear (to look for multinucleated giant cells).

Rx: Conservative management in most patients. In significant cases, consider antiviral valacyclovir, famciclovir, or acyclovir.

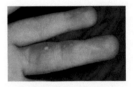

This 19-year-old immunocompetent patient had recurrent episodes.
Source: Brkljac M, Bitar S, Naqui Z. A Case Report of Herpetic Whitlow with Positive Kanavel's Cardinal Signs: A Diagnostic and Treatment Difficulty. Case Rep Orthop. 2014; 2014: 906487.

13.3.3 Herpes Zoster a.k.a. Shingles

Background: After getting chicken pox (primary varicella zoster virus infection), the virus can remain dormant in sensory nerve ganglia for years. Precipitating factors such as immunosuppression can lead to reactivation of virus and eruption of rash along a sensory nerve root distribution.

Presentation:

• Vesicles are in classical dermatomal distribution and unilateral (i.e., does not cross the mid-line). The rash is painful and itchy.

• Some patient can present only with neuropathic pain in dermatomal distribution (preherpetic neuralgia). *Pain can precede rash for days to weeks!*

• Severe postherpetic neuralgia (after onset of rash) can also occur.

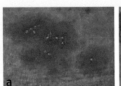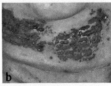

(a) Early zoster with grouped vesicles on an erythematous base. (b) More severe zoster, clearly showing dermatomal limitation.
Source: Zoster (Herpes Zoster, Shingles). In: Sterry W, Paus R, Burgdorf W, eds. Thieme Clinical Companions—Dermatology. 1st ed. Thieme; 2006.

Rx: Antiviral valacyclovir, acyclovir, or famciclovir (+clovir). In immunocompromised patients consider varicella zoster immune globulin.

Preventive measures:

Situation	Type of precaution in a health care setting (e.g., hospitals)	Indication for postexposure prophylaxis in patients who lack immunity[a]
Primary infection (chicken pox), disseminated zoster (when zoster involves more than 1 dermatome), and immunocompromised patient with dermatomal zoster	Airborne[b] + contact precautions	Yes
Uncomplicated herpes zoster	Standard precaution, including covering active lesions.	**Only for** close contacts of patients with open, weepy lesions NOTE: crusted zoster lesions are not infectious.

[a]Individuals with no immunity to VZV (varicella zoster virus) are:

• Those who *have not had* two doses of zoster vaccine, or

• Who *have no* laboratory evidence of immunity, or

• Who *have no* verified chicken pox infection.

[b]Requires negative-pressure room. Same type of precaution is used for active tuberculosis.

Postexposure prophylaxis is recommended with two doses of zoster vaccine. Since it is a live vaccine, it is contraindicated in newborns, pregnant, or immunocompromised individuals. In these patients, use varicella zoster immune globulin instead.

Unique presentations of Varicella Zoster (aka Herpes Zoster) virus reactivation

When herpes zoster reactivates in particular distribution of cranial nerves		Presentation
Herpes zoster oticus (Ramsay Hunt syndrome)	Reactivation in geniculate ganglion (facial nerve ganglion)	Unilateral facial nerve paralysis with painful vesicles in auditory canal and/or external ear Note: Due to the ganglion's proximity to other cranial nerves, it can also affect cranial nerves 8 (hearing loss, tinnitus), 9, 10, etc.
Herpes zoster ophthalmicus	Reactivation in ophthalmic division of trigeminal nerve	Conjunctivitis, keratitis (**corneal** involvement), and iritis. This can cause corneal scar or blindness, if severe. Topical ocular steroid + antiviral therapy is recommended.

 In a nutshell

Treatment for herpes infection

Condition		Rx
Herpes simplex virus		Any of "+clovir".[a] If resistant, use foscarnet.
Herpes zoster or chicken pox	In immunocompetent host	Any of +clovir[a]
	In immunocompromised host	Any of +clovir[a] + Varicella zoster immune globulin

[a]Acyclovir, famciclovir, or valacyclovir (except ganciclovir, which is used for cytomegalovirus).

13.4 Parasitic Skin Infections

13.4.1 Scabies

Background: Skin infection due to *Sarcoptes scabiei*, which is transmitted by close contact.

Presentation: Scattered papules and/or pustules ± underlying erythema found particularly in digital webs (interdigital space of hands or feet), palms, and intertriginous areas. These are very itchy. Look for history of exposure to patients with similar symptoms. Patients with HIV can develop extensive scabies with severe crusting, known as Norwegian scabies.

NSIDx: Find parasite in skin scrapings.

Rx: Topical permethrin or oral ivermectin. With crusted scabies, combine both oral and topical treatment.

Complication: Secondary bacterial skin infection can develop (e.g., impetigo, cellulitis).

Itchy papules and burrows.
Source: Scabies. In: Sterry W, Paus R, Burgdorf W, eds. Thieme Clinical Companions—Dermatology. 1st ed. Thieme; 2006.

13.4.2 Pediculosis (Head Lice)

Background: Infestation by lice can occur in hair-bearing areas; usually in head, but can occur in genital or axillary area.

Presentation: Prominent itching and skin excoriations. Secondary bacterial infection can develop.

NSIDx: Direct examination of hair-bearing areas.

Rx: Permethrin or lindane solution.

13.5 Intertrigo

Definition: Intertrigo is an umbrella term for inflammatory conditions located in skinfolds (intertriginous areas). It can develop due to mechanical skin-on-skin friction/irritation alone or become complicated by superimposed fungal or bacterial infection.

Risk factor: Diabetes, obesity, advancing age, and other forms of immunosuppression.

Presentation: Erythematous lesions that can be painful and pruritic. Secondary spongiosis can occur (formation of vesicles and pustules which can weep, ooze, and crust). Intertrigo can also present as diaper rash in children.

General treatment: Minimize friction (barrier creams) and prevent moisture buildup (absorptive powders such as corn starch).

Look for Secondary infection with dermatophytes, *Candida, Corynebacterium* (erythrasma), staphylococcus and streptococcus.

		Erythrasma due to Corynebacterium infection	Candidal intertrigo
Differentiating feature		**Sharply demarcated** red to **brown** patches ± scales	Can have whitish film. Look for satellite lesions (red papules or pustules) around the rash area.
		Source: Erythrasma. In: Sterry W, Paus R, Burgdorf W, eds. Thieme Clinical Companions—Dermatology. 1st ed. Thieme; 2006.	Intertriginous candidal infection, with typical satellite lesions Source: Oral Candidiasis. In: Sterry W, Paus R, Burgdorf W, eds. Thieme Clinical Companions—Dermatology. 1st ed. Thieme; 2006.
NSIDx		Wood lamp light typically reveals coral-red fluorescence.	Usually a clinical dx. Skin KOH preparation can be used.
Rx	Localized disease	Topical erythromycin, clindamycin, or fusidic acid	Topical azoles (e.g., clotrimazole, ketoconazole) or nystatin
	Widespread disease	Oral erythromycin or clarithromycin	Oral fluconazole

Primary skin disorders

Presentation	Condition	Additional points	Rx
Papules or plaques that can be of various colors. Rash can have overlying white lacy to net-like lines. Flat-topped papules to plaques 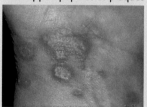 Source: Lichen Planus. In: Sterry W, Paus R, Burgdorf W, eds. Thieme Clinical Companions—Dermatology. 1st ed. Thieme; 2006.	**Lichen planus**[a] Oral lichen planus can present with white lacy or net-like reticular lesions inside oral cavity. 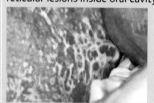 Source: Lichen Planus. In: Laskaris G, ed. Color Atlas of Oral Diseases. Diagnosis and Treatment. 4th ed. Thieme; 2017.	• Associated with Hep C infection • Can also be drug-induced	• **Localized form**: topical steroids • **Generalized form:** phototherapy, acitretin, or oral steroids.
Initial oval or round herald patch (looks like rash of tinea corporis), followed by development of maculopapular eruptions that occur in a Christmas-tree-pattern • Can be pruritic 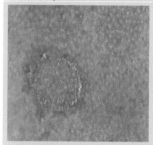 Typical herald patch. Source: Pityriasis Rosea. In: Sterry W, Paus R, Burgdorf W, eds. Thieme Clinical Companions—Dermatology. 1st ed. Thieme; 2006.	**Pityriasis rosea** 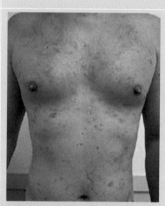 Source: James Heilman, MD, CC BY-SA 3.0, via Wikimedia Commons.	If rash is atypical do VRDL or RPR test to screen for syphilis (palms and soles' involvement points toward secondary syphilis)	Benign condition that usually resolves on its own. Topical steroids can be used for very itchy lesions.
Name giveth all. • Rosacea = facial redness, pronounced flushing reaction, and/or telangiectasias (visible superficial vessels) • Acne = superficial papules and/or pustules that look like pustular acne.	**Acne rosacea** 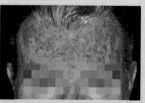 Source: Rosacea. In: Sterry W, Paus R, Burgdorf W, eds. Thieme Clinical Companions—Dermatology. 1st ed. Thieme; 2006.	Differential dx is with acne vulgaris (absence of comedones points toward acne rosacea)	**For rosacea:** First line includes avoidance of triggers of flushing, sun-protection, and skin care. Second line includes topical brimonidine and/or light therapy. **Papulopustular disease** • For mild cases, use topical metronidazole, azelaic acid, or ivermectin. • For severe disease, use one of the oral tetracyclines (tetra-/doxy-/mino-cycline). If this fails, consider oral isotretinoin.

[a]Ps: Planus lichen has pruritic, papules, or plaques of plural color (purple, violaceous, or red–pink).

13.6 Acne Vulgaris

Background: It is a common condition. Pathophysiologic factors include the following:

- Increased stress, *lack of sleep*, poor diet, sedentary life-style, etc.
- Bacterial infection with *Propionibacterium acnes.*
- Increased adeno-sebaceous secretion due to genetic factors or hormonal excess (Cushing's syndrome, partial 21-α-hydroxylase deficiency, etc.)

Type	Exam	Initial treatment[a]	
Comedonal acne[b]	Only comedones are present	Topical retinoids (TR) Other options are topical glycolic or salicylic acid.	
Inflammatory acne	Papules, pustules, or small nodules (< 5 mm) ± erythema 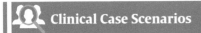 Source: Acne. In: Sterry W, Paus R, Burgdorf W, eds. Thieme Clinical Companions—Dermatology. 1st ed. Thieme; 2006.	Mild (few pustules only)	**TR** (± benzoyl peroxide)
		Moderate	**TR** + topical antibiotics[c] (e.g., erythromycin)
		Severe (e.g., large pustules)	**TR** + oral antibiotics[c,d]
Nodulocystic acne	> 5 mm nodules which can appear cystic	Mild to moderate	
		Severe	Oral isotretinoin as a monotherapy[e]

[a]If no response to initial treatment, step up therapy.

[b]Comedones are skin-colored papules that commonly occur in the face, neck, and back areas.

[c]Topical benzoyl peroxide is recommended with either topical or oral antibiotics to decrease emergence of resistance.

[d]Oral antibiotic choices are tetracyclines, tetra-/doxy-/mino-cycline erythromycin, etc.

[e]Potential side effects of "oral" isotretinoin include hepatotoxicity, intracranial hypertension, photosensitivity, and most importantly teratogenicity. Patients on oral isotretinoin should be on two different contraceptive methods (initiated 1 month prior and continued until 1 month after completion of therapy) and have pregnancy testing done routinely. They should also have at least two negative pregnancy tests prior to initiation of therapy.

Abbreviation: TR, topical retinoids.

Clinical Case Scenarios

1. A 25-year-old male presents with moderate inflammatory acne not responsive to combination of topical antibiotics, benzoyl peroxide, and retinoic acid. What is the NSIM?

13.7 Bullous Disorders

Types of bulla	Causes
Tense and hard bulla = deep-seated bulla	Bullous pemphigoid or Cicatricial pemphigoid
Flaccid and easily peeled off bulla = superficial bulla • After peeling off, it leaves behind a weepy erosion or ulcer.	Pemphigus disorder (pemphigus vulgaris, pemphigus foliaceus), staphylococcal scalded skin syndrome, and toxic epidermal necrolysis. • Nikolsky sign can be found in all of them (gentle rubbing of the area near to bulla results in skin peeling off easily). • Unlike bullous pemphigoid, these conditions can be life-threatening, as they can act like burns.

13.7.1 Primary Bullous Disorders

Condition	Typical patient profile	Typical rash	Presence of autoimmune antibody against	Biopsy findings	Rx
Pemphigus vulgaris Blisters that have already peeled off and have left behind multiple, crust-covered, erosions. Source: Pemphigus Vulgaris. In: Laskaris G, ed. Color Atlas of Oral Diseases. Diagnosis and Treatment. 4th ed. Thieme; 2017.	Middle-aged adults (in their 30–40s)	• Flaccid blisters • Unlike foliaceus, this involves mucous membrane (e.g., oral or conjunctival ulcer)	Antibody against desmosomes (desmoglein); this leads to loss of cell-to-cell adhesion (acantholysis)	Intercellular deposits of IgG	Oral steroids ± adjuvant immunosuppressant[a]
Pemphigus foliaceus		• Flaccid blisters • No mucosal involvement			
Bullous pemphigoid Bullous pemphigoid with large blisters, erosions, and hemorrhagic crusts. Source: Bullous Pemphigoid (BP). In: Sterry W, Paus R, Burgdorf W, eds. Thieme Clinical Companions—Dermatology. 1st ed. Thieme; 2006.	Old age (60–70s)	• Tense blisters • There is no residual scarring (as opposed to cicatricial pemphigoid)	Hemidesmosome	Linear deposits of IgG and/or C3 along the basement membrane zone (dermoepidermal junction)[b]	High-potency topical steroids or oral steroids
Cicatricial pemphigoid (aka mucous membrane pemphigoid)		• Tense blisters • Unlike bullous pemphigoid, this can cause scarring leading to various complications (ocular scarring can lead to corneal blindness)	Several basement membrane antigens		

[a]Methotrexate, azathioprine, and mycophenolate mofetil. They are also used as steroid sparing agents for significant pemphigoid disorders.
[b]Cicatricial pemphigoid can also have immunoglobulin A (IgA) or IgM deposits.

MRS ☺
- Tense **bulla** = **bullous** pemphigoid. On the other hand, pemphigus vulgaris/foliaceus do not have word "bullous" in it; pemphigus may not have any bulla at the time of presentation, as the bulla in pemphigus are typically flaccid and rupture easily.
- Cicatricial is sCarring, whereas bullous pemphigoid is not.
- Unlike pemphigus foliaceus, pemphigus vulgaris is "vulgar": it can involve vagina and any other mucosal membranes.

Drug-induced pemphigus or pemphigoid disorders can occur with highly allergenic drugs such as NSAIDs, ACE inhibitors, penicillamine, sulfa drugs, etc.

13.8 Dermatitis (Eczema)[5]

Eczema (aka dermatitis) is an umbrella term for inflammatory skin conditions due to various factors. There are different kinds of eczema (dermatitis), typically named after the inciting factor, but they can have the following common factors:

- A positive feedback cycle of inflammation —>itching —>damaged skin by excessive itching —> more inflammation (picture)
- Severe forms can lead to spongiosis, with **intercellular edema** in epidermis followed by development of vesicles or pustules. As these vesicles/bulla or pustules rupture it results in weeping, oozing, and crusting lesions. Underlying erythema may also be present.
- **Complications:**
  - Skin damage increases risk of infection (impetigo, erysipelas, cellulitis, etc.).
  - Scaly patches are also common.
  - *Recurrent and/or persistent* process leads to lichenification and lichen simplex chronicus.

[5] FYI: Some people consider eczema synonymous with dermatitis (which we will use in this book). Others consider eczema as the chronic form of dermatitis.

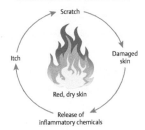

Type of dermatitis	Pathophysiology	Features	Rx
Xerosis aka asteatotic eczema	Older patients in winter months are susceptible to dry skin (xerosis). This typically occurs in extensor surfaces (e.g., pretibial area).	• Dry flaky skin Severe forms can present with spongiosis	Moisturizers
Seborrheic dermatitis Source: Roymishali, CC BY-SA 3.0, via Wikimedia Commons.	Sebaceous gland secretion may play a role in *proliferation of Malassezia* (a.k.a. *Pityrosporum* ovale). This leads to a hypersensitivity reaction to the fungal elements.	Erythema, scales (dandruff), particularly in eyebrows, nasolabial folds and scalp. • It is associated with HIV and Parkinson's disease. • Consider HIV testing in new onset severe or refractory cases, especially in young patients.	• Low-potency topical steroids ± topical antifungals • Shampoo that contains zinc, selenium, or an antifungal agent (e.g., ketoconazole shampoo)
Contact dermatitis (a) Acute allergic contact dermatitis with vesicles. (b) Allergic contact dermatitis to nickel in jeans button. Source: Allergic Contact Dermatitis. In: Sterry W, Paus R, Burgdorf W, eds. Thieme Clinical Companions—Dermatology. 1st ed. Thieme; 2006.	• Type IV hypersensitivity reaction to any chemicals or metals • Common allergens are nickel (used in jewelry, belt buckle), topical medications (neomycin, hydrocortisone), detergents, poison ivy, etc.	Signs of spongiosis occur in areas where there is contact with allergens: • Linear-streaked vesicles = contact with leaves of poison ivy • Rash around wrist = nickel bracelet allergy • Rash around the pocket area of pants = allergy to coins in the pockets	• Avoidance of allergens • Topical steroids or tacrolimus • In severe cases, oral steroids can be given

Type of dermatitis	Pathophysiology	Features	Rx
Atopic dermatitis Typical (**a**) facial, (**b**) flexural, (**c**) nuchal involvement, and (**d**) lichenification. Source: Clinical Features. In: Sterry W, Paus R, Burgdorf W, eds. Thieme Clinical Companions—Dermatology. 1st ed. Thieme; 2006.	Postulated to be due to IgE-mediated hypersensitivity reactions **Look for:** • hx of atopy (coexistent asthma and allergic rhinitis) • clustering of similar symptoms in family members (take caution as this history might make you think of scabies instead of atopic dermatitis)	Intensely pruritic rash along with spongiosis, that may lead to lichenification • Typically involves flexor joint surfaces (popliteal fossa or anterior elbow), but can involve any other areas • In infants look for sparing of diaper area	1st line- Topical steroids or emollients (non-cosmetic moisturizers) 2nd line –topical tacrolimus Phototherapy or oral immunosuppressives in severe cases.
Stasis dermatitis Source: Prof. Dr. med. Gerd Hoffmann, CC BY-SA 3.0 DE, via Wikimedia Commons.	• Venous stasis due to chronic venous incompetence (varicose veins, venous valve insufficiency, etc.) • Obesity is a significant risk factor	• Lower extremity pitting edema • Circumferential lower extremity erythema and/or hyperpigmentation (due to buildup of hemosiderin) • Acute spongiosis can occur.	• Treat underlying cause (e.g., treat varices). • Advise elevation of legs and use compression stockings. • Use topical steroids for acute spongiosis.
Dermatitis herpetiformis associated with celiac sprue Skin bullae in a child with dermatitis herpetiformis and celiac sprue. Source: Celiac Disease. In: Laskaris G, ed. Color Atlas of Oral Diseases. Diagnosis and Treatment. 4th ed. Thieme; 2017. Slightly lichenified version of dermatitis herpetiformis in an adult. Source: BallenaBlanca, CC BY-SA 3.0, via Wikimedia Commons.	• It is a cutaneous manifestation of gluten hypersensitivity. Antibodies against epidermal transglutaminase are present.	• Extremely pruritic papules, pustules, or vesicles—bulla (spongiosis) that typically occur in extensor surfaces. • Dx is made with biopsy, which will reveal **granular** deposits of IgA in papillary dermis.	Start dapsone along with gluten free diet when patients have active lesions. Later on, it can be tapered off if no remission.
Dyshidrotic eczema (aka pompholyx aka foot-and-hand eczema) Source: Maslesha, CC BY-SA 3.0, via Wikimedia Commons.	• Unknown etiology	Chronic or recurrent: • Intensely pruritic vesicular dermatitis, which occurs in palms, soles, or lateral aspects of fingers. Clear vesicles with clear base are early signs, followed by development of spongiosis (crusting and erythema).	Topical steroids. Use oral steroids in refractory cases

Type of dermatitis	Pathophysiology	Features	Rx
Nummular eczema 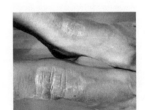Source: Topaz2, CC BY-SA 4.0, via Wikimedia Commons.	Unknown etiology	• Coin-like lesion (that is why it is called nummular) • May later develop spongiosis—vesicles, pustules, or papules that ooze over the coin-like lesion.	
Photodermatitis	Photosensitivity can occur due to: doxycycline, minocycline, griseofulvin (antifungal), oral retinoic acid, etc. Niacin deficiency (pellagra) Systemic lupus erythematosus	Signs of spongiosis in sun-exposed areas such as the face or distal upper extremities.	Avoid sun-exposure, avoid medications that can cause photosensitivity and treat underlying cause.

🪐 In a nutshell

Eczema in a nutshell

Forms of dermatitis (eczema)	Disease features
Xerotic (asteatotic)	Dry skin and itching. It may lead to signs of spongiosis.
Seborrheic	Mostly dry flaky skin with underlying erythema. • Prominent signs of spongiosis are usually absent.
Contact	Prominent spongiosis and itching in the contact area
Nummular	Prominent spongiosis and itching in coin-shaped patches
Stasis dermatitis	Mostly lower extremity circumferential erythema and hyperpigmentation. • Acute signs of spongiosis can occur.
Atopic dermatitis	Prominent spongiosis and itching: look for other signs of atopy
Dermatitis herpetiformis	Prominent spongiosis and itching: look for celiac sprue
Dyshidrotic eczema (aka pompholyx)	Vesicles with clear base that occur in palms and soles, followed by prominent spongiosis and itching

13.9 Lichen Simplex Chronicus

Background: It is a sequela of chronic itching. Look for underlying causes of chronic itching, such as narcotic abuse, chronic spongiosis (e.g., atopic dermatitis), psychiatric illness, insect bites, and trauma leading to perpetual cycle of itching, skin damage, inflammation, and more itching.

Physical Exam: Lichenified (thickened and hyperkeratotic) plaques or nodules and excoriations due to excessive itching. Look for features suggestive of primary disorder (e.g., features of atopic dermatitis).

Rx: Break the cycle of more itching and more damage by using topical steroids or anesthetics. Address underlying cause.

Source: Mohammad2018, CC BY-SA 4.0, via Wikimedia Commons.

13.10 Porphyria Cutanea Tarda

Background: Acquired accumulation of porphyrins due to things like oral contraceptives, alcoholism, liver disease, chronic hepatitis C, and iron overload in a genetically susceptible individual.

Presentation: Nonhealing painless blisters that typically occur in sun-exposed areas. May lead to hyper- or hypopigmentation, scarring, or infection. Increased facial hair growth may be present.

Workup: NSIDx is urinary and plasma porphyrin level. After confirming diagnosis, additional tests such as iron panel, serology for Hep C/HIV, genetic testing are done.

Rx: Stop exposure to offending agents such as alcohol, smoking, and oral contraceptive pills, and use sun-protective clothing. In patients with evidence of iron overload, screen for hemochromatosis and treat with phlebotomy. In patients with no evidence of iron overload, use either phlebotomy or hydroxychloroquine (this increases excretion of porphyrins).

Miscellaneous benign nonulcerative skin lesions (dermatofibroma, molluscum contagiosum, epidermal inclusion cysts, cherry angioma, erythema nodosum)

Picture	Description	Dx and pathophysiology	Rx
Source: Mohammad2018, CC BY-SA 4.0, via Wikimedia Commons.	Nontender and discrete nodules. Look for central dimpling when pinched.	**Dermatofibroma** due to benign fibroblast proliferation	For asymptomatic lesion, no need for treatment. It may be removed for cosmetic reasons with cryotherapy or surgical excision.
Multiple epidermoid cysts. Source: Epidermoid Cyst. In: Sterry W, Paus R, Burgdorf W, eds. Thieme Clinical Companions—Dermatology. 1st ed. Thieme; 2006.	Skin-colored, freely movable nodule. Look for firm cyst with central punctum (umbilicated)	**Epidermoid cyst (a.k.a. epidermal inclusion cyst or sebaceous cyst)** Can develop when epidermis (which produces keratin) becomes dislodged inside skin due to trauma or comedones. Some cysts may enlarge, rupture, and cause surrounding area inflammation.	• If asymptomatic, no need to treat; however, it can be removed for cosmetic reasons. • Inflamed lesion, can be treated with intralesional steroids.
Source: Evanherk, CC BY-SA 3.0, via Wikimedia Commons.	Flesh-colored, dome-shaped umbilicated papules	**Molluscum contagiosum** • Caused by infection with molluscum contagiosum virus (part of a family of pox viruses). If widespread disease, look for underlying immunosuppression (e.g., HIV)	**Various options**—curettage, cryotherapy, podophyllotoxin, or cantharidin (cantharidin is avoided in genital areas).
Source: Jmarchn, CC BY-SA 3.0, via Wikimedia Commons.	Look for central crater that has keratin-like material. Large keratin deposition in the center crater can make it look dramatic (google images)	**Keratoacantho**ma occurs due to benign squamous proliferation with increased keratin production. Usual natural history is rapid growth, followed by stable phase and spontaneous resolution.	Although spontaneous resolution might occur, surgical excision and pathology exam are recommended in all cases to differentiate it from squamous cell cancer of skin.
Source: Lee Wrigley, Public domain, via Wikimedia Commons.	Red vascular papules • Occasionally may bleed profusely after trauma	**Cherry angiomas:** They typically increase in number with age.	Reassurance

Picture	Description	Dx and pathophysiology	Rx
In this patient recurrence followed excision, and led to huge keloid formation. Source: Earrings. In: Bull T, Almeyda J, eds. Color Atlas of ENT Diagnosis. 5th ed. Thieme; 2009.	They grow outside of boundaries of wounds (as opposed to hypertrophic scars, which do not).	**Keloids** • Can occur in previous wounds (e.g., surgical incision) or de novo, in areas which are prone to injury or excessive stretch (e.g., back)	Use intralesional steroids or 5-fluorouracil. Surgical removal can be done for large earlobe keloids.
Flesh-colored lesions (black arrows) and lesions with classic "stuck-on" appearance (red arrows) Source: Seborrheic Keratosis. In: Sterry W, Paus R, Burgdorf W, eds. Thieme Clinical Companions—Dermatology. 1st ed. Thieme; 2006.	Classically have "stuck-on" appearance	Seborrheic keratosis • Due to benign *keratinocyte proliferation* with no malignant potential, but sudden appearance of multiple lesions has been associated with *lung or GI malignancy*. • It has no relationship with seborrheic dermatitis or actinic keratosis.	May be removed for cosmetic reasons with cryotherapy or surgical excision

13.11 Erythema Nodosum

Background: Panniculitis (inflammation of subcutaneous fat tissue) due to type IV delayed hypersensitivity, which can be incited by various conditions:

- Infection (recent strep infection, tuberculosis, coccidioidomycosis, histoplasmosis, syphilis, Epstein–Barr virus, etc.)
- Autoimmune disease (inflammatory bowel disease, sarcoidosis, etc.)
- Pregnancy
- Drugs (sulfonamides, penicillin, etc.)
- Malignancy

Presentation: Red painful nodules usually found in the anterior surface of legs + malaise, arthralgia ± fever.

Workup:

- Routine blood tests such as complete blood count (CBC) and complete metabolic profile.
- CXR (chest X-ray) to look for sarcoidosis and other fungal or atypical infection such as TB, histoplasmosis, etc.
- ASO (antistreptolysin O) titer (erythema nodosum is frequently associated with streptococcal pharyngitis).
- PPD (purified protein derivative), if TB risk factors present.

Rx: Treat underlying cause.

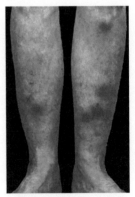

Source: Fever with Associated Cardinal Symptoms. In: Siegenthaler W, ed. Siegenthaler's Differential Diagnosis in Internal Medicine: From Symptom to Diagnosis. 1st ed. Thieme; 2007.

13.12 Miscellaneous Ulcerative Lesions (Necrobiosis Lipoidica, Pyogenic Granuloma, Pyoderma Gangrenosum)

Picture	Presentation	Dx and pathophysiology	Rx
Source: Warfieldian, CC BY-SA 3.0, via Wikimedia Commons.	Initially slightly raised plaque → flattens to become a patch (skin layers thin out, underlying veins become visible) → can later ulcerate. It commonly occurs in lower extremities, but can occur anywhere.	**Necrobiosis lipoidica** • It is a rare chronic granulomatous cutaneous lesion *strongly associated with diabetes*. • Dx is made with clinical and biopsy findings.	For nonulcerative disease, may use topical or intralesional high-potency steroids. For ulcerative disease, multimodality treatment.
Absence of surrounding skin thinning can help differentiate this from ulcerative necrobiosis lipoidica Source: Crohnie, Public domain, via Wikimedia Commons.	Rapid development of papule, pustule, or vesicle, followed by painful ulceration (typically has an irregular and violaceous border).	**Pyoderma gangrenosum** • It is due to neutrophilic inflammation associated with underlying autoimmune diseases such as inflammatory bowel disease, hematological malignancy, and seropositive/seronegative arthritis. • Dx is made with clinical scenario, exclusion of other ulcerative diseases, and biopsy findings.	For mild localized disease, use high-potency steroids or topical tacrolimus. If this fails, use minocycline or dapsone. For severe or wide spread disease, use systemic immunosuppressants (e.g., systemic steroids).
Source: Localized. In: Laskaris G, ed. Pocket Atlas of Oral Diseases. 2nd ed. Thieme; 2005.	Enlarging friable, vascular-appearing red lesion that frequently ulcerates and bleeds.	**Pyogenic granuloma** (a.k.a. lobular capillary hemangioma) • This typically develops at the site of minor injury (gums, skin, nasal septum, tongue, etc.). • Histologically it represents excessive granulation tissue.	Surgical excision, cryotherapy, or electrocauterization

13.13 Decubitus Ulcer

Background: Pressure-induced skin atrophy and necrosis that occurs in patients with significant immobilization (bedbound or wheelchair-bound patients). It commonly develops in pressure-prone areas of tail bone and heels (but can develop in other areas too).

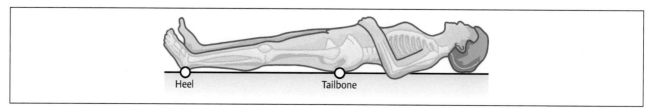

Presentation: Persistent erythema that does not blanch and progresses on to ulceration.

Management: Reposition every 2 hours, use pressure-offloading or pressure-reducing devices such as air mattress and waffle-boots, and consult wound care.

Complications: Wound infection, osteomyelitis, etc.

13.14 Premalignant and Malignant Skin Lesions

13.14.1 Actinic Keratosis

Pathology: Squamous dysplasia most commonly due to excessive sun exposure. It is also associated with arsenic exposure.

Presentation: Scaly, white-to-yellow, flaky rash with sandpaper texture ± red base. Horn-like structures can also occur.

Rx:

Localized and isolated	⇒	Nitrogen cryotherapy
Multiple thin lesions	⇒	Topical immunosuppressive therapy (5-fluorouracil, imiquimod) or phototherapy
Multiple hyperkeratotic/hypertrophic lesions	⇒	Nitrogen cryotherapy to remove prominent lesions and then use topical immunosuppressive therapy (5-fl uorouracil, imiquimod).

Complications: Actinic keratosis (squamous dysplasia) → Bowen's disease (squamous cell cancer in situ) → squamous cell cancer. Immunosuppression increases risk of transformation.

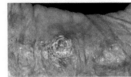

Actinic keratosis of hand
Source: James Heilman, MD, CC BY-SA 4.0, via Wikimedia Commons.

Close-up picture of actinic keratosis
Source: Actinic Keratosis. In: Sterry W, Paus R, Burgdorf W, eds. Thieme Clinical Companions—Dermatology. 1st ed. Thieme; 2006.

Etiologies of cutaneous horns which are made up of compact keratin:

- Seborrheic keratosis
- Keratoacanthoma
- Viral warts
- Actinic keratosis
- Squamous cell carcinoma

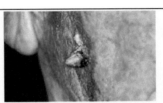

Source: Epithelium. In: Laskaris G, ed. Color Atlas of Oral Diseases. Diagnosis and Treatment. 4th ed. Thieme; 2017.

13.14.2 Skin Cancer

Skin cancer is the MC form of cancer.
MC skin cancer is basal cell carcinoma.

	Basal cell cancer	Squamous cell cancer
Presentation	This can have different morphologies: Shiny, pearly, or waxy nodular skin lesion Source: M. Sand, D. Sand, C. Thrandorf, V. Paech, P. Altmeyer, F. G. Bechara, CC BY 2.0, via Wikimedia Commons. Ulcerating pearly nodule Red beefy lesion that bleeds Source: Klaus D. Peter, Gummersbach, Germany, CC BY 3.0 DE, via Wikimedia Commons.	Nonhealing atypical skin lesion or ulceration. Can also arise from chronic nonhealing structures, such as ulcers, fistulas, sinuses, or from scar tissue[a] (e.g., from burns). Source: Unknown photographer, Public domain, via Wikimedia Commons.
Location	• Mostly found on sun-exposed areas such as the head, neck, and face. • Might be present in the upper lip (but never in lower lip).	Often develops in sun-exposed areas (lips and face), but can occur anywhere.

Immunosuppression and sun exposure are important risk factors for both squamous and basal cell carcinoma.

	Basal cell cancer	Squamous cell cancer
Spread	Does not metastasize, but can extend locally.	Can metastasize to local lymph nodes and can rarely spread to distant sites.
NSIDx	Shave, punch, or excisional biopsy	
Biopsy findings	Clusters of spindle cells surrounded by basal cells	Invasive squamous cells (keratinocytes) with keratin pearls
Rx	Surgical excision[b]	Surgical excision[b] • Other treatment options include cryotherapy, electrosurgery, or radiation treatment.

[a]All chronic ulcers, fistula, and sinuses need to be biopsied to rule out malignancy.

[b]In cosmetically sensitive areas (e.g., face) or if high risk for recurrence, Mohs surgery is recommended. It is least disruptive to surrounding tissues, but requires sequential thin excision with microscopic exam during the procedure to ensure removal of all malignant cells.

Significant arsenic exposure increases risk of:

• Arsenical hyperkeratosis: presentation is similar to actinic keratosis

• Basal cell carcinoma

• Squamous cell carcinoma

Similarly, sun exposure increases risk of actinic keratosis, <u>melanoma</u>, and basal-cell and squamous-cell carcinomas.

13.15 Nevus

Definition: Nevus (a.k.a. mole) is a benign lesion that contains increased number of melanocytes.

13.15.1 Acquired benign nevus

Types of nevus	Location of clusters of benign melanocytes
Junctional nevus	Dermal–epidermal junction
Intradermal	Dermis only
Compound nevus	Dermis + dermal–epidermal junction
Lentigo	Increased number of melanocytes occurs in linear arrangements (hence called lentigo)

Halo nevus: Autoimmune destruction of melanocytes in the area surrounding the nevus results in hypopigmentation around the nevus.[6]

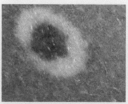

[6]Halo nevus.

Source: Halo Nevus. In: Sterry W, Paus R, Burgdorf W, eds. Thieme Clinical Companions—Dermatology. 1st ed. Thieme; 2006.

13.15.2 Atypical or dysplastic nevi

Background: It tends to run in families. Histologically, it has cytological atypia and dysplastic features. There is increased risk of melanoma.

Presentation: Single nevus or multiple nevi. They may have some asymmetry and variable color.

Management: Careful monitoring with dermoscopy and serial photographs is recommended. Suspicious lesions are excised and sent for biopsy.

13.16 Malignant Melanoma

Definition: Malignant transformation of melanocytes.

Risk factors: Sun exposure and fair-skinned individuals.

Different types of melanoma

Superficial spreading melanoma (MC type of melanoma)	• As name implies, it grows along the top layer of the skin for a long period of time before it penetrates deeper (hence better prognosis) • Commonly occurs in sun-exposed areas (e.g., trunk or legs). Occurrence of multiple nevi is additional risk factor.

Lentigo maligna melanoma	• Typically found in chronically sun-exposed areas, such as the face, neck, and scalp (melanoma on sun-damaged skin) and typically occurs in elderly. • Similar to superficial spreading melanoma, this tends to grow radially (more like a patch growth than a nodular growth), but this one is not associated with multiple nevi.
Nodular melanomas	• Tends to grow vertically, penetrating basement membranes (hence poorer prognosis). • The whole mole is nodular.[a]
Acral lentiginous	• Location is unique in that it is found in acral areas, such as palms, soles, or under the nail bed.

[a]Caution: Morphologically any type of melanoma can have small nodules, not only the nodular type. The type of melanoma is determined by biopsy.

Presentation: Look for the following features in a mole:
- **A**symmetry
- **B**orders are irregular
- **C**olor changes
- **D**iameter increase
- **E**volution (changing mole—e.g., recent changes in color or size)

Diagnosis: If suspected, NSIM is excisional biopsy (!). We need to remove the whole mole. We also need a full-thickness biopsy to find out the depth of tumor invasion, which is the most important prognostic factor.

After diagnosis is confirmed, additional excision with at least 1-cm margin is done (during excisional biopsy 1-cm margin excision is not necessary). Also, tumors with ≥0.75 mm depth or high-risk features will require sentinel lymph node biopsy.

Rx: For metastatic melanoma, there are various treatment options such as surgical excision of metastasis and immunotherapy (various monoclonal antibodies are available against different cancer pathways).

Preventive measures: Protective clothing is most important. Avoid sun exposure in the middle of the day and use sunscreen.

13.17 Congenital Melanocytic Nevus

- Found at birth.
- Can have ABCD features, especially as it can enlarge in tandem with child's growth.
- Can have malignant potential. Surgical removal is recommended for large lesions.

13.18 Vitiligo

Background: Acquired skin hypopigmentation due to autoimmune destruction of melanocytes in discrete areas. It is associated with other autoimmune disease such as systemic lupus erythematosus, Hashimoto's disease, Graves' disease, autoimmune adrenalitis (Addison's disease), diabetes mellitus type I, pernicious anemia, etc.

Presentation: White patches typically affecting hand and perioral area.

Rx: Topical or oral corticosteroids, topical tacrolimus, or UV light therapy.

Differential dx: Congenital albinism involves hairs and iris along with skin (i.e., hair and iris are also white), whereas vitiligo typically does not affect hairs and iris.

MRS

ABCDE

⚠ **Caution**

(!) Do not choose incisional biopsy as an answer: doing an incision and taking only a portion of the mole is not acceptable, as it can miss a malignant focus in a benign nevus.

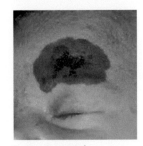

Source: Congenital Melanocytic Nevus. In: Sterry W, Paus R, Burgdorf W, eds. Thieme Clinical Companions—Dermatology. 1st ed. Thieme; 2006.

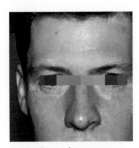

Source: External Appearance. In: Siegenthaler W, ed. Siegenthaler's Differential Diagnosis in Internal Medicine: From Symptom to Diagnosis. 1st ed. Thieme; 2007.

13.19 Hair Loss without Signs of Inflammation and Scarring (!)

⚠ Caution

(!) In patients with hair loss and signs of inflammation (e.g., erythema), think of tinea capitis or discoid lupus.

Condition	Pathophysiology	Features	Management
Telogen effluvium	Severe stress or change in hormonal status (e.g., child birth) may lead to a large number of growing hairs entering the **Te**logen stage (**Te**rminal hair-fall stage)	Diffuse shedding of normal hairs leads to diffuse thinning of hair	• Must rule out thyroid disorder and nutritional deficiencies (especially iron or zinc deficiency). • Evaluate for medication use that might cause alopecia and discontinue it if possible. • For idiopathic and chronic cases, minoxidil[a] can be tried.
Androgenetic alopecia	Genetic disorder thought to be caused by increased sensitivity of hair to effects of testosterone, resulting in change of hair to small thin forms. It is polygenic in nature with variable penetrance.	**Male pattern baldness** (recession of the anterior scalp line, or loss of hair starting from the center of scalp)	• Oral finasteride or topical minoxidil[a] • Hair transplantation can lead to permanent improvement
Alopecia areata	• Autoimmune antibodies that attack hair follicles • Associated with other autoimmune conditions such as thyroid disease, atopic dermatitis, etc.	• Discrete areas of hair loss • May be recurrent • In some cases, it may lead to complete loss of hair in scalp (called alopecia totalis), or even all over body (alopecia universalis).	**For localized disease:** intralesional corticosteroid or topical corticosteroid. **Second-line** treatments include topical minoxidil,[a] anthralin, or immunotherapy (a potent topical contact allergen is used to induce contact dermatitis, which stimulates hair growth). **For extensive disease: use** phototherapy combined with oral or topical psoralen.
Traumatic alopecia	• Due to prolonged or repetitive tension (e.g., tension due to dreadlocks or tighter ponytail hair style). This is known as traction alopecia.	• In hair damage due to dreadlocks or ponytail hairstyles, the small hairs in front of the scalp are not affected but the longer/larger hair fibers which are typically included to make these hairstyles are affected (known as the fringe sign).	Avoidance of underlying cause
	• Mechanical pulling (*trichotillomania*—a psychological disorder that involves pulling off one's hair)	• Look for broken hairs and irregular outline	

[a]MC side effect of minoxidil is allergic contact dermatitis.

13.20 Inherited Ichthyosis[7]—Low Yield

[7] Ichthyosis = fish-like scaly skin.

Condition	Features	Picture
Ichthyosis vulgaris	• Most common of inherited ichthyosis • Affects extensor surfaces more than flexor surfaces	 Source: Siegfried EC, Hebert AA. Diagnosis of Atopic Dermatitis: Mimics, Overlaps, and Complications. J Clin Med. 2015 May; 4(5): 884–917.
X-linked ichthyosis	• Occurs in males only • Affects extensor surfaces more than flexor surfaces	 Source: X-linked Recessive Ichthyosis. In: Sterry W, Paus R, Burgdorf W, ed. Thieme Clinical Companions—Dermatology. 1st ed. Thieme; 2006.
Lamellar ichthyosis	Most severe and rare condition that manifests at birth with plate-like scales all over the body	 Source: Autosomal Recessive Lamellar Ichthyosis. In: Sterry W, Paus R, Burgdorf W, eds. Thieme Clinical Companions—Dermatology. 1st ed. Thieme; 2006.

Answer

1.   Add oral antibiotics.

14 Emergency Medicine

"Before running the code, check your own pulse"
- Dr Paul L. Bernstein, Rochester, NY

14.1 Basic Life Support

When a person is found unresponsive:

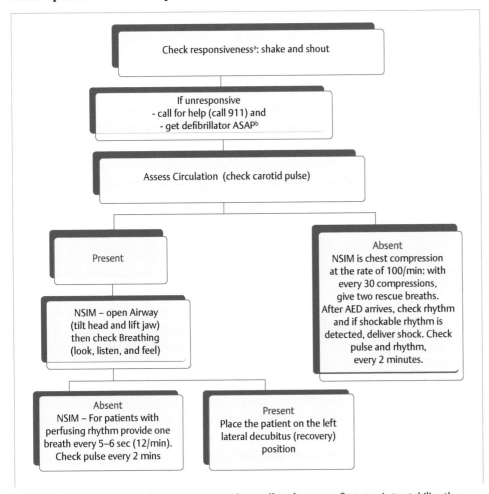

Check responsiveness[a]: shake and shout

If unresponsive
- call for help (call 911) and
- get defibrillator ASAP[b]

Assess Circulation (check carotid pulse)

Present

NSIM – open Airway
(tilt head and lift jaw)
then check Breathing
(look, listen, and feel)

Absent
NSIM is chest compression
at the rate of 100/min: with
every 30 compressions,
give two rescue breaths.
After AED arrives, check rhythm
and if shockable rhythm is
detected, deliver shock. Check
pulse and rhythm,
every 2 minutes.

Absent
NSIM – For patients with
perfusing rhythm provide one
breath every 5–6 sec (12/min).
Check pulse every 2 mins

Present
Place the patient on the left
lateral decubitus (recovery)
position

[a]In patients found unresponsive with suspected **spine/head trauma**, first step is to stabilize the neck and then only follow the algorithm given below (head tilting is contraindicated in this case).

[b]This scenario can have multiple causes, but one common cause is an arrhythmia. Nowadays, automated external defibrillators (AEDs) are widely available (e.g., shopping malls) and can be life-saving.

Abbreviation: AED, automated external defibrillator.

Circulation and airway are very important

- When you see "IV fluids" among answer choices in any question, **immediately** look at the blood pressure and heart rate. If BP is low (SBP ≤ 90), heart rate is >90/min and/or there are other features of volume depletion (e.g., dry oral mucosa, orthostatic drop in BP), then IV fluid resuscitation is **always** the right answer.[1]

- Similarly, apply this strategy when an exam-question has "intubation" as an answer choice. Look at the respiratory rate, arterial blood gas, etc.

14.1.1 Initial Empiric Treatment in Altered Mental Status[2]

Dextrose	For possible hypoglycemia (if blood glucose testing is not available)
Naloxone	Given to patients with signs of opiate poisoning (look for low respiratory rate)
Thiamine	IV dextrose can precipitate acute thiamine deficiency (due to increased consumption of thiamine). This is more likely to occur in patients with low thiamine levels (e.g., alcoholism, severe malnutrition).

 MRS

When found unresponsive
check call CAB:
- **C**heck
  unresponsiveness
- **C**all 911
- Address **c**irculation,
  airway, and **b**reathing

[1]Fluids most commonly used for resuscitation are normal saline and lactated ringers. In profoundly acidotic patient (blood pH ≤ 7), IV bicarbonate is preferred for volume resuscitation.

[2]This is typically done by emergency medical technicians outside of hospital.

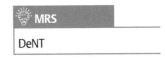 **MRS**

DeNT

14.2 Wernicke–Korsakoff Syndrome

Background	• Typically occurs in alcoholics or severely malnourished patients, due to thiamine deficiency. • Can be precipitated by administration of IV glucose without thiamine.	
Presentation	**Wernicke's syndrome or encephalopathy**	• Delirium (confusion). • Oculomotor dysfunction: nystagmus, lateral rectus palsy (almost always bilateral), and conjugate gaze palsy (due to involvement of oculomotor nerve). • Gait ataxia. • Imaging may reveal small lesions in midline brain structures.
	Korsakoff syndrome	After acute features of Wernicke improve, patients may develop chronic memory impairment. **Presentation:** Retro-anterograde amnesia, apathy of amnesia, and confabulation (patient typically makes up for what they cannot remember: an *"honest" lie*). Common imaging finding is atrophy of mammillary bodies.
Management	• Thiamine replacement. • Supportive treatment.	

14.3 Causes of Circulatory Collapse

For pulseless ventricular tachycardia or v-fib, please refer to Chapter 4, cardiology for further details
• Pulseless electrical activity

14.3.1 Pulseless Electrical Activity (PEA)

Definition: Electrocardiography (EKG) or telemetry shows electrical activity, but patient does not have a pulse.

Etiology:

4H		4T	
Hypovolemia	NSIM volume resuscitation[a]	Toxins	For example, overdose with sedatives, tricyclic antidepressants, heroine, etc.
Hyperkalemia or Hypokalemia	Hyperkalemia is common in dialysis patients who have missed treatment.	Tamponade (cardiac)	NSIM: pericardiocentesis
Hypoxia	For example, PEA arrest due to hypoxia can occur in patients with acute aspiration event.	Thrombosis (in pulmonary or cardiac vasculature)	For example. large pulmonary embolus or severe heart attack.
High acid (acidosis)	Missed dialysis treatment is a double trouble: acidosis and hyperkalemia.	Tension pneumothorax	NSIM: bedside needle thoracocentesis

[a]To address severe hypovolemia (e.g., in an ongoing bleeding), adequate IV access is necessary (at least two large-bore peripheral IV lines, or a central venous catheter/introducer[3] needs to be placed ASAP).

Abbreviation: TCA, tricyclic antidepressant.

[3]Introducer is a large bore central-venous catheter.

14.4 Shock

You have just admitted a patient with profound hypotension to ICU. Invasive hemodynamic monitoring is established. The cause of shock needs to be identified.

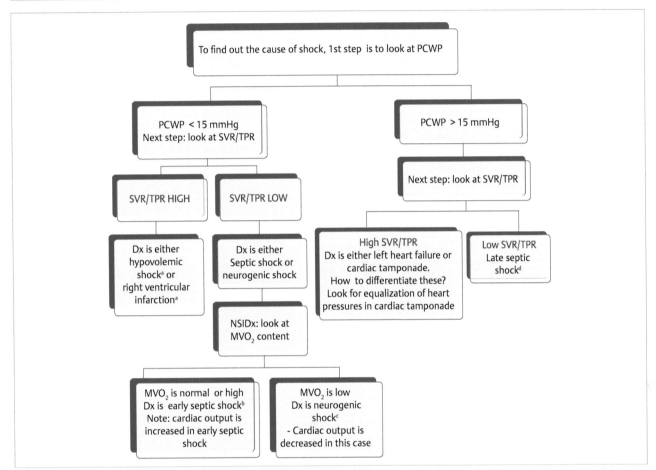

[a]There is compensatory increase in SVR/TPR (alpha-1 mediated vasoconstriction) in an effort to maintain BP and tissue perfusion.

Legend: "→" = leads to

[b]In early septic shock, inflammatory cytokines lead to primary vasodilation (low TPR/SVR) and compensatory increase in cardiac output (increased cardiac index) → increased blood flow and velocity → decreased oxygen extraction by tissues → normal or high **M**ean **V**enous **O**xygen content.

[c]In neurogenic shock (e.g., cervical or high thoracic spinal cord injury), there is sudden loss of sympathetic stimulation, which leads to primary vasodilation and a decrease in preload and cardiac contractility → low cardiac output → decreased velocity of blood flow → increased extraction of oxygen by tissues → low MVO_2.

[d]In late septic shock the heart starts failing (with development of decreased cardiac output, increased PCWP, and low MVO_2).

Abbreviations: MVO_2 content, mean venous oxygen content; NSIDx, next step in diagnosis; PCWP, pulmonary capillary wedge pressure (which is an indirect measurement of left heart pressure); SVR/TPR, systemic vascular resistance (a.k.a. total peripheral resistance).

14.4.1 Hemodynamic Parameters in Different Causes of Shock

	Cardiac output (cardiac index) and MVO$_2$	PCWP	SVR/TPR	Management
Hypovolemic shock	↓	↓, or **N**	Increased	IV fluid resuscitation
Right ventricular failure[a]	↓	↓	Increased	IV fluid ± dobutamine
Left ventricular failure	↓	Increased	Increased	Inotropic vasopressors (dobutamine, dopamine) and if refractory, IABP[b]
Pericardial tamponade[c]	↓	Increased	Increased	Pericardiocentesis
Anaphylactic shock	Increased	↓, or **N**	↓	IV fluids + epinephrine + antihistamines + IV steroids
Early septic shock (hyperdynamic stage of sepsis)	Increased	↓	↓	IV fluids, antibiotics, and vasopressors
Late septic shock	↓	Increased, or **N**	↓ [d]	
Neurogenic shock[MRS-1]	↓	↓	↓	Vasopressors like norepinephrine

[a]Clues to dx are elevated right atrial and right ventricular pressures with low PCWP.

[b]IABP = intra-aortic balloon pump. IABP is timed to inflate during diastole to augment coronary perfusion (**primary mechanism of action**) and deflate during systole, which increases the forward flow by creating a vacuum effect. IABP is contraindicated in patients with severe acute aortic regurgitation.

[c]In pericardial tamponade, look for equalization of pressures in the right and left sides of the heart.

[d]SVR/TPR will differentiate cardiogenic shock from late septic shock.

Abbreviations: IABP, intra-aortic balloon pump; MVO$_2$, mean venous oxygen; N, normal; PCWP, pulmonary capillary wedge pressure; SVR/TPR, systemic vascular resistance.

MRS

[MRS-1]In neurogenic shock, all systems are down.

Clinical Case Scenarios

[4]Trick is to look at diastolic pressures only.

Patient is in shock and is admitted to ICU. Pulmonary catheterization reveals the following pressure (in mmHg). What is the dx in each case?[4]

Right atrial pressure (normal is 2–6)[a]	RV pressure (normal is <25/8)[a]	PCWP (normal is <12–15)[b]	Diagnosis
18	25/18	18	Pericardial tamponade (there is equalization of pressure in all cardiac chambers)
25	30/20	8	Right ventricular infarction (cardiogenic shock with low PCWP but high right-sided heart pressures)
16	26/14	23	LV failure (cardiogenic shock)

[a]Do not memorize these values. They will be provided on exam.

[b]PCWP is an important number to know. Would recommend to memorize this value.

14.5 General Management of Poisoning or Acute Drug Overdose

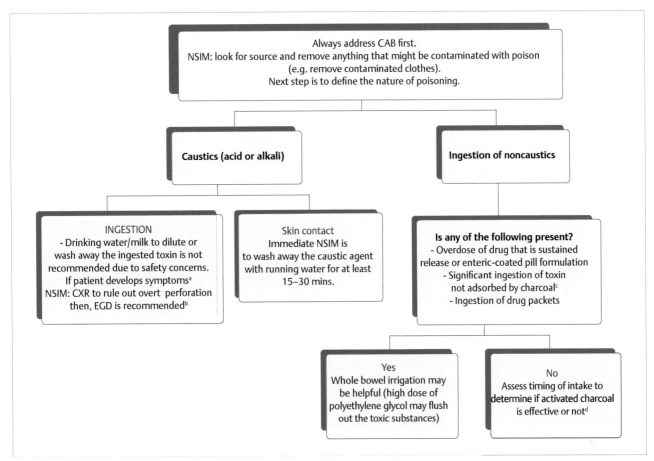

[a]Look for oral burns, heavy drooling of saliva, odynophagia, or inability to eat. Patients might also complain of retrosternal and epigastric pain.

[b]EGD is contraindicated in patients with suspected perforation or with severe upper airway edema.

[c]Activated charcoal is not effective for the following:

- **Heavy metals**: Iron, lead, mercury, arsenic, etc.

- **Inorganic ions**: Cyanide, lithium, fluoride, etc.

- **Caustics** (acid or alkali).

- Any form of alcohol ingestion.

[d]The more hours have passed the less the benefits of activated charcoal. It is not effective in situations where absorption is considered complete. This depends on what poison, drug, or chemical was ingested.

- In acetaminophen overdose, it can be used up until 4 hours after ingestion.

- For organophosphates, it is ineffective after 1 hour of ingestion.

Also, use of activated charcoal is contraindicated in patients with **altered mental status** as there is increased risk of aspiration.

Abbreviations: CAB, circulation, airway, breathing; EGD, esophagogastroduodenoscopy.

Patients with hx of caustic ingestion can present years later with mechanical dysphagia due to formation of peptic stricture related to scar tissue. Also, this scar tissue can predispose to squamous cell carcinoma of esophagus.

Gastric lavage: It includes placement of a large-bore orogastric tube, followed by repeated fluid instillation and aspiration. This is rarely used nowadays because evidence shows limited benefit and potential risk. It can however be performed in instances when a large amount of toxin has been known to be ingested within 1 hour.

14.6 Identification of Poison or Drug Overdose

Sometimes the cause of poisoning or ingested substance is unknown. Identifying the drug/poison responsible for presentation is very important.

Pupil size can be an important clue:

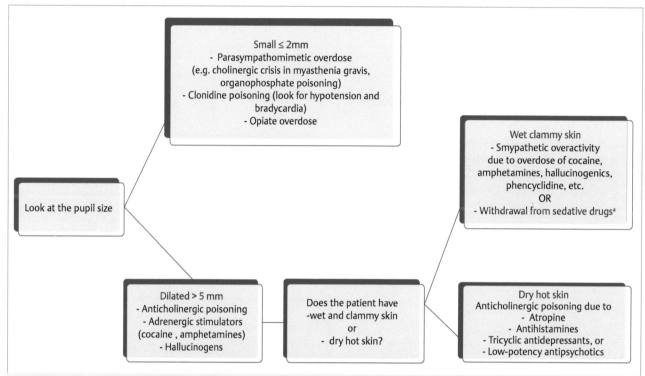

^aWithdrawal from most sedative drugs results in sympathetic hyperactivity (dilated pupils, hypertension, tachycardia, and wet and clammy skin).

14.7 Cholinergic and Anticholinergic Poisoning

	Cholinergic poisoning (muscarinic agonists)	Anticholinergic poisoning (muscarinic blockers)
Confusion/seizures/coma	May be present	Present
Skin (sweat glands)	Diaphoretic (clammy)	• Dry • Impaired heat-loss mechanism may lead to hyperthermia
Urine/bowel	• Incontinence (wet) • Diarrhea (watery)	• Urinary retention • Constipation
Pupils	Constricted ≤ 2 mm	Dilated > 5 mm
Drugs	Organophosphate or carbamate poisoning^a	Atropine and other anticholinergics^b
Antidote	• Give atropine, if there is evidence of bronchoconstriction or increased respiratory secretions. • 2-PAM (**Pr**Alidoxi**Me**) is an antidote for organophosphate or carbamate poisoning. It acts slowly.	• Physostigmine is used for significant symptoms. • Benzodiazepine is indicated for agitation and seizures.

[a]**Organophosphates and carbamates** are found in chemical pesticides and work by inhibiting acetylcholinesterase enzyme.

- Organophosphates = malathion, parathion, etc.
- Carbamates = methomyl, carbofuran, etc.

For treatment of poisoning, avoid further exposure by removing the clothes and washing the body thoroughly. If ingested, administer activated charcoal within 1 hour. Give pralidoxime, if evidence of cholinergic toxicity.

[b]**Other anticholinergics (muscarinic receptor blockers) are discussed below.**

The following drugs and chemicals can present with symptoms of anticholinergic (atropine-like) poisoning:

Most have sedating properties and can cause confusion, seizures, and coma	Drugs
Tricyclic antidepressants[a]	Amitriptyline, clomipramine, desipramine, imipramine
Older generation antihistamines[a]	Diphenhydramine, hydroxyzine (used for itching), chlorpheniramine
Antipsychotics[a]	Chlorpromazine, thioridazine
Antispasmodics	• Dicyclomine (used for irritable bowel syndrome) • Oxybutynin (used for bladder hyperactivity) • Cyclobenzaprine (a.k.a. flexeril) used for muscle spasms
Anti-parkinsonian drugs	Benztropine, trihexyphenidyl
Hallucinogenic plants	Jimson weed, deadly nightshade (Atropa belladonna), angel's trumpet, etc.

[a]They also have alpha-blocking properties and can cause hypotension.

14.8 Poisoning with Tricyclic Antidepressants

Presentation: Mydriasis, confusion, and seizures that can progress to coma. Tricyclic antidepressants (TCAs) also increase QRS interval and can lead to life-threatening arrhythmias.[5]

Management:

- Always address CAB first.
- If ingestion occurred < 2–4 hours ago, activated charcoal can be administered.
- NSIDx is serial EKGs. QRS interval is the most important indicator of severity of poisoning.
- If QRS is wide (> 100 ms) or patient develops ventricular arrhythmia, NSIM: IV NaHCO3 infusion (abates depressant action of TCA on cardiac Na+ channels).

14.9 β-Blocker Overdose

Background: Think about this poisoning in patients who are more likely to have access to this drug, e.g., hx of hypertension or coronary artery disease.

Clinical features: Bradycardia (PR prolongation on EKG) and hypotension. Additional features may include wheezing and prolonged expiratory phase due to β2 receptor blockade.

General management: Activated charcoal, if recent ingestion. Consider whole bowel irrigation if sustained release drug was ingested.

[5]TCAs block Na+ channels in cardiac tissues, similar to quinidine.

 MRS

ID 3Cs of TCA poisoning
- **ID** = **I**mipramine, **D**esipramine.
- **TCA** = **T**ricyclics are **C**lomipramine and **A**mitriptyline.
- **3Cs** = **C**oma, **C**onvulsions (seizure is very common), and **C**ardiotoxicity.

Very similar presentation can occur with thioridazine (antipsychotic drug) poisoning.

Specific antidote:

- For mild **hypotension or bradycardia**, give **IV** fluids ± **At**ropine (for symptomatic bradycardia).
- If no response to **IV fluids and still hypotensive**, try the following treatment in succession:

First: **Gl**ucagon bolus followed by infusion	Increases cardiac contractility via a different receptor than β-1
Second: **CA**lcium chloride or calcium carbonate	Increases cardiac contractility, thus indirectly negates the effect of excessive β-blockade
Third: **VA**sopressors	For example, epinephrine (positive chronotropic and inotropic drug)
Fourth: **IN**sulin bolus followed by infusion + glucose	Both β-blocker and calcium channel blockers decrease cardiac myocyte metabolism and glucose uptake by myocytes. Insulin negates this by increasing myocyte glucose uptake and myocyte energy production, thus increasing cardiac contractility.
Fifth: **LI**pid emulsion therapy	Intravenous lipid emulsion has micelle-like structures that draw in lipophilic drugs and thus lowers serum drug concentration, creating a concentration gradient that drives excess drug from tissues into blood.

> **MRS**
>
> **IVAT GLUCA VAIN LI**
>
> In patients with severe symptoms (profound hypotension or bradycardia), may give all of the above at once.

14.10 Differential diagnosis of β-blocker overdose

Calcium-channel blocker overdose/poisoning (e.g., diltiazem, verapamil)	It has similar features to B-blocker poisoning (hypotension + bradycardia), but without wheezing and prolonged expiratory phase.
	The treatment is similar to β-blocker overdose, but succession is a little bit different (use **IVAT CAGLU INVALI**). For example, try calcium salts prior to glucagon, in nonsevere poisoning.
Clonidine poisoning	It can also have similar features to B-blocker poisoning. Presence of miosis points toward clonidine poisoning.

14.11 Iron Poisoning

Background: Iron pills are readily available, so accidental ingestion/overdose is relatively common.

Toxic effects	Clinical features
Direct injury to GI mucosa causes mucositis	Abdominal pain, hematemesis, melena, diarrhea, nausea, and vomiting, etc.
Hypotension due to • direct GI fluid losses • distributive shock due to iron-mediated increased vascular permeability • cardiogenic shock: due to direct cardiodepressant effect of excessive iron	Shock-like phase with multiorgan failure syndrome: • shock liver • ARDS • acute renal failure, etc.

Abbreviations: ARDS, acute respiratory distress syndrome; GI, gastrointestinal.

[6]Note that activated charcoal binds poorly with iron, hence it is not an effective treatment.

General management: NSIDx is plain X-ray (iron is a radiopaque substance and can be easily seen). If a large number of radiopaque pills are seen on abdominal X-ray, NSIM is gastric lavage with a large-bore orogastric tube and/or whole bowel irrigation.[6]

Antidote: In patients with severe symptoms or a large number of radiopaque pills in X-ray, NSIM is IV deferoxamine (iron chelator).

Long-term sequelae: Permanent scarring of GI tract can occur. This can later present as GI obstruction.

14.12 Acetaminophen Poisoning

Mechanism of toxicity: Acetaminophen is metabolized by liver's phase II reduction reaction with the help of reduced glutathione. If a large amount of acetaminophen is ingested, liver's reduced-glutathione storage gets depleted and acetaminophen ends up being metabolized by the phase I oxidation reaction, which changes the drug into a substance which is toxic to liver.[7]

Clinical presentation: Acute hepatitis to acute liver failure. In very severe cases, patient may need liver transplant.

Management:

Administer activated charcoal, if within 4 hours of ingestion of toxic dose[8]
Indications for N-acetyl cysteine:
• Toxic level of acetaminophen 4 hours after ingestion
• Single ingestion of toxic dose,[8] in circumstances where the serum acetaminophen level cannot be checked within 8 hours
• In patients with unknown time of ingestion, and a random acetaminophen level of > 10 mcg/mL
• History of excessive acetaminophen ingestion with LFT abnormalities

Abbreviation: LFT, liver function test.

[7]Chronic alcoholics are more likely to develop severe toxicity, as alcohol induces phase I oxidation enzymes and depletes reduced-glutathione storage in the body.
Similarly malnourished patient are also at risk for tylenol toxicity, because they have decreased reduced-glutathione storage.

[8]Toxic dose of acetaminophen = either > 7.5 g or > 150 mg/kg

14.13 Aspirin Toxicity

Clues to diagnosis in test question: poisoning in a patient with a history of chronic pain syndrome.

Common presentation	• Gastritis: Nausea/vomiting and epigastric pain • Tinnitus
Severe presentation	• Noncardiogenic pulmonary edema • CNS toxicity: altered mental status and seizures

Work-up	• NSIDx—check blood aspirin level (the most specific test).
	• ABG finding:
	  – Mixed primary respiratory alkalosis (due to direct stimulation of the respiratory center) and primary metabolic acidosis (due to accumulation of anions such as lactate and ketones)
	  – Pure metabolic acidosis can be seen in children
	  – In late stages of severe poisoning, as patient develops altered mental status, respiratory acidosis can ensue.

Management: (always start with CAB)	• Activated charcoal for recent ingestion
	• Alkalinize urine to promote urinary excretion by using IV sodium bicarbonate infusion
	• Indications for hemodialysis
	  – Severe presentation, such as pulmonary edema, altered mental status, acidosis (pH ≤ 7.2).
	  – Significantly elevated creatinine that signals poor aspirin excretion (eGFR < 45 mL/min)
	  – Aspirin level of > 80–90 mg/dL
	  – Clinical deterioration despite optimal management

14.14 Sedative Overdose

	Opiate poisoning	GABA agonists (benzodiazepines, alcohol, phenobarbital) poisoning
Respiratory depression (slow and weak respiratory effort despite hypoxemia)	Present	Present
Varying levels of altered consciousness (*slurred speech → altered mental status → coma?*	Present	Present
Pupils	Pin-point[a]	Normal
NSIM	IV/IM naloxone, especially when respiratory effort is inadequate (e.g., respiratory rate < 12/min)	**Rx:** supportive. • The antidote of benzodiazepine, flumazenil, is only used to reverse excessive anesthesia in selected patients. Flumazenil can increase risk of seizures in patients who have been using benzodiazepine on a regular basis. • For barbiturates, use forced alkaline diuresis.

[a]Absence of miosis does NOT exclude opiate poisoning, as some opiates (meperidine or propoxyphene) do not cause miosis. Moreover, patients may have coingested other substances which make the pupil large (e.g., co-ingestion of opiates with diphenhydramine).

14.15 Other Alcohols

Alcoholics can ingest anything that smells like alcohol (methanol) and children can ingest anything that tastes sweet (methanol, ethylene glycol, and isopropyl alcohol all taste sweet).

	Methanol	Ethylene glycol	Isopropyl alcohol
Metabolism (first step requires alcohol dehydrogenase)	**Methanol** → formaldehyde → formic acid	Ethylene glycol → → oxalic acid	Isopropyl alcohol → acetone
Found commonly in	Antifreeze (used commonly in windshield washer fluid), coolants, solvents, and **moonshine whiskey.**	Antifreeze and coolants	*Antifreeze, solvents, cleaning fluids, and "rubbing alcohol."*
	All these alcohols can be used to make antifreeze. They make fluid resistant to freezing by lowering its freezing point.		
End-organ damage	Formic acid is toxic to optic nerve. Hence, methanol poisoning can cause visual impairment and even blindness.	Oxalic acid in urine can promote formation of calcium oxalate crystals, which can acutely precipitate in renal tubules and produce symptoms similar to a urinary tract stone (e.g., renal colic, hematuria) When this poisoning is suspected, NSIDx is urinalysis: look for needle-shape or envelop-shaped crystals.	Similar to ethanol intoxication
Varying levels of altered consciousness (**slurred speech → altered mental status → coma**)	Present	Present	Present
High anion gap acidosis	Yes (They may not have respiratory compensation, especially if obtunded)		No (Acetone is a neutral ketone)

High osmolal gap[a]	Yes	Yes (acetone is an active osmole)
NSIDx	Most specific test is serum assay for direct detection of the alcohol, e.g. serum methanol, ethylene glycol levels	
Management (always address CAB first)	• If a large amount is ingested less than 1 hour ago, gastric lavage may be beneficial. • Fomepizole, which inhibits alcohol dehydrogenase, is commonly used. If fomepizole is not available, ethanol infusion can be used, which is a substrate for alcohol dehydrogenase and acts as a competitive inhibitor. • Hemodialysis is recommended in severe cases; especially in patients with severe metabolic acidosis and/or evidence of end-organ damage.	• Supportive treatment • Manage as per alcohol intoxication. • There is no specific role for fomepizole.

[a]Osmolal gap = measured osmolarity (obtained by laboratory osmolarity detectors) – calculated serum osmolarity.[9]

[9] *FYI*: Calculated serum osmolarity =

$$2 \times [Na^+](meq/L) + \frac{Glucose\ (mg/dL)}{18} + \frac{BUN\ (mg/dL)}{2.8}$$

• Do not memorize this formula; it is not needed on exam.

An increased concentration of unaccounted osmoles leads to an increased osmolal gap.

Unaccounted osmoles	Increased concentration can be found in
Ketones	Diabetic ketoacidosis, alcoholic or starvation ketosis, Isopropyl alcohol ingestion
Lactate	Seizures, hypoperfusion states, carbon monoxide or cyanide poisoning, etc.
Protein	Hyperproteinemia
Various lipids	Severe dyslipidemia

A major source of loss of mark in exam is due to confusion in between different types of alcohol:
• Remember this MRS ☺ : MOP Floor = **M**ethanol = **Op**tic nerve damage by **For**mic acid. *"You can't drink the fluid that we use to MOP the floor with."*
• For ethylene glycol, I used to call it ethylene "glyco**X**ylate." It causes formation of **Ox**alate crystals.
• Additional MRS ☺ : o**X** = ✉ = envelope-shaped crystals (do you see the big "X" inside the envelope?)

MRS

Isopropyl = Iso-pH = same pH = does not cause acidosis.

14.16 Sedative Withdrawal[10]

Background: Common test question scenario might not give you specific drug intake history (otherwise the question would be too easy). It may give clues such as:
• "No hx could be obtained."
• The patient is homeless.
• May give elevated GGT in the lab results section (this suggests chronic alcohol use).
• Physical exam reveals track marks in arms (this suggests IV drug abuse and possible heroine withdrawal).

[10]Typically, sedative withdrawal occurs in patients after hospitalization as they lose access to abused substance and after few days of abstinence.

	Features[a]	Treatment
Alcohol withdrawal syndrome	**Scenario:** Typically occurs in a habitual heavy drinker after 2–3 days of alcohol abstinence or 2–3 days after hospitalization. **Presentation:** Acute onset delirium (confusion and disorientation) with or without hallucinations. • Classic hallucination is described as seeing insects and feeling them crawling all over the body. • Seizures can occur in severe cases.	Use benzodiazepines (e.g., lorazepam, diazepam, chlordiazepoxide), or phenobarbitals Hospitals commonly use alcohol withdrawal protocols, in which nurses assess the severity of withdrawal symptoms (using a chart) and depending on the calculated score, they give either IV or PO, high- or low-dose benzodiazepine, or phenobarbitals.
Opiate withdrawal	**Scenario:** May occur suddenly after administration of naloxone or naltrexone which are opiate antagonists, or may occur after hospitalization. **Presentation[b]:** • Features of GI stimulation (nausea, vomiting, diarrhea), • Restlessness • Rhinorrhea, lacrimation • Piloerection	Oral buprenorphine–naloxone[c] combination or methadone
Benzodiazepine withdrawal	It presents similarly to alcohol withdrawal. But the unique feature is that it can occur up to 3 weeks after stopping benzodiazepine (especially with long-acting forms).	Benzodiazepine

[a]All withdrawal states from sedatives are associated with features of increased adrenergic stimulation (hypertension and tachycardia). This can be treated with clonidine ± benzodiazepines.

[b]Unlike in alcohol or benzodiazepine withdrawal, opiate withdrawal is less likely to have seizures and hyperthermia.

[c]FYI, naloxone is added to prevent **injection** misuse. Oral naloxone has low bioavailability and is not absorbed into circulation, but if crushed and injected, naloxone blocks the euphoric effect of buprenorphine.

14.17 Miscellaneous Drugs of Abuse

	Cocaine/amphetamines	Hallucinogens like - Psilocybin ("magic mushroom") - LSD (lysergic acid diethylamide) - Mescaline - MDMA (ecstasy)	Phencyclidine (PCP)
Pupils	Dilated	Can be dilated	Can be dilated
Biochemical mechanism	Increased adrenergic transmission	Serotonin receptor agonist	NMDA—receptor blocker
Psychotic symptoms (hallucination, delusions)	May be present	Yes	Yes
Differentiating feature	Generalized hyperadrenergic symptoms	Flashbacks or hallucinations can occur with chronic use	**V**ertical nystagmus **V**iolent—agitated/loud[a]
Additional findings	As amphetamine is longer-acting, it mostly presents with prolonged wakefulness (awake for several days). Since cocaine is short-acting, the presentation is usually acute intoxication and rebound low mood after the drug effect wears off (on–off effect).	Profuse sweating, high blood pressure Acute presentation can be similar to cocaine use	Ataxia

[a]Another drug of abuse that can make patient very violent is **bath salts.**

14.18 Marijuana Use

Acute effect: Conjunctival injection (red conjunctiva), delayed reaction time, impaired orientation to time, slurred speech, etc.

Chronic effect: Regular marijuana use may lead to cognitive impairment, increased risk of infections, etc.[11]

[11]*FYI:* In a young patient with pneumonia, always inquire about marijuana use.

14.19 Exertional Heat

Disorders[12]

[12]Nonexertional heat disorders (unrelated to hot temperature environment) are malignant hyperthermia and neuroleptic malignant syndrome, which are discussed in Psychiatry chapter.

All are precipitated by hot environment	Heat cramps **(mild)**	Heat exhaustion **(moderate)**	Heat stroke **(severe)**
Main features to look for	• Only muscle cramps • No systemic features	• Weakness and lightheadedness • May have tachycardia and hypotension	• Hyperthermia + persistent cerebral dysfunction Other features include: • Acute kidney injury • Acute muscle injury (rhabdomyolysis)
Brain dysfunction	Not present	Mild confusion, but not persistent	• Persistent confusion and/or altered consciousness (may have coma) • May have seizures
Body temperature	Normal	Minor temperature elevation (≤ 104°F)[a]	High fever (> 104°F)[a]
Sweating	Present	Present	Skin is dry (loss of autoregulation and heat-losing mechanism)
NSIM	Oral fluids and electrolytes	• Oral fluids and electrolytes • May use any cooling method (e.g., cold-water immersion, cool shower)	Immediate step is cold-ice water immersion with continued cooling, IV fluids, and supportive treatment.

[a]Use rectal temperature to know the core temperature.

14.20 Hypothermia

Background: Hypothermia can occur as a result of exposure to very cold temperature.[13] Following drugs can impair body's temperature regulation and predispose to hypothermia:

● All the sedative drugs: alcohol, benzodiazepines, opiates, barbiturates, etc.

● High-potency antipsychotics (e.g., fluphenazine, haloperidol).

Work-up:

● Use thermometers that can read low temperatures.[14]

● EKG—may reveal Osborn waves, which is pathognomonic of hypothermia.[15] The MCC of death in hypothermia is cardiac arrhythmias, so EKG should be done ASAP.

Management:

	Definition in °F (in °C)	Management	
Mild hypothermia	90–95 (32–35)	**Passive** external warming (regular blankets, remove cold source)	Use warmed IV fluids, if hypotensive.
Moderate hypothermia	82–90 (28–32)	**Active** external warming (e.g., warming blankets)	

[13]Hypothermia unrelated to exposure to cold temperatures can occur in conditions like myxedema coma and Addisonian crisis.

[14]*FYI:* Standard thermometers can only read up to the minimum of 34°C (94°F).

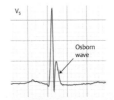

[15]Looks like a camel hump wave
Source: By Jer5150 - .', CC BY-SA 3.0, https://commons.wikimedia.org/w/index.php?curid=19566138.

Severe hypothermia (increased risk of ventricular arrhythmia and cardiovascular collapse)	< 82 (< 28)	• Start with warmed IV fluids and warming blankets. • If no response, NSIM is invasive warming measures, such as warmed pleural or peritoneal irrigation.

Other complications of hypothermia: Rhabdomyolysis and hyperkalemia.

14.21 Major Burn

First aid: Always address CAB first.

[16]Hoarse voice is due to development of laryngeal edema. It can develop suddenly and signals impending airway obstruction.

- Best initial management is 100% oxygen (due to common exposure to carbon monoxide)
- Consider intubation if any of the following present:
  - Dyspnea or shortness of breath
  - Hoarseness of voice[16]
  - Stridor
  - Wheezing
  - Cough
  - Burns or soot inside the nose or mouth
- NSIM: IV fluids (lactated Ringer's solution is preferred over normal saline in this case).

[17]Do not include superficial burns in this calculation.

How much fluid to start with? To calculate the amount of fluid replacement needed for initial 24 hours, use the following formula: $4 \, mL \times (\% \, body \, surface \, area \, burned^{17}) \times weight \, in \, kg$.

How to calculate burn area size?

In adults		In infants and small children
The rule of "multiple of 9's".		
Head and each upper extremity (anterior and posterior surfaces both)	9%	
Each leg (anterior and posterior surfaces)	18%	
Whole torso (anterior and posterior surfaces)	36%	
The width of the hand is 1% of the body surface area. This can be used to assess patchy burns.		

What is the rate of fluid administration?

- Half of the total calculated fluid requirement is given in the first 8 hours and the next half in the next 16 hours.
- Increase or decrease IV fluid administration to maintain hourly urine output of > 0.5 mL/kg, at the same time making sure that central venous pressure does not exceed 10 to 15 cm H20.

Other treatment considerations:

Other complications of major burns are hyperkalemia (due to major tissue breakdown) and hypothermia (due to heat loss).

- Circumferential burns require serial examination: progressive edema can lead to compartment syndrome, requiring urgent escharotomy.
- Most common cause of death in burn patients is septicemia. Use prophylactic topical antibiotics (silver sulfadiazine). There is no indication for **prophylactic** systemic antibiotics.
- Pain control.
- Tetanus prophylaxis.

14.21.1 Burn Patients, Especially Exposed to Fire in Closed Spaces, Have a High Risk of Carbon Monoxide and Hydrogen Cyanide Exposure

	Carbon monoxide (CO) poisoning	Cyanide poisoning
Additional situations where exposure can occur	• Car left running inside a garage • Gas heaters, wood burning stoves, or barbecuing in a closed space • Fireplace in unventilated areas	• Produced by combustion of synthetic polymers (e.g., silk, paint, cotton) in **a closed space** • Other notable cause includes prolonged nitroprusside infusion
Pathophysiology	CO binds with hemoglobin to create carboxyhemoglobin (CO-Hb). CO-Hb has high affinity for oxygen and binds with O2 readily, but does not release O2 to the tissues.	It is a mitochondrial poison that disrupts oxidative phosphorylation and aerobic metabolism. Presentation is similar to carbon monoxide, but symptoms are more severe as tissue hypoxia is more pronounced.
Common features	• Tissue hypoxemia without cyanosis. Skin may actually look pink. Pulse oximeter may detect 100% oxygen saturation.[a] **Depending on severity, the following can occur:** • Symptoms of cerebral hypoxia (altered mental status, confusion, seizures, coma) • Cardiac ischemia (chest pain, acute coronary syndrome, etc.) • Generalized hypoxemia (e.g., acute kidney injury, lactic acidosis[b])	
Differentiating features	• N&V and headache are the earliest signs	• Features of hypoxia are often more severe with very high lactate levels and acidosis.
Management	• First step is 100% oxygen • NSIDx is serum carboxyhemoglobin level (most specific test). • Severe cases may be treated with hyperbaric oxygen.	• If cyanide was ingested orally, activated charcoal can be used. • Give antidote hydroxocobalamin + sodium thiosulfate (Hydroxocobalamin avidly binds with cyanide and sodium thiosulfate donates sulphur to an enzyme that detoxifies cyanide). • If hydroxocobalamin not available, use a combination of amyl nitrite + sodium nitrite + sodium thiosulfate. (Nitrites induce formation of methemoglobin, which avidly binds with cyanide.)

[a]The following conditions can lead to generalized tissue hypoxia despite adequate oxygen saturation (or PaO$_2$):

• Anemia (absolute decrease in Hb).

• Carbon monoxide/cyanide poisoning or methemoglobinemia.

[b]Metabolism is diverted towards anaerobic glycolysis, causing lactic acidosis and resultant high anion gap metabolic acidosis.

Abbreviation: N&V, nausea and vomiting.

14.22 Methemoglobinemia

Etiology	• **Acquired:** Dapsone, nitrite drugs (e.g., inhaled nitric oxide), topical benzocaine, etc. • **Congenital:** (presentation: newborn appears blue)
Pathophysiology	When iron in hemoglobin gets abnormally oxidized to the ferric state (Fe^{3+}), it reduces hemoglobin affinity for oxygen.
Clinical features	Similar to above with symptoms of tissue hypoxia
Laboratory	• Suspect this in patients with cyanosis[a] and normal PaO$_2$. • Most specific test is the blood methemoglobin level.
Management	• Stop drugs that cause methemoglobinemia. • Antidote is methylene blue.

[a]In CO poisoning blood looks red and patient is not cyanotic, but in methemoglobinemia blood may look blue and patient appears cyanotic.

[18]Nowadays the distinction between salt water and fresh water is not considered clinically important.

14.23 Drowning

Background: Drowning can cause noncardiogenic pulmonary edema, hypothermia, etc. Most clinical pathophysiologic effects are related to hypoxemia or hypothermia.[18]

First-aid management:

- In an unresponsive patient, first SIM is two rescue breaths (the only situation in which two rescue breaths should be done first).
- Second SIM: If no spontaneous breathing, start cardiopulmonary resuscitation (CPR) and call 911.
- Maintain adequate ventilation: Use supplemental oxygen, non-invasive positive pressure ventilation or intubation as needed.

14.24 Spider Bites

	Black widow spider	Brown recluse spider
Pathophysiology and clinical features	It has neurotoxin[a] • Symptoms may look like tetanus with muscle spasm and/or pain involving various muscle groups. • Local pain at the bite site is present, but there is usually **NO** tissue necrosis. • Can cause hypertensive crisis.	Necrotoxin causes local skin necrosis
Treatment	– For severe pain or spasms, use antispasmodic such as IV benzodiazepine. – IV calcium is no longer recommended.	In patients with skin necrosis, use dapsone.[b] Once lesion has demarcated, surgical debridement may be done. Use antibiotics if features of cellulitis are present.

[a]MRS ☺ BLACK **WIDOW** IS NEUROTIC because she lost her husband to tetanus. Neurotic = neurotoxin.

[b]Prior to using dapsone (for any indication), screen for G6PD deficiency.

14.25 Snake Bites

Background: Snake venoms can be neurotoxic (similar to botulinum toxin), hemotoxic (can cause disseminated intravascular coagulation and hemolysis), and/or necrolytic (can cause significant local necrosis).

[19]Tourniquet should never be used as it cuts off arterial blood flow.

First-aid treatment:

- Immobilize the injured part of the body. This will help decrease the spread of the venom.
- Apply compression bandage[19] with a temporary splint fashioned out of things that are available in the environment (pressure immobilization). Apply bandage only so tightly and make sure the distal pulses are palpable so as not to cause tissue ischemia.

Antidote: Immediate transfer to the nearest hospital for administration of antidote (snake antivenom).

14.26 Over-the-Counter Supplements and Important Side Effects or Drug Interaction

This is a high yield topic for exam.

Herbal supplement	Commonly used for	Important side effect or drug interaction
Dong quai	Female health boosting effects	Prolonged INR
Kava kava	Anxiety and insomnia	Abnormal LFTs/liver damage
St. John's wort	Depression	– Cytochrome P450 inducer (decreases warfarin effects) – Can increase the risk of serotonin syndrome
Ginkgo biloba	Memory boosting effects	Prolonged bleeding time (similar to aspirin)
Ginseng	Used for lowering cardiovascular risk profile	
Feverfew	Pain (e.g., migraine, arthritis)	

Abbreviations: INR, international normalized ratio; LFT, liver function test.

Clinical Case Scenarios

CCS: Cover the last column for practice.

CCS	Choices	Answer
Patient who had a spider bite now presents with significant local black-colored necrotic area.	Brown recluse or black-widow spider bite?	Brown recluse spider bite
Unknown ingestion of drug with the following features: • Wheezing • Hypotension + bradycardia • Pupils are small	What is the likely drug? a) B-blocker b) Clonidine c) Verapamil	Clonidine (small pupils point towards this).
A person is found down on the ground.	What is the NSIM? a) Shake and shout b) Call 911 c) Get help	First step is to check responsiveness.
After a drowning accident, the person is unresponsive.	What is the NSIM? a) Check pulse b) Immediate two rescue breaths	Immediate two rescue breaths should be done first.
Patient took unknown quantity of home-made alcohol. This morning he woke up with visual blurring in both eyes.	What is the likely cause of poisoning? a) Methanol b) Ethylene glycol c) Isopropyl alcohol	Methanol.

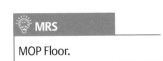

MRS

MOP Floor.

15. Ophthalmology

"Cataract *is an easily treatable condition*, but, unfortunately, it is the most common cause *of blindness in the world because of decreased availability of health-care. In developed countries, the three leading causes of blindness are glaucoma, age-related macular degeneration (AMD), and diabetic retinopathy.*"

15.1 Eye Infections

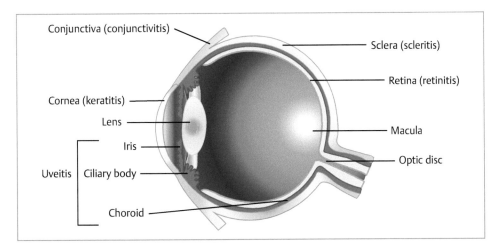

15.1.1 Conjunctivitis

Etiology

- **Infectious**—viruses, bacteria, fungi, and parasites (amoeba)
- **Noninfectious**—allergic or chemical conjunctivitis

Physical examination

Red conjunctiva (conjunctival injection) plus discharge.[1]

[1]Conjunctivitis alone does not cause visual impairment. Presence of decreased visual acuity in a patient with apparent conjunctivitis indicates involvement of cornea (keratoconjunctivitis).

	Viral	Bacterial	Allergic
Clues	Flu-like symptoms may be present	Other sites may also be infected (e.g., coexistent otitis media)	Coexistent allergic rhinitis, atopic dermatitis, asthma, etc.
Discharge	Mostly clear, but can be yellow	Mucopurulent discharge (yellow to white)	Watery, clear discharge (never mucopurulent)
Laterality	Unilateral or bilateral		Almost always bilateral
Management[a]	**Supportive:** • Use combination of topical antihistamine plus vasoconstrictor-decongestant (e.g., naphazoline + pheniramine) • Use warm or cold compresses, as needed	Topical antibiotic options are: • macrolides (erythromycin, azithromycin, etc.) • trimethoprim + polymyxin • bacitracin + polymyxin • sulfacetamide, etc.[b]	**Acute (< 2-week duration):** Use combination of topical antihistamine plus vasoconstrictor-decongestant eye drop (e.g., naphazoline + pheniramine) **Frequent episodes (> 2 days/ month) or lasting longer than 2 weeks:** Use topical antihistamine with mast cell stabilizing properties (Ketotifen, epinastine, azelastine, olopatadine, alcaftadine, etc.)[c]

[a]Drops are generally preferred in adults, as ointments may blur vision. Ointments are preferred in children and noncompliant patients, as they typically remain in contact longer.

[b]Use quinolone eye drops to cover pseudomonas in patients using contact lenses (e.g., ofloxacin, ciprofloxacin). It is very important to rule out keratitis in such patients.

[c]Oral antihistamines can worsen dry eyes and should be avoided.

Conjunctivitis in newborns

Etiology	Usual time of appearance	Rx
Chemical conjunctivitis (reaction to silver nitrate eye drops)[a]	Within the first 24 hours	Symptomatic treatment with eye lubricants as needed
Gonococcal conjunctivitis	1–5 days	Single dose of intramuscular ceftriaxone[b]
Chlamydial conjunctivitis	> 5 days	Oral erythromycin[b]

[a]All newborn babies routinely get erythromycin ointment (or silver nitrate) within the first few hours of birth to prevent gonococcal conjunctivitis.

[b]Topical treatment is not necessary when systemic is given. One can use saline irrigation until the discharge clears up.

Trachoma

Microbial cause: certain subtypes of Chlamydia Trachomatis, which is the bacteria commonly known to cause sexually transmitted infections

Background: it is easily treatable with run-of-the-mill antibiotics, but unfortunately it is one of the leading causes of preventable blindness in developing countries, due to decreased availability of health care.

Disease features: persistent follicular conjunctivitis (usually accompanied by nasal discharge) followed by corneal neovascularization and opacification.

Rx: single-dose oral azithromycin or topical tetracycline.

15.1.2 Corneal Injury

Etiology

Infectious keratitis, ulcer, abrasion, foreign body, direct trauma, etc.

Common Presentation to All Forms of Corneal Injury

Eye pain (may be severe) and foreign body sensation in the cornea	
Miosis	In corneal injury, sensory trigeminal nerve gets irritated, which initiates a miotic reaction
Photophobia	• Exposure to light dilates irritated miotic pupil, which results in pain and photophobia • Cycloplegics (M blockers such as atropine, homatropine, and scopolamine) help alleviate the pain by paralyzing pupillary muscle
Blurred vision	Corneal involvement will result in vision abnormalities
Reactive conjunctival injection	Red conjunctiva

Eye Examination

- Start with the gross penlight examination first.
- The next step is a full eye examination. If a patient is uncomfortable or uncooperative, a topical anesthetic like tetracaine can be used to perform the examination.[2]
- Full eye examination includes visual acuity test and fundoscopic examination, followed by fluorescein dye examination (this dye stains only the exposed basement membrane of the cornea).[3] Use Wood's lamp (or slit lamp + cobalt-blue filter or ophthalmoscope + cobalt-blue filter) for better visualization.

[2]Use topical anesthetic only when necessary, as its use have been associated with local complications.

[3]Early dye examination can interfere with visual acuity and fundoscopic examination; hence it is done at the end.

Etiology of corneal injury	Additional information	Management (urgent ophthalmologic referral is recommended)
Corneal abrasion, ulcer, or presence of foreign body	Can occur as a result of blast injury or abrasion in contact lens wearers	• Foreign body removal, if present • Topical antibiotic to prevent secondary infection. For contact lens-related abrasions, give topical antibiotics that are effective against pseudomonas (e.g., moxifloxacin, ciprofloxacin) • Large abrasions and ulcers may require cycloplegics and an eye patch
Bacterial keratitis	Contact lens is the most common risk factor **Examination:** red eye + round white spot in cornea (corneal infiltrate)	Do Gram stain and culture of corneal scrapings before initiating topical antibiotics (e.g., topical quinolones)
Amebic keratitis	• Occurs in contact lens wearers • Causative organism is *Acanthamoeba*	Staining of corneal scraping can reveal the organism **Rx:** antiprotozoal eye drops
HSV keratitis	This can be recurrent (akin to recurrent herpes labialis). Episodes can cause corneal scarring, opacification and corneal blindness. **Examination:** vesicles can be seen. Fluorescein staining can reveal dendritic ulcers.	**Rx:** oral and topical acyclovir or valacyclovir. Chronic suppressive therapy may be indicated in patients with recurrent episodes
Epidemic adenoviral keratoconjunctivitis	Membranes and pseudomembranes can occur	• Self-limiting disease • Supportive treatment
Fungal keratitis	• Causative organism is *Fusarium* spp. • This typically occurs after a corneal injury involving plant material (e.g., palm branch hitting the eye); hence, it is more likely to occur in agricultural workers • Can also occur in contact lens wearers	Use topical voriconazole or natamycin. In immunocompromised patients or severe infections, add systemic voriconazole.

Abbreviation: HSV, herpes simplex virus.

Keratoconjunctivitis Sicca (Dry Eye Disease)

Risk factors: advanced age, lacrimal gland inflammation associated with autoimmune syndrome (Sjögren syndrome, systemic lupus erythematosus, rheumatoid arthritis, etc.).

Pathophysiology: decreased lubricating effect of tears may lead to conjunctival and corneal irritation, with subsequent development of conjunctival injection, sensation of foreign body in eye, and mild photophobia. Complications may include corneal abrasion, scar, and corneal blindness.

Rx: use artificial tears. For refractory ocular Sjögren's syndrome, use topical immunosuppressive (e.g., cyclosporine).

15.1.3 Uveitis

Definition	**Anterior uveitis:** inflammation limited to iris and ciliary body (iridocyclitis)—mostly anterior chamber
	Posterior uveitis: inflammation of the choroid (choroiditis) and other adjacent structures (commonly involved structures are retina and/or optic nerve head)
	Panuveitis: anterior + posterior uveitis

Type	Granulomatous	Nongranulomatous
Differentiating feature (slit-lamp examination)	• Large and greasy-looking keratic precipitates[a] • Presence of iris nodules	No iris nodules
Etiology[b]	It can be a part of systemic granulomatous disease, such as Lyme disease, tuberculosis, syphilis, or autoimmune (sarcoidosis)	Associated with autoimmune conditions related to HLA-B27 (e.g., seronegative spondyloarthropathy, ulcerative colitis)

Presentation	• **Anterior uveitis:** eye pain, photophobia, miosis, and conjunctival injection (presentation is similar to corneal injury)
	• **Posterior uveitis:** floaters and/or visual impairment (in contrast to anterior uveitis, it is less likely to have red eye or eye pain)
Work up	• **NSiM** is immediate referral to ophthalmologist for slit-lamp and fundoscopic examination
	• **Anterior uveitis:** pus or leukocytes in the anterior chamber (hypopyon) makes the dx of uveitis and differentiates it from keratitis
	• **Posterior uveitis:** direct visualization of choroiditis + leukocytes in vitreous humor
Management	**Infectious cause:** treatment is directed against underlying microbial cause
	Noninfectious uveitis:
	• **Anterior uveitis**—topical steroids[c]
	• **Posterior uveitis or panuveitis**—observation (in mild cases), or periocular and/or sometimes intraocular steroids[d] **For refractory cases,** give oral steroids
	Use cycloplegics for severe pain

[a]Keratic precipitates are clusters of inflammatory cellular deposit on cornea, seen as white spots when examined with a slit lamp.[4]

[b]Patients with Crohn disease (granulomatous inflammation of colon) can have both granulomatous and nongranulomatous uveitis.

[c]Topical steroids should only be prescribed by ophthalmologists, as they can be associated with significant local side effects.

[d]Topical steroids do not reach posterior portions of uvea; hence they are not helpful.

Abbreviation: HLA, human leukocyte antigen.

[4]Slit-lamp view of anterior granulomatous uveitis in sarcoidosis, showing "mutton fat" granulomatous keratic precipitates.

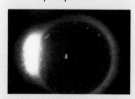

Source: Sarcoidosis. In: Biousse V, Newman N. Neuro-Ophthalmology Illustrated. 2nd ed. Thieme; 2015.

15.2 Severe Eye Infection

Risk factor: Patients with high-grade immunosuppression (HIV with low CD4 count, immunosuppressive therapy, organ transplant recipients) may develop eye infection that progresses faster or have higher risk of complications.

Features	Diagnosis	Management[a]
• Immunosuppression + features of only retinitis (e.g., floaters,[b] photopsia,[c] visual impairment) • Patients may or may not have symptoms of other organ involvement (e.g., pneumonitis, diarrhea)	**CMV retinitis** (This usually doesn't have conjunctivitis or keratitis). • In HIV patients, it occurs with **CD4 count of** < 50 cells/µL	**If sight threatening infection**—use intravitreal ganciclovir or foscarnet + systemic oral valganciclovir. **If non-sight threatening infection**—use oral valganciclovir (preferred).
Immunosuppression + features of retinitis + features of encephalitis (e.g. changes in the personality, altered mental status)	**Toxoplasmosis** • In HIV patients, it occurs with **CD4 count** of < 100 cells/µL	Oral pyrimethamine + sulfadiazine (with folinic acid)

Infection of all internal eye structures (scleritis, choroiditis, uveitis and retinitis) including infection of vitreous and aqueous humor	**Endophthalmitis**
	Etiology:
	• Fungal or bacterial infection due to:
	  ○ Complication of eye surgery, intravitreal injection, penetrating eye trauma, keratitis, etc.
	  or
	  ○ Blood-borne microbial seeding into the eye from systemic infection (e.g., from candidemia).
	• Virus (e.g., HSV, CMV) can do it but it is very rare.
		Systemic and intravitreal antimicrobial treatment, directed against underlying pathogen

Hx of progression in the following manner: conjunctivitis and keratitis → uveitis→ scleritis → retinitis and acute retinal necrosis → *Endophthalmitis*—infection of all internal eye structures (scleritis, choroiditis, uveitis, and retinitis) • Fluorescein examination may reveal dendritic ulcers and vesicles.	Does the patient have **vesicular rash** in the distribution of ophthalmic branch of trigeminal nerve? • If yes, then dx is Herpes **zoster ophthalmicus.** • If no, then think of **herpes simplex keratitis**.	• Topical and oral acyclovir or valacyclovir. • In herpes **zoster ophthalmicus**, consider varicella-zoster immunoglobulin.

[a]Specific intravitreal therapy can be considered in all cases of severe or sight threatening infections.

[b]Debris in vitreous humor are seen as floaters.

[c]Irritation of retina can result in abrupt firing of retinal nerve cells causing photopsia (seeing flashes of light). This irritation can be due to vitreous pathology (e.g., vitreous detachment) or retinal pathology (e.g., retinitis).

Abbreviation: HSV, herpes simplex virus.

15.3 Infection Involving the Preseptal Area, Orbit, and Cavernous Sinus Thrombosis

	Preseptal cellulitis	Orbital cellulitis	Cavernous sinus thrombosis
	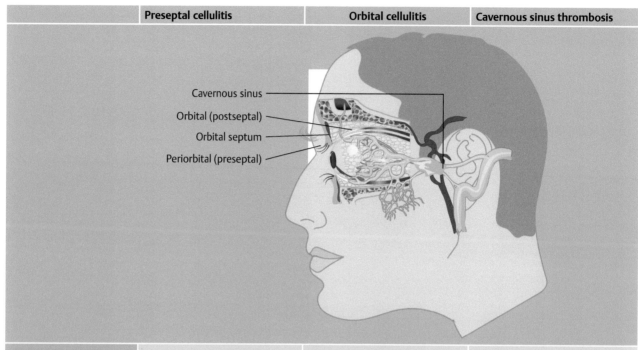 Cavernous sinus — Orbital (postseptal) — Orbital septum — Periorbital (preseptal) —		
Pathophysiology and etiology	Mild infection involving the structures anterior to the orbital septum **Etiology:** local trauma (e.g., insect bite, trauma, surgery, etc.) or contiguous site infection (e.g., facial cellulitis, sinusitis, dental abscess, etc.)	More severe infection that involves the structures posterior to the orbital septum (fat and ocular muscles) **Etiology:** common underlying conditions include contiguous site infection (e.g., sinusitis), orbital trauma, local surgery, etc. • Etiology is similar to preseptal cellulitis	• The cavernous sinuses receive blood from the face area (nose, tonsils, orbits, etc.) • Infections in these areas (e.g., sinusitis and furuncles) can spread to and involve the cavernous sinus • Most clinical features are due to venous obstruction/congestion and nearby cranial nerve impairment
Common features: periorbital edema, erythema, swelling, chemosis (conjunctival edema), increased warmth and/or tenderness with systemic signs of infection/fever	No ophthalmoplegia, no diplopia, and no pain with eye movements.	• Ophthalmoplegia (cranial nerves 3, 4, and 6 may be involved) ± diplopia • Pain with eye movements • Proptosis might be very subtle • Absence of features of increased intracranial pressure (e.g., papilledema, headache)	• Ophthalmoplegia (cranial nerves 3, 4, and 6 may be involved [6 is the earliest involved]) ± diplopia • Proptosis is more prominent • Less likely to have pain with eye movements • Look for signs of increased intracranial pressure (e.g., papilledema and headache)
	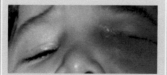 Dacryocystitis, of left lacrimal sac with associated preseptal cellulitis. Source: Lacrimal System Disorders. In: Agarwal A, Jacob S. Color Atlas of Ophthalmology. The Quick-Reference Manual for Diagnosis and Treatment. 2nd ed. Thieme; 2009.	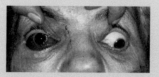 Chemosis (conjunctival edema) plus ophthalmoplegiain the right eye. (Note that the right eye is not moving with the left eye.) Source: Orbital Cellulitis. In: Lang G. Ophthalmology. A Pocket Textbook Atlas. 3rd ed. Thieme; 2015.	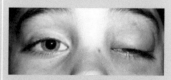 There is subtle proptosis and ophthalmoplegia. Source: Carotid Cavernous Thrombosis. In: Biousse V, Newman N. Neuro-Ophthalmology Illustrated. 1st ed. Thieme 2009.

	Preseptal cellulitis	Orbital cellulitis	Cavernous sinus thrombosis
Management	• **Mild infection in a patient > 1 year old**—outpatient treatment with oral antibiotics that covers MRSA and streptococci: ○ Oral trimethoprim-sulfamethoxazole, doxycycline,[a] or clindamycin + ○ Amoxicillin (± clavulanate) or cefdinir[b] Treatment is similar to cellulitis • **< 1 year or more severe infection**—manage as orbital cellulitis[c]	• **NSiM:** blood cultures and Gram stain/culture of drainage (if present), and IV antibiotics that cover MRSA, streptococci, and gram negatives (e.g., IV vancomycin + ampicillin–sulbactam) • After this, NSiM is urgent ENT and ophthalmologic consultation and further diagnostic test, such as a CT scan or MRI scan with contrast, to define the extent of infection • Anticoagulation is controversial in cavernous sinus thrombosis	

[a]Avoid doxycycline in children.

[b]Clindamycin has inadequate H. influenza coverage. Trimethoprim/sulfamethoxazole and doxycycline do not reliably cover group A streptococci.[5]

[c]Orbital septum is not completely developed in infants, so infection can spread rapidly into the orbital area, meninges, and brain.

Abbreviations: ENT, ears, nose, and throat; IV, intravenous; CT, computed tomography; MRI, magnetic resonance imaging.

[5] MRSA resistance to clindamycin is on the rise (check your local hospitals' or community's antibiogram), but for board-purposes, clindamycin is still the right answer. In my hospital, around 40% of MRSA isolates are resistant to clindamycin.

Clinical Case Scenarios

Patient with hx of eye surgery comes in with the following complications	Diagnosis
Swollen eyelids	Blepharitis
Red and swollen conjunctiva	Conjunctivitis
Severe photophobia plus floaters. Slit-lamp examination shows pus in the anterior chamber	Uveitis
Decreased vision, flashing lights and floaters	Retinitis

1. What would the diagnosis be if patient has all of the above complications?

2. Patient had Hx of severe trauma to the right eye 6 weeks ago. He now presents with blurred vision and severe photophobia.
   Slit-lamp examination shows pus in the anterior chamber in both eyes. What is the likely dx?

The answers are given at the end of the chapter.

15.4 Glaucoma

Background: Increase in intraocular pressure (IOP) leads to pressure on the optic nerve causing pressure atrophy (cupping of optic disc) and vision loss.

	Open-angle glaucoma	Closed-angle glaucoma
Primary pathology that leads to increased IOP		
	Pathogenesis isn't clear; it may be related to increased aqueous humor production by ciliary body and/or decreased absorption through trabecular meshwork	In patients with preexisting anatomic abnormality (narrow-angle), the following sequence can be precipitated by mild dilatation of pupil—increased opposition between iris and lens → relative blockage of pupillary outflow → increased aqueous humor collection in posterior chamber, which pushes the iris anteriorly (iris bombe) → increased contact of iris with cornea → blockage of trabecular meshwork → decreased drainage of aqueous humor
Risk factors	Advancing age, family history	
	Black race, myopia (nearsightedness)	Asian race, hyperopia (farsightedness), female
Presentation	**Chronic** painless slowly progressive vision loss that affects peripheral vision earlier (tunnel vision) Tunnel vision Dx is made by tonometry	Can be **acute** or **chronic** (chronic closed-angle glaucoma presents similar to open-angle glaucoma)
Diagnosis	Made by combination of tonometry (IOP > 23–24 mmHg), fundoscopy (evidence of optic-disc cupping), visual field testing, pachymetry (measure of corneal thickness—patients with thin cornea are at higher risk of development of open-angle glaucoma) and gonioscopy (a special lens is used with slit lamp to visualize the angle). See table in Section 15.4.1 Acute Angle-Closure Glaucoma	
Treatment	Initiate treatment if IOP is > 25 mm Hg in two office visits • **First-line agents:** topical prostaglandins (e.g., bimatoprost, latanoprost, travoprost) or laser therapy (trabeculoplasty) • Other second-line agents for combination therapy include a topical beta-blocker (e.g., carteolol, bisoprolol) and a carbonic anhydrase inhibitor (e.g., dorzolamide, brinzolamide)[a] • Surgery is advised, if medical therapy or laser trabeculoplasty fails to control IOP	• See next page for Acute Angle-Closure Glaucoma • For chronic angle-closure glaucoma, first-line treatment is laser peripheral iridotomy (making a hole in the iris to drain aqueous humor). If not responsive, treat similarly to open-angle glaucoma
Screening	Comprehensive eye examination starting at age 40	

[a]Alpha-adrenergic agents such as apraclonidine and brimonidine have been associated with higher risk of allergic conjunctivitis, so they are not used as first- or second-line agents.

Abbreviation: IOP, intraocular pressure.

15.4.1 Acute Angle-Closure Glaucoma

Presentation: sudden eye pain, blurred vision, photophobia with headache, nausea, and vomiting.[6]
Eye examination: the eye appears red with fixed and dilated pupils. On palpation the eyeball feels stony hard.

Exam-question scenario	Underlying reasons for acute angle-closure[a]
Recent upper respiratory tract infection	Decongestant use (which has M-blocking effect)
Watching movies in theater or going spelunking	Darkness-related pupillary dilatation
Recent onset nausea	Antiemetic use (which has M-blocking effect)
Motion sickness, COPD, bladder spasms, etc	Use of medicines that have anti-muscarinic effect (motion sickness—scopolamine or meclizine; COPD—tiotropium, ipratropium, etc.; bladder spasm—oxybutynin)
Symptomatic bradycardia	Atropine usage

[a]All of these reasons lead to pupillary dilatation.
Abbreviation: COPD, chronic obstructive pulmonary disease.

NSIDx is an indentation gonioscopy (using a special lens with slit lamp to visualize the angle). It is the gold standard for diagnosis.

Management

- First step is immediate instillation of topical eye drops that decrease IOP: timolol (B-blocker) + apraclonidine (alpha-2 agonist), and addition of pilocarpine (M-agonist that produces miosis).
- Second step is to add systemic diuretics—oral/intravenous (IV) acetazolamide. Second-line is IV mannitol.
- Definitive treatment is laser iridotomy.

Differential Diagnosis of Sudden Painful Visual Impairment Plus Red Eye

Visual impairment with the following features...	Keratitis	Anterior uveitis	Acute angle-closure glaucoma
Red eye, eye pain, and photophobia	Yes		
Pupil size		Small[a]	Fixed and dilated
Slit-lamp examination reveals pus cells in anterior chamber	No	Yes	No
Floaters	No	±	No

[a]In keratitis and uveitis, cycloplegics (M-blockers), which paralyze the pupils, relieve the pain. On the contrary, in acute angle-closure glaucoma, cycloplegics can precipitate an episode, and M-agonists are used for treatment.

Optic Neuritis and Multiple Sclerosis

Pathology: autoimmune inflammation of optic nerve.

Presentation

- Blurry vision and decreased visual acuity (patients may complain that colors look washed out).
- Pain with eye movements and/or pain behind the eye.
- Look for history of transient episodes of extremity weakness, numbness, or urinary incontinence, which may suggest multiple sclerosis.

[6]Secondary acute angle-closure glaucoma can be due to anterior uveitis, dislocation of lens, topiramate therapy, etc.

⚠ **Caution**

Cluster headaches and acute angle-closure glaucoma can have similar presentation with retrobulbar pain, tearing of eyes, and conjunctival injection. There is however no blurred vision in cluster headaches.

Treatment: treat as multiple sclerosis exacerbation with short course of IV steroids.

Differential dx: neuromyelitis optica is a rare demyelinating condition similar to multiple sclerosis, but in this case the disease is confined to spinal cord (myelitis) and optic nerve (optic neuritis). It is also treated with IV steroids.

15.5 Sudden Painless Loss of Vision

The following conditions can cause sudden painless loss of vision and majority of them must be treated in an emergency setting to prevent permanent visual loss. Next step in management is emergent ophthalmology referral with full eye examination (including fundoscopy).

	CRAO	CRVO	Retinal detachment	Vitreous hemorrhage
Pathophysiology and risk factors	**Pathology:** emboli from ipsilateral internal carotid artery or ophthalmic artery **Risk factors** are same as they are for a stroke—ASCVD, vasculitis, thrombophilia, etc.	Virchow's triad of hypercoagulability: • **Thrombophilic disorders** • **Inflammation**— local infection and vasculitis • **Stasis**—compression of vein due to local causes such as glaucoma, inflammatory optic disc swelling, atherosclerotic plaques/thickening in retinal artery causing compression of adjacent veins (hence risk factors include ASCVD)	**Pathology**—retina peels off from underlying supportive connective tissue **Risk factors:** • Proliferative retinopathy due to diabetes, wet-type AMD (heavy retina), etc. • Trauma (e.g., surgical extraction of cataract) • Myopia	**Rupture of abnormal blood vessels**—proliferative retinopathy due to diabetes, AMD, CRVO, sickle cell retinopathy, etc. **Rupture of normal vessels**—trauma, retinal tear or detachment, etc.
Additional history points	Look for hx of amaurosis fugax ("black curtain falling in front of the eye" and return of vision) • Amaurosis fugax is an equivalent of TIA • CRAO is an equivalent of a stroke	Nonspecific	• Patients may describe visual loss as "curtain falling in front of the eye," "flashes of light" (photopsia) • Floaters	• Visual impairment • Floaters ± photopsia (flashing lights)
Fundoscopy (most important examination)	With artery occlusion, everything looks pale (retina and optic disc looks pale), except the macula (cherry-red spot), because macula is supplied by an artery other than central retinal artery. Box-car segmentation of vessels may be seen.	Congested retina with disc swelling, venous dilatation, tortuosity, and/or hemorrhage	• Pale detached retina with tears on it • **Fundus is usually easy to visualize** • Floating debris may be present	Fundus is **hard to visualize** (**loss of fundal details**) and there is floating debris
	Source: Retinal Artery Occlusions. In: Biousse V, Newman N. Neuro-Ophthalmology Illustrated. 2nd ed. Thieme; 2015.	Source: Central and Branch Retinal Vein Occlusion(CRVO and BRVO). In: Tabandeh H, Goldberg M. The Retina in Systemic Disease: A Color Manual of Ophthalmoscopy. 1st ed. Thieme; 2009.	Source: Tabandeh H, Goldberg M. The Retina in Systemic Disease: A Color Manual of Ophthalmoscopy. 1st ed. Thieme; 2009.	Source: Cerebrovascular Disease. In: Biousse V, Newman N. Neuro-Ophthalmology Illustrated. 2nd ed. Thieme; 2015.

(Continued)

	CRAO	CRVO	Retinal detachment	Vitreous hemorrhage
Management	The following measures were not proven to improve visual outcomes, but are commonly tried: • Ocular massage[a] and/or maneuvers to reduce IOP (anterior chamber fluid aspiration, IV acetazolamide, IV mannitol, etc.) • High-flow oxygen ± hyperbaric therapy • Thrombolytic can be considered • To find the source of a clot, TIA/stroke work up is done (e.g., EKG, TTE, carotid ultrasound)	• In patients with macular edema or visual impairment, give intravitreal anti-VEGF[b] • Second-line treatment—dexamethasone implant or intravitreal triamcinolone	One of the following procedure can be done: Retinopexy (laser-, pneumatic-, or cryo-retinopexy) scleral buckle, or vitrectomy	Treat the underlying cause

[a]During ocular massage, intermittent ocular pressure and release is done. This induces pressure changes that may potentially dislodge the clot, taking the clot further downstream and decreasing the area of ischemia.

[b]Examples of anti-VEGF are aflibercept, bevacizumab, ranibizumab, etc. They decrease macular edema and risk of neovascularization.

Abbreviations: ASCVD, atherosclerotic cardiovascular disease; AMD, age-related macular degeneration; CRVO, central retinal vein occlusion; TIA, transient ischemic attack; CRAO, central retinal artery occlusion; IV, intravenous; VEGF, anti-vascular endothelial growth factor.

15.6 Age-Related Macular Degeneration

Background: Degenerative disease of retina and macula, which presents with central vision loss. Smoking and aging are major risk factors. Genetics also seem to play a role. Eye involvement is always bilateral, but the disease progression or type is not always the same in both eyes (e.g. a patient may have dry-type in one eye and wet-type in the other). There are two major types of age-related macular degeneration (AMD):

	Dry (atrophic) type of AMD	Wet (exudative) type of AMD	
Pathology	Areas of patchy depigmentation in the retina (known as drusen), particularly in the macular region Drusen—multiple, nonrefractile, yellow subretinal deposits with indistinct margins in nonexudative "dry" age-related macular degeneration. Source: Age-Related Macular Degeneration. In: Tabandeh H, Goldberg M. The Retina in Systemic Disease: A Color Manual of Ophthalmoscopy. 1st ed. Thieme; 2009.	• Neovascularization with increased risk of vascular leakage and/or bleeding • Retinal tear and detachment can also occur Intraretinal serous fluid (arrows), which is extravasating from the choroidal neovascularization. Source: Age-Related Macular Degeneration. In: Lang G. Ophthalmology. A Pocket Textbook Atlas. 3rd ed. Thieme; 2015.	Intraretinal and subretinal hemorrhage (arrows) from choroidal neovascularization. Source: Age-Related Macular Degeneration. In: Lang G. Ophthalmology. A Pocket Textbook Atlas. 3rd ed. Thieme; 2015.

Presentation	• Early loss in *fine visual acuity* (patients may need bright light or magnifying glass to read)
	• Gradual loss of central vision
		• Earlier during the course, patients may complain of straight lines or objects appearing curved or zigzagged
		• Gradual loss of central vision
		or
		• Might present with acute deterioration of vision in one eye due to:
		  - Acute rupture of small blood vessels,
		  - Leakage of fluid in subretinal macular space, and/or
		  - Retinal detachment	

Management	AREDS supplementation (a combination of antioxidant vitamins and zinc) has been shown to improve outcome. In smokers, do not use beta-carotene containing AREDS supplementation as beta-carotene has been associated with increased risk of lung cancer	• AREDS supplementation • Treatment commonly includes intravitreal VEGF-inhibitors or laser photocoagulation of abnormal vessels (*Fluorescein angiography* is done to visualize the blood vessels and then laser photocoagulation is done)	

Abbreviations: AMD, age-related macular degeneration; AREDS, age-related eye disease study.

15.7 Differential Diagnosis of Gradual Onset of Visual Impairment

	Cataract	Optic nerve glioma	Open-angle glaucoma, or chronic close-angle glaucoma	AMD
Pathology	Lens opacification related to aging and oxidative damage to the lens	Low-grade astrocytomas that occur in the optic nerve • Associated with neurofibromatosis (look for café-au-lait spots and axillary freckling)	Increased IOP leads to pressure atrophy of optic nerve	See the previous display table
Typical vision loss	• Blurry vision • Hard to drive at night (think of it like a dirty windshield of a car)	• Several months' history of slowly progressive decrease in visual acuity • May also have proptosis or strabismus Tunnel vision	Chronic slowly progressive peripheral vision loss (tunnel vision)	Central vision loss **Dry type** of AMD—slowly progressive **Wet type** of AMD—over weeks to months
Fundoscopy	Loss in transparency of affected eye, so retinal details are difficult to visualize	Optic disc can be normal, swollen (papilledema),[a] or atrophied, depending on various stages of compression of optic nerve by the tumor. This is unilateral	Cupping of optic disc[b]	**Dry type** of AMD—yellowish deposits in macula (drusen) **Wet type** of AMD—neovascularization
Management	• Lens extraction and implantation of artificial lens. • BP should be controlled prior to surgery in hypertensive patients	Neurosurgical referral	See the previous display table	See the previous display table

[a]Early papilledema: the disk borders are blurry and elevated. There is a peripapillary halo.

[b]Optic disc cupping due to glaucoma.

Normal optic disc.

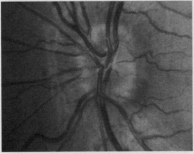

Source: Classification and Progression of Papilledema. In: Biousse V, Newman N. Neuro-Ophthalmology Illustrated. 1st ed. Thieme; 2009.

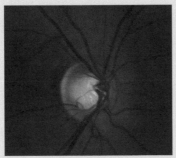

Source: Optic Disc Anomalies. In: Tabandeh H, Goldberg M. The Retina in Systemic Disease: A Color Manual of Ophthalmoscopy. 1st ed. Thieme; 2009.

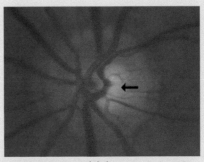

Source: Optic Disc Ophthalmoscopy. In: Lang G. Ophthalmology. A Pocket Textbook Atlas. 3rd ed. Thieme; 2015.

Abbreviations: AMD, age-related macular degeneration; IOP, intraocular pressure; BP, blood pressure

15.8 Visual Impairment Related to Medication Use

> **MRS**
>
> **IT CLAIMED** to cause optic neuropathy

> **MRS**
>
> **PICA** has iron deposits in cornea

Toxic optic neuropathy	Corneal deposits
Drugs that can cause optic neuropathy are given as follows: • Isoniazid • Tamoxifen • Chloroquine and other quinine-based drugs (hydroxychloroquine, quinidine, etc.) • Linezolid • Amiodarone • Isotretinoin • Methanol • Ethambutol • Ethylene glycol (*Optic neuritis is more common with methanol than with ethylene glycol.*) • Digitalis **Presentation:** painless visual impairment in a patient taking one of the above medications	• Phenothiazines such as thioridazine (antipsychotic) • Indomethacin • Chloroquine and hydroxychloroquine • Amiodarone

15.9 Papilledema

Definition: optic disc swelling due to increased pressure in the brain or around the eye.

Causes

Malignant HTN, pseudotumor cerebri, intracranial tumor	⇒ These cause increased intracranial pressure leading to bilateral papilledema
Mass lesion in the orbit, or a mass compressing the optic nerve sheath (optic nerve glioma)	⇒ These cause unilateral papilledema

Presentation: symptoms of increased intracranial pressure (headache, nausea, vomiting). Earlier in the disease course visual symptoms are minimal (minor blurring of vision and enlarged blind spot). Chronic papilledema may lead to permanent blindness, if left untreated.
Rx: address underlying cause.

[7] On the other hand, excessive vitamin A has been associated with pseudotumor cerebri, which can lead to papilledema.

15.10 Effects of Vitamin A Deficiency on Vision[7]

Etiology: fat malabsorption, poor diet in developing countries, etc.

Clinical Effects

[8] Bitot's spots

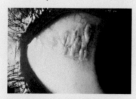

Source: Conjunctival Xerosis. In: Lang G. Ophthalmology. A Pocket Textbook Atlas. 2nd ed. Thieme; 2006.

Decreased production of rhodopsin in cones (which are active in low-light conditions)	⇒ Leads to decreased visual acuity during low-light conditions (night blindness)
Dry eyes (xerophthalmia)	⇒ Can lead to corneal ulceration and/or necrosis
Bitot's spots	⇒ White plaques made up of built-up keratin that occurs on conjunctiva[8]

Other features include dry skin, follicular hyperkeratosis (multiple red–brown follicular papules on the skin), etc.

15.11 Miscellaneous Eye Problems

	Presentation	Dx and pathophysiology	Management
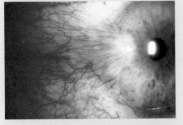 Source: Subconjunctival Hemorrhage. In: Lang G. Ophthalmology. A Pocket Textbook Atlas. 3rd ed. Thieme; 2015.	This may develop after coughing fits (e.g., in patients with whooping cough)	**Spontaneous conjunctival hemorrhage** (it looks very deadly but does not affect vision and regresses spontaneously.)	• Next step in management is to review bleeding history and take blood pressure (this can be caused by bleeding disorder and malignant hypertension) • If secondary causes are ruled out, then only observation is recommended
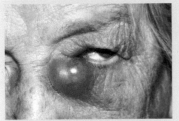 Source: Pterygium. In: Lang G. Ophthalmology. A Pocket Textbook Atlas. 2nd ed. Thieme; 2006.	Triangular plaque on conjunctiva with the apex of the triangle pointing toward the cornea	**Pterygium** It is a benign lesion of collagen degeneration and fibrovascular proliferation due to excessive exposure to sun, wind, and dust	• If it encroaches into cornea causing visual difficulties, do surgical treatment • If there is no visual impairment, Next step in management is reassurance
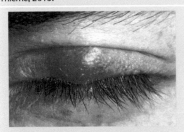 Source: Acute Dacryocystitis. In: Lang G. Ophthalmology. A Pocket Textbook Atlas. 3rd ed. Thieme; 2015.	Acute pain and swelling over lower inner aspect of eye **Eye examination**—localized tenderness, swelling, and redness over the lower inner aspect of eye. Pressure over that area may cause expression of purulent material	**Dacryocystitis** (lacrimal gland infection) Most likely causative organisms are *Strep. pyogenes* and *Staph. aureus*	• Culture of pus, then next step in management is empiric antibiotic (e.g. amoxicillin clavulanate)[a]
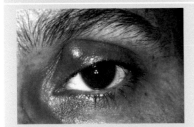 Source: Hordeolum. In: Lang G. Ophthalmology. A Pocket Textbook Atlas. 3rd ed. Thieme; 2015.	**Acute** painful, tender, red, nodular swelling over a localized area of the eyelid	**Hordeolum (also known as a stye)** is a localized infection of the eyelid, which may involve: - Hair follicles of the eyelashes = **external hordeolum** - Meibomian glands = **internal hordeolum**	• Symptomatic treatment with warm compresses to decrease swelling. • If there are no signs of resolution within the next 48 hours, the next step in management is incision and drainage
Source: Chalazion. In: Lang G. Ophthalmology. A Pocket Textbook Atlas. 2nd ed. Thieme; 2006.	Hard **painless rubbery nodule** in eyelid that has been present over weeks to months (**chronic**)	Dx is **Chalazion** due to chronic granulomatous inflammation precipitated by obstruction of Meibomian glands	• Expectant management with warm compresses • Symptomatic patients with persistence of lesion might require incision and drainage. Other options include intralesional steroids • **Recurrent or persistent chalazion** could be due to Meibomian gland sebaceous carcinoma or basal cell carcinoma. Do biopsy in this case

(Continued) **521**

	Presentation	Dx and pathophysiology	Management
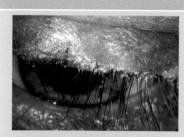Source: Seborrheic Blepharitis. In: Lang G. Ophthalmology. A Pocket Textbook Atlas. 3rd ed. Thieme; 2015.	Acute pain, erythema, and **diffuse** swelling of **bilateral**[b] eyelids. Usually have hx of recurrence	**Blepharitis** (inflammation of eyelid) is a recurrent chronic eye condition associated with *Staph. Aureus* colonization, seborrheic dermatitis (inset image), or Meibomian gland dysfunction	• The first step includes warm compresses, gentle lid massage, and washing • If there is no response, then the second step is topical or systemic antibiotics

[a]If acute dacryocystitis occurs in an infant, this is an emergent situation, requiring hospitalization and IV antibiotics. Remember that orbital septum is not completely formed in infants, so infection can spread rapidly into the brain and meninges. Dacryocystitis in infants can occur due to congenital dacryostenosis (congenital lacrimal duct obstruction).

[b]If unilateral blepharitis is persistent or recurrent, suspect malignancy (e.g., sebaceous carcinoma). Biopsy is indicated.

Answers

1. Postoperative endophthalmitis (usually occurs within 6 weeks of surgery).

2. Sympathetic eye (sympathetic ophthalmia) also known as spared eye injury. Pathology is due to uncovering of hidden ocular antigen that incites an autoimmune response and granulomatous uveitis in a genetically susceptible individual. Manifestation can range from anterior uveitis to panuveitis, and can result in blindness.

16. Ear, Nose, and Throat

"How great was the humiliation when one who stood beside me heard the distant sound of a shepherd's pipe, and I heard nothing; or heard the shepherd singing, and I heard nothing. Such experiences brought me to the verge of despair; but little more and I should have put an end to my life. Art, art alone deterred me."

Ludwig van Beethoven on slowly losing his hearing. (By the age of 46 he was completely deaf, possibly due to a mixture of nerve deafness and a degree of otosclerotic bony deafness)

16.1 Causes of Hearing Loss

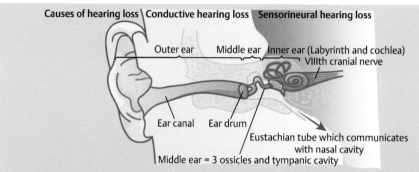

Causes of hearing loss | Conductive hearing loss | Sensorineural hearing loss

Outer ear | Middle ear | Inner ear (Labyrinth and cochlea)
VIIIth cranial nerve

Ear canal | Ear drum

Eustachian tube which communicates with nasal cavity

Middle ear = 3 ossicles and tympanic cavity

Causes of conductive hearing loss		Causes of sensorineural hearing loss[a]
Outer ear	**Middle ear**	**Inner ear[a]**
– Cerumen (ear wax) impaction – Bony lesions in ear canal (e.g., osteoma) – Infection and debris – Atresia of ear canal	– Otosclerosis, or damage to middle ear ossicles – Middle ear infection or fluid – Cholesteatoma – Tympanic membrane (TM) perforation or retraction	– Meniere's disease – Labyrinthitis – Cochleotoxicity[b] – Acoustic neuroma (eighth cranial nerve tumor) – Other neural lesions

[a]Tinnitus (ringing in ears) is common in patients with sensorineural hearing loss, but can also occur with middle ear issues.

[b]Drugs that are cochleotoxic (ototoxic)

- Quinine, chloroquine (antimalarials), quinidine (antiarrhythmic)[1]
- Aspirin
- Aminoglycosides
- Cisplatin
- Loop diuretics

[1]Overdose with these drugs can lead to cinchonism (tinnitus, hearing loss, blurred vision, confusion, nausea, vomiting, etc.).

16.2 Bedside Test for Hearing Loss

Rinne test

After vibrating the tuning fork, put it on the bone as pictured. After patient stops hearing the sound, then place the tuning fork in front of ear.

- If patient still hears the tuning fork, then air conduction (AC) is better than bone conduction (BC), which is normal, since air conducts sound better than bone.
- If BC (bone conduction) is better, it means that there is an abnormality in the conductive portion of the ear.

In sensorineural hearing loss, both AC and BC are decreased equally, thus AC > BC.

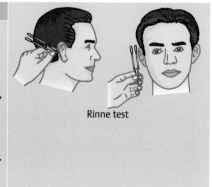

Rinne test

Weber test

After vibrating the tuning fork, it is placed right in the center of the top of the head (between the two ears), as pictured.

- To understand what happens in the Weber test with **conductive hearing loss**, we must understand the principle of external interference.

Example of external interference—we may be able to hear water drops in a silent cave where there is no other sound interference, but we may not be able to hear the whole fountain in a city center where there are a lot of ambient sounds interfering with your hearing.

In the affected ear with conductive hearing loss, external interference from conducted sound waves from air is absent or reduced, so the sound conducted through the bone is better heard in the affected ear.

- In **unilateral sensorineural hearing loss**, as both BC and AC are affected in an abnormal ear, the sound will be heard more in the normal ear (lateralizes to the normal ear).

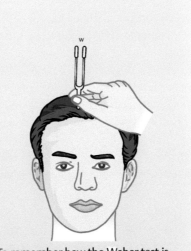

To remember how the Weber test is done, picture W in the center of the head.

 In a nutshell

	Rinne test	Weber test
Normal	AC > BC	No lateralization
Conductive hearing loss	BC > AC in the affected ear	Lateralizes to affected ear
Sensorineural hearing loss	AC > BC in all ears	Lateralizes to normal ear

16.3 Presbycusis

Background: Progressive bilateral hearing loss that occurs primarily with age due to degeneration of inner ear sensory structures. This is the MCC of hearing loss.
Presentation: Hearing loss that is more pronounced in noisy environments.[2]
Workup: Audiometry will reveal hearing function more preserved at high frequencies.
Management: Hearing aids and if severe, cochlear implant.

16.4 Otitis Externa

16.4.1 Uncomplicated otitis externa

Background: Infection of external ear canal is commonly due to *Pseudomonas* (MCC), *Staphylococcus epidermidis* or *Staphylococcus aureus.*
Presentation: Ear pain and discharge. Patients may have mild low-grade fever, but there are usually no other systemic symptoms.
Physical exam findings: Tenderness while pulling the ear. External ear canal will appear edematous and red. Otosocopy will reveal normal tympanic membrane.
Management: Topical antiseptic or antibiotic (e.g., ciprofloxacin) ± topical steroids (for significant itching or inflammation).

[2]When I am talking to my mother on the phone, I always make sure that she is in a very quiet environment (e.g., TV is not on).

16.4.2 Malignant (Necrotizing) Otitis Externa

Background: Think of this when patient with otitis externa has any of the following features:
- Persistent foul-smelling discharge not responsive to general measures.
- Granulation tissue in external canal.
- Severe pain out of proportion to exam findings.
- Systemic symptoms (e.g., high-grade fever).

Microbiological cause: Same as in uncomplicated otitis externa.

Risk factor: Occurs particularly in patients who have underlying immunosuppression (e.g., HIV, uncontrolled diabetes, active malignancy).

Workup: NSIDx is computed tomography (CT) scan (presence of bony erosions distinguishes this from severe otitis externa).

Rx: Systemic antibiotics that should cover *Pseudomonas* (e.g., oral or IV ciprofloxacin depending upon severity).

16.5 Middle Ear Issues

Condition	Presentation (all middle-ear issues can present with conductive hearing loss)	Otoscopic findings[a]	Management
Acute otitis media[b]		Red (erythematous) ± bulging TM (tympanic membrane)	• Use oral amoxicillin. • If symptoms persist after 3 days or if hx of recent antibiotic usage, then give amoxicillin + clavulanate.
Bullous myringitis	• Pus drainage from ear • Fever • Pain in the ear[c] • **No tenderness** when the pinna is pulled[d]	Painful vesicles in TM (tympanic membrane) + red (erythematous) TM ± bulging TM	Rx is the same as above, as the causative organism is similar to acute otitis media. • Additional causes include *Mycoplasma pneumoniae*, viral (e.g., influenza, herpes zoster), etc.
Serous otitis media (a.k.a. otitis media with effusion) This might be a complication of eustachian tube dysfunction or sequelae of acute otitis media.	• Painless hearing loss • No signs of active infection	• Dull hypomobile TM (tympanic membrane) ± air-fluid level in tympanic cavity • Best diagnostic test is tympanometry, which uses a probe to detect reflected sound waves. Stiff middle ear or TM reflects more sound.	• Conservative expectant management in uncomplicated cases. • Tympanostomy is indicated for persistent symptomatic effusion (> 12 wk) or in whom air travel cannot be deferred.
Chronic otitis media MC causes are *Pseudomonas* and *S. aureus*.	Recurrent or persistent ear discharge (major differentiating factor from acute otitis media is hx of > 6 weeks)	Calcific patches + perforation	• In uncomplicated cases, use ear irrigation with topical antibiotics (e.g., ciprofloxacin). • In complicated cases (e.g., with mastoiditis, systemic symptoms), do CT scan and give systemic antibiotics. Surgery might also be needed.

Condition	Presentation (all middle-ear issues can present with conductive hearing loss)	Otoscopic TM findings[a]	Management
Cholesteatoma (keratinized desquamated epithelial collection, with inflammatory and infectious component that can spread and destroy bones) **May be primary** **(due to chronic eustachian tube dysfunction) or secondary (due to acquired TM perforation)**	Presents similarly to chronic otitis media, but otoscopic findings are different	Debris, granulation tissue, and inflammatory polyps	NSIM is CT to determine the extent of disease. Rx: surgical removal/debridement.
Eustachian tube dysfunction **Look for hx of recent upper respiratory tract symptoms which can cause eustachian tube inflammation and edema.** **If persistent, look for secondary causes such as:** **• Obstructive tumors** **• Obstructive lymph nodes** **• (e.g., in HIV or lymphoma)** **• Nasal polyps**	Fullness and pain in ear, worsened by chewing food. Audible pop might also be heard when the tube opens intermittently.	Retracted TM	Treat underlying cause. Nasal decongestants, hydration.

[a]For all middle ear issues the best initial test is pneumatic otoscopy. Decreased mobility on air insufflation is the most sensitive finding and can be present in all the following conditions.

[b]Remember the MC bacterial cause of bronchitis and sinusitis; they are also the ones that commonly cause otitis media—they are **St**reptococcus pneumoniae, **Hae**mophilus influenzae, and **Mo**raxella catarrhalis.

[c]After TM ruptures, patients may feel less pain as the pressure inside the middle ear cavity is released.

[d]Absence of external ear tenderness is the major differentiating factor in between uncomplicated otitis media and otitis externa. Both can have pus coming out of ear.

Complication of acute or chronic otitis media, cholesteatoma, malignant otitis extern

Complications typically occur in patients with underlying immunosuppression or infection with a virulent organism. Complications occur due to local contiguous spread of infection that can eat through bones leading to the following:

- Bacterial infection spreads in a contiguous manner: mastoiditis → bony erosion[3] → septic thrombosis of sinuses → meningitis → subdural or epidural empyema → intracranial brain abscess.
- Labyrinthitis.
- Facial nerve palsy: due to direct bone erosions into the facial nerve canal.
- Osteomyelitis of skull base with involvement of other lower cranial nerves.

 MRS

St HeMo, or **S**weet **h**eart **M**ary (whichever you prefer)

[3]Bony erosions seen on CT scan can be present in all conditions.

16.6 Otosclerosis

[4]The stapedial reflex (a.k.a. acoustic or auditory reflex) has a protective role by attenuating loud sound. This reflex requires intact middle ear bones, sensorineural system, facial nerve, etc., thus absence of the stapedial reflex can be seen in many conditions and isn't specific for otosclerosis.

Pathophysiology: As the name giveth all; **otosclerosis**: oto = ear and sclerosis = hardening and nonfunction of the **st**apes. It is inherited in an autosomal-dominant pattern with incomplete penetrance.

Presentation: Slowly progressive hearing loss and tinnitus (may be bilateral). It usually occurs in the middle age. Exam may reveal attenuated or absent stapedial (acoustic) reflex.[4]

Management: Hearing amplification or surgical replacement of stapes with a prosthesis.

👥 Clinical Case Scenarios

A 30-year-old male presents to clinic with ear pain while chewing and sometimes this pain wakes him up at night. Upon further questioning his wife gives hx of teeth crunching during night (bruxism).

1. What is the likely dx?
   a) Eustachian tube dysfunction
   b) Temporomandibular joint dysfunction
   c) Chronic otitis media
   d) Cholesteatoma

2. What is the management?

16.7 Nose Problems

- When patient presents with **nasal stuffiness, fullness, rhinorrhea,** postnasal drip cough (± **congestion** ± hyposmia or anosmia), think of the following conditions:

	Allergic rhinitis	Viral rhinitis	Nasal polyps[a]	Rhinitis medicamentosa aka rebound rhinitis	Chronic nonallergic rhinitis
Differential features	**Hx is recurrent or persistent** • ± conjunctivitis • ± asthma Also look for transverse nasal crease in the lower half of the nose, which occurs due to repeated rubbing and pushing up of nose (allergic salute).	**Hx is acute** • ± conjunctivitis	**Chronic progressive**	**Look for nasal congestion alone** + use of • Nasal decongestant (e.g. pseudoephedrine, oxymetazoline, phenylephrine.) • Cocaine use. It is a rebound phenomenon, which occurs after stopping nasal decongestant, or cocaine use.	**Late onset (around 20s), recurrent, or persistent** • ± asthma • Conjunctivitis is absent (*there is allergic asthma and late-onset nonallergic asthma. Just like that there is allergic rhinitis and late-onset nonallergic rhinitis*)
Nasal mucosal findings	• Pale bluish or gray edematous mucosa or turbinates (*Image*) • Cobble stoning of mucosa	Red edematous mucosa or turbinates (*image*)	Polyps are visible in rhinoscopy	Beefy-red nasal mucosa	Turbinates are boggy and edematous

	Allergic rhinitis	Viral rhinitis	Nasal polyps[a]	Rhinitis medicamentosa aka rebound rhinitis	Chronic nonallergic rhinitis
Management	• Avoidance of exposure to allergens[b] • Topical intranasal steroids • Second-line: antihistamine nasal spray (e.g. azelastine spray)	Supportive management	• Intranasal steroids • If nonresponsive to above, NSIM is surgical removal.	Discontinue offending agent and use intranasal steroids.	Intranasal steroids ± intranasal antihistamines

[a]Polyp formation is usually due to chronic inflammation from sinusitis or allergy symptoms. Triad of chronic rhinosinusitis, nasal polyps, and asthma can occur with the use of nonsteroidal anti-inflammatory drugs (NSAIDs) or aspirin in certain individuals.

[b]Allergen-specific immunoglobulin E (IgE) are present in serum, and can be useful for diagnosis and focused exposure - prevention.

Clinical Case Scenarios

3. A 25-year-old male presents with whistling noise during respiration. He has hx of cocaine abuse. What is the likely dx?

A 10-year-old child presents with symptoms of nasal obstruction. He has hx of recurrent epistaxis. Exam may reveal mass in the nasal cavity.

4. What is the likely dx?

5. What is the NSIDx?

16.7.1 Acute Rhinosinusitis

Definition: Infection of nasal cavity and paranasal sinuses.

Presentation: Recent-onset sinus congestion, nasal discharge (purulent or clear) +/- headaches +/- sinus tenderness. Hyposmia (decreased smell) or dysosmia (qualitative alteration of perception of smell) is present.

Workup: Usually a clinical diagnosis, no imaging is needed in uncomplicated cases. Important differentiating features are shown below.

Viral rhinosinusitis	Bacterial rhinosinusitis[a]
< 10 days of symptoms	> 10 days of symptoms
Low-grade fever	Higher grade fever
No associated complications	Presence of complications
If all of the above present, antibiotics are not indicated. NSIM: symptomatic treatment (analgesics, saline irrigation)	Antibiotics likely needed: First-line: amoxicillin alone or amoxicillin-clavulanate Second-line: doxycycline or respiratory fluoroquinolones

[a]Often occurs as a complication of viral rhinosinusitis. The same bacteria that cause otitis media and bronchitis also can cause bacterial rhinosinusitis. Nasal swabs and culture of secretions are not helpful. Endoscopic cultures of sinuses (done by ENT specialist) can be obtained when patient is not responding to empiric antibiotics or in serious complications.

Complications of bacterial rhinosinusitis: Similar to malignant otitis externa or severe otitis media: septic thrombosis of sinuses → meningitis → subdural or epidural empyema[5] → intracranial brain abscess. Another complication is orbital cellulitis.

[5]Management of subdural empyema or epidural empyema requires combination of broad-spectrum IV antibiotics and surgical drainage.

16.8 Sore Throat + Drooling

- Uncomplicated throat infection is common, but presence of signs like dysphagia, odynophagia, and drooling often point toward more complicated disease, as following.
- These conditions typically occur in children, adolescents, or in immunosuppressed adults.

529

MRS

MRS-1Alphabetical progression of mnoPQ. So Peritonsillar abscess = quinsy.

	Peritonsillar abscess (Quinsy)MRS-1	Retropharyngeal abscess	Epiglottitis
Presentation (fever, lymphadenopathy, sore throat, odynophagia/dysphagia, and drooling may be present in all)	• Absence of neck stiffness, nuchal rigidity, and no neck pain with movement.	• Nuchal rigidity/ stiff neck, and/ or neck pain with movement	• **Stridor** (noisy harsh breathing) • Respiratory distress can develop early[a]
	Trismus (difficulty opening mouth) and hot potato or muffled voice can occur in both		
Exam findings	Swollen tonsils with deviated uvula **Or** bulging or fluctuance near the tonsil area	• Tonsils are usually normal. • Swelling and edematous changes can be visualized in the posterior aspect of pharynx.	• Normal tonsils • Laryngeal tenderness in the anterior neck area
Major causative organism	Polymicrobial: *Strep*, *Staph*, and anaerobes		• MCC is *H. influenzae* (typically occurs in under-vaccinated children) • Other potential cause includes: – Penicillin-resistant *Streptococcus* – Community-acquired MRSA
First SIM	Look for signs of impending airway obstruction[a,b] (e.g., tripod posturing, neck extension, stridor, and/or cyanosis) If present, NSIM is to secure airway before doing any diagnostic testing such as X-ray or CT scan.		
Second SIM Blood cultures and empiric IV antibiotic therapy should be given before doing any diagnostic test.	IV antibiotics that covers the above organism (e.g., ampicillin-sulbactam or clindamycin). If presence of MRSA risk factors, add vancomycin or linezolid.		IV antibiotics (third-generation cephalosporin + an antibiotic that covers MRSA, e.g., clindamycin or vancomycin)
NSIDx	CT scan with IV contrast is usually done. This will help differentiate cellulitis from abscess.		• In children who may not cooperate with direct exam, do X-ray of the neck soft tissue.[c] • In adults, direct visualization of epiglottis is recommended.
Surgical management	Usually requires drainage (needle aspiration or incision and drainage) OR Tonsillectomy (in patients with indication of tonsillectomy)[d]	Surgical drainage might be necessary in patients with larger abscess (> 3 cm²), impending airway compromise, OR failure to respond to antibiotic therapy	No specific surgical drainage required. Primary treatment is airway management.

[a]Airway obstruction in epiglottitis is so common that in children < 4–6 years of age, experts recommend prompt intubation even in the absence of signs of respiratory compromise.

[b]Impending respiratory compromise in retropharyngeal abscess and quinsy also requires immediate surgical intervention.

Abbreviations: MRSA, methicillin-resistant *Staphylococcus aureus*; SIM, step in management.

[c]X-ray of epiglottitis: the normal narrow contour of the epiglottis (**a**, *arrow*) is replaced by a round swelling (**b**, *arrow*).

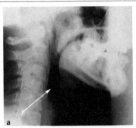
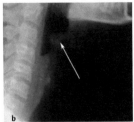

a   b

Source: Infections of the Tonsils, Pharynx, and Oropharynx. In: Bull T, Almeyda J, eds. Color Atlas of ENT Diagnosis. 5th ed. Thieme; 2009.

[d]Indication for tonsillectomy in Quinsy includes significant upper airway obstruction, prior hx of severe recurrent pharyngitis or Quinsy, or in patients with general indication of tonsillectomy.[6]

[6]**General indication of ton-sillectomy**
Acute tonsillitis frequency of at least

- 7 in 1 year
- 5 in 2 consecutive years
- 3 in 3 consecutive years

16.9 Oral Cavity Lesions

		Presentation	
White plaque anywhere in the oral cavity (e.g., the tongue) NSIM—try to scrape it off	Plaque is scraped off easily and reveals red mucosa underneath.	Source: Inflammations of the Lips and Oral Cavity. In: Probst R, Grevers G, Iro H, eds. Basic Otorhinolaryngology: A Step-by-Step Learning Guide. 2nd ed. Thieme; 2017.	Dx **is candidiasi**s. NSIM—oral nystatin or clotrimazole
	If it cannot be scraped off, ask the following: - Is patient HIV +ve? - Does the lesion look benign (no ulceration, necrosis, or pain)?	HIV positive *and* benign-appearing lesion. Source: Symptomatic HIV Infection, AIDS. In: Siegenthaler W, ed. Siegenthaler's Differential Diagnosis in Internal Medicine: From Symptom to Diagnosis. 1st ed. Thieme; 2007.	Dx is likely **oral hairy leukoplakia**. It is commonly found in lateral tongue area and is due to Epstein–Barr virus (EBV) virus replication. **Rx:** Usually specific treatment is not required. Treat underlying HIV.
		White plaque or patch in an immunocompetent patient, even benign-appearing, requires biopsy to rule out malignancy.	Precancerous hyperplasia or dysplasia is known as **leukoplakia** (leuko = white, plakia = plaque). **Risk factors are** similar to squamous cell cancer (smoking and alcohol are synergistic). NSIDx is biopsy (typical pathologic findings are hyperkeratosis, parakeratosis, with or without dysplasia. **Rx:** For high risk lesion, do surgical excision. Low-risk lesions may be managed with close follow-up and avoidance of alcohol and smoking.

Other oral cavity lesions	
Pigmented lesion in oral cavity with one of the ABCDE features[a]	⇒ **NSIDx is biopsy** to rule out melanoma.
Reticulated (net-like) or lacy white papules or plaques ± erythema around the lesions ± ulcers	⇒ **Dx is oral lichen planus.** It can be associated with cutaneous lichen planus or might present with oral lesions only. This can also cause scarring. **Rx:** For symptomatic lesions, give topical steroids.
Painful ulcer with red border, and whitish to pale-yellow base	⇒ **Dx is oral aphthous ulcer.** It sometimes can cause odynophagia if it occurs in upper esophagus or back of the throat. **Rx:** Conservative management mostly with reassurance.

[a]ABCDE = Asymmetry, Border irregularity, Color changes, Diameter is big, and Elevated borders.

16.10 Salivary Gland Pathology

16.10.1 Salivary Gland Stone

Risk factors: Dehydration, trauma, anticholinergic, etc.

Presentation: Hx of intermittent pain and/or salivary-gland swelling after eating food.

Workup: CT scan or ultrasound (US) can be done to detect nonpalpable stone.

Rx: Conservative management with adequate hydration, massaging/milking the salivary gland, NSAIDs as needed, and promotion of salivary flow with sucking on tart hard candies. If acute infection is suspected, use antibiotics with gram-positive coverage, such as cloxacillin or cephalexin. Interventions such as endoscopic removal of stone can be done after acute infection has subsided and if the stone does not pass spontaneously.

16.10.2 Acute Suppurative Parotitis

Other causes of salivary gland inflammation include viral infection (e.g. mumps, HIV), sarcoidosis, Sjogren's syndrome, etc.

Background: This can occur in elderly hospitalized patients, as a complication of acute significant stress (e.g., acute sickness or surgery). Underlying obstruction due to stone or tumor can predispose to this condition.

Microbiology: MCC is *S. aureus*. Other causes include oral anaerobes, aerobes, or gram negatives.

Presentation: Acute parotid area tenderness, swelling, and/or spreading erythema with signs of sepsis.

Workup: If purulent drainage from the salivary duct is present, do gram stain and culture. US or CT can be done to rule out abscess.

Rx:

Immunocompetent (cover *Staph* + anaerobes)		Immunocompromised (cover MRSA, gram negatives, *Pseudomonas*, and anaerobes)
MRSA risk factors present	MRSA risk factors absent	Vancomycin **+ either any one of the following:**
Vancomycin or linezolid + either metronidazole or clindamycin	Nafcillin or cefazolin + either metronidazole or clindamycin	• (Cefepime + metronidazole) • Piperacillin-tazobactam • Meropenem

Parotitis due to mumps virus	
It is usually bilateral. It can be associated with the following complications:	
	Clinical findings
Oophoritis	Lower abdominal pain and tenderness (in females)
Epididymo-orchitis	Testicular swelling and tenderness
Aseptic meningitis	Headache, stiff neck
Pancreatitis	Epigastric pain/tenderness

16.11 Squamous Cell Cancer of Head and Neck

Risk factors: MC ones are tobacco (smoking or chewing), alcohol, and radiation. Alcohol and tobacco have synergistic effects. Other risk factors include EBV (for nasopharyngeal cancer) or HPV infection (for oropharyngeal cancer).

Presentation: Depends on the location of tumor.

Location	Presentation
Nasopharyngeal or sinus tumors	• Hearing loss or recurrent otitis media • Symptoms of nasal obstruction • Sinus congestion
Oral cavity	• Nonhealing ulcerative or plaque lesion in oral cavity
Oropharyngeal tumor	Dysphagia, odynophagia, and/or new-onset snoring/sleep apnea
Laryngeal tumor	Hoarse voice, cough, stridor, etc.

Neck mass (due to lymph node enlargement) and bleeding due to primary lesion are common symptoms. As the disease progresses, it can involve contiguous structures (e.g., laryngeal tumor can locally metastasize to the esophageal–oropharyngeal area and can cause dysphagia, odynophagia, and hematemesis).

Workup:

● NSIM is thorough ENT examination to try to directly visualize the tumor (e.g., office-based flexible laryngoscopy).

● CT scan or MRI head or neck with IV contrast is done for initial staging of suspicious lesions.

● Panendoscopy (laryngoscopy,[7] bronchoscopy, and esophagoscopy) OR positron emission tomography (PET) scan combined with CT is usually done for further staging.

Rx: Surgery if localized, and chemoradiation if locally advanced.

[7]Usually tissue diagnosis is obtained by endoscopy under general anesthesia. In patients with neck mass (lymph node) with nonobvious primary, do fine-needle aspiration of lymph node.

Clinical Case Scenarios

Practice questions: Rinne and Weber Tests

CCS	Rinne	Weber
6.	AC > BC in both ears	Lateralizes to right ear
7.	BC > AC in right ear	Lateralizes to right ear
8.	AC > BC in left ear	Lateralizes to left ear

 MRS

To help with interpretation of the Rinne test, always think that A should come before B; if B comes before A it is abnormal. So, if AC > BC there is no problem with **conduction.**

Answers:

1. b) Dx is temporomandibular joint dysfunction. Patients can present with ear pain (*referred to as otalgia*) or pain just in front of tragus. This can be due to predisposing conditions like bruxism.

2. Treat underlying disorder (e.g., oral splints for bruxism). Use NSAIDs and antispasmodics (e.g., cyclobenzaprine) as needed.

3. Perforated nasal septum. This can be due to nasal trauma (surgical or nonsurgical) or due to cocaine use.

4. **Juvenile angiofibroma** (occurs exclusively in late childhood and adolescent population).

5. CT scan to evaluate the extent of tumor, which can also involve the bones. Avoid biopsy, because of risk of severe bleeding. Treatment is surgical removal.

6. Sensorineural hearing loss in the left ear (normal Rinne in both ears means normal conduction in both ears). Weber will lateralize to the normal ear in unilateral sensorineural hearing loss.

7. Right ear conductive hearing loss.

8. To interpret this, we must take it step by step: as BC > AC in the right ear, it means the right ear has conductive hearing loss. Now as the Weber test is lateralizing to the left ear, it means that right ear also has sensorineural hearing loss. The conclusion is that the right ear has combined conductive and sensorineural hearing loss. Possible causes include complicated ear infection (e.g., otitis media with inner ear involvement), tumors, head injuries, etc.

17. Ethics

We hold these truths to be self-evident **that all patients are created equal, that they are endowed by their Creator with certain unalienable rights, that among these are autonomy, informed consent, pursuit of health, and the right to peaceful death.**

17.1 Autonomy

Definition: An inherent right of a patient with **capacity or competence** to be responsible for and make decisions regarding one's life, health, and well-being.

Capacity	Medical determination	Can the patient make an informed decision **at this point in time**?	Loss of capacity occurs when the patient has acute deterioration in cognitive function (e.g., when patient is acutely psychotic[a] or has acute confusion due to encephalitis).
Competence	Legal determination (determined after legal proceedings)	Can the patient make an informed decision **at any point in time**?	Loss of competence occurs when one has **chronic** underlying cognitive dysfunction resulting in failure to make sound decisions (e.g., patients with mental disabilities or advanced Alzheimer's disease). They require guardianship for financial or health care-related decisions.

[a]Common red herring in a test question is a patient with a stable psychiatric diagnosis such as schizophrenia with no acute psychotic symptoms. These patients commonly have the capacity to make their own decisions.

In situations where a **patient with capacity** does not want to undergo recommended test, or hear about diagnosis, or is refusing treatment, do the following:

- First, always try to find out the underlying reason.
- If the answer choices in exam do not involve an open-ended question, the right answer is likely what the patient wants, even if it goes against your medical judgment.

A competent patient without loss of capacity has the right to refuse hearing the diagnosis and refuse life-saving treatment.

Patient loses autonomy when:	Example scenarios
The patient is deemed to likely harm others	- Refusing treatment or quarantine with communicable disease that presents high risk to community[a]: Cholera, diphtheria, active infectious TB, plague, small pox, yellow fever, viral hemorrhagic fever, severe acute respiratory syndrome (SARS), pandemic flu, meningococcal meningitis, etc. - Intent of rape or homicide
The patient is deemed to likely harm one-self	Suicide risk

[a]In patients with communicable disease, public health authorities and physicians must balance the magnitude of the public health risk against the rights of the individuals or groups.

A pregnant patient has the right of autonomy and can refuse treatment even if it puts fetus at risk.

17.2 Patient Confidentiality, Which Includes HIPAA (Health Insurance Portability and Accountability Act)

- Do not give patient's information to anyone else without his/her consent. Do not discuss patient's case in public spaces where it can be overheard.
- Disclosure of health information needed for patient care and other important purposes (e.g., specialty consultation service) is allowed.
- In cases where there is a risk to third party, patient loses the right of confidentiality, e.g., sexually transmitted disease (STD),[1] harm to others (intent of rape or homicide), or high-risk communicable disease as above.

[1]**STD (e.g., HIV) and confidentiality**

- First step is to encourage patient to inform all people at risk (e.g., all sexual partners).
- If patient declares unwillingness to inform his/her sexual partner/s, next step is to inform the local health department. They will subsequently identify the people at risk and inform them.

[2] A healthcare proxy is considered to represent patient themselves. They can withdraw life-saving measures, against physician's judgement. However a surrogate decision maker by themselves cannot withhold or withdraw lifesaving emergency measures against the judgment of physician.

For nonemergent cases, when a surrogate makes a decision that contradicts physician's judgment, NSIM is to get judicial or institutional (e.g., hospital ethics committee) review.

If there are disparate views in between family members, always try to arrange a family meeting to try to reconcile differences in opinion.

[3] Parents act in the capacity of "surrogate decision maker," but not "health care proxy" for their children.

17.3 Decision Making Process for an Adult Who Is Not Able to Make Decision for Self (e.g., Loss of Capacity Due to Acute Confusion)

First step is to look for the following (given below in order of preference):

- Previous written advanced directives, or "verified" prior oral directive (i.e., in presence of a "health care provider" and an adult witness).
- Designated health care proxy.

If none of the above is available, find out who makes health care-related decisions for the patient (i.e., who is the surrogate decision maker?).

The surrogates can be appointed from the following list, given in order of priority:

- **Legal** guardian (power of attorney = POA). This is different from health care proxy.[2]
- **S**pouse or **H**ouse partner (the one who lives with the patient).
- **O**ffspring >18 years of age.
- **P**arents.
- **S**iblings.
- Close friend.

17.4 Minors (Patients < 18 Years of Age)

- The parent is the de facto decision maker for minors. Parental presence and consent is necessary for medical decisions. Only one consenting parent is enough.
- **Exception:** Parental presence, consent, or knowledge is not needed for seeking medical treatment in the following situations:

Medical conditions where autonomy is provided **(limited autonomy)**	• STD, substance abuse treatment, **routine prenatal care**, and birth control[a] • Emergency
Emancipated minors (treated as adults who can make their own medical decisions)	Minors who are homeless, have given birth to a child, married, financially independent, high school graduates, and military service

[a] Therefore, patients of any age should have the opportunity to speak with the doctor alone.

- Also note that parents are not allowed to withhold life- or limb-saving measures.[3]
  - If emergency treatment is required, proceed. Informed consent is not required.
  - In nonemergent situations, continue to engage with parents with a multidisciplinary approach. If not successful, NSIM is to obtain court order for treatment.

17.5 Informed Consent

- All patients or decision makers have the right for informed consent.
- Informed consent involves explanation of the **P**rocedure, **A**lternatives, **R**isks, **A**nswering questions that the patient has, and allowing the patient to **PARA**phrase the given information to ensure understanding.

Informed consent is not necessary in the following situations:

- Emergency life- or limb-saving procedure (no need for consent, just proceed).
- Unexpected finding during surgery, where delaying surgery to obtain an informed consent will be harmful to the patient (e.g., laparotomy for possible appendicitis reveals about-to-rupture ectopic pregnancy).

17.6 Breaking Bad News (e.g., Informing a Patient of the Diagnosis of Cancer)

- Set a **setting** that patient is comfortable with. It may be a private conversation or patients may choose to have a partner with them.
- **Inquire** about the following (always use open-ended questions):
    - What does the patient already know about the diagnosis so far?
    - What does the patient want to know about the diagnosis in this visit or encounter?
- **Inform:** Tell about diagnosis in a clear way so that patient understands.
- **Respond** To the feelings that are brought upon by the bad news.
- **Establish** Further plan of action.
- **Summarize** the visit, with paraphrasing by the patient.

Setting → Inquire → Inform → Respond → Establish → Summarize.

Special situation: If a family member asks that the patient not be notified of the bad diagnosis, NSIM is to inquire the reason. Patient always has the right to know diagnosis, but here, getting more information from family members will help physician find an ideal way to inform the patient.

17.7 Conflict Issue or Dealing with Emotions in a Patient or Family Member

| First step | ⟹ | Acknowledge the emotion or conflict issue (be empathetic) | For example, I can see that you are angry |
| Second step | ⟹ | Get more information regarding the issue | For example, tell me more about this issue (an open-ended question?)[a] |

[a]Even if they imply that they are angry at you, they may have other reasons to feel that way, so it is important to pry further.

17.8 End of Life Issues

Futile care	When it is medically evident that interventions of any type will not benefit or prolong the quality or length of life. This is grounds for physician-determined withdrawal of care. For example, diagnosis of brain death; NSIM—remove all life support with no need for consent.
Hospice care	It is provided to patients **with estimated survival of < 6 months**. It involves providing symptom control, clinical and psychosocial support.
Terminal/comfort care	In an actively dying patient with a terminal illness under comfort care, examine patient regularly for any sign of discomfort, such as facial cues of pain, moaning, or increased respiratory rate. If these are present, start or increase dosage of morphine or other opiate (such as hydromorphone) ± benzodiazepines to make the patient comfortable.

17.9 Miscellaneous Ethics Issues

17.9.1 Physician–Patient Boundaries

The following are examples of unreasonable patient requests:

- Patient requesting to be seen immediately when your office is about to get closed and it is not an emergency.
- Asking for a medical advice when you are outside (e.g., during grocery shopping).
- When the patient is your friend and he keeps on texting you asking for a medication prescription.

In this case, the physician has the right to maintain a professional relationship and ask the patient to schedule an appointment in the office, or call during office hours.

17.9.2 Conscientious Objection

Health care professionals have the right to refuse to participate in any activity they find morally, religiously, or ethically against their beliefs. This is only considered acceptable when not coupled with patient abandonment. Arranging for their care by an equally licensed professional without similar concerns is necessary.

However, in the event of emergency, patient's safety and life take precedence over any objections or personal inconvenience.

[4]It is okay to accept information handouts (e.g., handouts explaining disease or treatment) and medicine samples, which will benefit patients. It is not okay to accept **pen, erasers, flash drives**, etc. (even though the monetary value is low). It is not okay to accept money as a part-time spokesperson for a drug company, or co-owning the imaging center you send your patients to.

17.9.3 Conflict of Interest

When a physician has something to gain from an interaction that can bias his/her judgment.

- Doctors cannot accept any form of gifts from pharmaceutical or medical-device companies that do not directly benefit patient care.[4]
- Disclose all potential conflicts of interest: being transparent about any potential or real conflicts of interest in lectures, contracts, research, etc.

17.9.4 Medical Negligence

When a medical professional does one of the following, and results in harm to a patient:

- Fails to demonstrate the level of skill,
- Is careless in care of a patient, or
- Fails to perform standard of care consistent with the best practices in the **LOCAL** medical community[5]

If confronted with a question of medical negligence/malpractice done by a colleague, the physician should first talk with the colleague to determine the circumstances.

[5]Unlike medical negligence, medical malpractice has an element of "intent"— when a doctor knows what should have been done, but was not done.

Clinical Case Scenarios

Situation	NSIM
Possible Jehovah's witness[a] with no advanced directives, or no prior oral directive is currently confused and needs life-saving **emergent** blood transfusion. Son and husband report that it is against their religious belief to get blood transfusion, but they do not have any written advanced directive and there is no official designated health care proxy.	Transfuse. In this case there is no clear-cut advanced directive and you cannot be sure that the wife shares their religious belief; so, when in doubt do what you think is best. Remember the caveat that surrogate decision makers by themselves cannot withhold life-saving **emergency** measures against the judgment of physician.
Adult Jehovah's witness has profuse life-threatening hemorrhage. Earlier, he had told the social worker and doctor that he does not want blood transfusion. Physician thinks patient needs **emergent** blood transfusion.	No transfusion. We have a clear-cut advanced oral directive witnessed by a health care professional and an adult.
Parent, who is a Jehovah's witness, does not want his son to get **emergent** blood transfusion that he really needs.	Transfuse. Parents cannot withhold **emergent** life-saving measures.
Parent, who is a Jehovah's witness, does not want his son to get nonemergent blood transfusion.	Get a court order when faced with parents refusing **nonemergent** recommended treatment.
A child needs **emergent** appendectomy.	No consent required. **Emergent** conditions do not require informed consent.
A child needs elective cholecystectomy. Mother agrees but father refuses.	Proceed to schedule surgery. Only one consenting parent is needed.
A homeless patient diagnosed with active TB wants to leave against medical advice. He does not seem to be acutely psychotic, and knows where he is and knows what will happen if he leaves against medical advice. Despite multiple efforts, patient still wants to leave the hospital.	He cannot leave the isolation unit. He has lost his autonomy (there is a high potential of harm to others).
A 14-year-old boy seeks STD treatment. He does not want his parents to know.	Give treatment. Do not tell parents. Treatment of STD is given limited autonomy.
A 15-year-old pregnant girl with 8 weeks' pregnancy seeks abortion. She does not want her parents to know.	Pregnancy is not included in one of the clauses of emancipation of minor. Most states require parental consent or notification for **nonroutine** prenatal care-related decisions.
An 18-year-old pregnant girl with 8 weeks' pregnancy seeks abortion. She does not want her parents to know.	18 is an adult age. Proceed with abortion and do not tell parents.

[a]Jehovah's witnesses have religious beliefs that recommend against blood transfusion.

Abbreviations: STD, sexually transmitted disease; TB, tuberculosis.

18. Disorders of Sexual Development

XXX

XXX

"....................We were working on puberty quote, but it's not fully-developed yet."

18.1 Introduction

- Genetic sex is determined at fertilization by the genetic content of the sperm cell.
- Gonadal sex (ovary vs. testes) is determined by hormones, as shown below:

	Factors/hormones	Present	Absent
	TDF (testis-determining factor) is a protein encoded by sex-determining region Y (SRY) gene located in Y chromosome.	Testes	Ovaries
The following hormones are secreted by the testes:	**Testosterone**	Male internal accessory system (e.g., epididymis, ductus deferens)	No male internal accessory system
	Testosterone converted to dihydrotestosterone (DHT) by 5α-reductase	Male external genitalia	Female external genitalia
	MIF (Müllerian-inhibiting factor)	Primordial uterus and fallopian tubes degenerate	Uterus, fallopian tubes and upper vagina

Note: Complete female sexual development requires absence of all the above-mentioned factors/hormones: TDF, testosterone, DHT, and MIF. In a rare case of loss-of-function mutation in SRY gene, there is absence of all the above-mentioned hormones/factors (leading to female internal and external organs in an XY genotype fetus). They also have failure of ovaries to develop, resulting in streak gonads (ovaries). This is called gonadal dysgenesis (a.k.a. Swyer syndrome).

18.2 Disorders of Embryonal Sexual Differentiation

Underlying condition	Gonads	Male internal organs	External organ	Müllerian structures (uterus, fallopian tube, and upper part of vagina)
Complete androgen insensitivity syndrome in genetic males (XY-genotype)[a]	As TDF is working, testes are present, and **ovaries are absent**.	No male internal organ	Female external genitalia (blind vaginal pouch)[d]	None (no uterus, no tubes, and no upper part of vagina)
Absolute testosterone deficiency due to 17-alpha hydroxylase deficiency in genetic males (XY-genotype)[b]	But DHT-dependent testicular descent **may not** occur, resulting in cryptorchidism[c]			
5-Alpha reductase deficiency (autosomal recessive disorder) in genetic males (XY genotype)[e]		Male internal organs are present (as the testosterone-dependent process is preserved).		
Müllerian agenesis (Mayer–Rokitansky–Kuster–Hauser syndrome) in XX fetus[f]	Ovaries	No male internal organs	Female external genitalia (blind vaginal pouch)	
Virilization in females (due to exposure to excessive androgen, e.g., in congenital adrenal hyperplasia, androgen-secreting tumors)			Clitoromegaly (ambiguous genitalia)	Present

[a]Complete androgen insensitivity syndrome is an X-linked mutation that results in defective androgen (testosterone/DHT) receptors that *do not* respond to androgens. Note: **Genetic females (XX genotype) are carriers of this disease**.

[b]It is a type of congenital adrenal hyperplasia. Note: In genetic females (XX genotype), deficiency of estrogen (due to decreased conversion of testosterone into estrogen) leads to failure/delay of sexual development (e.g., primary amenorrhea with ultrasound [US] revealing uterus).

[a,b]**Presentation:** an apparently normal phenotypically female fails to have menarche, and is found to have a blind vaginal pouch.

[c]Gonadectomy is recommended in cryptorchidism, as there is increased risk of dysgerminoma and gonadoblastoma. **When to do gonadectomy?** Wait until puberty (benefits of waiting until puberty for attainment of adult height likely outweighs gonadoblastoma risk).

[d]In less severe forms, external genitalia can be ambiguous or have decreased virilization of male parts (e.g., partial androgen insensitivity syndrome, incomplete 5-alpha-reductase deficiency or mild 17-alpha hydroxylase deficiency). The less severe forms are harder to make a diagnosis.

[e]

Mutation in 5-α-reductase

Testosterone ———×——→ D̶H̶T̶

Note: In genetic females (XX genotype) this has a subtler impact—e.g., delayed menstruation. Testosterone to estrogen conversion occurs in this case. In males, they might have blind vaginal pouch, or ambiguous genitalia with micro-penis.

[f]Defective embryogenesis resulting in absence of or very small Müllerian structure. They are phenotypically normal female with functioning ovaries and normal female hormonal levels. They present with amenorrhea (as no uterus) and a short vagina.

Defects of Müllerian Structures due to Abnormal Fusion

• Septate/arcuate uterus	• These are often incidentally found.
• Bicornuate uterus	• They may present with pelvic pain, endometriosis, hematocolpos (if uterus is
• Transverse vaginal septum	obstructed), dyspareunia, etc.

18.3 Sexual Maturation Stages

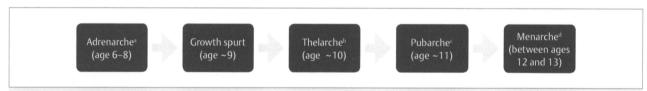

[a]**Adrenarche:** Maturation of the adrenal glands, between 6 and 8 years of age, leads to the production and secretion of sex steroids from the zona reticularis. This will lead to growth spurt.

[b]**Thelarche:** Initial breast bud formation occurs around age 10.

[c]**Pubarche:** Initial growth of pubic and axillary hair typically around age 11 (due to increased androgens).

[d]**Menarche:** Onset of menses occurs on average at the age of 12 to 13, approximately two and a half years after thelarche.

18.4 Tanner Stages of Sexual Development

Important for boards because this is very helpful in counseling parents on the development of their children.

Tanner stages	Median age of onset	Male external genitalia	Female breast		Male and female pubic hair
Stage 1	< 10 (prepubertal)	Prepubertal	Prepubertal elevation of breast papilla only	Papilla Areola	• No pubic hair • Only vellus hair, that is similar to that of arms/legs
Stage 2	10	Scrotal and testicular enlargement, **scrotal skin darkens/reddens**	First sign of puberty—breast bud forms with elevation of breast tissue (thelarche) and areolar enlargement		Sparse growth of long, slightly pigmented **straight hair**
Stage 3 (Peak height growth velocity)	11	Increase in penile length and growth of testes	Further enlargement of areola and breast, with no separation of their contour (single contour)		Hair becomes darker, coarser, and more **curled**
Stage 4	12	• Penile size increases, with development of glans penis • Testicular enlargement	Areola develops a secondary mound above the level of the breast (separate contours)		Hair is of adult type but covers smaller areas and there is no horizontal or medial spread to thighs
Stage 5	13	Adult genitalia	Mature stage		Adult-type pubic hair and there is horizontal and medial spread to thighs

Peak height growth velocity

18.4.1 Menarche-Related Issues

During early stages of menarche, as it takes time for hypothalamic–gonadal axis to mature, there might be insufficient gonadotrophin hormonal secretion. The first few menstrual cycles may be anovulatory and this exposes uterus to unopposed estrogen, which may lead to the following:

- Physical leukorrhea: Asymptomatic whitish to clear discharge
- Dysmenorrhea: Painful menstruation
- Dysfunctional uterine bleeding
- Irregular menstrual cycles

¹Prolactin and thyroid hormones are closely related to gonadotrophin hormones. Hypothyroidism can increase prolactin hormone secretion and hyperprolactinemia can subsequently:
- stimulate breast tissue (causing gynecomastia, galactorrhea)
- decrease gonadotrophin hormone secretion (causing amenorrhea, dysfunction uterine bleeding, delayed puberty, impotence, etc.).

So, first SIDx in amenorrhea or DUB (dysfunctional uterine bleeding) is to check β-hCG, prolactin, TSH along with LH/FSH.

18.5 Delayed Puberty

Etiology: Primary or secondary hypogonadism.

Definition/criteria:

- In females, no thelarche by age 12.
- In males, no increase in testicular size by age 14 (In males, the earliest sign of puberty is increase in testicular size).

Work-up: Full physical exam and check luteinizing hormone (LH)/follicle-stimulating hormone (FSH), prolactin, and thyroid stimulating hormone (TSH).[1] Also screen for chronic medical diseases.

18.6 Primary Amenorrhea

Definition/criteria: Failure of onset of menses at the age of:

- 13 with absence of secondary sexual characteristics, or
- 15, in patients with normal development of secondary sexual characteristics.

Etiology:

- Chromosomal (e.g., 45 XO Turner syndrome).
- Anatomical (e.g., absent vagina or uterus).
- Hormonal (e.g., gonadotrophin releasing hormone deficiency or hypopituitarism).

Diagnostic evaluation:

First SIDx is pelvic exam followed by pelvic US. Also check serum β-hCG, TSH, prolactin, and LH/FSH.

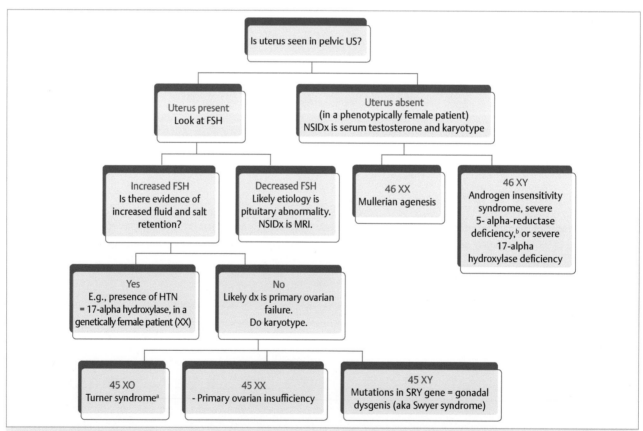

^a**Turner syndrome:** Triad of short stature, primary amenorrhea, and abnormal sexual development. Classic features like webbed neck might be absent. If suspected, NSIDx is FSH/LH and pelvic US (to look for streak ovaries).

^bFemale patients (XX genotype) with these conditions have only subtle features.

18.7 Gynecomastia in Males

Presentation: Initially may present as a mass or lump behind the areolar area and later progresses into diffuse breast enlargement (bilateral or unilateral). It can be tender and painful.

Management: Pubertal boys can have mild gynecomastia and they usually regress on their own, NSIM is reassurance. Indications for work-up include any of the following: rapid progression, diameter of ≥ 4 cm, persistence of >1 year, and occurrence after 17 years or in prepubertal age without development of secondary sexual characteristics.

18.8 Congenital Adrenal Hyperplasia

(Do not memorize the diagram below for exam purpose, just understand it. Deficient enzymes result in more substrate being available for reactions that occur upstream, e.g., 21-hydroxylase deficiency leads to elevated 17-OH progesterone and pregnenolone, which results in increased formation of testosterone).

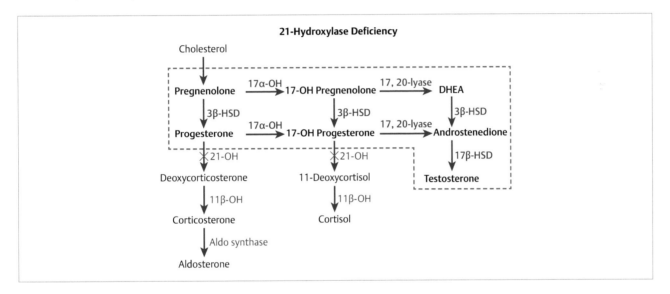

Enzyme deficiency	Biochemical effect	Clinical effects
21-Hydroxylase (most common type)	Increased testosterone	• In females: masculinization (enlarged clitoris and ambiguous genitalia) • In males: precocious puberty
	Decreased cortisol/aldosterone	Salt wasting due to decreased mineralocorticoid effect leads to **hypotension**, volume depletion, and hyperkalemia.
11-Beta hydroxylase	Increased testosterone	• In females: masculinization (enlarged clitoris and ambiguous genitalia) • In males: precocious puberty
	Increased deoxycortisone/deoxycortisol—has mineralocorticoid effect	Increased fluid and salt retention (hypertension)
17-Alpha hydroxylase	Decreased or absent testosterone	• In males, presentation can be similar to androgen insensitivity syndrome ("female from outside" = short vagina, "male from inside" = hidden testes) • In females, there is no sexual development (since estrogen are derived from androgens) • All patients (XX or XY) are phenotypically female (outside organs are female).
	Increased cortisol/aldosterone	Increased fluid and salt retention (hypertension)

MRS

To remember the table above, we only need to know what happens to testosterone and cortisol/aldosterone hormones. Is the effect increased or decreased?

			Testosterone effect	Cortisol/ aldosterone effect
11-Hydroxylase deficiency	☺ 11 looks like both are ⇧⇧; so both testosterone and cortisol are increased.		⇧	⇧
21-Hydroxylase deficiency	☺ There is only one "1", so only one of them is increased, and the other one is decreased.	☺ A 21 year old is older than 11 year old, so will have higher testosterone levels.	⇧	Decreased
17-Hydroxylase deficiency		☺ If in 21-hydroxylase deficiency, there is increased testosterone, this one has decreased testosterone, and the other one is increased.	Decreased	⇧

18.9 Precocious Puberty

Definition: Signs of pubertal development (breasts, scrotal or pubic hair development) in <= 7 years of age in girls, or <=8 years in boys.

Diagnostic evaluation: Check all gonad-related hormones (i.e., LH/FSH, testosterone, and estrogen). Look for other associated features.

Associated features	Likely diagnosis
HTN	11-Beta hydroxylase deficiency
Salt wasting/hypotension	21-Hydroxylase deficiency
Bone lesions and café-au-lait spots	Polyostotic fibrous dysplasia (a.k.a. McCune–Albright syndrome)
Ovarian mass	Granulosa cell tumor
Testicular mass	Leydig cell tumor

19. Obstetrics

The power of modern *medicine can never be understated:*

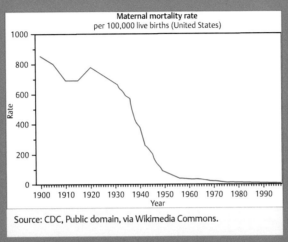

Maternal mortality rate
per 100,000 live births (United States)

Source: CDC, Public domain, via Wikimedia Commons.

19.1 Introduction

When a patient is planning to become pregnant

- Start folate supplementation (0.4 mg daily).
- In patients with prior hx of neural tube defects, use higher dose of folate (4 mg daily).
- Folate supplementation decreases risk of neural tube defects.

Diagnosing pregnancy

- Most common (MC) presentation is missed menstrual period in a sexually active female.
- Diagnostic test of choice is qualitative urine pregnancy tests. This detects β-hCG (human chorionic gonadotropin) in the urine.
- NSIDx is ultrasonography (US) of pelvis. If it shows intrauterine pregnancy, no further diagnostic steps are necessary.

19.2 Pregnancy Terminology and Timeline

19.2.1 Gravida and Parity

[1]A mother who has delivered twins is G1P1. Successful twin pregnancy is counted as 1.

Gravida	Number of pregnancies including current pregnancy.
Parity	Number of instances of delivery of viable fetus/es.[1]

What is gravida and parity in the following situation?
1) Hx of first-trimester abortion.
2) Pregnant mother with prior hx of twin delivery
Answer:
1) G1P0
2) G2P1

Terminology	Timeline
First trimester	Weeks 1–12
Second trimester	Weeks 13–27
Third trimester	Weeks 28–till birth
Spontaneous abortion	Loss of pregnancy prior to 20 weeks[a]
Intrauterine fetal death	Death in utero of fetus >20 weeks
Preterm pregnancy	Delivery between 24 and 36 weeks
Full-term pregnancy	Delivery between 37 and 41 weeks
Postterm pregnancy	Any pregnancy beyond 42 weeks

[a]20–24 weeks is the cut-off for a potentially viable pregnancy.

Exam tip: For all obstetric questions, categorize gestation into first, second, or third trimester. If third trimester, categorize further into preterm, term, and postterm.

[2]If LMP is September 8, 2016, what is the EDD?
EDD = – 3 months and + 7 days
9 – 3 = 6: 8 + 7 = 15
EDD = June 15, 2017

19.2.2 Dating Pregnancy

Naegele's rule: It is used to determine the estimated date of delivery (EDD) based on the first day of the last menstrual period (LMP).

EDD = LMP – 3 months and + 7 days[2]

Ultrasound dating:

Pregnancy dating using first trimester US is more accurate than LMP dating. Crown-rump length measurement is used in the first trimester.[3] After the first trimester, use combination of head and abdominal circumference and femur length.

US accuracy falls with the increase in pregnancy duration.

[3]Crown–rump length.

Crown to rump length

19.3 Physiological Changes in Pregnancy

Pregnancy hormones	• Soon after fertilization, the *embryo* starts making β-hCG that signals corpus luteum to continue producing progesterone and estrogen, which maintain uterine lining. • After placenta develops, it replaces corpus luteum for the job of supplying progesterone and estrogen to maintain pregnancy. • Relaxin, a hormone produced by placenta, plays a role in relaxation of pelvic girdle and cervical dilation in preparation of delivery.
Cardiac	• Decrease in blood pressure (BP; this is due to vasodilatory properties of female hormones). • Increased cardiac output: initially due to increase in stroke volume, and later in pregnancy, as a result of increased heart rate (HR). • Increased plasma volume.
Respiratory	• Increased tidal volume and resultant chronic respiratory alkalosis with metabolic compensation (this is progesterone-mediated). • Decreased total lung capacity due to elevation of diaphragm.
Gastrointestinal	• Morning sickness (typically resolves by 16 weeks). • Increased risk of gastric reflux and constipation.
Renal	• Increased renal plasma flow and GFR (glomerular filtration rate). • Decreased blood urea nitrogen (BUN)/creatinine (Cr) ratio. • Increased urinary frequency.
Skin	• Hyperpigmentation: linea nigra (straight black midline in the suprapubic region), melasma, and hyperpigmentation of the nipples and perineum. • Spider angiomata and palmar erythema may develop due to increased estrogen levels. • Varicose veins and venous stasis.
Endocrine	• Increased estrogen and progesterone. • Increased human placental lactogen. • Increased prolactin. • Elevation of "total T4" due to increase in thyroglobulin synthesis (stimulated by estrogen). • Slightly lower T3 and FT4 can occur in the latter half of pregnancy. • Slightly low or low–normal thyroid-stimulating hormone (TSH) in the first trimester.
Hematological	• Dilutional anemia. • Hypercoagulable state.
Musculoskeletal	• Increased lumbar lordosis occurs typically in the latter half of pregnancy and can cause lower back discomfort. • Relaxation of ligaments.

19.4 Prenatal Care

Pregnancy time line	Recommended routine/screening tests	What to do?
First visit	• Blood type: if Rh(D) −ve, do antibody screen (anti-D immunoglobulin screen). • CBC (complete blood count) to rule out anemia • Rubella and varicella antibody, Venereal Disease Research Laboratory (VDRL)/ Rapid Plasma Reagin (RPR), hepatitis panel, Chlamydia testing, HIV. (All pregnant women should have these tests.) • *Neisseria gonorrhoeae* testing only in women age < 25 or those at risk (multiple sex partners, history of sexually transmitted disease [STD], illicit drug use, etc.) • Pap smear, as per schedule • Influenza vaccination during flu season[a] and TDaP • Urine protein and culture[b] • US to confirm EDD • It is reasonable to offer genetic screening for cystic fibrosis to all pregnant patients or couples planning pregnancy (especially to white couples)	If rubella and varicella antibodies are negative, they may be candidates for postpartum immunization. If VDRL or RPR is positive, NSIDx is specific treponemal testing (e.g., MHA-TP, FTA-ABS)
24–28 weeks	If Rh(D) −ve, repeat antibody screen.	If antibody screen is negative, prevent sensitization (give 300 mcg dose of RhoGAM at 28 weeks' gestational age [GA]).
	One hour oral glucose tolerance test	See in gestational diabetes section
36th–37th week	Group B streptococci (GBS) rectovaginal culture	If positive, give prophylactic intravenous (IV) penicillin during labor

[a]If an exam question of routine pregnancy follow-up mentions one of the months in-between October to May, then the likely answer is to give flu vaccination.

[b]Asymptomatic bacteriuria in pregnancy needs to be treated promptly. Without treatment, it is likely to cause clinical UTI (urinary tract infection), acute pyelonephritis, and various feto-maternal complications (e.g., preterm labor, low birth weight). (!)
DOC is nitrofurantoin. Other antibiotic options include amoxicillin-clavulanate, cephalexin, cefpodoxime (an oral third-generation cephalosporin), or single-dose fosfomycin.[4]

⚠ **Caution**

(!) do not choose chorioamnionitis as a complication of asymptomatic bacteriuria in pregnancy, as it is not related to chorioamnionitis.

[4]Avoid Bactrim in the first trimester and at term.

19.4.1 Prenatal Screening for Common Aneuploidies

Background: Aneuploidy occurs due to abnormal cell division (most commonly due to meiotic nondisjunction). This results in daughter cells having **wrong number** of chromosomes. The commonly encountered non-sex chromosomal aneuploidies are Down (trisomy 21), Edward (trisomy 18) and Patau syndrome (trisomy 13). **Edward and Patau** are universally fatal.

Screened population: Pregnant women ≥35 years old are offered screening for detection of chromosomal abnormalities. There is a 1/200 risk for any chromosomal abnormality in this age group.

Screening method: Use the following test as per GA[5]:

	GA	What screening test to offer?	
Late first trimester	9–13 weeks	Nuchal translucency (US), free β-hCG, and PAPP-A (pregnancy-associated plasma protein A)[a,b]	
	> 10 weeks	**Cell-free fetal DNA**[a]: Placental fetal DNAs are present in maternal circulation, which can be used for the detection of chromosomal abnormalities (e.g., trisomy 21, 18, or 13).	Not recommended for sex chromosome aneuploidies due to a high rate of false-positive results, despite claims of high accuracy in company-sponsored studies.
Early second trimester	10–14 weeks	**Chorionic villus sampling (CVS):** Removal of a small amount of placental chorionic villi using a transcervical or transabdominal approach under US guidance.	As these are invasive, it is usually performed after noninvasive testing.
	15–18 weeks	**Amniocentesis** involves transabdominal removal of amniotic fluid under US guidance.	
	15–18 weeks	Quadruple screening[a,b] measures maternal serum alpha-fetoprotein (AFP), β-hCG, estriol, and inhibin-A levels.	

[a]If noninvasive testing is abnormal, NSIM is a thorough US (to confirm GA and to look for anatomic abnormalities). Cell-free fetal DNA testing (for suspected trisomy) can be done. Confirmatory testing, such as chorionic villus sampling or amniocentesis, is done only if abnormal results are found in noninvasive testing.[6] Complications of invasive methods include spontaneous abortion, infection, fetomaternal hemorrhage, and fetal injury.

[b]Table

	First trimester testing		Quadruple screening			
Condition	PAPP-A	Nuchal translucency	AFP	β-hCG	Unconjugated estriol	Inhibin A
Trisomy 21 (Down syndrome)	Low	↑ ↑	Low	↑ ↑	Low	↑ ↑
Trisomy 18 (Edwards syndrome)	Low	↑ ↑	Low	Low	Low	n/a
Open neural tube, ventral-wall defects	n/a	n/a	↑ ↑	n/a	n/a	n/a
Multiple gestation	n/a	n/a	↑ ↑	↑ ↑	n/a	n/a

Abbreviation: n/a, not applicable.

19.5 Vaginal Bleeding during Pregnancy

19.5.1 Abortion

Definition: Fetus loss of < 20 weeks' gestation.
Etiology: The (MCC) spontaneous abortion in the first trimester is chromosomal abnormalities. During the second trimester, etiologies of abortion include infection/teratogen exposure, incompetent cervix, trauma, etc.

MRS

Down APE = Down syndrome has low (or down) APE = AFP, PAPP-A, Estriol
Edward low HEAP = Edward syndrome has low HEAP = Hcg, Estriol, AFP and PAPP-A is low
Trisomy 13 (Patau syndrome) not included here as the quadruple screening results can be variable. But. PAPP-A is typically low and nuchal translucency is increased.

19.5.2 Types of Abortion

Types of abortion	Description		Main differentiating features			Management
			Cervical Os	Pain/ cramping	US findings	
Threatened	Vaginal bleeding or spotting *without any cervical changes* and a viable fetus.		Closed	**Absent or mild**	Alive and viable fetus	Reassurance and outpatient follow-up.
Inevitable	Vaginal bleeding and cramping with dilated open cervix, without passage of POC (products of conception).		Open	Present	POC visualized in uterus	If heavy bleeding, hemodynamic instability or infection, surgical evacuation (D&C) is performed.
Incomplete	Passage of some POC, with some POC remaining in the uterine cavity.		Open	Present	Some retained POC in uterus	If the above not present, any of the following can be done: • Expectant management is reasonable in stable patients. (Here we need to make sure the abortion is complete.)[a] or • Medical abortion (use misoprostol[b] alone or in combination with mifepristone[c]). Note that medically induced abortion is less effective in late first trimester. Or • Surgical evacuation

MRS

Think of this as the **first stage of abortion.**

MRS

Think of this as the **second stage of abortion.**

Complete	Final stage of abortion: POC completely evacuated from the uterine cavity		Closed	**Absent or mild**	Empty uterus	Usually no intervention
Missed	Death of fetus in utero, with a closed cervix and no passage of POC. This is equivalent to intrauterine fetal death.[e]		Closed	**Absent or mild**	Dead fetus in utero[d]	Manage as inevitable or incomplete abortion[d]

[a]In management of expectant or medical abortion, some experts recommend follow-up US and/or β-hCG testing until undetectable.

[b]Misoprostol (a prostaglandin agonist) causes cervical ripening, dilation, and uterine contractions.

[c]Mifepristone (progesterone antagonist) is rarely used alone, probably because the progesterone level in abnormal pregnancy is already low, thus it is less effective.

[d]In some cases, there might be an empty gestational sac with no fetal tissue development inside the sac. This condition is known as empty gestational sac (blighted ovum), which presents in a similar manner to missed abortion and is managed the same way. It likely occurs due to spontaneous fetal regression.

[e]Fetal death in utero < 20 weeks of GA (gestation age) = missed abortion; > 20 weeks GA = intrauterine fetal death.

19.5.3 Septic Abortion

Definition: Abortion + intrauterine infection.

Risk factors: Induced abortion, uterine instrumentation, STD, etc.

Presentation: Recent abortion or ongoing active abortion with symptoms of uterine infection (e.g., fever, foul-smelling discharge, uterine tenderness).

Management: Get blood and endometrial cultures, start broad-spectrum antibiotics, and perform emergent surgical evacuation.

19.5.4 Recurrent Abortions

Definition: Three or more **consecutive** pregnancy losses.[7]

Potential causes and diagnostic evaluation:

[7]For healthy women who had 1–2 spontaneous abortions in the first or early second trimester, no extensive workup is needed.

Uterine abnormalities (cervical incompetence, bicornuate uterus, etc.)	Sonohysterography is preferred (transcervical saline infusion into the uterine cavity followed by transvaginal US [TVUS]) • Other tests, which may be needed, include hysterosalpingography, magnetic resonance imaging (MRI), laparoscopy, hysteroscopy, etc.
Antiphospholipid syndrome	• Look for hx of deep-vein thrombosis (DVT) or arterial embolism, and elevated activated partial thromboplastin time (APTT). • If suspected, NSIDx is to check anticardiolipin antibodies and lupus anticoagulant. • **Rx:** LMWH (low-molecular-weight heparin) throughout pregnancy.
Thyroid disorders	TSH and free T4
Chromosomal disorders	Do cell karyotyping in parents to look for chromosomal abnormalities (translocations, deletions, etc.)
Thrombophilia	MCC of thrombophilia is factor V Leiden.

19.5.5 Cervical Incompetence

Etiology:

Cervical tissue trauma	Hx of forceful delivery, multiple gestation, dilation and curettage, etc.
Cervical tissue removal	LEEP (loop electrosurgical excision procedure), cone biopsy, etc.
Collagen disease	Ehlers–Danlos syndrome
Uterine abnormalities	• Diethylstilbestrol (**DES**) exposure • Congenital conditions

Pathophysiology: Weak cervix may not be able to support the enlarging fetus and increasing uterine pressure, leading to preterm prelabor rupture of membranes and preterm labor.

Presentation: Painless cervical dilatation typically in the latter half of pregnancy. Exam may reveal membranes bulging into vagina.

Management:

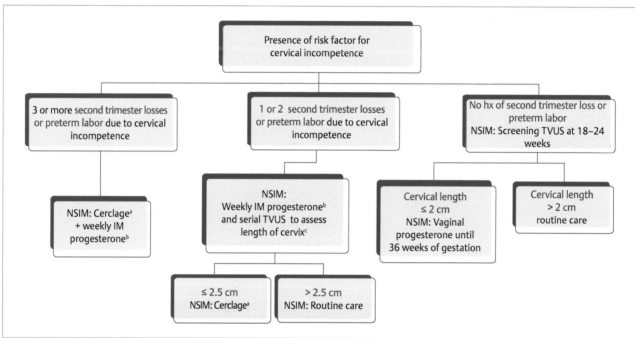

[a]Cervical cerclage (bands or suture) is placed at *12–14 weeks* and removed at term (*37th week*).

[b]Progesterone is started at *16–20 weeks* and continued until *36 weeks of pregnancy*.

[c]Start TVUS at 14–16 weeks and end screening at 24 weeks.

Exam tip: Know the timing of various interventions.

Abbreviation: TVUS, transvaginal ultrasound.

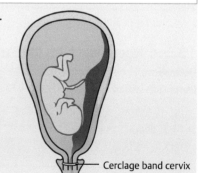

Cerclage band cervix

19.5.6 Ectopic Pregnancy

Definition: Any pregnancy that occurs outside of the uterus.[8]

Risk factors: Sexually transmitted diseases (STDs), pelvic inflammatory disease (PID), Intrauterine devices (IUDs), tubal ligation, etc.

Presentation: Abdominal pain, lower abdominal tenderness ± vaginal bleeding ± hx of amenorrhea. Ruptured ectopic pregnancy can present with hemodynamic instability due to bleeding and hypovolemic shock.[9]

Diagnosis: Pelvic exam may reveal a palpable, tender mass (can be absent in ruptured ectopic pregnancy), cervical motion tenderness, and/or adnexal tenderness ± gross bleeding.

Management:

[8]MC location is *fallopian tube.*

[9]Any woman of reproductive age presenting with abdominal pain should be evaluated for ectopic pregnancy.

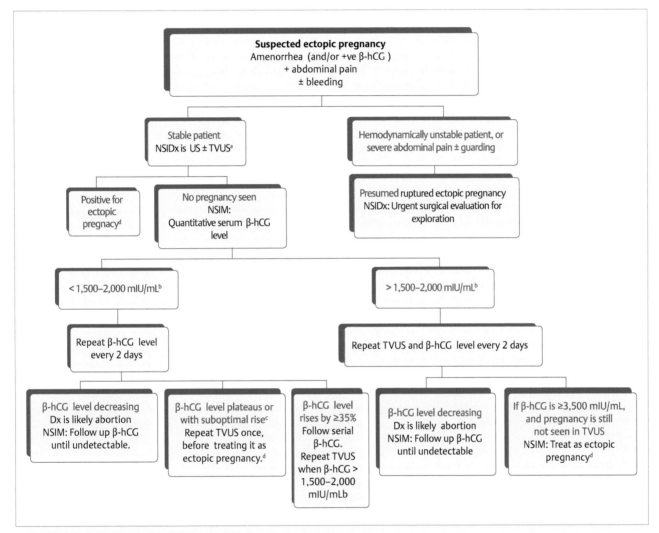

[a]If transabdominal US is negative, NSIDx is TVUS.[10]

[b]This cut-off of β-hCG (>1,500–2,000 mIU/mL) is used because at this β-hCG level, TVUS should be able to visualize intrauterine pregnancy.

[c]In intrauterine pregnancy, β-hCG levels rise by ≥35% by every 2 days.

[d]In stable patients with unruptured ectopic pregnancy, treatment may be surgical (laparoscopy) or medical (methotrexate or similar agent). If medically managed, closely follow β-hCG levels. If β-hCG is not trending down, a second round of methotrexate dose can be given. If still not responding, NSIM is laparoscopy.

[10]In early pregnancy, transabdominal US may not reveal an intrauterine sac, so use TVUS.

Abbreviations: TVUS, transvaginal ultrasound; US, ultrasound.

19.5.7 Third-Trimester Bleeding

Condition	Key features	Management
Placenta previa Complete previa Partial previa Normal placenta	Abnormal placental implantation in the *lower uterine segment*, overlapping the cervical os: • **Partial placenta previa:** Covers a portion of the internal cervical os. • **Complete placenta previa:** Covers the entire surface of the internal cervical os. **MC risk factor:** Scarring as a result of previous cesarean delivery **Presentation:** *Painless* bleeding in third trimester (bleeding occurs due to separation of anchoring villi in the lower uterine segment).	• The following are contraindicated due to risk of bleeding: digital vaginal exam, intercourse, excess physical activity, and vaginal delivery. • When low-lying placenta is seen in the first or second trimester, NSIM is abdominal US in the third trimester. Usually as the uterus stretches, placenta migrates upwards. • If persistent in the third trimester, schedule cesarean section at **36–37 weeks**. • For acutely bleeding patients, NSIM is hospitalization and close fetomaternal surveillance. In < 34 weeks' pregnancy, expectant conservative management is appropriate (give steroids too). If > 34 weeks, cesarean delivery is indicated.

Placental abruption aka abruptio placenta
 	
• **Look for retroplacental clot.**
	This occurs when a portion of the placenta prematurely separates from the uterine wall.
	
	Risk factors:
	
	• Chronic pathologic vascular processes such as hypertensive disorders of pregnancy, cigarette smoking, maternal old age, etc.
	
	• Can also occur due to trauma,[a] acute vasoconstriction (such as cocaine use), or sudden decompression (such as polyhydramnios with rupture of membrane)
	
	Presentation: Presents beyond 20 weeks with *painful* bleeding, abdominal and back pain. If hematoma is contained within the uterine cavity, there may be no frank bleeding.
	
	• Large separation leads to decreased oxygen delivery to fetus (this can be detected by abnormal heart tracing).
	
	• Maternal complications include hemorrhagic shock, disseminated intravascular coagulation (**DIC**), and Couvelaire uterus.[b]
	
	• Chronic abruptio placenta can result in intrauterine fetal growth restriction (IUGR), oligohydramnios, and pre-eclampsia.
		NSIDx is abdominal US.
		
		• First step is continuous fetal and maternal monitoring and supportive management (blood products and/or IV fluids as needed).
		
		• If maternal or fetal *instability*, prompt delivery is indicated (cesarean section, if vaginal delivery *is not imminent*) + aggressive supportive treatment.
		
		• If mother and fetus are *stable* and no evidence of worsening abruption, look at the GA (gestational age):
		
		  – In < 34 weeks' pregnancy, expectant conservative management is appropriate (give steroids too).
		
		  – If > 34 weeks, delivery is indicated.

Placenta accreta/increta and percreta • Placenta normally should be attached only to decidua, so it can easily separate from uterine wall after delivery. 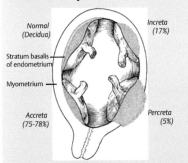 Source: TheNewMessiah at English Wikipedia, Public domain, via Wikimedia Commons.	**Definition:** • Accreta is when placental villi attach to myometrium. • Increta is when it invades myometrium. • Percreta is when it penetrates the myometrium to reach the serosa and into the peritoneal cavity. If it invades the bladder, it might cause hematuria. **Risk factors:** MC risk factor is *placenta previa with hx of cesarean delivery*; other risk factor includes prior uterine surgery (such as myomectomy) **Presentation:** Placenta fails to delivery spontaneously and when manual placental separation is attempted, profuse massive bleeding occurs (morbidly adherent placenta).	• Best case scenario is when it is discovered during a screening US. • Elective hysterectomy with cesarean section is recommended in most cases, at 34–36 weeks with predelivery steroids. Rarely, if further childbearing is desired, uterus conservation may be attempted (e.g., placental resection). • If discovered during cesarean delivery, NSIM is hysterectomy (cannot risk trying to remove placenta because of risk of massive hemorrhage).
Uterine rupture	**Risk factors**: Uterine scarring (due to prior cesarean deliveries—particularly vertical cesarean section, or myomectomy), multiple gestation, trauma, excessive use of oxytocin during labor, etc. **Presentation:** Typically presents with sudden acute *pain*, signs of fetal distress, and the fetal-presenting part may withdraw into the abdomen (*loss of fetal station*). Most often occurs during labor.	*Emergent* surgery with cesarean delivery, followed by either hysterectomy or repair (in women who desire further pregnancies).
Vasa previa 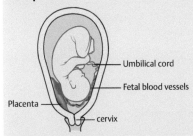	**Description:** Aberrant fetal vessel near the cervical os **Presentation of bleeding:** *Painless* bleeding with significant fetal distress. Pulsating vessels may be palpated on clinical exam.	All women with low-lying placenta or placenta previa should get screening for vasa previa with TVUS and Doppler flow assessment. If found to have vasa previa, schedule cesarean section at *34–37 weeks*.

[a]When pregnant patients present with hx of significant trauma in late-pregnancy, NSIM is close fetomaternal surveillance and US.

[b]This is when the retroplacental hemorrhage penetrates the myometrium. The uterus becomes atonic, very painful, and prone to severe postpartum bleeding. This may progress to bleeding into the peritoneal cavity.

• All of the above can present with bleeding during labor. Placenta previa *can have* abdominal pain and bleeding, but is usually mild to moderate. Severe pain points toward abruptio placenta or rupture, but these can also present with mild to moderate pain. So, an important differentiating factor is US (ultrasound).

• Look for loss of fetal station in uterine rupture.

• Normal delivery does not have vaginal bleeding; however, there may be the passage of a small amount of blood or blood-tinged mucus through the vagina near the end of pregnancy (which is called the bloody show).

• Also look for management of Rh(D) incompatibility.

19.5.8 Rhesus (Rh) Incompatibility

Rh(D) is an antigen found in RBCs. Most people are Rh(D) +ve, but some people can be Rh(D) negative. When an Rh(D)-negative person is exposed to Rh(D) +ve RBCs, this will stimulate production of anti-Rh(D) antibodies. Exposure to Rh(D) antigen occurs with incompatible blood donation (which rarely occurs), or when the Rh(D)-negative female is pregnant with an Rh(D) +ve fetus and there is fetomaternal hemorrhage.

Immunoglobulin G (IgG) antibodies against Rh(D) produced as a result of exposure to Rh(D) +ve antigen is called Rh(D) sensitization (*alloimmunization*). These IgG antibodies can cross the placenta and cause hemolytic disease of the fetus and newborn.

Screening for antibody:

All pregnant patients who are Rh(D) −ve	Screen for antibody: • During the initial prenatal visit • At 24–28 weeks' GA (gestational age) • After delivery	If Rh(D) antibody is −ve	**Prevention of sensitization** (alloimmunization) is important; use RhoGAM (anti-RhD immunoglobulin) when indicated.
		If Rh(D) antibody is +ve	Fetus is at **risk for hemolytic diseases of newborn.** There is no use of giving RhoGAM to already alloimmunized patient.

Prevention of sensitization:

- In uncomplicated pregnancy give the standard 300 mcg dose of RhoGAM is at 28 weeks.
- RhoGAM is also given in situations where there is increased risk of fetomaternal hemorrhage occurs: **after delivery**, amniocentesis, chorionic villus sampling, abortion (even threatened), ectopic pregnancy, blunt abdominal trauma, external cephalic version, antepartum bleeding, molar pregnancy, and fetal death (*in all these situations, look at the following algorithm to determine the dose of RhoGAM*).

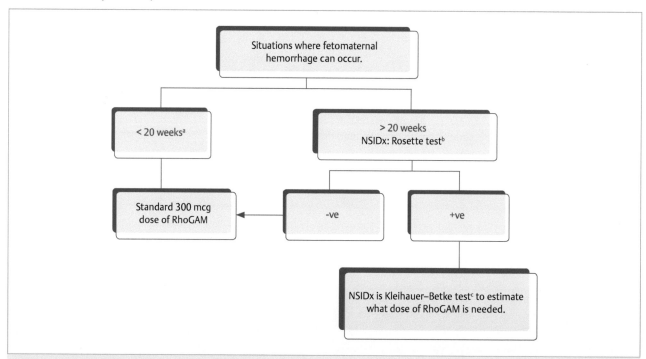

[a]With a small fetus, it is rare that we need anything more than 300 mcg of RhoGAM.

[b]Screen for fetomaternal hemorrhage (qualitative test).

[c]It estimates volume of fetomaternal hemorrhage (quantitative test).

19.5.9 Management of Pregnancy at Risk for Hemolytic Diseases of Newborn

If a woman already has been exposed and carries anti-Rh antibodies, then NSIM is to determine the probability of the fetus being Rh(D) positive:

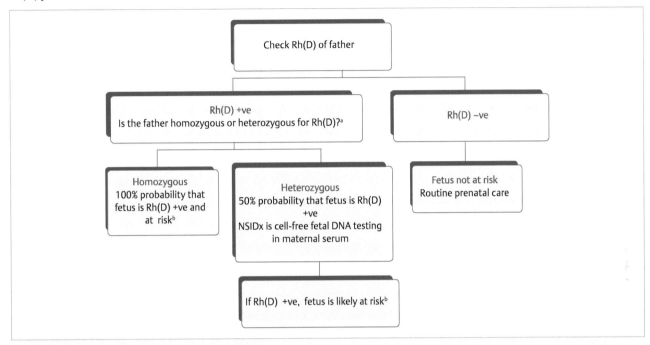

[a]Rh(D) has an autosomal-dominant pattern of inheritance.

[b]After determining that the fetus is at risk, NSIDx is to check serial maternal anti-Rh(D) titers (by indirect Coombs test); management depends on the titer (as shown below).

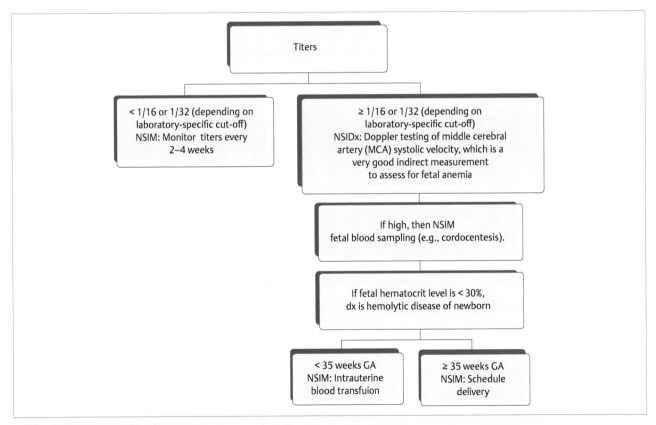

Abbreviation: GA, gestational age.

> **ABO incompatibility:** Pregnant patients with blood type O, carrying fetus with blood type A, B, or AB, only have mild hemolysis and reassurance is recommended.

19.5.10 Chronic Uteroplacental Insufficiency (Sick Placenta)

Background/risk factors: When a mother is sick, the placenta is sick too. This may be due to a variety of causes, such as maternal smoking, cocaine use, chronic medical conditions (e.g., systemic lupus erythematosus, severe diabetes, advanced kidney, heart, liver disease), hypertensive disorders of pregnancy, etc.

Clinical sequelae:

- Higher risk of pre-eclampsia and eclampsia.
- Fetal abnormalities (asymmetric IUGR, oligohydramnios, fetal death, etc.).
- Higher risk of placental abruption (chronic placental abruption can in turn cause the placenta to be sicker).
- Premature delivery.
- Increased rate of cesarean delivery.
- Mortality risk.

19.5.11 Hypertensive Disorders of Pregnancy

Condition	Definition	Treatment
Chronic hypertension (HTN)	Elevated BP of ≥ 140 systolic and/or ≥ 90 diastolic at < 20 weeks of GA	• No need to treat BP of < 150/100 mmHg in the absence of complications
Gestational HTN	• New-onset elevated BP (≥ 140 and/or ≥ 90) at ≥ 20 weeks' GA in a previously normotensive woman. • *NO* edema or proteinuria.	• Treat only if BP is ≥ **150–160** systolic and/or ≥ **100–110** diastolic and/or evidence of ongoing end organ damage. • Use oral antihypertensives[a]
Pre-eclampsia	Gestational HTN[b] (≥ 140/or ≥ 90) + proteinuria (≥ 300 mg/24 hours, 1+ or more in urine dipstick test and/or protein/creatinine ratio of ≥ 0.3). Dipstick test of 1+ needs to be confirmed by either urine spot protein/creatinine ratio or 24-hour urine protein test.	• Hospitalize and manage expectantly with close monitoring • Delivery at ≥ 37 weeks' GA. • For < 34 weeks' GA, give steroids to mature fetal lungs. • Treat with IV meds if BP is ≥ 160 systolic and/or ≥ 110 diastolic. (Note that this BP fulfills criteria for severe pre-eclampsia.)
Severe pre-eclampsia	HTN + presence of any of the following: • Sustained BP of ≥ 160 systolic and/or ≥ 110 diastolic (on at least two occasions 4 hours apart) • New onset headache unresponsive to conservative therapy • New onset severe epigastric or RUQ pain not attributed to another cause • End organ damage: Vision changes, altered mental status, liver function abnormalities ≥ 2 times upper limit of normal, acute kidney injury (doubling of serum creatinine, or absolute value of > 1.1 mg/dL), pulmonary edema. • Thrombocytopenia (platelet count < 100,000)	• Antihypertensive drugs as above • Magnesium sulfate[c] for seizure prophylaxis • For ≥ 34 weeks' GA, prompt delivery is recommended.[d] • For < 34 weeks' GA, expectant management **may** be attempted.
Eclampsia	Pre-eclampsia + tonic-clonic seizure	Control BP and seizures with the same medications as for severe pre-eclampsia, and deliver the infant[c,d]
HELLP syndrome (hemolysis, elevated liver enzymes [AST/ALT], and low platelets)	Variant of severe pre-eclampsia • Systemic inflammation and activation of the coagulation cascade result in microangiopathic hemolytic anemia, platelet consumption, and liver damage.	Stabilize the mother and deliver the infant. DIC-like picture in severe cases makes surgical treatment very challenging.

[a]The following antihypertensives are safe to use in pregnancy:

- DOC: labetalol (IV or PO)
- Methyldopa
- Nifedipine (extended-release)
- Hydralazine (IV or PO).

In severe cases (e.g., pre-eclampsia/eclampsia), use IV labetalol (DOC), IV hydralazine, or PO nifedipine.

[b]Patients with **chronic HTN** and *new/or increased* proteinuria are said to have pre-eclampsia superimposed on chronic HTN.

[c]MgSO4 is given at the onset of labor or induction of labor. Watch out for magnesium toxicity. MC risk factor for Mg toxicity is renal insufficiency (toxicity rarely occurs in women with normal kidney function). To diagnose Mg toxicity, look for *absent reflexes*, cardiovascular instability (hypotension, rarely pulmonary edema), and/or neurologic effects (muscle weakness, headache, visual disturbances). Antidote is calcium gluconate.

[d]Induce labor if > 32–34 weeks' GA or <32–34 weeks GA with favorable cervix. Do cesarean section for unfavorable cervix and <32–34 weeks' GA (see the delivery section in this chapter for further details).

19.5.12 Liver Pathology in Pregnancy

Condition	Key features	Treatment
HELLP syndrome	A variant of severe pre-eclampsia with **h**emolysis, **e**levated **l**iver enzymes (AST/ALT), and **l**ow **p**latelets	Stabilize the mother and deliver the infant
Acute fatty liver of pregnancy	• Severe condition that occurs due to mitochondrial dysfunction, resulting in abnormal oxidation of fat in the liver cells and microvesicular fatty infiltration of liver cells. • Many features are similar to HELLP (both can have HTN + proteinuria). • Features that point toward acute a fatty liver are the presence of acute liver failure (e.g., hyperammonemic encephalopathy, hypoglycemia, elevated INR and absence of hemolysis.	Stabilize the mother and deliver the infant
Intrahepatic cholestasis of pregnancy	Most common pregnancy-related liver disorder. Presents with intense pruritus, jaundice, and elevated LFTs (liver function tests). As it is a dx of exclusion, rule out other causes of cholestasis.	Ursodeoxycholic acid and early delivery
Acute hepatitis E during pregnancy	For reasons unknown, acute Hep E virus infection can be very severe in pregnancy. Fulminant hepatic failure may occur.	Supportive treatment

Clinical Case Scenarios

1. A pregnant patient at 21 weeks' GA presents with BP of 150/60. 10 weeks ago her BP was 120/60. Urine dipstick reveals 3+ proteinuria. Is dx of pre-eclampsia confirmed?

2. A pregnant patient at 21 weeks' GA presents with BP of 190/100. Urine dipstick reveals 2+ proteinuria. Is dx of pre-eclampsia confirmed?

3. A pregnant patient at 21 weeks' GA presents with BP of 155/105. Urine dipstick is negative for proteinuria. Her platelet count is 90,000/mcL. At 16 weeks of GA her platelet count was 160,000/mcL. What is the likely dx?

   a) Pre-eclampsia
   b) Severe pre-eclampsia
   c) Gestational HTN with idiopathic thrombocytopenia
   d) Chronic HTN

19.5.13 Amniotic Fluid Embolization

Definition: A rare but life-threatening condition, which occurs when amniotic fluid enters maternal circulation. It can cause cardiogenic shock, respiratory failure, and anaphylactoid reaction.

Risk factors: Advanced maternal age, uterine or cervical trauma, conditions that cause hemorrhage during pregnancy (e.g., abruptio placenta), eclampsia, etc.

Clinical presentation: Shock, respiratory failure, DIC, and/or coma. It usually occurs during labor and delivery or in immediate postpartum period.

Treatment: Supportive.

19.5.14 Gestational Diabetes

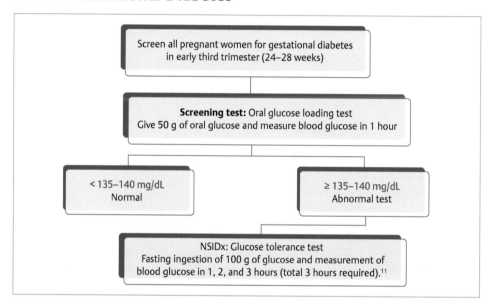

Goals for glucose control are stricter in pregnancy[11]:

	Normal values (also target blood sugar level during therapy)[11]
Fasting glucose	≤ 95 mg/dL
1-hour postprandial glucose	≤ 140 mg/dL
2-hour postprandial glucose	≤ 120 mg/dL

[11]Note that these cut-offs for normal values and target blood sugar are lower for gestational diabetes than in diabetes mellitus.

Management:

First step: Start with diet and exercise.

Second step: If target blood glucose not achieved, start insulin (DOC) or oral hypoglycemic agent (such as metformin or glyburide).

Complications of maternal uncontrolled hyperglycemia in pregnancy	
When fetus is exposed to hyperglycemia in 1st trimester (occurs in patients with pre-existing diabetes only)	When fetus is exposed to hyperglycemia in 2nd and/or 3rd trimester (can occur in patients with either pre-existing diabetes or gestational diabetes)
Diabetic embryopathy[a] (May present with severe congenital abnormalities): • Neurologic: anencephaly, microcephaly, neural tube defects • Cardiovascular: ventricular septal defect, transposition of the great vessels, coarctation of aorta, patent ductus arteriosus, atrial septal defect • Gastrointestinal: duodenal atresia, situs inversus • Genitourinary: renal agenesis, hydronephrosis • Skeletal abnormalities	Diabetic fetopathy: • Respiratory distress syndrome (MC) • Macrosomia and subsequent high risk of birth-related injury (e.g., shoulder dystocia, fracture of clavicle) • Preterm delivery • Neonatal hypoglycemia • Polycythemia and hyperviscosity syndrome • Hypertrophic cardiomyopathy

Maternal:	Maternal:
• Spontaneous abortions • Increased risk of infections	• Pregnancy-related hypertensive disorders (HTN, pre-eclampsia) • Preterm and/or prolonged labor • Polyhydramnios • Increased risk of infections • Risk of perineal injuries (due to macrosomia) • Lactation failure • Women with gestation diabetes are more likely to develop diabetes later on

[a]Unlike pre-existing diabetes, gestational DM **is not** associated with embryopathy and fetal anomalies, as gestational diabetes occurs in the latter half of pregnancy.

19.6 Other Medical Disorders in Pregnancy

19.6.1 Thyroid Disease and Pregnancy

Two hormones affect thyroid function in pregnancy:

- High levels of β-hCG weakly stimulate the thyroid gland: slightly low or low to normal TSH can be seen in the first trimester and has no clinical significance.
- Estrogen increases thyroid-binding protein (thyroglobulin) synthesis leading to an increase in total thyroid hormone levels (free levels are normal).[12]

Hypothyroidism:

- Maintaining the euthyroid state is critically important for both mother and fetus.
- In women with pre-existent hypothyroidism, levothyroxine requirements often increase by 25 to 30%, due to an increase in thyroxine-binding globulin. If patient is pregnant, NSIM is to increase the dose of levothyroxine by 25 to 30% and follow up TSH and FT4.

Maternal hyperthyroidism:

- Causes include Graves' disease, hCG mediated hyperthyroidism (in gestational trophoblastic disease) and others.
- Treat moderate to severe symptomatic maternal hyperthyroidism with antithyroid drugs (thionamides - propylthiouracil in the first trimester, transition to methimazole in 2nd trimester).[13]
- Thionamides will also prevent fetal hyperthyroidism. Add short-term β-blockers for maternal symptoms.[14] If thionamides are not well tolerated, consider surgery.
- Fetal monitoring: monitor regularly fetal heart rate and growth rate. In mother with Graves' disease, check fetal thyroid US and maternal thyroid-stimulating antibodies (thyrotrophin receptor antibody) titres.
- Pregnant mothers with active or history of Graves' disease (e.g., hx of thyroidectomy or radiation, and currently euthyroid) may have significant titers of thyroid-stimulating antibodies. These can cross placenta and stimulate fetal thyroid, causing fetal/neonatal Graves' disease and hyperthyroidism (pathophysiology is similar to RhD-associated hemolysis).
- Fetal US revealing fetal goiter, hear rate >160/min, intrauterine growth restriction suggest fetal hyperthyroidism. If these features develop, thionamides may be given to the mother to control fetal hyperthyroidism and mother may need levothyroxine is she develops hypothyroidism.
- Neonatal effects: neonates with hyperthyroidism may have prematurity, goiter, exophthalmos, and signs of hypermetabolic state (low birth weight, microcephaly, irritability, restlessness, tachycardia, etc.). Treat the hyperthyroid infant with thionamides and β-blockers.

Venous thromboembolism (VTE) in pregnancy:

- Pregnancy and postpartum period are risk factors for VTE.
- DOC for VTE in pregnancy is low-molecular-weight heparin. Warfarin is contraindicated due to its teratogenic effects. DOACs (direct-acting oral anticoagulants) are also avoided as little is known about their effects on pregnancy.

[12]In the follow-up of thyroid disorders in pregnancy, check FT4 only. Do not check total thyroid hormones.

[13]All thionamides are potentially teratogenic, but methimazole is associated with more severe defects. Methimazole is more potent than propylthiouracil, hence preferred after the fi rst trimester.

[14]Do not treat mild symptoms: β-blockers have been associated with uteroplacental insuffi ciency. Once hyperthyroidism is controlled with thionamides, attempt should be made to discontinue β-blockers.

19.6.2 Fetal Growth Abnormalities

Macrosomia

Definition: Infant weighing ≥ 4,500 g at birth.

Risk factors: Diabetic mothers, mother aged > 35 years, pregnancy of >42 weeks.

Complications: Hypoglycemia of the newborn, shoulder dystocia, and birth injuries.

Screening/management: Weight can be estimated by US.

Do elective cesarean section if estimated fetal weight is ≥ 5 kg or (≥ 4.5 kg in infants of diabetic mothers).

Shoulder dystocia

Description: Following delivery of the head, the shoulder becomes lodged behind the pubic symphysis. It increases risk of birth-related injuries.

Risk factor: Large fetus (due to maternal diabetes, obesity, postterm pregnancy) and/or small pelvis (cephalopelvic disproportion).

Management steps: How to dislodge the shoulder?

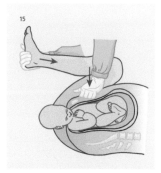

- First step: Ask patient to stop pushing and drain bladder if distended. Enlarge vaginal opening with episiotomy if not adequate.
- Second step: McRoberts maneuver is the *first-line maneuver*—flex hip/knee against abdomen and apply suprapubic pressure (**NOT** on the fundus).[15]
- If it fails and patient is well anaesthetized, NSIM—try to deliver the posterior arm. If good regional anesthesia is not present, try other maneuvers (trying to deliver the posterior arm in the absence of anesthesia is very painful). Intentional clavicular fracture might be necessary.
- Last resort is cesarean delivery after getting the presenting part back inside the pelvis.

Birth-related injuries:

Clavicular fracture	• Exam may reveal a tender mass near the newborn's neck.
	• **Rx:** Observation is usually sufficient. Immobilization of the affected arm for comfort by using a long-sleeve wear can be done.
Humeral fracture	Immobilization
Perinatal asphyxia	Presentation depends on the degree of hypoxic injury; cerebral palsy may occur in rare situations.
For Erb–Duchenne palsy (upper-brachial plexus injury) and Klumpke's palsy (lower-brachial plexus injury), see Chapter 22, pediatrics for further details.	

19.7 Intrauterine Fetal Growth Restriction (IUGR)

Definition: Estimated fetal weight by US is below the 10th percentile for GA (gestational age).

[16]Acronym TORCH stands for the causative pathogens of congenital infections:
- Toxoplasmosis
- Others = syphilis, varicella zoster, Zika virus, etc.
- Rubella
- Cytomegalovirus (CMV)
- Herpes virus

Types	Features	Etiology
Primary (symmetric) IUGR	All organs are reduced in size and in equal ratio.	Usually due to problem with the fetus itself (genetic disorders, congenital TORCH infections,[16] congenital heart disease, etc.)
Secondary (asymmetric) IUGR	Head and brain are spared, but other organs are smaller. US will typically reveal a small abdominal circumference and a normal head size.	Occurs due to sick placenta, usually due to maternal factors such as substance abuse, autoimmune diseases, anorexia, vascular insufficiency due to hypertensive disorders of pregnancy, etc.

Management steps:

- First step is to ensure accurate GA (first trimester US is the best test to determine this).
- After delivery, it is important to send placenta for histopathologic exam. Consider karyotyping and testing for TORCH infections, especially for symmetric IUGR.

19.8 Intrauterine Fetal Demise (IUFD)

Definition: Fetal death in utero after 20 weeks of gestation.

Etiology: Multiple causes ranging from perinatal infection to maternal illness, such as HIV, severe HTN, SLE, thyroid disease, and trauma. Many remain unexplained.

Presentation: Absent[17] fetal movements and decrease in uterine growth.

Workup:

- First SIDx is fetal Doppler to detect fetal heartbeat.
- If fetal heartbeat not detected, NSIDx is real-time US.

Additional tests recommended after dx of IUFD:

Rosette–Kleihauer–Betke test	If Rh(D)-negative pregnant women at risk for Rh(D) sensitization
Antiphospholipid antibody, TSH	Possible etiology
DIC screening	Possible complication
STD screening	If STD risk factors are present

Management: Evacuate the fetus (when patient is emotionally ready) and perform autopsy to determine the cause. Watchful waiting can result in DIC and chorioamnionitis.

Modes of delivery to evacuate the fetus			
20–23 weeks	Dilatation and evacuation (preferred), or induction of labor		
≥ 24 weeks	Induction of labor	24–28 weeks	Induction with misoprostol ± mifepristone.
		>28 weeks	• If favorable cervix, use oxytocin. • If unfavorable cervix, use misoprostol for ripening prior to oxytocin.

Complication:

Most-threatening complication is DIC. Woman presenting with IUFD needs to have coagulation profile checked. If abnormal, immediate delivery with induction is recommended.

[17] As opposed to absent fetal movements, decreased fetal movements point toward fetal distress, which can be further investigated by doing a nonstress test.

19.9 Amniotic Fluid Abnormalities

	Polyhydramnios	Oligohydramnios
Definition	Excess of amniotic fluid	Paucity of amniotic fluid
Dx is by US	≥ 8 cm at the deepest pocket or Amniotic fluid index ≥ 24 cm	≤ 2 cm at the deepest pocket or Amniotic fluid index ≤ 5 cm
Etiology	• **Decreased fetal ingestion of amniotic fluid:** Due to gastrointestinal obstruction (e.g., duodenal stenosis) or anencephaly. • **Increased fetal production of amniotic fluid:** Multiple gestations, gastroschisis, fetal anemia (hydrops fetalis), increased fetal urination (e.g., due to fetal hyperglycemia in uncontrolled maternal diabetes).	**Decreased production** • **By sick placenta (uteroplacental insufficiency):** e.g., due to hypertensive disorders of pregnancy • **By fetus (decreased urination):** Often a result of congenital malformations of the renal system (often leads to severe IUGR)
Potential complications	Preterm labor or early ROM, fetal malposition, cord prolapse, postpartum uterine atony or rupture	Severe oligohydramnios may manifest as *Potter's sequence* (facial and limb deformities and fetal lung hypoplasia)

	Polyhydramnios	Oligohydramnios
Management	Treat only if significant maternal discomfort or preterm labor. Do amnioreduction (needle aspiration of amniotic fluid). If < 32 weeks, consider indomethacin[a] for periprocedural discomfort or as a tocolytic for preterm labor.	• Do complete fetal structural survey to assess fetal anatomy • For idiopathic cases, schedule delivery at 37–38 weeks (with induction).

[a]NSAIDs (nonsteroidal anti-inflammatory drugs) reduce amniotic fluid volume. They are contraindicated in ≥ 32 weeks' pregnancy, because of increased risk of premature closure of ductus arteriosus.

19.10 Preterm Labor

Definition: Onset of labor between week 20 and 37.[18]

Risk factors: *Previous preterm labor*, multiple gestation, placental abruption, infection, pre-eclampsia, preterm prelabor rupture of membranes (PPROM), cervical incompetence, *bicornuate uterus*, etc.

Presentation: Contractions *with* cervical changes (dilation, effacement) between week 20 and 37 GA.[19]

Diagnostic evaluation:

First step: Cervical exam to assess for any cervical changes. If cervical changes are not significant enough to diagnose labor, next step is TVUS (to assess the cervical length; smaller the cervical length the more imminent is delivery). Fetal fibronectin test can also be done.[20]

Management of confirmed preterm labor:

Gestational age (weeks)	Treatment		
≥ 34	Delivery		Antibiotics prophylaxis is usually indicated as Group B streptococcus (GBS) status is typically not known at this time (GBS screening is done at 36th–37th week)
32–33	Tocolytics[a]—nifedipine (first line) or terbutaline (second line)	+ Corticosteroids, if delivery is not imminent[c]	
24–31	Tocolytics[a]—indomethacin[b] (first line), nifedipine (second line), or terbutaline (third line) + magnesium sulfate for neuroprotection (for < 32 weeks)		

[a]Tocolytics are drugs used to reduce uterine contractions, to try to delay delivery for 48 hours and let corticosteroids work in utero to mature lungs. Tocolysis is contraindicated when risk of prolonging pregnancy is higher than risk of preterm birth (e.g., severe pre-eclampsia/eclampsia, intra-amniotic infection, severe bleeding).

[b]NSAIDs (cyclooxygenase inhibitors) increase the risk of premature ductus arteriosus closure, so avoid after 32 weeks of pregnancy.

[c]Corticosteroids start working after 24 hours, hence it is used with tocolytics. But if delivery is likely to be immediate, they are not going to work. IM betamethasone and dexamethasone are commonly used.

[18]Onset of labor before 20 weeks is termed as abortion as the fetus is nonviable.

[19]Differential diagnosis is false labor (a.k.a. Braxton Hicks contractions): **irregular**, infrequent contractions with no cervical change, and no rupture of membranes. NSIM is reassurance.

[20]Fetal fibronectin is a protein produced by fetal cells that acts like a biological adhesive, which binds fetal sac to the uterus. In true labor it starts leaking into the vagina and can be detected.

19.11 Prelabor Rupture of Membranes (ROM)- Previously Known as Preterm ROM

Definitions:

Prelabor ROM (rupture of membranes)	ROM without coexistent contractions at ≥ 37 weeks' GA
Preterm prelabor ROM (PPROM)	ROM without coexistent contractions at < 37 weeks of GA

Diagnostic evaluation: When a woman presents complaining of her "water breaking," a sterile speculum examination should be performed. Amniotic fluid flowing from cervical os and pooling in vagina confirms ROM. Avoid doing a digital pelvic exam to decrease risk of infection. Note: involuntary loss of urine can also present as a sudden gush of fluid. If equivocal speculum exam, NSIDx is to do ultrasound. If US shows oligohydramnios, it is highly suggestive of ROM. If amniotic fluid volume is normal, it rules out ROM. If amniotic fluid volume is low normal, commercially available testing can be done to confirm presence of amniotic fluid in vagina.

The following diagnostic signs are also helpful:

- A fluid sample placed on a nitrazine paper results in a blue color, indicating alkaline amniotic fluid.
- A ferning pattern occurs when a dried amniotic fluid sample is examined under a microscope.[21]

[21]In pregnancy, a ferning pattern can be seen in cervical mucus and amniotic fluid. This ferning pattern in cervical mucus occurs due to changes brought upon by high estrogen during pregnancy. This ferning pattern also occurs just before ovulation. Looking for a ferning pattern might also be useful in fertility testing.

Fertile   Infertile

 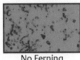

+ve Ferning   No Ferning

Risk factors are similar to those of preterm labor.

Management

For PROM, NSIM prompt induction of labor (routine antibiotic prophylaxis not indicated). For PPROM, look at algorithm below:

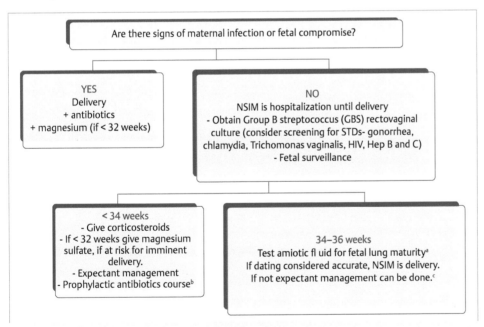

[a]Amniocentesis to test for lung maturity is rarely done rarely nowadays.

[b]Azithromycin at admission.+ IV Ampicillin for 2 days followed by amoxicilin for 5 more days.

[c]Take samples of amniotic fluid from either the vaginal vault, or amniocentesis. The following measurements are taken:

Note that for patients with GBS culture positive screening and undergoing elective cesarean section with intact membrane do not need antibiotic prophylaxis.

Indications for Antibiotics prophylaxis against Group B streptococcus (GBS) during labor

- Positive GBS screening (culture)
- Hx of delivery of GBS-affected neonate
- Unknown GBS status with any one of the following factors: Preterm labor (< 37 weeks), Prolonged ROM (≥ 18 hours), preterm prelabor ROM undergoing expectant management, Maternal fever, or if rapid nucleic acid amplification test (NAAT) is positive for GBS

Antibiotic choices: Use penicillin or ampicillin. If mild penicillin allergy, use IV cefazolin (first-generation cephalosporin). If severe penicillin allergy, use clindamycin if sensitivity results available, if not, use vancomycin.

Chorioamnionitis

Definition: Intra-amniotic infection usually due to *ascending vaginal flora*.

Risk factor: Prolonged ROM is the most important risk factor.

Presentation: Maternal fever + any one or more of the following: uterine tenderness, fetal tachycardia ≥ 160/min, malodorous amniotic fluid, and/or purulent vaginal discharge.

Management: IV antibiotics that cover gram positives, gram negatives ± anaerobes (e.g., piperacillin-tazobactam), and expedited delivery (e.g., oxytocin-induced labor or cesarean section)

19.12 Late-Term (Post-Term) Pregnancy

Definition: Pregnancy that extends ≥ 42 weeks.

Potential complications:

In fetus	Intrauterine infection, macrosomia, uteroplacental insufficiency (placenta ages and eventually fails), fetal dysmaturity, meconium aspiration syndrome, oligohydramnios, etc.
In mother	Increased rate of cesarean delivery, infection, postpartum hemorrhage, and macrosomia-related birth issues (e.g., perineal trauma)

Preventive measures: At 41 weeks of GA, induction of labor is recommended. Induction is indicated earlier for complicated pregnancies (e.g., oligohydramnios). If patient opts for watchful waiting and has uncomplicated pregnancy, close fetal monitoring by nonstress testing (NST) and amniotic fluid volume assessment is recommended. Do induction if no spontaneous labor by the end of the 42nd week.

19.13 Induction of Labor and Cervical Ripening

Exam tip: In a question "What is the most important risk factor for this condition?", always answer previous occurrence of that condition. For example, the most important risk factor for post-term pregnancy is previous postterm pregnancy.

	Management
Unfavorable cervix	Ripen cervix first: • **Medical method:** Preferred is prostaglandin E1 analog (e.g., misoprostol), or prostaglandin E2 analogs (e.g., **di**noprostone). • **Mechanical methods:** Insertion of laminaria or an inflatable balloon are acceptable alternatives.
Favorable cervix	**Oxytocin**[a] ± amniotomy[b]

[a]Oxytocin can be used to jump start contractions or intensify weak contractions.

[b]Artificial rupture of the amniotic sac can induce uterine contractions. It is imperative to do a pelvic exam prior to rupture, to ensure that the fetal head is the presenting part and is well applied to the pelvis. If the cord is palpated, amniotomy should not be done, as it can precipitate acute cord prolapse.

19.14 Uterine Hyperstimulation (Tachysystole)

Definition: Overstimulation and overcontraction of uterus, which may be caused by oxytocin or PGE1 analog (e.g., misoprostol).

Criteria: > 5 contractions in 10 minutes, or contractions lasting ≥ 2 minutes.

Management steps: NSIM is to look at fetal tracing.

- If reassuring, reduce dosage of oxytocin.
- If nonreassuring, stop oxytocin, left lateral maternal position, and give IV fluids. If still not responding, give terbutaline.

Complication: Uterine rupture and amniotic fluid embolism.

Other adverse effects of oxytocin:

- **Hyponatremia:** Oxytocin can act like its cousin ADH (antidiuretic hormone).
- **Cardiovascular instability**: In high doses it acts as a vasodilator, causing hypotension, tachycardia, and cardiac hypoperfusion (which can result in myocardial ischemia and arrhythmias).

19.15 Fetal Monitoring

19.15.1 Fetal Movement Count by Mother

All pregnant patients are asked to monitor fetal movement with "kick count" logs after 24 weeks' GA. At least 10 fetal movements in 2 hours is reassuring. Any decreased perception of movement by the mother warrants further investigation of fetal well-being.

- First step is to document fetal heartbeat by using Doppler.
- If positive, NSIDx is NST (non-stress test).
- If negative, NSIDx is US (possible fetal death).

19.15.2 Antenatal/Antepartum Fetal Surveillance

Indication: High-risk pregnancies in which there is increased risk of fetal death, such as in hypertensive disorders of pregnancy, diabetes, significant chronic medical disorders in mother, complicated multiple gestation, postterm pregnancy, IUGR, oligo/polyhydramnios, etc. Additional indication is decreased fetal movement.

Timing: Start surveillance at ≥ 32 weeks' GA. Can be done earlier (≥ 26 weeks' GA) in patients with multiple worrisome features.

Method of surveillance: Regular (typically weekly) nonreactive stress test or modified biophysical profile (BPP).[22] Abnormal test is followed by either full BPP or contraction stress test (CST, again done weekly, or twice weekly if higher risk).

[22]Modified BPP is NST + US for amniotic fluid index.

19.15.3 Nonstress Test (NST)

Test description: Measurement of fetal HR and frequency of fetal movements.

Test result: Criteria for reactive NST

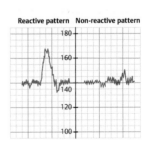

Reactive pattern   Non-reactive pattern

GA	Reassuring if following is present during a 20-minute evaluation period (in the absence of decelerations)
≥ 33 weeks	Two fetal HR accelerations of at least 15 bpm, each lasting at least 15s
< 32 weeks	Two fetal HR accelerations of at least 10 bpm, each lasting at least 10s

Nonreactive NST is when accelerations do not fulfill the above criteria or are simply absent.	MCC of nonreactive NST is a sleeping fetus. **NSIM is either** • Extend the test to 40–120 min (*wait for the fetus to wake up spontaneously*), or • Vibroacoustic stimulation (*wake up the fetus*). **If still nonreactive or if initial NST showed decelerations,** NSIDx is contraction stress test (CST) or full biophysical profile (BPP).

19.15.4 Contraction Stress Test (CST)

Test description: Fetal heart is monitored while inducing uterine contractions (by giving oxytocin or by nipple stimulation). During uterine contractions, if oxygen delivery to the fetus is decreased, fetal hypoxemia will manifest as a decrease in heart rate and late decelerations (similar in pattern to intrapartum surveillance graphs as shown below).

Contraindications to CST: Placenta previa, vasa previa, twin pregnancy, cervical incompetence, and suspected uteroplacental insufficiency.

19.15.5 Biophysical Profile (BPP)

Test description: It consists of the following five elements[23]:

- NST.
- One or more fetal breathing movements lasting 30 seconds in a 30-minute period.
- Fetal movement—three or more movements in 30 minutes.
- Fetal tone—extension and flexion of a limb or opening and closing of a hand.
- Amniotic fluid level > 2 cm determined by US.

[23]No need to remember all the points, as exam is likely not going to ask you to calculate the BPP. The question will give you the computed score and ask you the NSIM.

Each is worth two points. If a criterion is not fulfilled, the score is 0. The lower the score, the higher the risk of fetal asphyxia.

Score	Management
10/10	Reassuring
8/10 without oligohydramnios[a]	Repeat BPP in 1 week, or in higher risk pregnancy, twice weekly
8/10 due to oligohydramnios	• If ≥ 37 weeks' GA, NSIM is delivery.
6/10	• If < 37 weeks' GA, do 24 hourly BPP (steroids[b] if < 34 weeks). May do CST.
4/10	• If ≥ 32 weeks' GA, consider delivery (± steroids[b]) • If < 32 weeks' GA, individualize decision. May consider extending time of the test or performing CST.
0, or 2/10	Consider extending time of the test. If still low, may need to do delivery regardless of GA.

[a]Score of 8 without oligohydramnios is considered reassuring.

[b]Abnormal BPP in < 34 weeks' GA gets steroids for the preparation of imminent delivery.

19.15.6 Umbilical Artery Doppler Velocimetry

It is used in pregnancies with fetal growth restriction to assess fetal well-being. If diastolic flow is absent or reversed, it is a nonreassuring finding.

19.16 Intrapartum Fetal Surveillance

Indicated for complicated pregnancies (e.g., antepartum hemorrhage, oligo/polyhydramnios, post-term pregnancy, insulin-dependent diabetes).

Normal HR accelerations

Criteria: Two fetal HR accelerations of at least 15 bpm within a 20-minute period, each lasting at least 15 seconds (same as the NST).

Note: Each small horizontal box represents 10 seconds; In fetal HR graph, each small vertical box represents HR of 10 bpm.

Tip: First always look at the baseline HR, and then only look at decelerations

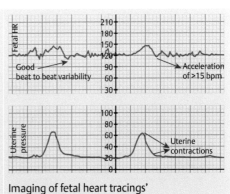

Imaging of fetal heart tracings' acceleration—normal

HR decelerations

Early decelerations

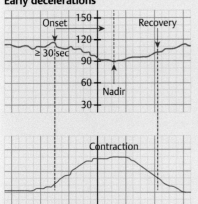

Criteria: The deceleration lasts the duration of the contraction and onset to nadir is ≥ 30s. (*Note: "Early" is a misnomer, as it starts with the contraction.*)

Cause: Autonomic response to fetal head compression during uterine contractions.

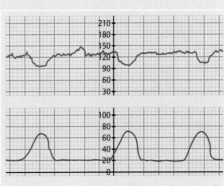

NSIM: Continue monitoring (this can be normal)

Variable deceleration (VD)

Criteria: Abrupt decrease in HR of at least 15 bpm (abrupt = onset to nadir is in < 30s)

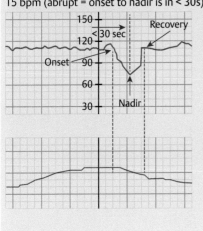

Intermittent VDs are VDs associated with < 50% of contraction. This is well tolerated by fetus.

Predictors of negative fetal outcome:

Recurrent VD = VD seen in > 50% of contractions

Severe VD = Decrease of ≥ 60 bpm in HR

Cause: *Umbilical cord compression* due to cord prolapse, oligohydramnios, etc.

NSIM: Continue monitoring

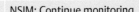

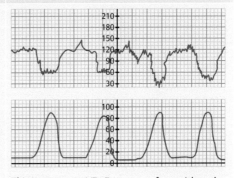

This is recurrent VD. Do not confuse with early decelerations, here the onset to nadir is abrupt *(VD looks like a tomb stone rather than a wave).*

NSIM: Initiate resuscitative measures.

The orange boxes in the table above represent non-reassuring fetal monitoring; the latter ones being more severe than the earlier ones.

> ⚠ **Caution**
>
> (!) If lasting for > 10 min, it is considered a change in baseline.

Late deceleration

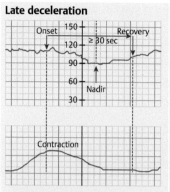

Criteria: Onset to nadir in ≥ 30 secs and unlike early decelerations, does not occur synchronously with contractions.

Recurrent late deceleration is indicative of *uteroplacental insufficiency* (insufficient blood supply to fetus through placenta).

Severe (drop of > 45 bpm) is suggestive of severe fetal acidemia with myocardial depression.

Causes: Maternal hypotension, hypoxia, or severe bleeding

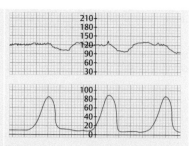

NSIM: Initiate resuscitative measures.

Prolonged deceleration

Criteria: Decrease in HR of at least 15 bpm, lasting at least 2 min, but not more than 10 mins. (!)

Causes: Multiple, but importantly this can be due to cord compression from oligohydramnios or cord prolapse.

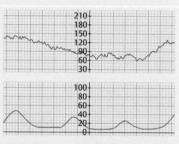

NSIM: Initiate resuscitative measures.

Bradycardia (fetal HR of < 110 bpm)

Causes: High-grade heart block or serious fetal compromise (could be from cord compression)

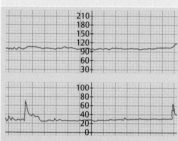

NSIM: Initiate resuscitative measures.

Sinusoidal pattern

Multiple causes

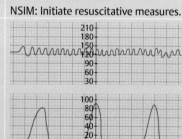

Think of saw-tooth waves

NSIM: Initiate resuscitative measures.

No baseline variability

No accelerations and beat-to-beat variability

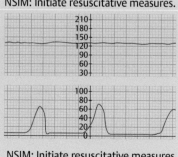

NSIM: Initiate resuscitative measures.

19.16.1 Management of Nonreassuring Intrapartum Fetal Monitoring

NSIM is to initiate resuscitative measures ASAP:

- Change maternal position (left or right lateral).
- Oxygen administration.
- IV fluids.
- Reduction of contraction frequency.
    - Remove application of uterotonic prostaglandin (if it was applied for induction).
    - Stop oxytocin.
    - Might have to give terbutaline to stop contraction.
- Abrupt onset of recurrent/severe VDs or prolonged deceleration/bradycardia can be due to umbilical cord compression from oligohydramnios or cord prolapse. Do quick exam to feel for cord presentation.
    - If cord prolapse is palpated, the examiner should keep the finger in the vagina and continue to gently elevate the fetal presenting part and rush the patient to the operating room. Do not try to push it in.
    - If oligohydramnios is suspected, NSIM is to consider amnioinfusion and elevate the fetal presenting part.

If initial resuscitative measures do not correct the problem and *scalp stimulation* does not cause reflex fetal HR acceleration, then the baby may need to be delivered right away.

- If vaginal delivery is imminent (cervix completely dilated and fetal station is low enough), then forceps or vacuum delivery may be attempted.
- If not, NSIM is cesarean delivery.

Fetal scalp sampling:

Performed rarely nowadays but know the following numbers:

pH	Management
> 7.25	Expectant management with continued observation.
7.2–7.25	Repeat test in 15–20 min.
< 7.2	This is severe fetal acidosis due to severe hypoxemia. Expedite delivery (forceps/vacuum or cesarean section).

19.17 Delivery[24]

Indications for elective cesarean delivery:

- Macrosomia—fetal weight of ≥ 5 kg (≥ 4.5 kg in infants of diabetic mothers).
- HIV with viral load of ≥1,000 copies/mL.
- Hx of classical cesarean section (vertical incision).
- Hx of myomectomy with entry into the uterine cavity.
- Previous two or more low-cesarean sections.[25]
- Active maternal genital herpes infection.
- Breech presentation with failed external cephalic version.

[24]In this chapter, wherever NSIM says delivery, it either means vaginal delivery (± induction of labor) or cesarean section.

[25]After one cesarean section, vaginal birth may be attempted in uncomplicated pregnancies.

19.17.1 Vaginal Delivery

Stages of labor:

Stage		Problems that can occur during this stage and management
I **Lasts from onset of labor until the cervix is completely dilated (10 cm)**	**Latent:** Lasts from onset of labor till 5-cm cervical dilation Cervix = 0–5 cm	**Protracted latent phase** = ongoing latent phase for ≥20 hours in a primiparous woman, or ≥ 14 hours in a multiparous woman. ∟ NSIM: Therapeutic rest (sedatives and analgesics as needed). Oxytocin is not indicated. ∟ If still no progression after adequate rest, oxytocin can be given (± amniotomy). Cesarean delivery is not recommended. If allowed to rest, the vast majority of these women will eventually progress to normal labor.
	Active: Lasts from 6-cm cervical dilatation to fully dilated cervix (this is a more rapid phase) Cervix = 6–10 cm	**Protracted active phase** = progression of cervical dilatation is ≤ 1cm over 2 hours. ∟ NSIM: Oxytocin and if adequate fetal descent is present, amniotomy. ∟ If still no change after 4–6 hours, NSIM is amniotomy if membranes not yet ruptured, regardless of fetal head position. ∟ If still no change, NSIM is cesarean delivery.
		Arrested labor = no increase in cervical dilation in a patient with ruptured membranes for ≥ 4 hours despite adequate contractions, or ≥6 hours with inadequate contractions. ∟ If no change despite oxytocin and adequate contractions, NSIM is cesarean section. (Instrumental delivery cannot be attempted if cervix has not completely dilated.)
II	Lasts from complete cervical dilation until the infant is delivered	After 60–90 min of entering stage II, if there is no fetal descent/rotation and uterus is hypocontractile, NSIM is oxytocin. **Arrest of the second stage** = no fetal descent/rotation in 2 hours in multiparous women or 3 hours in nulliparous women; add 1 hour for women who received epidural anesthesia. ∟ When arrest is diagnosed, NSIM is instrumental or cesarean delivery.
III	Time between infant delivery and placental delivery (lasts approximately 30 min)	Proactive management is recommended in this stage to prevent complications: • IV infusion (or IM administration) of oxytocin, AND • Securing of uterine fundus by one hand, and giving a gentle traction on the umbilical cord by the other hand. **Signs of placental detachment:** Surge of fresh bleeding and lengthening of the umbilical cord.

All of the above may result from sedation, insufficient contractions, or due to abnormal cervix anatomy.

• In the first stage, most common cause is inadequate contractions of uterus.

• Protracted/arrested second stage is more likely due to cephalopelvic disproportion: disproportion between presenting fetal part (due to macrosomia, malposition, or malpresentation) and pelvic dimensions (due to small and/or nulliparous pelvis).

 In a nutshell

• Protracted = Slow change.

• Arrest = No change.

• For protracted or arrested labor, NSIM is oxytocin (± artificial ROM, which is amniotomy). After oxytocin, if there is still no change, NSIM is instrumental or cesarean delivery.

19.18 Malpresentation

Definition: Presenting part of the fetus is other than the head (e.g., breech, transverse).[26]
Diagnosis is made by pelvic exam or US.

19.18.1 Breech Presentation

Definition: Presenting part is the buttocks.
Management: Most of breech presentation self-corrects by the 37th week of gestation. If persistent at 37 weeks or more, external cephalic version can be attempted in normal pregnancy in the absence of complications such as oligohydramnios, significant fetal or uterine anomaly, placental abruption, placenta previa, multiple gestation, etc.
If external cephalic version fails or is contraindicated, plan cesarean section.[27]

19.18.2 Twins with One of Them in the Breech Position

For delivery of the second twin with breech:
- Breech extraction of the second twin can be attempted if all of the following present:
    - Adequate pelvis.
    - Fetal weight of > 2 kg.
    - Flexed fetal head.
    - General anesthesia and experienced physician available
      OR
- External cephalic version can be attempted after the birth of the first twin.
  OR
- Elective cesarean delivery of both twins.

Cesarean section is recommended in all other fetal "malpresentation" (e.g., transverse position)

19.19 Postpartum Issues

19.19.1 Postpartum Hemorrhage

Criteria: > 500 mL of blood loss after vaginal delivery, or > 1,000 mL after cesarean delivery.
Cause:
- MCC is uterine atony (uterine contractions are not sufficient to compress blood vessels). Risk factors of uterine atony include increased uterine distension (large fetus, twins, polyhydramnios), uterine fatigue (prolonged labor), etc.
- Less common causes include placenta accrete/increta/percreta, unrepaired lacerations, coagulopathy, etc.

[26]As opposed to malpresentation, malposition is when the presenting part is head, but it is not in the occiput-anterior position (MC malposition is occiput posterior).

[27]There is less risks with planned C-section than with attempted vaginal breech delivery.

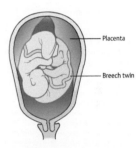

Source: C.Monck, CC BY-SA 4.0, via Wikimedia Commons.

Management:

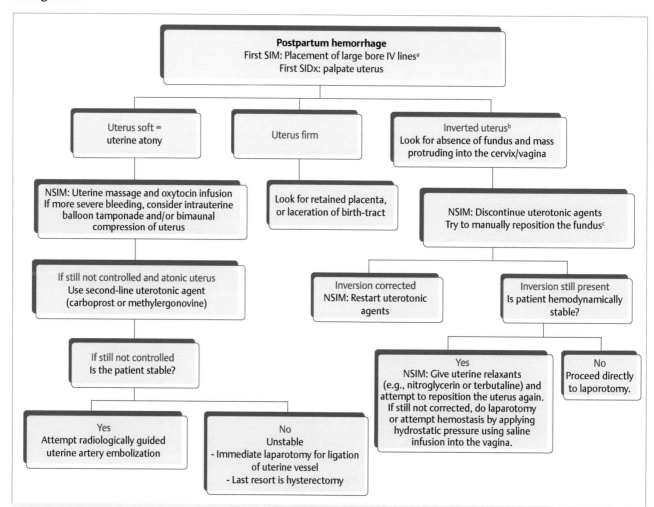

Postpartum hemorrhage
First SIM: Placement of large bore IV lines[a]
First SIDx: palpate uterus

Uterus soft =
uterine atony

Uterus firm

Inverted uterus[b]
Look for absence of fundus and mass
protruding into the cervix/vagina

NSIM: Uterine massage and oxytocin infusion
If more severe bleeding, consider intrauterine
balloon tamponade and/or bimaunal
compression of uterus

Look for retained placenta,
or laceration of birth-tract

NSIM: Discontinue uterotonic agents
Try to manually reposition the fundus[c]

If still not controlled and atonic uterus
Use second-line uterotonic agent
(carboprost or methylergonovine)

Inversion corrected
NSIM: Restart uterotonic
agents

Inversion still present
Is patient hemodynamically
stable?

If still not controlled
Is the patient stable?

Yes
Attempt radiologically guided
uterine artery embolization

No
Unstable
- Immediate laparotomy for ligation
of uterine vessel
- Last resort is hysterectomy

Yes
NSIM: Give uterine relaxants
(e.g., nitroglycerin or terbutaline) and
attempt to reposition the uterus again.
If still not corrected, do laparotomy
or attempt hemostasis by applying
hydrostatic pressure using saline
infusion into the vagina.

No
Proceed directly
to laporotomy.

[a]Do not choose diagnostic testing for an answer in an actively bleeding patient. First step is securing good large bore IV access and proactively replacing ongoing losses (crystalloids and blood transfusion as needed).

[b]Rare condition when uterine fundus collapses into the uterine cavity after a vaginal or cesarean delivery. This is a life-threatening emergency, as it can cause severe hemorrhage, shock, and death. Risk factors include placenta accreta, short umbilical cord, uterine anomalies (e.g., tumors), rapid labor, etc.

[c]Manual reposition of uterus shown below.

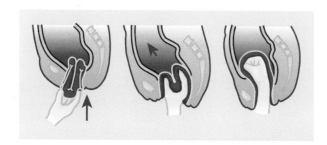

Differential diagnosis: Placenta accrete/increta/percreta

Look for failure of spontaneous delivery of placenta and massive bleeding after attempted manual removal of placenta.

 In a nutshell

Bleeding during pregnancy (timeline and differential dx):

Hemorrhage during early pregnancy	Abortion and ectopic pregnancy
Hemorrhage (third trimester)	Placenta previa, abruptio placenta, vasa previa
Hemorrhage during labor	Uterine rupture, placenta previa, abruptio placenta, vasa previa
Hemorrhage after attempted delivery of placenta	Placenta accrete/increta/percreta
Hemorrhage after delivery	Uterine atony, uterine inversion

Potential complication of severe hemorrhage during late pregnancy: Sheehan's Syndrome–Severe hemorrhage during late pregnancy may result in pituitary tissue infarction and panhypopituitarism. Hypertrophied pituitary in pregnancy is particularly vulnerable to hypoperfusion. Typical question will involve a woman returning for postpartum appointment and complaining of inability to lactate. Other symptoms resulting from the loss of hormone include signs of adrenal insufficiency (fatigue, low blood pressure), loss of pubic hair, cessation of or irregular/infrequent menstrual periods, etc. Imaging may reveal an empty sella. Treatment consists of hormonal replacement.

Rosette test followed by Kleihauer–Betke test is recommended for Rh(D)-negative pregnancies > 20 weeks' GA who are at risk for sensitization.

19.20 Other Postpartum Issues

19.20.1 Bladder Atony

Presentation: Lower abdominal tenderness or fullness and inability to urinate after delivery
Management:
First step: Ambulation and analgesia.
Second step: Bladder catheterization.
It is usually temporary and resolves on its own.

19.20.2 Postpartum Endometritis

Presentation: Fever, painful uterus, and/or foul-smelling discharge 2 to 3 days after delivery.
Risk factors: Cesarean delivery, prolonged labor, prolonged ROM, vaginal infection, immunosuppression, etc.
Treatment: This is usually of polymicrobial infection and treatment is similar to chorioamnionitis. Use antibiotics that cover anaerobes and gram negatives (e.g., clindamycin + gentamicin)

19.20.3 Postpartum Breast issues

Condition	Presentation	Management
Breast engorgement	• Breast fullness, tenderness and warmth • Usually bilateral • No fever	• May use cold compresses, NSAIDs, acetaminophen and manual milk expression or pumping for symptomatic relief. • Women who desire lactation suppression (e.g., neonatal death) should not use frequent breast pumping as this stimulates more lactation. Do not use medications to suppress lactation, as their risk outweigh benefits.
Mastitis without abscess	Fullness, tenderness and warmth + fever Usually unilateral	Dicloxacillin or cephalexin • Important to continue lactation (mastitis usually happens due to inadequate milk drainage)
Mastitis with breast abscess	Mastitis + area of fluctuance	Needle aspiration + antibiotics (as above) • If aspiration fails, NSIM is incision and drainage.

19.21 Hyperemesis Gravidarum

Definition: Severe nausea and vomiting during pregnancy, resulting in weight loss, dehydration, dizziness, and/or ketosis.

Background: It is theorized to be due to the surging β-hCG levels during the first trimester, as most patients improve as pregnancy advances. Patients with multifetal pregnancy and gestational trophoblastic disease are at a higher risk.

Criteria: Significant nausea and vomiting + 5% or more loss of prepregnancy weight, or evidence of presence of ketones, dehydration, and/or electrolyte and acid-base derangements.

NSIDx, when pregnant patients present with symptoms of severe nausea/vomiting, is to check serum electrolytes and ketone.

Management of nausea and vomiting during pregnancy:

- If evidence of volume depletion, NSIM is to hospitalize and give IV fluids + IV thiamine. Use IV ondansetron, as needed.
- In mild cases, first try conservative measures (e.g., ginger-containing foods, small frequent meals). If not responsive or for moderate cases, use doxylamine + Vit b6 (pyridoxine).
- Other treatment options include diphenhydramine, meclizine, or promethazine.

19.22 Gestational Trophoblastic Disease—Benign (Hydatidiform) Mole and Gestational Trophoblastic Neoplasia

19.22.1 Molar Pregnancy (Hydatidiform Mole)

Background: *Benign tumor* of pregnancy that occurs due to abnormal fertilization, causing placenta to develop into abnormal mass of cysts. Most important risk factor includes *previous molar pregnancy* and advanced age.

There are two types of molar pregnancy:

	Partial	Complete
Karyotype	69 XXY or XXX (two sperm cells fertilize an ovum)	46 XX or XY (one or two sperm cells fertilize an empty ovum that is lacking genetic material. In the case of one sperm, the sperm duplicates its chromosomes to make it 46)
β-hCG	Usually low	High Typically presents with hyperemesis gravidarum, and may have theca-lutein cysts.
Embryonic or fetal tissue	Present There is an embryo, but it is abnormal and cannot survive (may present as spontaneous abortion)	No embryo or normal placental tissue
Malignant transformation	May occur but rare	Yes (higher rates than partial)

Diagnosis: Higher than expected β-hCG level suggests this dx. To confirm dx, best test is pelvic ultrasound, which typically reveals "honeycombed," "snow-storm," or "cluster of grapes" appearance.

Management: Dilatation and suction curettage. Offer hysterectomy in patients with higher risk for malignant transformation (i.e., patients aged ≥ 40 years) or who have completed childbearing.

Follow-up: Follow β-hCG until no longer detectable (to ensure clearance). For β-hCG follow-up to be accurate, it is important to send the patient home on a contraceptive (oral or barrier). IUD is contraindicated as it increases risk of molar pregnancy.

Complication: If the β-hCG level is persistent, remains detectable, and/or goes higher, this is classified as persistent gestational trophoblastic disease (a.k.a. gestational trophoblastic neoplasia).

19.22.2 Gestational Trophoblastic Neoplasia (GTN)

Background: May arise from apparently normal pregnancy, abortion, or molar pregnancy.[28]

Types: Invasive mole, choriocarcinoma, placental site trophoblastic tumor, epithelioid trophoblastic tumor.

Clinical presentation:

- **Due to excess β-hCG stimulation:** Hyperthyroidism, ovarian theca-lutein cysts, nausea, and vomiting, and/or
- **Metastatic disease:** E.g., friable vaginal mass that bleeds, cough due to pulmonary metastasis, etc.

Diagnosis: Most important finding is persistent detectable serum β-hCG (after other causes such as normal pregnancy or molar pregnancy are excluded). Do cervical speculum exam, routine blood test (thyroid function testing, complete metabolic profile) and imaging (US of pelvis and chest X-ray: CT scan of chest is not needed). If no evidence of metastasis, no further testing needed. If abnormal lab test, consider CT scan of abdomen and pelvis or whole body PET-CT scan. If new onset headache, do MRI of brain. Unlike other cancers, a tissue diagnosis is not required before initiating treatment. Also, as the tumor is highly vascular, life-threatening bleeding can occur if biopsy is attempted.

Treatment:

Low risk	Without distant metastasis	Methotrexate + leucovorin
	With lung metastasis only (CXR-positive)	
High risk	With extrapulmonary metastasis, or in higher risk patients	• Leucovorin, Actinomycin D, Methotrexate, Etoposide **alternating with** • Cyclophosphamide + Vincristine

Follow-up: Serial measurement of β-hCG levels.

> The general rule is that **carcinomas** are more likely to metastasize through lymphatic channels and **sarcomas,** hematogenously. The few exceptions to this rule are:
> - **Choriocarcinoma**
> - Follicular carcinoma
> - Renal cell carcinoma
> - Hepatocellular carcinoma
>
> } These carcinomas are more likely to metastasize hematogenously.

🔍 Clinical Case Scenarios

A 41-year-old female presents at your clinic with severe nausea and vomiting. She has hx of amenorrhea for 2 months. Exam reveals palpable uterus.

4. What is the first SIDx?

5. If pregnancy test is positive, what is the likely dx for severe nausea and vomiting?

Patient is admitted to the hospital with evidence of dehydration. US reveals the following[29]:

6. What is the best SIM?

7. Patient refuses hysterectomy and undergoes dilatation and suction curettage. Before discharge from the hospital, what should be done?

β-hCG remains persistently detectable during follow-up. Patient also starts complaining of cough. Patient does not have any other symptoms.

8. What is the likely dx?

9. What is the NSIDx?

10. Chest X-ray shows the following.[30] What is the NSIM?

[28]In some cases, there may be no hx of pregnancy, as patients might not have detected the pregnancy that had culminated in spontaneous abortion (bleeding may be mistaken for menses).

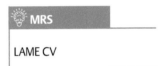

MRS

LAME CV

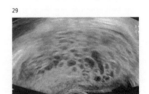

Looks like a cluster of grapes
Source: By Mikael Häggström, used with permission. CC0, via Wikimedia Commons.

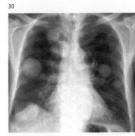

Source: Imaging signs. In: Galanski M, Dettmer S, Keberle M et al., eds. Direct Diagnosis in Radiology. Thoracic Imaging. 1st ed. Thieme; 2010.

19.23 Luteoma and Theca-Lutein Cysts in Pregnancy

Luteoma	Theca-lutein cysts
Occurs during normal pregnancy	Associated with abnormally high β-hCG, which occurs with multiple gestation, molar pregnancy, ovulation induction, etc.
Bilateral or unilateral	Usually bilateral

- Both can lead to increase in sex hormones (mostly progesterone and testosterone), masculinization of mother (acne and increased facial hair) and, sometimes, fetus.
- Both are usually benign and resolves after delivery.

19.24 Multiple Gestation

Background: With the advent of in-vitro fertilization multiple gestations are becoming more common.

Identical (monozygotic) twins	A single egg is fertilized by one sperm, but the zygote splits early in development.
Fraternal (dizygotic) twins	Two eggs are fertilized by two separate sperm (more common with in-vitro fertilization)

Features: Uterine size may be larger than expected for GA. In addition, β-hCG and AFP levels are higher than expected.

Potential complication: Excessive uterine distension may lead to preterm labor, postpartum atony, etc.

19.25 Appendix

19.25.1 Practice questions

Tip: Cover Cover the last column and try to answer the question first, before looking.

Problem	Situation	NSIM or NSIDx
Preterm pregnancy with the need for early delivery	< 34 weeks	Give steroids
	< 32 weeks	Give magnesium sulfate + steroids
Preterm labor	≥ 34 GA	Delivery + GBS prophylaxis
	32–33 GA	Nifedipine (preferred tocolytic) + corticosteroids + GBS prophylaxis
	24-31 weeks' GA	Indomethacin (preferred tocolytic) + corticosteroids + GBS prophylaxis + IV magnesium sulfate
PPROM without sign of maternal infection or fetal compromise	34–36 weeks	If dating considered accurate, deliver baby.
	< 34 weeks	obtain GBS culture + Antibiotics + corticosteroids + fetal surveillance + IV magnesium sulfate if < 32 weeks, if at risk for imminent delivery.

Problem	Situation	NSIM or NSIDx
High-risk cervical incompetence (hx of three or more second-trimester pregnancy loss or preterm labor)	At what GA is cerclage done? When to remove cerclage?	Place cerclage at *12–14 weeks'* GA and remove it at the *37th week* GA
	Is IM progesterone indicated and when to stop giving progesterone?	Start regular interval IM progesterone at 16–20 weeks' GA and continue it until 36 weeks' GA
Intermediate-risk cervical incompetence (hx of one or two trimester pregnancy loss or preterm labor)	Is IM or vaginal progesterone indicated and when to stop giving progesterone?	Give IM progesterone. Timing as above.
	At what GA do we begin TVUS screening and when do we stop?	Start TVUS at 14–16 weeks and end screening at 24 weeks.
	When is cerclage indicated?	If TVUS shows cervical length of ≤ 2.5 cm
Presence of risk factor for cervical incompetence	When to do screening TVUS to assess cervical length?	18–24 weeks
Mode of delivery of IUFD	> 28 weeks	If favorable cervix, use oxytocin.
		If unfavorable cervix, use misoprostol for ripening prior to oxytocin.
	24–28 weeks	Induction of labor with misoprostol ± mifepristone.
	20–23 weeks	Dilatation and evacuation (preferred), or induction of labor

Answers:

1. No. When BP is < 160/110, we must have at least two readings 4 hours apart to make the dx of HTN and pre-eclampsia.

2. Yes.

3. (b) Severe pre-eclampsia. The dx of pre-eclampsia can be made in the absence of proteinuria, if there are one or more features of severity.

4. Urine pregnancy test, serum electrolytes, and ketones.

5. Hyperemesis gravidarum.

6. Offer hysterectomy (higher risk of malignant transformation in patients aged ≥ 40).

7. Initiate contraception (barrier or oral).

8. Persistent gestational trophoblastic disease/neoplasia.

9. Chest X-ray + ultrasound of pelvis.

10. Chest X-ray shows classic canon-ball metastasis. Treatment is with methotrexate + leucovorin.

20. Gynecology

Ninety-five percent of ovarian cancers arise from the epithelial portion and only 5% are germ-cell tumors. As opposed to this, 90% of testicular cancers arise from germ cells.

The reason germ-cell tumors are less common in females is because a female germ-cell system only produces one egg per month (approximately 300–400 in a female's life), whereas a male germ-cell system produces about 525 billion sperm cells over a lifetime. Less active cell multiplication means smaller chance of abnormal cell division.

20.1 Normal Menstrual Cycle

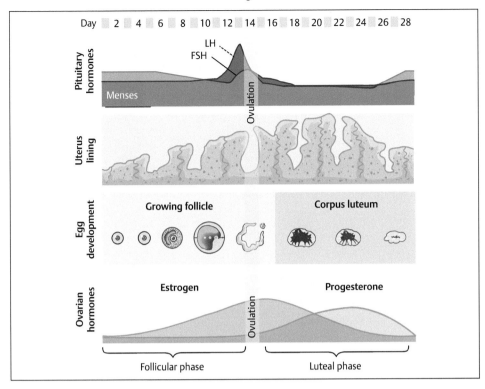

Day 1 of menstrual cycle is the first day of menses.

There are two phases, each lasting approximately 14 days in a 28-day cycle:

- **Follicular phase:**
    - Follicle-stimulating hormone (FSH) stimulates the growth of ovarian follicles and secretion of estrogen by follicles.
    - A luteinizing hormone (LH) and FSH surge leads to release of a mature ovum from the ovarian follicle (ovulation), ending the follicular phase.
- **Luteal phase:**
    - After ovulation, the remains of the follicle develop into the corpus luteum that produces **estrogen and progesterone,** which prepare uterine lining for implantation.[1]
    - If fertilization does not occur, the corpus luteum withers away, and with decreasing progesterone, menstruation results (end of the cycle).
    - If fertilization occurs, the *embryo* starts making *β-hCG*, which signals the corpus luteum to continue producing progesterone and estrogen (which maintain the uterine lining).

[1]Anovulatory cycles result in unopposed estrogen secretion, as there is no formation of corpus luteum that secretes progesterone.

20.2 Menstrual Pathologies

Terminology	Description
Secondary amenorrhea	No menses for: • >3 months in a previously regular menstrual cycle, or • > 6 months in previously irregular menstrual cycle
Oligomenorrhea	Prolonged menstrual cycles > 35 days in length, or < 9 menstrual cycles per year
Menorrhagia	Heavy and prolonged menstrual bleeding
Hypomenorrhea	Light menstrual bleeding or spotting
Metrorrhagia	Bleeding between menstrual periods
Menometrorrhagia	Irregular bleeding that is prolonged or excessive

20.3 Abnormal Uterine Bleeding

Etiology:

MRS

PALM CONE
that bleeds

Structural causes	Functional causes
• Polyp (uterine), **P**regnancy-related • Adenomyosis • Leiomyoma • Malignancy and hyperplasia	• Coagulopathy • Ovulatory dysfunction • Not yet classified • Endometrial
Ovulation is usually normal. Thus, presentation is usually menorrhagia (i.e., cyclical heavy bleeding)	MCC of functional bleeding is ovulatory dysfunction leading to anovulatory cycles, which presents as irregular and noncyclical bleeding.

Management:
- In reproductive age patients, the first step is to rule out pregnancy.
- Control bleeding and treat anemia if present and look for bleeding disorders (e.g., von Willebrand disease).
- Oral contraceptive pills (OCPs) with estrogen and progesterone are first-choice agents. (In ovulatory dysfunction, it is important to decrease the risk of endometrial hyperplasia and cancer, by counteracting the effect of unopposed estrogen.)[2]
- If patient does not want hormonal treatment:
    - **Mild symptoms**—nonsteroidal anti-inflammatory drugs (NSAIDs) or tranexamic acid (anti-fibrinolytic agent).
    - **Significant bleeding**—endometrial ablation, or in women who do not desire further pregnancy, hysterectomy.

[2]Other choices include oral or injectable progesterone and levonorgestrel containing hormonal IUD. These also decrease risk of endometrial hyperplasia and cancer.

Management of acute severe bleeding
- Address hemodynamics first—IV fluid resuscitation and transfusion as needed. Treat underlying blood disorder if present (e.g., give von Willebrand factor concentrate for von Willebrand disease).
- **For hemodynamically unstable patient,** NSIM is intrauterine tamponade (balloon or gauze packing), then uterine curettage. For persistent bleeding, start IV estrogen. Emergency hysterectomy might be needed in refractory cases.
- **For hemodynamically stable patient,** NSIM is high-dose oral estrogen.

20.3.1 Secondary Amenorrhea

Criteria: No menses for > 3 months in a previously regular menstrual cycle, or > 6 months in previously irregular menstrual cycle.

Diagnostic evaluation:

MCC is pregnancy, so first do β-hCG testing. If pregnancy is ruled out, look at the following algorithm for workup.[3]

[3]The following algorithm can also be used for workup of hypo/oligomenorrhea with some minor changes.

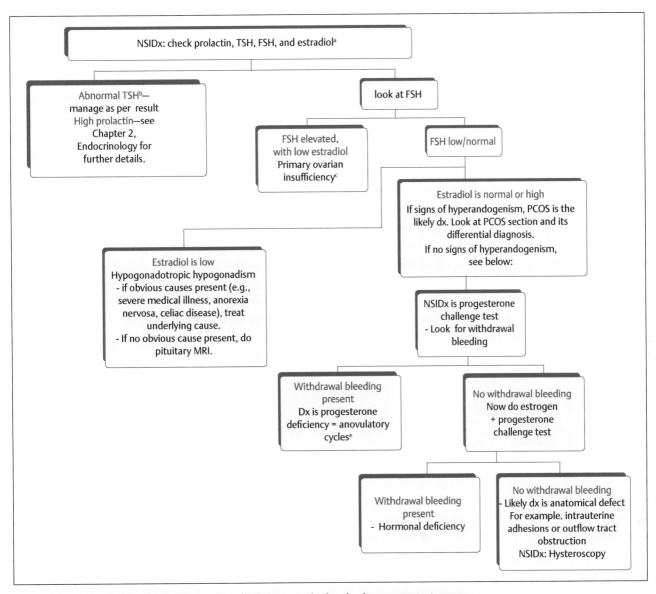

[a]If there is evidence of hyperandrogenism (e.g., hirsutism, acne), also check serum testosterone level. Think of polycystic ovary syndrome (PCOS).

[b]Both hypo- and hyperthyroidism can cause amenorrhea. In hypothyroidism, thyrotropin-releasing hormone stimulates both thyroid-stimulating hormone (TSH)[4] and prolactin secretion. Prolactin inhibits gonadotropin-releasing hormone (GnRH; low FSH and LH).

[c]This results in hypergonadotropic hypogonadism. Look for symptoms of hot-flashes and/or atrophic vaginitis.

[d]Causes of hypogonadotropic hypogonadism are:

• Bulimia nervosa

• Significant chronic illness

• **Excessive exercise** or weight loss

• Starvation

• If there is no obvious etiology, NSIDx is MRI to look for pituitary disorders. Sheehan's syndrome (postpartum pituitary necrosis) is a potential cause, if there is a history of pregnancy-related hemorrhage.

[e]The idea behind progestin challenge is that a woman with sufficient estrogen level will have withdrawal bleeding after a dose of progesterone, indicating that amenorrhea is likely due to progesterone deficiency, e.g., chronic anovulation in conditions such as PCOS.

[4]Remember to check TSH in any patient presenting with irregular menses.

Condition	Estrogen	FSH	LH
Hypergonadotropic hypogonadism (menopause or premature ovarian failure)[a]	Low	↑	↑
Hypogonadotropic hypogonadism = pituitary dysfunction	Low	Low	Low
PCOS	Normal or slightly high[b]	Usually falls within normal limits—as estradiol is normal.	↑ ↑[c]

[a]Premature ovarian failure can be due to chemotherapy/radiation, autoimmune conditions, Turner's syndrome, etc.
[b]PCOS patients are typically obese and have a higher testosterone level. Peripheral conversion of testosterone into estrogen in the adipose tissues maintains the estrogen level.
[c]In PCOS, LH/FSH ratio is typically > 1.

20.4 Polycystic Ovary Syndrome (PCOS)

Background: Exact etiology is unknown. Main problem is abnormal steroidogenesis in ovaries with *increased androgen production*. It is the MCC of infertility in women.

Presentation:

Typical features[5]:

- Hyperandrogenism (hirsutism, acne, androgenic alopecia).
- Irregular menstrual cycle, amenorrhea, and anovulation.
- Due to issues with follicular development and regression, there are multiple immature follicles in ovaries. These *look like* cysts in ultrasound (polycystic-looking ovaries).
- Insulin resistance, acanthosis nigricans, weight gain, obesity, and type 2 diabetes.

Diagnostic evaluation:

Pelvic US will show ovaries that look like they have multiple cysts in them.

- PCOS is a diagnosis of exclusion: rule out conditions that present similarly to PCOS (i.e., other causes of late-onset virilization and **hyperandrogenism**). Check 17-OH progesterone level, TSH, prolactin, IGF-1, cortisol, and testosterone levels.[6]

[5]Usually presents in puberty and gradually worsens.

[6]Remember, not all women with US findings of multicystic ovaries have PCOS. Other causes of hyperandrogenism can also lead to similar picture in ultrasound.

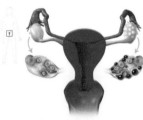

Polycystic ovary syndrome
Source: BruceBlaus, CC BY-SA 4.0, via Wikimedia Commons.

Differential dx of PCOS	Key features	Laboratory findings
Nonclassic congenital adrenal hyperplasia, due to **mild 21-hydroxylase deficiency** with some 21-hydroxylase activity present	• May present in late childhood to early adulthood, unlike severe ones which present at birth • May also have polycystic ovaries and hypo/amenorrhea	• Elevated 17-OH-progesterone level
Ovarian hyperthecosis (idiopathic hyperplastic increase of luteinized thecal cells that overproduce androgen)[a]	• Primarily seen in postmenopausal women	• High testosterone • Normal DHEA[b]
Ovarian or adrenal virilizing tumors	• These are typically rapid in onset • Pelvic and adrenal US may reveal the tumor.	• Markedly elevated androgens (testosterone and/or DHEA[b]) • Low LH
Cushing's syndrome (they may have hirsutism and oligo/amenorrhea)	• Centripetal obesity • Diabetes • Other features of corticosteroid excess	• High cortisol
Hyperprolactinemia	• Hypogonadism and oligo/amenorrhea • Galactorrhea	• High prolactin
Acromegaly	• Increased bone growth	• Increased insulin-like growth factor-1

[a]This is thought to be due to genetic mutation. Similar in pathophysiology, **luteoma** (which can occur with normal pregnancy) and **hyperreactio luteinalis** (associated with abnormally high β-hCG, which occurs with multiple gestation, molar pregnancy, ovulation induction, etc.) can result in transient hyperandrogenism.
[b]Normal DHEA with elevated testosterone suggests extra-adrenal sources (typically ovaries). Elevated DHEA suggests adrenal virilizing tumors.
Abbreviations: DHEA, dehydroepiandrosterone; LH, luteinizing hormone.

Management of PCOS:

- First step is weight loss (this not only decreases insulin resistance and risk of diabetes, but may also restore ovulation).
- Second step depends upon the patient's goal.

Women who do not desire pregnancy	Women who wish to get pregnant
• Combination OCP (this will decrease risk of endometrial hyperplasia/cancer,[a] menstrual abnormalities, and decrease androgenic symptoms). • For persistent hyperandrogenic symptoms, second line is spironolactone.	Induce ovulation: • Clomiphene, or • Letrozole[b] (preferred in women with BMI of > 30)
Metformin is used as an adjunctive treatment in patients with obesity, diabetes mellitus (DM), or impaired fasting glucose.[c]	

[a]Remember that chronic anovulation is associated with increased risk of endometrial hyperplasia and cancer due to unopposed estrogen effect.

[b]Letrozole is an aromatase inhibitor that decreases estrogen production and thus removes negative feedback effect on FSH.

[c]Studies have not shown protective effect of metformin on endometrium.

20.5 Contraception

FYI: Given in order of somewhat effective to highly effective (e.g., failure rate of spermicides is ≈25–33%; failure rate of vasectomy is ≈0.15%).

Method	Considerations
Spermicide use	• Can cause irritation of genitalia, and allergic reaction • Inexpensive • May INCREASE risk of STD transmission due to mucosal irritation • High failure rate
Calendar method (avoid intercourse near predicted ovulation days)	• Requires couple to predict ovulation • High failure rate
Withdrawal method (ejaculate outside the vagina)	• High failure rate
Female or male condom	• Best contraception that protects against STDs (including HIV)
Diaphragm (barrier method)— used with spermicide	• *Does not protect against HIV* • Potential for toxic shock syndrome (TSS) if left in place too long • Not commonly used nowadays
Vaginal ring (hormonal method)	• Remains in place for 3 weeks and in the fourth week of menstrual cycle it can be removed (ring-free week). Reinsert after the end of the fourth week. • Does not need to be removed for intercourse • Fertility returns in 1 month after discontinuation • No STD protection
Oral contraceptive pill (OCP)	• Requires daily ingestion • Reduces incidence of ovarian cancer, endometrial cancer, ectopic pregnancy, pelvic inflammatory disease (PID),[a] etc. • Increased risk of benign hepatic tumors, gallbladder disease, hypercoagulability, cervical cancer, hypertension • Increased triglycerides • No STD protection • *Does not cause weight gain (the dose is typically low)*
Hormonal transdermal patch (combined estrogen/ progesterone)	• Apply weekly for 3 weeks; the fourth week is patch-free week. • Possible skin irritation • If patch detaches from skin for > 24 hours, it needs to be replaced with a new one. • Same advantages and disadvantages as OCPs (e.g., no STD protection, higher risk of venous thromboembolism)

Method	Considerations
Hormonal progesterone injection—depot medroxyprogesterone acetate (DMPA)	• High efficacy and requires injection only every 3 months • If late by > 2 weeks, do pregnancy test before giving q3 monthly injection • Reduction in risk of endometrial cancer, PID,[a] and amount of menstrual bleeding • May have irregular bleeding or hypo/amenorrhea, weight gain, depression. • There is a delay of return to menstruation once injections are stopped and return to fertility may take longer ($\approx$1–1.5 year)
Intrauterine device (IUD) **Two types—copper IUD and hormonal IUD (hormone is levonorgestrel—a progesterone agonist)**	• This is the most effective nonsurgical contraception • Requires physician to place and remove • *Rapidly reversible and cost-effective* • Hormonal IUD lasts $\approx$5 years; copper IUD$\approx$10 years • Hormonal IUD may decrease menses (useful in menorrhagia and dysmenorrhea), and decreases risk of PID[a] • There is no weight gain with levonorgestrel-containing IUD • Copper-containing IUD may cause heavy/painful menses (which often improves after some time) • Copper IUD may be used as emergency contraception • Higher risk of ectopic pregnancy if woman becomes pregnant with IUD in place • Not to be placed within 3 months of dx of STD • Previous hx of STD or ectopic pregnancy **IS NOT** a contraindication for IUD
Female sterilization (tubal ligation)	• Permanent • High efficacy, however if pregnancy results, there is increased risk of ectopic implantation. • Risks associated with surgery: infection, hemorrhage, anesthesia complications, etc. • *Tubal ligation with complete salpingectomy may decrease risk of ovarian cancer*
Male sterilization (vasectomy)	• Permanent • High efficacy • Safer and less costly than female sterilization • Can be performed in the outpatient setting

[a]Possibly due to thick impenetrable mucus.

20.5.1 Short Note on Oral Contraceptive Pills (OCP)

Formulary: A 28-pill OCP pack has 21 hormone pills (known as active pills). The additional seven pills are placebo pills (containing sugar or iron) to help the user stay in the habit of taking a pill every day.

Mechanism of action: Combination of estrogen and progesterone prevents mid-cycle LH surge and follicular maturation. Progesterone also works by making endometrium less suitable for implantation, and by making cervical mucus thick (this might be the reason for the decreased risk of PID).

Absolute contraindications to OCP:

- History or risks of venous thromboembolism.
- Tobacco use (more than half a pack per day) and age $\geq$ 35.
- Liver disease (cirrhosis, liver cancer, etc.).
- Clinical history of atherosclerotic cardiovascular disease (ASCVD; e.g., coronary artery disease), or high ASCVD risk (e.g., uncontrolled diabetes).
- Hypertension (systolic of $\geq$ 160 mmHg or diastolic of $\geq$ 100 mmHg).
- Migraine with aura.
- Migraine without aura in > 35 years of age or with tobacco abuse.
- Breast cancer.
- Systemic lupus erythematosus.
- Complicated valvular heart disease.

Clinical Case Scenarios

1. Patient calls with an issue of two missed active pills. What is the NSIM?

Emergency contraception

Most effective	Very effective	Effective
Copper IUD (not hormonal IUD)	Ulipristal (antiprogestin)	Levonorgestrel
Needs to be inserted within 5 days after unprotected sex	• Can be used up to 5 days after unprotected sex • Requires prescription	• Can be used up to 3 days after unprotected sex • Available over the counter

20.6 Differential Diagnosis of Dysmenorrhea[7] and Pelvic Pain

[7]Dysmenorrhea refers to uterine pain that occurs with the menstrual cycle.

Condition	Features	Management
Primary dysmenorrhea (most common) **Pathophysiology:** Due to prolonged uterine contractions likely mediated by prostaglandins	**Presentation:** recurrent crampy suprapubic pain that occurs *with or just* before the menses • Normal pelvic exam	• First step is to rule out pregnancy and infection. **Rx:** Exercise and heat application is 1st line. If not responding, 2nd line is NSAIDs like ibuprofen or hormonal therapy (combination OCPs or progestin-only pills). If 1st line NSAIDs fail, 2nd line NSAIDs is mefenamic acid (a specific type of NSAIDs for menstrual pain). For patients who desire contraception, use combination OCPs or progestin-only pills.
Secondary dysmenorrhea usually presents in adulthood		

Endometriosis
 	
Pathophysiology: presence of endometrial stroma and glands outside the uterus
	Presentation depends on location of endometriosis:
	• **Pelvic:** Dysmenorrhea, dyspareunia
	• **Bladder:** Urinary frequency, urgency, dysuria
	• **Others:** Constipation, hematochezia, infertility, etc.
	Typically, pain is cyclical with/without menses.
	Pelvic exam: May reveal fixed retroverted uterus (endometrial cells "glue" the uterus to posterior pelvic structures), tender nodular masses along uterosacral ligaments or in cul-de-sac, etc.
		Abdominal/transvaginal US may show ectopic endometrial tissue.
		Rx:
		• First line is NSAIDs + hormonal contraception.
		• Laparoscopy (diagnostic and therapeutic) is indicated for any of the following:
		  – Severe symptoms
		  – Patients who have failed medical therapy or have contraindications
		  – Hx of infertility
		• Second-line agents are GnRH agonist.[a] Third-line treatment is aromatase inhibitor (before giving second- or third-line agents, diagnostic laparoscopy is recommended.)
		• Definite treatment is hysterectomy with oophorectomy.

	• Ovarian endometriosis = endometriomas – It is the MC site of endometriosis.	For symptomatic or enlarging endometriomas, first SIM is laparoscopic management (it is important to rule out ovarian malignancy).

Condition	Features	Management
Leiomyomas (uterine fibroids) **Pathology:** Benign tumor arising from smooth muscles in uterus. It is the MC pelvic tumor in women. It is more common in African-American women.	**Presentation:** Can be asymptomatic and often an incidental finding on US. Symptomatic patients may have any of the following: • Cyclical pelvic pain • Heavy/or prolonged menstrual bleeding • Dysmenorrhea • Infertility • Fibroids can push on the bladder or colon and cause symptoms (e.g., frequent urination, constipation). • Fibroids can also protrude through vagina. • Acute pain can occur due to degeneration or torsion. **Pelvic exam:** May reveal *asymmetrically* enlarged uterus with an irregular surface.	NSIDx: is pelvic ultrasound. For asymptomatic patients, just follow up. For most patients with *symptomatic* fibroids, treatment of choice is surgery. • For patients who wish to preserve fertility, consider myomectomy (abdominal approach for subserosal or intramural, and hysteroscopic approach for submucosal). For patients who do not desire to preserve fertility, consider hysterectomy. • In severe cases, GnRH agonist can be used to reduce the bulk of disease prior to surgery. • Patients who have symptoms due to excessive/painful bleeding and do not want to undergo surgery, consider *hormonal IUD*.
Adenomyosis **Pathology:** Endometrial glands within myometrium	**Presentation:** Painful, heavy, prolonged menses, and chronic pelvic pain. **Pelvic exam:** Symmetrically enlarged **tender** uterus on pelvic exam.	NSIDx: Transvaginal US reveals symmetrically enlarged uterus; **cystic areas can be seen within the myometrium.** Rx: Hysterectomy is curative and provides a definitive dx. Because of diffuse involvement, myomectomy is usually not feasible.
Pelvic inflammatory disease (can cause secondary dysmenorrhea)	**Presentation:** Fever, nausea, abnormal vaginal discharge, dyspareunia, etc. **Pelvic exam:** Cervical motion tenderness, uterine/adnexal tenderness	NSIDx: Cervical specimens for microscopy, nucleic acid amplification tests (NAATs) for *C. trachomatis* and *gonorrhoea* (+/-*Mycoplasma genitalium*). Do not forget pregnancy test and screening for other STDs (HIV, HBV, HCV). Rx: Antibiotics (see PID section, later in this chapter for further info)

[a]GnRH agonists are leuprorelin, nafarelin, buserelin (+ relin), etc. Continuous stimulation by GnRH agonist paradoxically results in downregulation of gonadotropin secretion.

Abbreviations: HIV, human immunodeficiency virus; HBV, hepatitis B virus; HCV, hepatitis C virus; STDs, sexually transmitted diseases.

20.7 Premenstrual Syndrome (PMS) and Premenstrual Dysmorphic Disorder (PMDD)

PMS	⟹	Presence of any symptom (physical and/or behavioral) that occurs regularly or repetitively in relation to menses (bloating, abdominal pain, breast pain, headache, hot flashes, irritability, fatigue, etc.)
PMDD	⟹	A psychiatric form of PMS disorder with more prominent anger and irritability.

Workup: Ask patient to keep a menstrual diary to record symptoms; the symptoms should occur in the second half of menstrual cycle, **impair daily functioning,** and improve after menses.

Management:

Mild symptoms	⟹	Lifestyle modifications (e.g., regular exercise, avoiding excessive caffeine, alcohol, tobacco use).
Severe symptoms	⟹	Selective-serotonin reuptake inhibitor (SSRI; sertraline, fluoxetine, etc.), or in patients who desire contraception, use OCPs that contain drospirenone.

20.8 Menopause

Definition: Expected cessation of menstrual cycle in old age (ovarian senescence); usual age of onset is > 45 years. (!)

Presentation[8]:

- Early signs may include menstrual irregularities and anovulatory cycles (menopausal transition).
- Hot flashes, irritability.
- Pain during intercourse due to atrophy or dryness of the vagina and cervix.
- Increased frequency of urination/dysuria due to atrophic urethritis.

Workup: It is a clinical diagnosis, but can be confirmed by elevated FSH and low estrogen level.

Treatment: Hormone replacement therapy (HRT) for short-term management of *moderate to severe* menopausal symptoms (most importantly hot flashes).

- Combination estrogen/progesterone for patients with uterus and estrogen only for patients without uterus (see the table below).
- Topical lubricants and/or topical estrogen for atrophic vaginitis.

HRT increases risk of:	Decreases risk of:
• Venous thromboembolism (DVT/PE)	• Colorectal cancer
• Endometrial cancer (risk with estrogen-only HRT)	• Fractures/osteoporosis
• Stroke	
• Breast cancer[a]	
• Coronary artery disease[a]	

[a]No risk when only estrogen is used; hence, estrogen alone is preferred in patients with no uterus.

⚠ **Caution**

(!) Women 40–45 years may have symptoms of menopausal transition, but in this age group workup of oligo/amenorrhea is done.

[8]Obese women usually have milder symptoms, as fat tissue aromatase converts androgen into estrogen.

20.9 Vaginitis

Definition: Inflammation of the vagina due to infection, atrophy, or in rare cases cancer.

Presentation: Itching, burning, discharge, or may be asymptomatic.

Etiology: Majority of infectious vaginitis is caused by bacterial vaginosis (MCC), candidiasis, and trichomonas vaginalis.

Diagnosis	Differentiating features[9]	Management
Bacterial vaginosis (infection due to *Gardnerella vaginalis*)	• Thin, malodorous gray discharge • Vaginal exam: usually no or mild inflammation only • Vaginal pH is alkaline (> 4.5) • "Clue cells"[a] on microscopy • +ve "whiff test"[b] • Dx can also be made by PCR testing, but is usually not necessary.	• In nonpregnant patients, use either oral or intravaginal metronidazole or clindamycin.[c] • In pregnant patients, use oral metronidazole or clindamycin. Upper genital infection may occur in pregnancy where topical will be ineffective. • It is not an STD, hence no need to treat partner.
Vulvovaginal candidiasis	• Thick, nonodorous, cottage-cheese discharge • Vaginal pH is acidic (pH < 4.5)[d] • Yeast and hyphae on microscopy	• In nonpregnant patients, use oral fluconazole—150 mg single dose (DOC), or topical antifungals (miconazole/clotrimazole). • In pregnant patients, topical is preferred.

[9]First diagnostic step is vaginal discharge analysis, including microscopy.

Diagnosis	Differentiating features	Management
Trichomonas vaginalis	• Any kind of discharge (frothy, white, yellow, green, etc.) • Vaginal pH is alkaline (> 4.5) • Motile organism with flagella may be seen on microscopy (this finding is specific but not sensitive). • Dx can also be made by DNA probe	• It is an STD—MUST treat all partners whether symptomatic or asymptomatic. • Use single-dose oral metronidazole or tinidazole in uncomplicated patients (e.g., without immunosuppression), and in pregnant and nonpregnant patients. • Longer duration might be needed in complicated cases (e.g., immunosuppression).

[a]Microscopic exam.

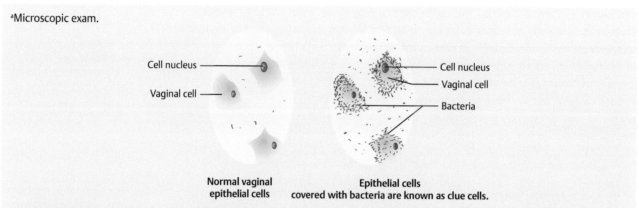

Normal vaginal epithelial cells

Epithelial cells covered with bacteria are known as clue cells.

[b]Whiff test: Addition of KOH to vaginal discharge results in a **strong fishy odor**. This is strongly positive in bacterial vaginosis and may be positive in trichomoniasis.

[c]Sometimes bacterial vaginosis is detected in cultures done for other reasons. The only indication for treating an asymptomatic patient is when the patient is undergoing hysterectomy or medical termination of pregnancy.

[d]Major differentiating factor from the other two (*G. vaginalis* and *T. vaginalis*).

20.10 Other Causes of Vaginal Discharge

Diagnosis	Features	Management
Physiologic leukorrhea This is due to unopposed estrogen: • In newborns, this can be due to maternal estrogen exposure. • Anovulatory cycles (e.g., during early stage of menarche)	• May have mild irritative symptoms of pruritus and burning. • Small to copious white discharge. • Microscopy: no or rare white cells with a lot of squamous cells. • Vaginal exam will reveal no inflammation.	Reassurance
Vaginal cancer	• Suspect this if symptoms are chronic, and especially in older patients. • Foul smelling discharge ± bleeding. • Exam will likely reveal a vaginal lesion.	Dx is confirmed with biopsy of suspicious lesion. **Rx:** Surgical excision ± radiation ± chemotherapy (similar in strategy to cervical cancer)
Atrophic vaginitis This is due to estrogen deficiency (occurs after ovulation stops, e.g., after menopause)	• Vaginal dryness, itching, and pain. • Atrophic urethritis can produce symptoms similar to UTI (CCS—increased frequency of urination and dysuria in a postmenopausal woman with negative urinalysis). Urinary incontinence can also occur. • Small yellow or white discharge. If there is change in symptoms or color/amount of discharge, look for infection.	First SIM—vaginal moisturizer and lubricant. Second step, if no improvement, is topical vaginal estrogen.

Diagnosis	Features	Management
Foreign body	• Most commonly it is a retained toilet paper or tampon. • Discharge can be foul smelling and purulent.	• Irrigation with warm fluid and removal of foreign body. • If large foreign body or unsuccessful retrieval, sedation or general anesthesia might be required.

Abbreviation: UTI, urinary tract infection.

20.11 Pelvic Inflammatory Disease

Definition: Infectious process that starts from cervix and goes up to involve the upper genital tract (uterus, oviducts, ovaries). In rare cases, pelvic abscess or peritonitis can develop.

Etiology: MCC is *Neisseria gonorrhoeae* and *Chlamydia trachomatis*. Other causes include enteric gram-negative rods, anaerobes, streptococci, G. vaginalis, etc.

Presentation: Main symptom is lower abdominal pain that can range from mild to severe + vaginal discharge. Intermenstrual bleeding or dysmenorrhea can occur. Some women can have subtle or no symptoms and present with infertility.[10]

[10]Infertility is due to tubal adhesions/dysmotility.

Signs and symptoms supporting diagnosis of PID
• Cervical motion tenderness
• Abnormal cervical or vaginal discharge
• Red, friable cervical tissue
• Fever
• Elevated C-reactive protein (CRP), erythrocyte sedimentation rate (ESR)
• WBCs are seen on microscopy of vaginal secretions

Diagnostic work-up: Pelvic exam can reveal cervical and adnexal tenderness. Cervical specimens for microscopy, nucleic acid amplification tests (NAATs) for *C. trachomatis* and *gonorrhoea* (+/-*Mycoplasma genitalium*) need to be obtained. (!)

Management:

Hospitalize patients if any of the following is present:

● Pregnancy.

● Inability to maintain oral intake (nausea and vomiting).

● Severe infection (sepsis, pelvic abscess, peritonitis, etc.).

Antibiotics should generally cover chlamydia and gonorrhea given the high likelihood of infection with these organisms.

⚠ **Caution**

(!) Do not forget pregnancy test and screening for other STDs (HIV, HBV, HCV).

If patients are acutely ill or not responding to therapy, do pelvic imaging (transvaginal ultrasound or CT) to look for abscess.

Inpatient antibiotic therapy	• Cefotetan or cefoxitin + doxycycline • Alternative therapy: clindamycin + gentamicin (use this in pregnant patients)	Followed by outpatient doxycycline[a] or clindamycin (total of 14 days)
Outpatient therapy	• Ceftriaxone single dose IM + doxycycline[a] (for 14 days). • In pregnant patients, use single-dose 2 g azithromycin instead of doxycycline.[a]	

[a]Add metronidazole (if doxycycline is used) for anaerobic coverage in patients with history of gynecologic instrumentation in the last 2–3 weeks or complicated with abscess, or T. vaginalis or bacterial vaginosis coinfection. Note: Clindamycin covers anaerobes, but doxycycline does not.

Complications: Infertility, chronic pelvic pain, and dyspareunia.

Fitz-Hugh–Curtis syndrome: It is a complication of PID that results from ascending infection leading to a perihepatitis. Patients present with right upper quadrant (RUQ)[11] pain and elevated liver function tests (LFTs) in addition to symptoms of PID.

[11]**Exam tip:** Board favorite is to include the RUQ pain in a CCS that sounds like PID.

20.12 Differential Dx of Acute Pelvic or lower abdominal pain in Women (!)

Condition	Key points in history and exam	Workup	Treatment
Mittelschmerz	• Pain associated with ovulation which occurs in the middle of menstrual cycle. • Usually unilateral and may be recurrent. • Usually last for few hours, but can last for few days.	• Detailed history and normal findings on pelvic exam are sufficient to make the diagnosis. • US may reveal a small amount of fluid in the cul-de-sac area.	• NSAIDs in mild cases. • OCPs to prevent ovulation in severe cases.
Ectopic pregnancy	• Hx of missed period may or may not be present. • Sudden-onset abdominal/pelvic pain with vaginal bleeding. • Syncope, hypotension, severe pain (if ectopic pregnancy has ruptured). • **Localized** guarding and rebound tenderness. • **Generalized** guarding/rigidity may occur due to ruptured ectopic and hemoperitoneum.	• Pregnancy test and transvaginal US.	• Medical or surgical abortion (see the ectopic pregnancy section).
PID (pelvic inflammatory disease)	• Unilateral or bilateral pelvic pain. • Abnormal per-vaginal discharge. • Cervical motion tenderness ± painful adnexa. • **Localized** guarding/rebound tenderness; **generalized** guarding/rigidity may occur due to abscess leakage and peritonitis. • Look for signs of sepsis.	• Pelvic exam. • PCR and culture of vaginal discharge.	• Antibiotics. • Tubo-ovarian abscess may require surgery.
Ovarian torsion	• Sudden-onset unilateral pain.[a] • Primary risk factor is enlarged ovary (cyst, mass). • Occurs mainly in women of reproductive age. • May have **localized** guarding/rebound tenderness; **generalized** guarding/rigidity may occur due to necrosis.	• US will reveal unilaterally enlarged ovary ± mass. • Decreased or absent Doppler flow within the ovary suggests impaired blood flow. • Surgery provides definitive diagnosis.	• Do surgery (laparoscopy with detorsion) ASAP in an effort to salvage the ovary. • Salpingo-oophorectomy is done in cases of suspected malignancy, clearly necrotic ovary/tube and in postmenopausal women.
Ovarian cyst rupture (ovulation induction can be a risk factor)	• Sudden-onset unilateral pain, usually in a woman of reproductive age • Can present after a physical activity (e.g., after vaginal sex or exercise). • Usually **localized** tenderness, but **generalized** guarding/rigidity may occur due to complicated cyst rupture and this may look like ruptured ectopic pregnancy but hemodynamic compromise is rare.	• Pelvic US can reveal an ovarian cyst; however, the cyst may not be visualized if collapsed.	• Observation in uncomplicated cases. • Laparoscopy in unstable patient or if clinical evidence of ongoing hemorrhage.

[a]Pain in ovarian torsion occurs due to edema, internal hemorrhage, or infarction of the twisted ovary (ischemic necrosis).

In a nutshell

Don't forget other causes of acute pelvic or lower abdominal pain that are outside of the gynecological spectrum:

Gastrointestinal	Appendicitis, diverticulitis, inflammatory bowel disease, colitis, irritable bowel syndrome
Urinary	UTI, nephrolithiasis
Vascular	Mesenteric venous thrombosis, dissecting aortic aneurysm

20.13 Urinary Incontinence

20.13.1 Acute Urinary Incontinence

Causes:

Delirium	MCC of acute delirium is infection.
Infection—urinary tract	First step in acute retention is always UA (urinalysis).
Atrophic vaginitis/urethritis	Occurs in postmenopausal women or with premature ovarian failure.
Pharmacological cause	Meds such as M-antagonists (e.g., amitriptyline, first-generation antihistamines).
Psychological	–
Excess urine output	For example, due to hyperglycemia, diabetes insipidus.
Restricted mobility	You will see this a lot in clinical rotations:
Stool impaction	Immobility → constipation → urinary retention[12] → increased risk and development of UTI → acute delirium.

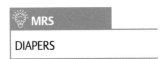 **MRS**

DIAPERS

[12]In lower pelvis, fecal impaction can press on bladder causing urinary retention.

20.13.2 Chronic Urinary Incontinence in Women

Definition: Chronic loss of bladder control.

	Stress incontinence	Urge incontinence	Overflow incontinence
Pathophysiology	Weak pelvic floor muscles and resultant urethral hypermobility. **and/or** weak urethral sphincter.	Bladder muscle (detrusor) spasms and overactive bladder due to irritation or loss of inhibitory neurons.	Bladder muscle (detrusor) weakness or bladder outlet obstruction leading to incomplete bladder emptying/full bladder and urine leakage by overflow.
Presentation	Urine leakage with increased intra-abdominal pressure (e.g., during coughing or laughing).	• Sudden urge to void followed by passage of urine. • Urinary frequency. • Nocturia.	• Constant or intermittent urine leakage/dribbling. • No urge is felt. • Sometimes when bladder is full stress leakage can occur.
Etiology	Multiparity, obesity, age-related (menopause and atrophic changes), prostatectomy (in men)	Spinal cord injury, stroke, dementia, or bladder irritation (due to cystitis, atrophic vaginitis, prostatitis, etc.).	• **Underactive/weak bladder due to neuopathy** (e.g., vit B12 deficiency, diabetes, multiple sclerosis), muscarinic blockers, etc. • **Bladder outflow obstruction** due to cystocele, uterine prolapse.
NSIDx after pelvic exam + UA[a] **+ Keep a urination diary (keeping a log when urine leaks during the day)**	• **Bladder stress test:** Look at urethra for urine leakage when patient is asked to cough with full bladder. • **Provocative testing:** Q-tip is inserted in urethra and patient is asked to cough. If ≥ 30 degrees movement of the Q-tip, it suggests urethral hypermobility.	• Nonspecific. • Postvoid residual volume is normal (< 200 cc).	Check postvoid residual volume with bedside bladder scanner (best noninvasive test).

	Stress incontinence	Urge incontinence	Overflow incontinence
Initial treatment	**Pelvic floor exercises (Kegel exercises):** Practice holding urine in the middle of urination. This same act when repeatedly done, while not urinating, is Kegel exercises.		
	• Bladder training (e.g., frequent scheduled voiding while awake) is useful in all cases of URGE type. This can also be helpful in stress type, if incontinence occurs in high bladder volumes. • In postmenopausal women, if atrophic vaginitis is present, treat with vaginal estrogen.		
Second-line treatment options[b]	If above fails, NSIM urethral sling surgery vs. pessaries.	M-blockers (e.g., oxybutynin, tolterodine). If not responding or significant side effects with M-blockers, use mirabegron (beta-3 agonist).	Depends upon cause: • If bladder outlet obstruction is due to cystocele or uterine prolapse, treat with surgery or pessary. • If detrusor inactivity, stop M-blockers. Sometimes sacral nerve stimulation may be pursued. • Intermittent self-catheterization.

[a]First step in management of any form of chronic incontinence is pelvic exam and UA. Pelvic exam is helpful to evaluate for conditions that can cause chronic incontinence. UA is helpful to detect infection. We also need to evaluate for all potentially reversible causes.

[b]**Urodynamic study** is done when dx is not clear and before surgical treatment in all causes of chronic incontinence. (Pressure catheter is introduced into the bladder and vagina. Pressures and urine flow are monitored. If bladder is empty it may be filled with fluid via the catheter.) Other test that is commonly employed is cystoscopy.

20.14 Breast Tumors and Cancer

20.14.1 Evaluation of Solitary Breast Mass

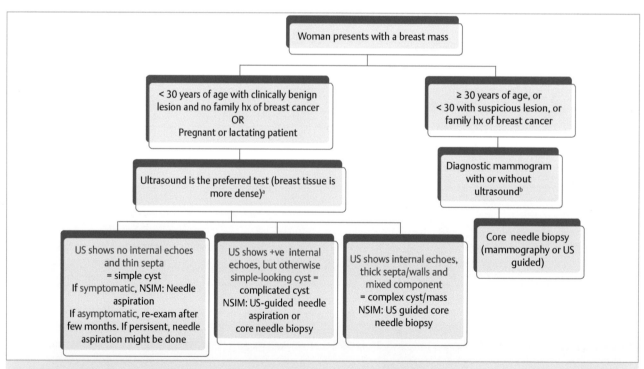

[a]Screening mammogram generally NOT recommended in < 30 years of age. In adolescents, small breast lesions with no worrisome features can be followed clinically without doing a US. US is indicated only if lesion persists.

[b]Add ultrasound in patients with denser breast tissue.

Options for obtaining tissue sample in breast mass:

Fine-needle aspiration (FNA)	Less invasive, but not a lot of information is obtained. It is done usually for low-probability cystic masses. If aspirated fluid is **not** clear, it should be sent for cytology.
US-guided core needle biopsy	More invasive and larger sample can be obtained. Sensitivity and specificity are comparable to surgical biopsy.
Surgical biopsy	Only done if core needle biopsy is nondiagnostic or reveals high-risk abnormality (e.g., atypical hyperplasia or *lobular* in situ carcinoma). Surgical biopsy can be incisional (a portion of mass is removed), or excisional (whole lesion with some margin is removed). Usually excisional biopsy is done, but incisional can be done if mass is too large to be excised.

Clinical tips:
- A high-risk patient with a palpable breast mass still requires a mammogram to complete evaluation due to possibility of nonpalpable lesions.
- In palpable breast masses, negative mammogram still warrants further evaluation with US ± biopsy.

20.14.2 Benign Breast Pathology

	Additional information and features	Management
Simple breast cyst	**Pathophysiology:** fluid-filled cystic mass at the end of the duct, which usually occurs because of obstruction. • Can be solitary or multiple.	• US is usually sufficient, but aspiration can be done if symptomatic. • Usually no further intervention is required. • Solid, complex, or complicated lesions are suspicious and should be aspirated and/or biopsied.
Fibrocystic changes	**Pathophysiology:** increase in stromal elements of the breast tissue, which occurs in premenopausal women and is thought to be due to progesterone/estrogen imbalance. • It is often associated with the menstrual cycle (typically painful before menses). • **Exam:** "lumpy bumpy" breast—multiple, painful breast masses that fluctuate in size and/or palpable fibrotic tissue. • Serosanguineous discharge may be present. • It is not associated with increased risk of cancer.	**NSIDx**—breast US **Rx:** • NSAIDs as needed. • OCPs may be helpful. • Advise to avoid caffeine and to wear supportive bras.
Fibroadenoma	**Pathophysiology:** Benign tumor containing glandular and fibrous tissue. It is the MC breast lesion in adolescents. **Features:** • Typically solitary and found in women in their 20s. • They are nontender, mobile, firm, and have a rubbery texture when palpated. • US reveals solid mass with benign features.	NSIM is either core needle biopsy or short-term follow-up with repeat US. • If rapid growth, NSIM is surgical excision. Depending on histology, this may be associated with breast cancer, but is not a premalignant lesion by itself. • **Complex fibroadenoma, proliferative type, and family history of breast cancer** are associated with increased risk of breast cancer.
Giant fibroadenoma	> 5 cm fibroadenomas	Best SIM is excisional biopsy.
Fat necrosis	• Occurs due to breast trauma or surgical intervention. • May mimic malignancy on physical exam, or by radiographic appearance on mammogram or US (calcification with spiculation).	• For typical appearance on US/mammogram, NSIM is reassurance, as it is not a premalignant lesion. • If atypical appearance on imaging, biopsy can be done.

20.14.3 Breast Cancer[13]

Risk factors: Age is the most important risk factor; other factors include personal or family history of breast cancer, gene mutation (p53 or BRCA), obesity, alcohol use, early menarche or late menopause, nulliparity, first child over age 30,[14] exposure to ionizing radiation, white race.

Screening:
- At age 40, all women **can be offered** screening mammography.
- At age 50 (earlier if family history of breast cancer) all women **should** begin screening.
- Frequency of screening is every 1–2 years.

Presentation: Breast cancer is often found during screening mammography or incidentally as a painless, hard, immobile (tethered) mass on physical exam.

Breast cancer management

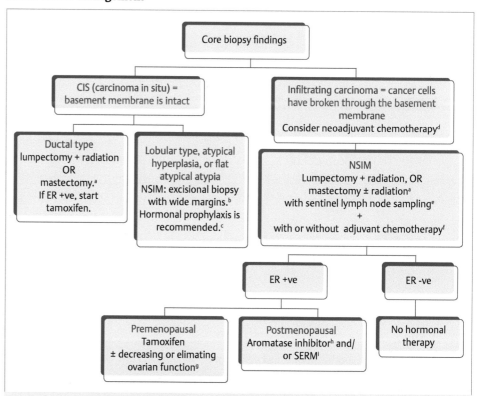

^aMastectomy is preferred over lumpectomy in the following situations: diffuse or multicentric tumor, large tumor (in comparison to breast size), pregnant patients, and persistently positive margin despite re-excision.
^bThese high-risk lesions can be associated with locally invasive cancers, so we must perform a biopsy of the whole lesion.
^cThese lesions are also typically ER +ve.
^dNeoadjuvant chemotherapy is the chemotherapy given before surgery to reduce tumor bulk and in patients with temporary contraindication to surgery, who are expected to have surgery later (e.g., pregnancy, recent pulmonary embolism). (!)
^eContrast dye is injected into the area of breast mass during lumpectomy or mastectomy, and the first few lymph nodes that light up are the sentinel lymph nodes that drain that area.
^fConsider systemic chemotherapy in the presence of any negative prognostic factor (discussed below).
^gThis can be achieved by GnRH analogues or oophorectomy.
^h**Aromatase inhibitors** are anastrozole, letrozole, exemestane, etc.
ⁱSERM = selective estrogen receptor modulator (tamoxifen or raloxifene).
Factors that predict poor prognosis in infiltration carcinoma are given below in order of importance (need to know the order for exam):

- **A**xillary lymph node status.
- **S**ize > 2 cm.
- **G**rade of tumor is high.
- **G**ene expression: HER2/neu overexpressed due to overexpression or amplification of ERBB2 oncogene.
- **R**eceptors **negative** (ER/PR −ve): ER +ve indicates responsiveness to hormonal therapy.

Abbreviation: ER, estrogen receptor.

Sidebar (left column):

[13]
- MC cancer in females is breast cancer.
- MC breast cancer is infiltrating ductal breast carcinoma.

[14]Higher number of **ovulatory cycles** increases the risk of ovarian and breast cancer (e.g., early menarche or late menopause, nulliparous, first child over age 30).
On the other hand, increased **anovulatory cycles** decrease the risk of ovarian cancer (and maybe breast cancer) but increase risk of endometrial cancer (due to unopposed estrogen).

⚠ **Caution**

(!) In patients with HER2 positive disease, consider trastuzumab (Herceptin). This is a monoclonal antibody against HER2 receptors. Patient needs transthoracic echocardiogram before initiation of treatment, as trastuzumab is associated with heart failure.

MRS

AS-graded genes receive negative news.
Note that BRCA is not included in this list.

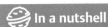 **In a nutshell**

Tamoxifen	Raloxifene
Indication: used for treatment and prevention of recurrence of ER +ve breast cancer in pre- and postmenopausal women.	**Indication:** • Only used in postmenopausal women with ER-positive breast cancer (no studies have been carried out in premenopausal women). • Also, used for treatment of osteoporosis (postmenopausal).
Increased risk of endometrial hyperplasia/cancer.	No risk of endometrial hyperplasia as it does not activate estrogen receptors in uterus.
Other **common side effects** include: • Irregular periods, hot flashes (menopausal-like effects). • Weight loss. • Increased risk of venous thromboembolism. **Beneficial effect:** Decreases LDL level. Abbreviation: LDL, low-density lipoprotein.	

Unique Forms of Breast Cancer

	Features	Management
Mammary Paget's disease Ulcerative form of mammary Paget's disease Source: Ductal Carcinoma (70 % of all cases). In: Riede U, Werner M, eds. Color Atlas of Pathology: Pathologic Principles, Associated Diseases, Sequela. 1st ed. Thieme; 2004	It is a type of cancer that looks like eczema involving the nipple ("itchy and scaly," eczematous or ulcerative superficial lesion).	NSIDx is full-thickness skin biopsy or punch biopsy[a] (will reveal malignant intraepithelial adenoma-carcinomatous cells). After dx bilateral mammography is usually done. It is commonly associated with underlying invasive or in-situ carcinoma. **Rx:** As shown above in breast cancer management.
Inflammatory breast cancer Source: Levine PH, Zolfaghari L, Young H, et al. What is inflammatory breast cancer? Revisiting the case definition. Cancers (Basel). 2010 Mar; 2(1): 143–152.	It is the most aggressive type of breast cancer where cancer cells block lymph ducts and the breast appears red, swollen, and inflamed (peau d'orange appearance). Presentation is like breast cellulitis, which does not respond to antibiotics.[a]	NSIDx is bilateral mammography. Best SIDx is core needle biopsy. If core needle biopsy is suggestive of cancer, NSIDx is full-thickness skin biopsy of at least two sites (to evaluate for dermal lymphatic invasion). After dx, full metastatic workup is done. **Rx:** Neoadjuvant chemotherapy followed by modified radical mastectomy + radiation.

[a]Any female that has a persistent rash around the breast area for more than few weeks or breast cellulitis that does not respond to antibiotics should have mammogram and skin biopsy.

Nipple Discharge

	Pathologic discharge	Physiologic discharge
Laterality	Usually unilateral	Usually bilateral
Color of discharge	Bloody or serous (clear or straw-colored)	Can be of any color (e.g., green, straw-colored, clear, blue, etc.)
NSIDx	Cytology of discharge and mammogram/US of breast	Check medication list that can cause hyperprolactinemia and check prolactin level, TSH and pregnancy test.
Potential causes	• Intraductal papilloma (benign)—may be bilateral.[a] • Breast cancer.	Hyperprolactinemia due to any of the following: • Due to chronic use of drugs such as metoclopramide. • Hypothyroidism. • Prolactinoma. • Pregnancy.

[a]In intraductal papilloma, exam may reveal a nodule. Best SIDx is excisional ductal biopsy, which is curative too.

[15]Lynch syndrome (aka hereditary nonpolyposis colorectal cancer) is an autosomal-dominant genetic condition that increases risk of cancer in colon, endometrium, ovary, and other organs.

BRCA mutation

Indications for BRCA1/BRCA2 mutation testing

- Strong family history of ovarian cancer or ovarian cancer in a first-degree relative.
- Breast cancer in women <30 years of age, or with triple-negative disease in < 50-year-old women (i.e., negative ER, PR, and Her2/neu).
- Breast cancer in men.
- Tubal or primary peritoneal cancer.
- Ovarian cancer with family hx.

In patients with BRCA mutation positive:

- Offer bilateral salpingo-oophorectomy (when child bearing is completed) and bilateral mastectomy.
- If mastectomy is not done, regular screening with MRI (at younger age) and mammography (at older age) is recommended. Also, tamoxifen should be offered.

20.15 Ovarian Cancer

Background: Majority of ovarian cancers arise from the epithelial portion (MC is serous epithelial carcinoma). The minority are germ-cell tumors.

Risk factors: Age > 60, family history, BRCA1/BRCA2 gene mutation, history of breast cancer, PCOS, Lynch syndrome,[15] cigarette smoking, nulligravity, and anovulatory cycles.

Protective factors: OCPs, hysterectomy, and breast feeding.

Presentation: Often presents in advanced stage with ascites, pleural effusion, bowel obstruction. Sometimes may be diagnosed earlier if adnexal mass is found on exam.

Management steps:

- NSIDx in patients with suspected ovarian mass is to do transvaginal US and check serum CA-125 level.
- Treatment is usually surgical—**explorative laparotomy** with hysterectomy, bilateral salpingo-oophorectomy, and removal of local lymph nodes and omentum.
- Chemotherapy is not very effective. Unfortunately, the prognosis is very poor as the disease is usually advanced when diagnosed.

Screening for ovarian cancer: Routine screening for low-risk general population is not recommended. In patients with a strong family history of ovarian cancer or in patients with known BRCA or Lynch mutation, screening can be offered with regular transvaginal US and serum CA-125 level.

In a nutshell

Gonadal Tumors (Ovarian and Testicular) and Their Markers

Tip: *To remember the following table, focus on negatives marker status*

	β-hCG	LDH	AFP
Dysgerminoma (equivalent of seminoma in males)	Can be elevated	↑ ↑	−ve
Other germ-cell tumors: e.g., *immature teratomas,*[a] *embryonal carcinoma, yolk sac tumor.*	Can be elevated	Can be elevated	Can be elevated
Choriocarcinoma (*trophoblastic tumor*): *a variant of germ-cell tumor.*	↑ ↑	Can be elevated	−ve
Non-germ-cell tumors (a.k.a. sex cord-stromal tumors): e.g., Sertoli–Leydig cell tumor,[b] granulosa cell tumor,[c] thecoma-fibroma.	−ve	−ve	Can be elevated in Sertoli–Leydig cell tumor

[a]A distinct type of teratoma made of up thyroid tissue is called struma ovarii. It can present with hyperthyroidism.
[b]Can secrete androgens, leading to precocious puberty in males, or virilization in females.
[c]Can secrete estrogen, leading to increased risk of endometrial hyperplasia or cancer in females, or gynecomastia in males.

20.16 Endometrial Hyperplasia and Cancer[16]

Pathogenesis: Abnormal proliferation of endometrial glands due to chronic estrogen stimulation, unopposed by progesterone

(hyperplasia with nuclear atypia → dysplasia → cancer).

Risk factors are conditions associated with increased and/or unopposed estrogen: PCOS, obesity, anovulation, estrogen-producing tumors, long-term estrogen therapy without progesterone, nulliparity, tamoxifen, etc. Additional risk factor is genetic mutations (e.g., Lynch syndrome).

Presentation: Abnormal uterine bleeding usually in middle age or postmenopausal women. Sometimes the presentation can be abnormal adenomatous or glandular cells seen in Pap smear (note, cervical cancer is squamous cell cancer).

Workup:

Start workup, if any of the following present:

- Any bleeding in postmenopausal women (even spotting).
- Any abnormal uterine bleeding in females aged >45.
- Abnormal uterine bleeding in females aged <45, which persists despite medical treatment, or presence of risk factors for endometrial cancer (e.g., oligomenorrhea, obesity).
- Abnormal adenomatous or glandular cells seen in Pap smear.

[16]MC female reproductive-tract cancer in developed countries is endometrial. carcinoma.

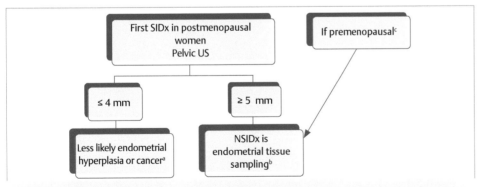

[a]Presence of thin and homogenous endometrium can exclude hyperplasia and help to avoid invasive testing. However, if bleeding persists, endometrial tissue sampling needs to be done.
[b]Dx is confirmed with tissue sample. Sometimes US or hysteroscopy-guided biopsy may be needed for localized lesion.
[c]In premenopausal women, measuring endometrial lining thickness with US is not helpful in assessing risk of endometrial hyperplasia or cancer. However, US can reveal other causes of abnormal uterine bleeding.

Management:

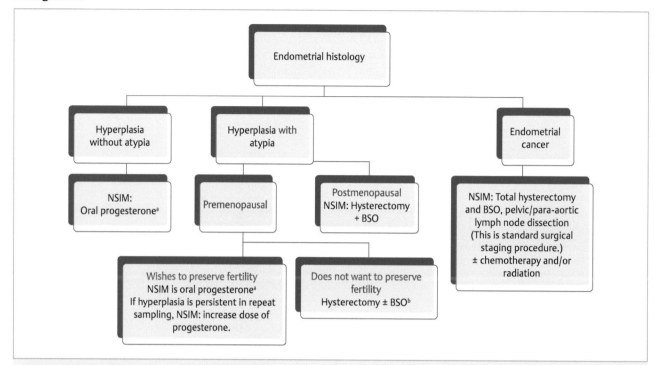

^aIf on tamoxifen, stop it.

^bIn this age group, BSO will lead to menopausal symptoms. Hence, ovarian conservation needs to be considered.

Abbreviation: BSO, bilateral salpingo-oophorectomy.

20.17 Cervical Cancer

[17]Many HPV serotypes have been associated with cervical cancer. The MC ones are 16 and 18.

Risk factors: Most important risk factor is infection with high-risk human papillomavirus (HPV) serotypes.[17] Others include smoking, early onset of sexual activity, multiple sexual partners, history of STD, immunocompromised states, etc.

Presentation: Early cancer is usually asymptomatic. MC symptoms are heavy vaginal or postcoital bleeding or pain during intercourse.

Screening test: Pap smear ± HPV testing is the screening test of choice for cervical cancer. Pap smear involves taking cervical cells and doing cytology tests. HPV testing involves DNA testing for high-risk serotypes (usually read as positive or negative for high-risk serotype). *"Co-testing" refers to doing Pap smear cytology + HPV testing at the same time.*

Patient group	Screening
Age 21–29^a	Pap smear every 3 years.
Age 30–65	"Co-testing"^b every 5 years.
Age > 65	Stop testing if low risk and negative testing with three consecutive Pap smear or two consecutive "co-testing" within the previous 10 years. Offer continuous screening in patients with risk factors such as recent new partner or hx of abnormal Pap tests.
Special risk population: HIV^c	Begin with "co-testing" at diagnosis (with colposcopy the first time) and repeat "co-testing" after 6 months (should get it twice in the first year). • If HPV testing is −ve, do Pap smear cytology yearly. • If HPV testing is +ve, do Pap smear cytology every 6 months.
Special risk population: patients on immunosuppressive therapy	Begin 1 year after patient becomes sexually active, or at age 21 and then repeat annually.

^aScreening is NOT recommended in women < 21 years of age (regardless of onset of sexual activity), unless immunocompromised.

^bHPV testing is not recommended in women aged < 30 years.

^cThey should also get annual visual inspection of the genital area.

20.17.1 Management of Abnormal Pap Smear Findings

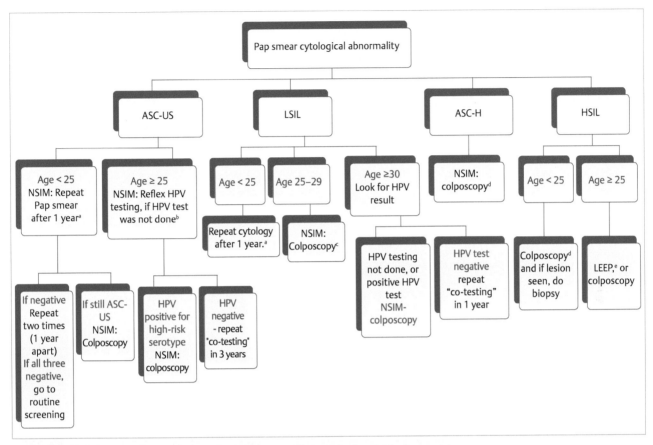

[a]In age 21–24, do not do HPV testing as risk of transient HPV infection is high and risk of cancer is low.

[b]In women ≥ 30 years of age, usually HPV testing is already done with Pap smear. In women 25–30 years of age, request a HPV testing on the Pap-smear sample.

[c]HPV testing is not an option in the LSIL work-up, as opposed to ASC-US work-up in this age group.

[d]Also, perform endocervical curettage (scraping of mucus membrane of cervix). **Indications for endocervical curettage:** ASC-H, HSIL, atypical glandular cells,[18] adenocarcinoma in situ, and *LSIL with no visible lesion in colposcopy.*

[e]Loop electrosurgical excision procedure (LEEP) is diagnostic and curative. LEEP is not recommended in *pregnant and postmenopausal* women.

Abbreviations: **ASC-H,** atypical squamous cells, cannot exclude high grade lesion; **ASC-US,** atypical squamous cells of undetermined significance (! MC abnormal finding); **HSIL,** high-grade squamous intraepithelial lesions; **LSIL,** low-grade squamous intraepithelial lesions.

[18]In patients with atypical glandular cells. also recommended is endometrial sampling.

 In a nutshell

- For ASC-US and HSIL, there are two categories: age ≥ 25 and < 25.

- For LSIL, there are three categories: age < 25, ≥ 25, and ≥ 30.

- For ASC-H, there is only one outcome: colposcopy.

Practice questions are given at the end of this section.

20.17.2 Colposcopy and Subsequent Management

Following findings can be seen after performing colposcopy with biopsy:
- Cervical intraepithelial neoplasia (CIN): can be grade 1, 2, or 3.
- Glandular neoplasia.
- Cervical cancer.

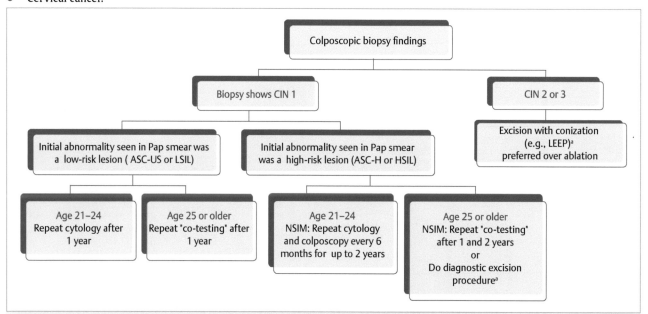

[a]Diagnostic and therapeutic excisions are pretty much the same. It involves conization (removal of cone-shaped cervical tissue including the transformation zone). Conization can be done in three different ways (LEEP, cold-knife or laser). LEEP is preferred, as it is easier to perform.

Abbreviation: CIN, cervical intraepithelial neoplasia.

Clinical Case Scenarios

Type of Pap smear abnormality	Age	NSIM
ASC-US	24	Repeat Pap smear cytology in 1 year
	25	Obtain HPV testing from the sample
	30	
ASC-H	24	Colposcopy
	25	
	30	
LSIL	24	Repeat Pap smear cytology in 1 year
	25	Colposcopy
LSIL and HPV testing was not done	30	Colposcopy
LSIL and HPV testing was negative	30	Repeat co-testing in 1 year
HSIL	24	Colposcopy
	25	Colposcopy or LEEP
Other CCS	**Age**	**NSIM**
No endocervical[a] cells in Pap smear	≥ 30	Depends upon HPV testing. If HPV -ve, return to regular schedule. If HPV +ve, NSIM is either do genotype of high risk HPV serotype (16,18) , or repeat co-testing in 1 year. If high risk serotype is positive, do colposcopy.
No endocervical cells and no risk factors	**< 30**	Follow regular screening schedule, or repeat testing in 1 year.
No endocervical cells in previously abnormal Pap smear	**Any age**	Repeat it
Pap smear showed HSIL. Colposcopic biopsy shows CIN1	24	Repeat cytology and colposcopy every 6 months for up to 2 years
	25	Offer either repeat co-testing after 1 and 2 years or, diagnostic excision procedure
Pap smear showed LSIL. Colposcopic biopsy shows CIN1	**24**	Repeat Pap smear cytology after 1 year
	25	Repeat "co-testing" after 1 year

[a]Usually cervical cancer originates from the area of transformation zone, where the squamous architecture ends and the glandular endocervical architecture begins. Pap smear is considered adequate when both glandular (endocervical) and squamous cells are seen.

20.17.3 Management of Cervical Abnormalities in a Pregnant Patient

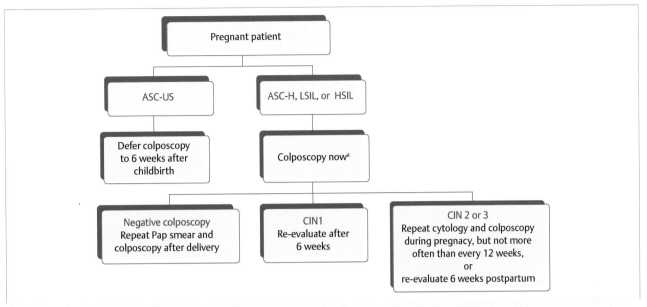

ᵃDo not do endocervical curettage during pregnancy. Do biopsy only for lesions that appear high grade or cancerous.

20.17.4 Management of Cervical Cancer

Early-stage tumor: tumor size < 4 cm	Microinvasive disease (no clinically visible lesion) and low-risk features (i.e., stromal invasion of ≤ 3 mm depth or horizontal spread of ≤ 7 mm)	⟹ Simple hysterectomy (extrafascial hysterectomy)—lymph-node dissection not required	**Further management depends upon pathologic findings:** **For high-risk disease (**positive lymph nodes, positive surgical margin, or microscopic involvement of structures near the uterus—parametria), *do chemoradiation.* **For intermediate-risk disease (**lymphovascular or deep cervical stromal invasion, but without high-risk features as above), **do radiation.**
	Lesion ≤ 2 cm who want to preserve fertility	⟹ Conization and removal of cervix	
	Clinical visible lesion ≤ 4 cm, or microinvasive disease with stromal invasion of > 3 mm	⟹ Modified radical hysterectomy with pelvic lymphadenectomy	
Locally advanced cancer	Tumor size of > 4 cm or not localized to cervix (e.g., invades vagina, side walls)	⟹ Primary chemoradiation ± posttreatment hysterectomy	

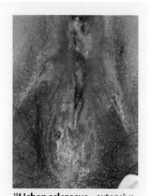

[19]**Lichen sclerosus—extensive involvement of female genitalia.**

Source: Lichen Sclerosus. In: Sterry W, Paus R, Burgdorf W, eds. Thieme Clinical Companions–Dermatology. 1st ed. Thieme; 2006

> ⚠ **Caution**
>
> (!) For any vulvar pruritus, unresponsive to treatment, NSIM is biopsy.

20.18 Diseases of Perineal Area

20.18.1 Lichen Sclerosus

Background: It is a chronic inflammatory dermatosis of skin in the anogenital area, associated with increased risk of squamous cell carcinoma and is considered premalignant.

Presentation: Chronic white plaques, dryness, and itching.[19] This can also occur in males.

Management: Perform punch biopsy to rule out cancer. (!) Treat with topical high potency steroids.

20.18.2 Vaginal Cancer

Two notable forms of vaginal cancer:

- **MC form is squamous cell cancer:** Risk factors are the same as in cervical cancer.
- **Rare form is clear cell adenocarcinoma:** Main risk factor is exposure to diethylstilbestrol (DES).

Presentation: MC symptom is bleeding.

Work-up: First SIDx is vaginal speculum exam. Dx is confirmed with biopsy of suspicious lesion.

Rx: Surgical excision ± radiation ± chemotherapy (similar in strategy to cervical cancer).

20.18.3 Bartholin's cyst (Greater Vestibular Gland Cysts)

Presentation: Cyst in the 4 or 8 o'clock position of labia majora. It may cause symptoms such as dyspareunia. Infection and abscess can develop.

Management:

Bartholin area mass	Signs of infection (tender, red and warm mass)	Management
< 3 cm	YES	Incision and drainage (I&D). Treat with antibiotics if there are signs of surrounding area cellulitis, or systemic involvement (e.g., fever). If it recurs, repeat I&D, add antibiotics, and if possible insert Word catheter.[a]
	NO	Dx is Bartholin cyst. NSIM is Sitz baths and warm compresses. If the cyst persists beyond 1 month, offer expectant management or biopsy or removal.
≥3 cm 1st step is I&D and Word catheter placement[a] for a big mass like this.	YES (or I&D reveals clear pus)	Do culture, and treat with antibiotics if there are signs of surrounding area cellulitis, or systemic involvement (e.g., fever). If 2nd recurrence, repeat the same process (I&D, Word catheter placement, and antibiotics) If 3rd recurrence, NSIM is marsupialization (a new ductal orifice is surgically created). And if it fails gland excision.
	NO	NSIM is Word catheter placement. If the cyst persists beyond 1 month, do biopsy. If benign, offer expectant management or surgical removal.

[a]It is catheter with a balloon at the end which promotes continuing drainage and epithelization of the tract to promote future drainage.

20.19 Infertility

Criteria:

- No pregnancy after more than 6 months of trying to conceive in women age > 35, or in patients with risk factors for infertility (e.g., hx of oligo/amenorrhea), or
- After 1 year of frequent sex in women with no risk factors and <= 35 years of age.

Etiology[20]:

Female causes	
Ovulatory dysfunction	• Thyroid dysfunction, prolactinoma, significant medical disease (e.g., uncontrolled diabetes). • Anovulation due to eating disorders and intense exercise regimen (these patients typically also have oligo/amenorrhea).
Anatomical abnormalities	Fallopian tube obstruction, uterine leiomyomas. • Hysterosalpingogram is used for dx.
Premature ovarian failure	**Etiology:** Mumps, oophoritis, chemotherapy, and diseases associated with female predominant autoimmune disorder (Hashimoto's disease, pernicious anemia, etc.). **Presentation:** Amenorrhea, hypoestrogenism, and markedly increased FSH in <40-year-old women. FSH/LH increased, as FSH is more elevated than LH. **Rx:** These patients lack oocytes, and in-vitro fertilization (IVF) with donor oocytes is typically needed.
Decreased ovarian reserve	Women > 35 years of age might have a hard time conceiving.

[20]The etiology remains unknown in almost half of the cases.

Male causes of infertility	
Decrease in sperm quantity, quality, or both (this is the MC etiology of male infertility)	Due to primary hypogonadism: androgen insensitivity, Klinefelter syndrome, cryptorchidism, orchitis, varicocele, trauma, exogenous steroid and anabolic hormone use (testosterone analog use mostly by body builders).
Anatomic	Altered sperm transport (duct obstruction, retrograde ejaculation). • If retrograde ejaculation is suspected, examine urine for sperm after ejaculation.

- History and physical exam are important: look at sexual history, medications, potential STD, hernia, varicocele, etc.
- If there is no apparent cause, look at the following algorithm for workup:

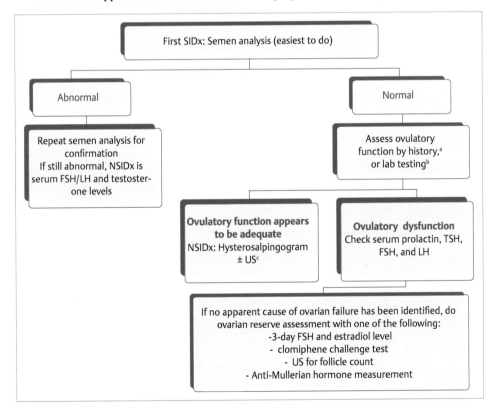

[a]If hx of regular cycles and progesteronic symptoms (e.g., bloating, breast tenderness) prior to menses, the patient likely has normal ovulation.
[b]If no such hx, do lab testing to check ovulatory status: check mid-luteal phase progesterone level (i.e., 1 week before expected menses in a 28-day menstrual cycle), or may use an over-the-counter mid-cycle LH kit.[21]
[c]For suspected endometriosis, diagnostic laparoscopy is indicated.

[21]The most accurate test for ovulation is daily US to monitor follicular maturation. This can be done as a confirmatory test. Also, clear cervical mucus at cervical os is a sign of ovulation.

Management: Treat underlying cause. Management options include hormone injections to induce ovulation (e.g., clomiphene), intrauterine inception (e.g., for hostile cervix), and in vitro fertilization.

20.20 Ovarian Hyperstimulation Syndrome

Background: Exaggerated ovarian response to ovulation induction with gonadotrophins (e.g., recombinant hCG, LH, or FSH). Milder forms can occur with clomiphene citrate.

Primary pathophysiology: Increased capillary permeability. In rare instances, generalized increase in capillary permeability can even result in distributive shock.

Presentation: Severe cases can present with abdominal pain, ascites, pleural effusion, hypoxia, and ± hypotension.

Management: Supportive treatment is the mainstay along with withdrawal of induction therapy.

Answers:
1. Use back-up contraception for 7 days. During these 7 days, patient should take daily active pills.

---

21. Male Reproduction

The continuity of any species **requires an efficient system for multiplication. It is not only survival of the fittest, but also survival of the most efficient reproducers.**

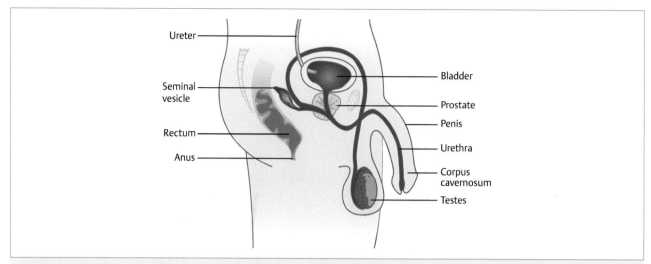

A sagittal view of the major structures of the male reproductive system. (Modified with permission from Male reproductive system. In: Gunderman R, ed. Essential Radiology: Clinical Presentation, Pathophysiology, Imaging. 3rd ed. Thieme; 2014.)

21.1 Congenital Anomalies of the Male Genitalia

21.1.1 Cryptorchidism

Pathology: Fetal testes must descend from their intra-abdominal location into the scrotal sac before birth. One or both testes may stop at any point along this path, remaining hidden inside the abdomen or protruding out just slightly.

Presentation: Unilateral is not uncommon, especially in preterm males, but they usually descend by 6 months of age. Bilateral is usually due to an underlying genetic disorder.

Diagnosis: It is made by physical exam, where nonpalpable or partially descended testes and asymmetry can be detected. Ultrasound (US) can aid further in dx.

Management:

- If persistent beyond 6 months of age, NSIM is orchiopexy, which should be done before 2 years of age.
- Infants with other associated abnormalities or with bilateral cryptorchidism should be referred to a specialist.

Complications: Cryptorchidism increases the risk of subfertility, inguinal hernia (due to coexistence of persistent processus vaginalis), testicular torsion, and testicular cancer. Orchiopexy has been shown to reduce the risk of these complications, except testicular cancer.

21.1.2 Hypospadias or Epispadias

Definition: Embryological malformation leading to abnormally located opening of urethral meatus and shortened urethra.

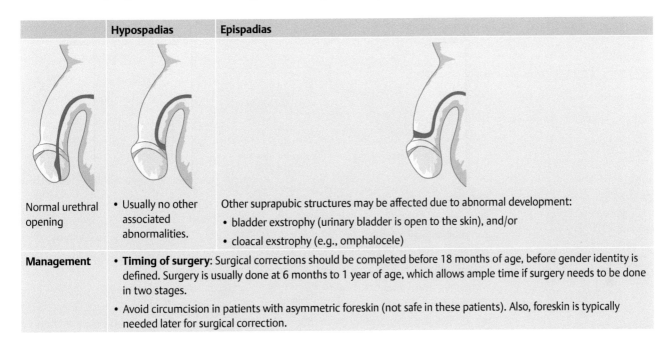

	Hypospadias	Epispadias
Normal urethral opening	• Usually no other associated abnormalities.	Other suprapubic structures may be affected due to abnormal development: • bladder exstrophy (urinary bladder is open to the skin), and/or • cloacal exstrophy (e.g., omphalocele)
Management	• **Timing of surgery**: Surgical corrections should be completed before 18 months of age, before gender identity is defined. Surgery is usually done at 6 months to 1 year of age, which allows ample time if surgery needs to be done in two stages. • Avoid circumcision in patients with asymmetric foreskin (not safe in these patients). Also, foreskin is typically needed later for surgical correction.	

21.2 Testicular Pathologies

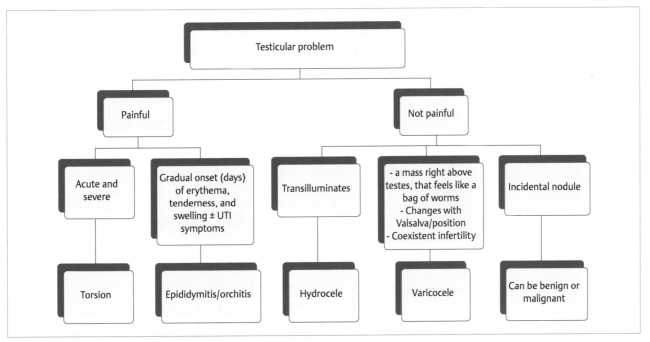

In most testicular pathologies, US (ultrasound) is a good diagnostic tool.

21.2.1 Hydrocele

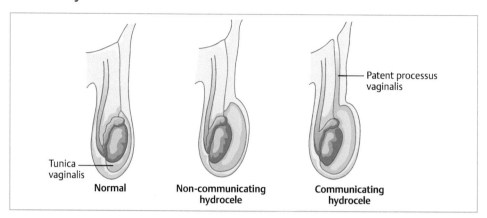

Normal   Non-communicating hydrocele   Communicating hydrocele

Patent processus vaginalis

Tunica vaginalis

Definition: Fluid collection in the tunica vaginalis.

Etiology: In pediatric population, MCC is failure of processus vaginalis to close which leads to communicating hydrocele. In adults, it is mostly idiopathic. It may be caused by parasitic infection (filariasis) but is rare in the United States.

Presentation: Gradually enlarging, painless swelling of scrotum.

Diagnosis: Trans-illuminates with a flashlight. US can confirm the diagnosis.

Management:

- **Communicating hydrocele in infants** generally resolves by 12 months. If persistent beyond 12 months of age or if diagnosed later, NSIM is elective surgical repair. Unrepaired communicating hydrocele increases the risk of incarcerated inguinal hernia.
- **For idiopathic hydrocele,** do surgical repair only if symptomatic. Simple aspiration does not work, as it frequently recurs.

21.2.2 Testicular Torsion

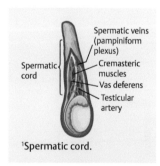

Spermatic cord

Spermatic veins (pampiniform plexus)

Cremasteric muscles

Vas deferens

Testicular artery

[1]Spermatic cord.

Pathophysiology: Twisting of the spermatic cord results in loss of blood flow and acute ischemia.[1]

Etiology: Majority of testicular torsion occurs due to congenital deformity (malformed processus vaginalis fails to attach the testicle to the scrotal surface leaving it free to rotate).

Presentation: Acute severe, unilateral testicular pain with nausea/vomiting.

Physical exam: Exam is often difficult due to pain, but typically reveals unilateral tender swelling of scrotum, absent cremasteric reflex and high-riding testis.

At times torsion can occur prenatally (before birth), and it might present within 24 hours of birth with **painless** firm enlarged testes and discolored hemiscrotum.

Management:

- **If diagnosis is certain**: emergent surgical detorsion and orchiopexy.
- **If diagnosis is not clear**, immediate diagnostic testing such as US with Doppler color flow needs to be done.

21.2.3 Varicocele

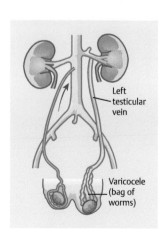

Left testicular vein

Varicocele (bag of worms)

Pathophysiology: Dilation of the pampiniform plexus, caused by various anatomical factors that prevent proper drainage of the plexus.

Similar to leg varicosities, the idiopathic cases develop usually due to venous valve incompetence. It is more commonly seen on the left side, since the left gonadal vein is longer as it empties into the left renal vein. It is also a smaller-caliber vessel.

Secondary causes: Obstruction due to renal cell carcinoma, IVC (inferior vena cava) thrombus, or any abdominal mass in the pathway of the vein.

Presentation: Most often asymptomatic but can cause some discomfort, especially in hot weather. It can present with infertility (MCC of correctable infertility in males).

Diagnosis: When palpating a varicocele, it might feel like a "bag of worms." Valsalva maneuver, by increasing abdominal pressure, will increase the size. A change in position from standing to lying flat will facilitate draining and decrease the size. Severe case may have visible swelling. Obstructive pathology needs to be ruled out with computed tomography (CT) scan in patients with varicocele that is acute in onset, fails to drain in supine position, or is right-sided.

Management: Surgical correction is done in patients with varicocele associated with low testicular volume or infertility. In older patients who no longer desire fertility and with minor symptoms can be managed conservatively with NSAIDs (nonsteroidal anti-inflammatory drugs) and scrotal support.

Complications: Subfertility and testicular torsion.

21.3 Testicular Cancer[2]

[2]It is the MC malignancy in men 20–35 years of age.

Risk factor: Cryptorchidism, HIV, family history, etc.

Presentation: Unilateral testicular swelling. It can also present with symptoms due to metastatic disease such as hemoptysis with chest X-ray revealing multiple nodules.

Physical exam: Unilateral, *hard, firm, nodular or mass-like* testicular, swelling, which is usually painless and does not transilluminate or change with position.

Work-up:

- **NSIDx** is testicular US, which can reveal *hypoechoic mass.* A homogenous, cystic, fluid-filled structure is likely not malignant.
- After US, NSIM is radical inguinal orchiectomy to obtain tissue diagnosis. Do not choose needle biopsy, as it may cause tract seeding. CT or magnetic resonance imaging (MRI) scan of chest, abdomen, and pelvis for staging and serology for tumor markers needs to be done. Semen cryopreservation should be offered.

Further management depends upon histological subtype. Testicular germ-cell tumors (the MC type of testicular cancer) are subclassified into two major categories:

	Seminomas	Nonseminomatous germ-cell tumor
Features	• Likely to be localized at presentation • Indolent and prolonged course • More common late relapses	• More likely to be metastatic at presentation • Tumor markers are useful in staging and treatment
	• Very radiosensitive • Radiation ± chemotherapy when indicated	• Not radiosensitive • Surgical lymph-node dissection and/or chemotherapy when indicated
Management after orchiectomy depends upon imaging finding or tumor markers	• No evidence of metastasis or lymphadenopathy: NSIM-Surveillance (may consider radiation or adjuvant chemotherapy to minimize risk). • Retroperitoneal lymphadenopathy, but all ≤ 2 cm: NSIM-radiation to regional (retroperitoneal) lymph nodes. • Any lymph node size is > 2 cm, or metastasis: NSIM-chemotherapy.	• No evidence of metastasis or lymphadenopathy: NSIM-Surveillance (may consider retroperitoneal lymph node dissection or adjuvant chemotherapy). • If evidence of metastasis or significant tumor-marker elevation: NSIM-chemotherapy. • Retroperitoneal lymphadenopathy in imaging, but all ≤ 2 cm and normal tumor markers: NSIM-retroperitoneal lymph-node dissection. • If any lymph node size is > 2 cm or retroperitoneal lymph-node dissection reveals > 4 lymph nodes involved, consider chemotherapy

Note: Testicular tumors are the most curable solid neoplasm, even if metastatic at diagnosis.

21.4 Gonadal Tumors (Ovarian and Testicular) and Their Markers[3]

Tip: To remember the following table, focus on negatives marker status.

	β-hCG	LDH	AFP
Seminoma (a type of germ-cell tumor)[a] (equivalent to **dysgerminoma** in females)	Can be elevated	↑ ↑	−ve
Nonseminomatous germ-cell tumors: E.g., immature teratomas,[b] embryonal carcinoma, yolk sac tumor.	Can be elevated	Can be elevated	Can be elevated
Choriocarcinoma (trophoblastic tumor): A variant of non-seminomatous germ-cell tumor.	↑ ↑	Can be elevated	−ve
Non-germ-cell tumors (aka sex cord-stromal tumors): E.g., Sertoli–Leydig cell tumor,[c] granulosa cell tumor,[d] the coma-fibroma.	−ve	−ve	Can be elevated in Sertoli–Leydig cell tumor

[a]MRS **HELPS** monitoring seminoma, which is the MC type of testicular tumor = HCG, LDH, and Placental alkaline phosphatase are Elevated in Seminoma.

[b]A distinct type of teratoma made of up thyroid tissue is called struma ovarii. It can present with hyperthyroidism.

[c]Can secrete androgens, leading to precocious puberty in males, or virilization in females.

[d]Can secrete estrogen, leading to increased risk of endometrial hyperplasia or cancer in females, or gynecomastia in males.

Abbreviations: AFP, alpha-fetoprotein; LDH, lactate dehydrogenase.

21.5 Cystic Testicular Swelling

Spermatocele	Extratesticular, fluctuant cystic swelling, which transilluminates	These almost always arise in the epididymal head.	May have internal echo on US.	**Rx:** Asymptomatic cyst can be observed. If large enough to cause discomfort, consider surgical removal. Cyst is likely to recur if aspirated.
Epididymal cyst		These may arise throughout the epididymis.	Usually does not have internal echoes.	

Clinical Case Scenarios

A 35-year-old male presents with painless left testicular swelling. Exam reveals hard nodular left testicle.

1. What is the NSIM?

2. What type of testicular cancer is it more likely to be?

3. What is the best NSIM after testicular US reveals hypoechoic mass?

4. A 3-year-old male is found to have left testicular swelling. US reveals heterogeneous collection with internal echoes. What type of testicular cancer is it more likely to be?

21.6 Penile Pathologies

21.6.1 Balanitis and Balanoposthitis

Definition: Balanitis—inflammation of the glans penis (or clitoris). When foreskin also gets involved, it is called balanoposthitis.

Etiology: MCC is candidal infection. Other causes include STDs (e.g., herpes, chlamydia), skin disorders (e.g., lichen planus, eczema), autoimmunity (e.g., reactive arthritis is associated with circinate balanitis).

Risk factors: Infections (with candida or other organisms) occur more commonly in uncircumcised males with poor hygiene and underlying immunosuppression (e.g., diabetes).

Presentation: Tenderness and/or erythema of glans penis ± plaques, itching, or discharge. It can also cause painful retraction of foreskin. In chronic or recurrent cases, formation of adhesions can result in inability to retract foreskin (phimosis).

NSIDx: Gram stain and culture, KOH prep, and screening for diabetes.

Management: Clean the area frequently. May give topical antifungal if *Candida* is suspected.

21.6.2 Phimosis and Paraphimosis

	Phimosis	Paraphimosis
Definition	Phimosis The foreskin cannot be retracted and is adhered to the glans. This can lead to painful erections and also increases risk of UTIs (urinary tract infections).	Edematous retracted foreskin — Strangulated glans penis Foreskin gets stuck behind the coronal sulcus. Associated edema can impede blood flow to the glans penis.
Etiology	May be physiologic in adolescents. Normal growth and erections will eventually break the adhesions. It might also occur from poor hygiene and/or recurrent balanitis.	Commonly occurs after penile manipulation (e.g., urinary catheterization, cystoscopy), direct injury, or after sexual activity or erection.
Management	• In pathologic phimosis, address underlying condition. • Physiologic phimosis is often benign. • If causing problems, recommend circumcision or preputioplasty.	Considered emergency, this must be manually reduced. If manual reduction is not successful, do emergent surgery.

21.6.3 Priapism

Definition: Painful prolonged erection.

	Ischemic	Nonischemic
Pathophysiology	Low-flow, anoxic, or veno-occlusive priapism	High-flow or arterial priapism (due to arteriovenous fistula or artery damage)
Work-up	To differentiate between ischemic and nonischemic, NSIDx is blood gas analysis of cavernosum aspirate or US Doppler.	
Findings	Blood gas will reveal hypoxemia, hypercarbia, and acidosis. US will reveal reduced blood flow.	Blood gas will show normal levels. US will reveal normal or high flow and may also reveal underlying cause such as fistula.
Etiology	• Drugs (e.g., prazosin, trazodone): due to venoconstriction. • Hematological disorder—*sickle cell disease*,[a] leukemia (e.g., chronic myeloid leukemia), plasma cell disorder, hyperviscosity, etc.	Due to direct trauma (e.g., blunt trauma due to bicycle)
Management	Phenylephrine injection[b] + blood aspiration from penis[c] • If priapism lasts for more than 24 hours, best SIM is surgery.	Conservative (they usually resolve spontaneously). If not resolving, arteriography with embolization can be tried.

[a]Recurrent (stuttering) priapism is a type of ischemic priapism, which occurs in sickle cell disease. Typical history includes few weeks of "on and off" episodes of spontaneous priapism. Ongoing episodes lasting more than 4 hours are treated as ischemic priapism.

[b]Sympathomimetics improve blood flow by inducing contraction of penile smooth muscles.

[c]If refractory to this treatment, consider exchange transfusion in sickle cell disease and leukapheresis in patients with hyperviscosity due to increased cell count.

21.6.4 Peyronie's Disease

Pathophysiology: Fibrosis of subcutaneous tissue of penis with resulting increased curvature of the penis. The etiology is not clear. It is associated with other subcutaneous fibrotic disorders such as Dupuytren's contracture.

Presentation: Painful or decreased strength of erection. Exam reveals palpable subcutaneous plaque and penile angulation.

Management: Observe if mild disease (many cases stabilize after 18–24 months, and some cases resolve on their own). Medical treatment (pentoxifylline) or surgery is done when severe.

21.6.5 Erectile Dysfunction/Impotence

Definition: Inability to achieve or maintain erection.

Risk factors: Diabetes, old age, smoking, obesity, alcohol, depression.

Etiology:

Psychogenic	In all cases of impotence, first step is to inquire about spontaneous erection (which usually occurs in the morning). If present, the diagnosis is most likely psychogenic.
Nonpsychogenic = organic	Vasculopathy, neurogenic, hormonal, drug-induced (e.g., β-blockers, centrally acting sympatholytic), or due to local factors (e.g., Peyronie's disease).

Work-up of organic impotence: If no obvious cause is identified, check CBC (complete blood count), CMP (comprehensive metabolic panel), HbA1c, and serum testosterone ± prolactin.

Management:

[4]PDE inhibitors (e.g., Sildenafil, tadalafil, vardenafil) used concomitantly with nitrates can cause severe hypotension.

- Treat underlying cause and advise lifestyle modifications. Prescribe phosphodiesterase (PDE) inhibitors[4] as needed.
- If patient is not responding, NSIM is vacuum devices or self-injectable drugs (e.g., alprostadil, papaverine).
- Third-line treatment is insertion of penile prosthesis.

Answers

1. Testicular ultrasound.

2. Seminoma is the MC type of testicular cancer in the postpubertal age group.

3. Surgical orchiectomy.

4. Teratomas are the MC testicular tumors in the prepubertal age group. In children they are usually benign, but in adults teratomas can be malignant.

22. Pediatrics

> *"The child is **the father of a man.**"*

Fontanels are space between the bones of the skull in an infant or fetus, where ossification is not complete and the sutures are not fully formed.

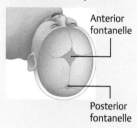

Anterior fontanelle

Posterior fontanelle

[1]*Just for your reference (no need to memorize)*

Age	Upper limit of normal heart rate/bpm
Newborn (<1 month)	190
1-11 months	160
2 years	130
4-6 years	120
8-12 years	110

22.1 Few Important Points in Pediatrics

- Parents bring in a child with concern for increased crying/irritability, decreased feeding, and playing:
  - If persistent—something is wrong (pathologic).
  - If transient (e.g., child gets fussy and irritable for 1 hour and later plays well), it is most likely physiologic. Reassure the parent.
- Examination of fontanels:

Full	Normal
Bulging	Increased intracranial pressure (ICP). NSIM is cranial imaging.
Sunken	Dehydration. NSIM is intravenous (IV) fluids.

- Pay attention to child's age in the exam question (very important clue).
- Sepsis in neonates can present with *hypothermia* (≤ 36 °C) *and/or jaundice*. In adults, jaundice as a presentation of sepsis is uncommon.
- **Heart rate (HR) and respiratory rate (RR):** Resting HR and RR of newborns can be as high as 190 and 60, respectively.[1] Resting HR and RR decrease as children get older. Be careful in interpreting tachycardia or tachypnea as a sign of sepsis, dehydration, or respiratory distress in newborns and children. Look for other danger signs.

22.2 Newborn Assessment

Immediately after delivery, the first step is to calculate the APGAR score. Calculate it again 5 minutes after delivery.

MRS

Note: Normal newborns typically get the score of 8-9. Nobody is a perfect 10.

APGAR Score	2 (Healthy baby score)	1	0
Appearance	All pink	Trunk is pink, but hands and feet are blue or pale	No part of body is pink (baby is blue and pale)
Pulse (beats per minute)	≥ 100	< 100	0
Grimace	Grimaces, coughs, and cries	Only grimaces, or weak grimace	0
Activity	Active	Some activity	Limp (zero movement)
Respiration	Regular	Irregular	0

APGAR score	Management
8–10	No resuscitation required
4–7	May require additional resuscitative measures
0–3	Immediate resuscitation

22.3 Neonatal Resuscitation

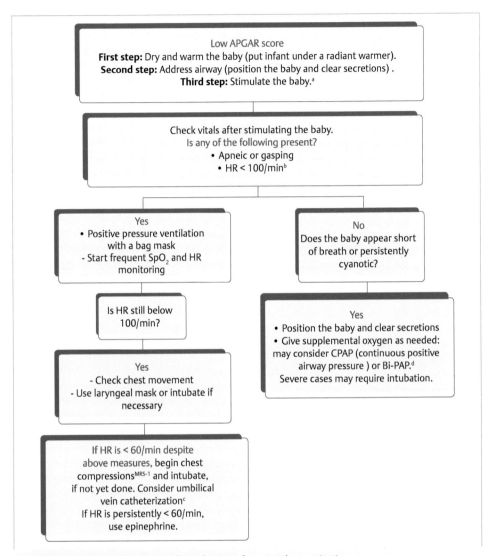

Low APGAR score
First step: Dry and warm the baby (put infant under a radiant warmer).
Second step: Address airway (position the baby and clear secretions) .
Third step: Stimulate the baby.[a]

Check vitals after stimulating the baby.
Is any of the following present?
• Apneic or gasping
• HR < 100/min[b]

Yes
• Positive pressure ventilation with a bag mask
- Start frequent SpO$_2$ and HR monitoring

No
Does the baby appear short of breath or persistently cyanotic?

Is HR still below 100/min?

Yes
• Position the baby and clear secretions
• Give supplemental oxygen as needed: may consider CPAP (continuous positive airway pressure) or Bi-PAP.[d]
Severe cases may require intubation.

Yes
- Check chest movement
- Use laryngeal mask or intubate if necessary

If HR is < 60/min despite above measures, begin chest compressions[MRS-1] and intubate, if not yet done. Consider umbilical vein catheterization[c]
If HR is persistently < 60/min, use epinephrine.

 MRS

[MRS-1]Newborn with HR of <60/min is treated in the same manner as asystole in adults.

[a]Remember the exact sequence of initial steps of neonatal resuscitation.

[b]HR < 100/min is an indicator of decreased cardiac output in neonates.

[c]It is a great IV access in neonates.

[d]See next page for differential Diagnosis of Respiratory Distress in a Newborn (nasal flaring, grunting, tachypnea, and hypoxemia).

Note: Normal respiratory rate is 30–60/min in neonates.

22.3.1 Routine Care in All Newborns (Within the First Few Hours of Birth)

- Topical antibiotic to the eyes (e.g., erythromycin or silver nitrate solution) to prevent gonococcal or chlamydial conjunctivitis.
- IM vitamin K—to prevent bleeding.
- Screening for hypothyroidism and other congenital conditions.
- Consider Hep B vaccination. Infant of mother with positive HBsAg (Hep B virus surface antigen) should also receive Hep B immunoglobulin.

Clinical Case Scenarios

A newborn baby is being assessed after a complicated delivery. She has a heart rate of 90 and her trunk is pink. The baby is coughing and has some activity. Her respirations are irregular and labored.

1. What is her APGAR score?

2. What is the immediate NSIM?
   a. Airway (position the baby and clear secretions)
   b. Stimulate the baby
   c. Dry and warm the baby (put infant under a radiant warmer)

22.3.2 Differential Diagnosis of Respiratory Distress in a Newborn (Nasal Flaring, Grunting, Tachypnea, and Hypoxemia)

Condition (and pathophysiology)	CXR (chest X-ray) findings	Other points
Transient tachypnea of the newborn (due to delayed resorption of fetal lung fluid)	Looks like congestive heart failure, with perihilar streaking and fluid in the fissures.	As the name giveth all, it is transient and resolves on its own.
Meconium aspiration syndrome (fetal asphyxia → intrauterine passage of meconium → aspiration). Look for meconium-stained infant at birth.	In initial stages, CXR may be similar to transient tachypnea. In later stages, CXR typically shows hyperinflation (with diaphragmatic flattening) and diffuse patchy opacities. Severe cases may appear similar to acute respiratory distress syndrome (ARDS). Source: Pathology. In: Gunderman R, ed. Essential Radiology: Clinical Presentation, Pathophysiology, Imaging. 2nd ed. Thieme; 2000.	Respiratory distress occurs within few hours of birth and does not resolve rapidly (unlike transient tachypnea of newborn). **Rx:** Supportive.
Respiratory distress syndrome (hyaline membrane disease) **of the newborn** • Occurs in premature infants due to decreased lung surfactant production	Diffuse bilateral reticulonodular or fine granular opacities + air bronchograms (*red arrow*) throughout lung Source: Pathology. In: Gunderman R, ed. Essential Radiology: Clinical Presentation, Pathophysiology, Imaging. 2nd ed. Thieme; 2000. Progression to "white out" of the lung. Modified from the source: snich, CC0, via Wikimedia Commons.	**Risk factors:** Infants of diabetic mother, cesarean delivery, prematurity, etc. **Rx:** Supportive (postnatal steroids may decrease mortality risk, but may also increase the risk of cerebral palsy). In severe cases, give surfactant therapy.

Congenital diaphragmatic hernia (developmental defect in diaphragm, which at times can be big enough to allow abdominal contents to enter the thorax, leading to pulmonary hypoplasia. Most commonly occurs on the left side).	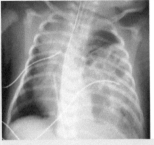 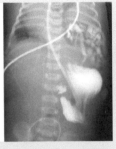Right CXR is taken after orogastric contrast administration. Source: Pathology. In: Gunderman R, ed. Essential Radiology: Clinical Presentation, Pathophysiology, Imaging. 2nd ed. Thieme; 2000.	**Prenatal presentation**: If esophagus is compressed, maternal polyhydramnios can develop due to inability of the fetus to swallow fluids. **Physical exam of neonate:** Scaphoid abdomen, absent breath sounds on one side (bowel sounds may be heard in the lung area) **Rx:** Once suspected, NSIM is intubation, followed by nasogastric suction (to decompress bowel). After initial stabilization, do surgical repair.
Congenital cardiovascular anomalies	CXR may show clear lung fields or increased pulmonary vascular markings, depending on anomaly.	Usually does not respond to supplemental oxygen, as opposed to pulmonary conditions.

Abbreviation: CXR, chest X-ray.

22.4 Birth-Related Injuries

Caput succedaneum	Cephalohematoma
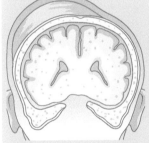	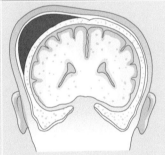
This is due to pressure effects of delivery. Physical exam will reveal soft-tissue swelling that crosses suture line. **Rx:** Benign and resolves on its own.	It is a birth-related injury, with blood collection under the periosteum of a skull bone. It does not cross suture line. **Rx:** Conservative management. It may take weeks or months to resolve.
Erb–Duchenne palsy (C5–6 nerve injury)	**Klumpke's palsy (C8–T1 nerve injury) ± Horner syndrome**
Mechanism of injury: Shoulder dystocia increases risk of injury to upper cervical nerve roots (or brachial plexus)	**Mechanism of injury:** Pulling arm too much during delivery may result in lower brachial plexus injury.
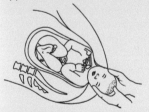	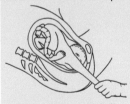
Presentation:	**Presentation:** Flexed elbow and closed, supinated fist (opposite of Erb–Duchenne palsy).
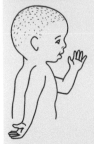 • Waiter's tip sign (supinator and abductor muscles are not working).	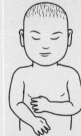
Rx: Physical therapy to prevent contractures; surgical therapy may be considered if no improvement in few months.	**Rx:** Physical therapy to prevent contractures; surgical therapy may be considered if no improvement in few months.

22.5 Pathologic Conditions More Commonly Seen in Preterm (Born before 37 Weeks of Gestation) and Low-Birth-Weight Infants (< 3.3 lbs or < 1,500 g)

In preterm infants (<34 weeks gestation age), antenatal corticosteroid therapy has been shown to reduce the incidence of respiratory distress syndrome, intraventricular hemorrhage, necrotizing enterocolitis, sepsis, and neonatal mortality by approximately 50 percent.

Condition	Additional information
Intraventricular hemorrhage	• Occurs due to immature autoregulation and increased capillary fragility. • **Presentation:** Signs of increased intracranial pressure (bulging fontanels, seizures, bradycardia, etc.). • It is the MC complication in very low birth-weight infants. • **Rx:** Mostly supportive. Infants with rapidly progressive hydrocephalus or signs of increased ICP will require neurosurgical intervention.
ARDS—aka hyaline membrane disease of newborn	• Occurs in premature infants due to decreased lung-surfactant production. • **Presentation:** Acute onset of respiratory distress **within minutes to hours** of birth. • **Rx:** Mostly supportive. In severe cases, give surfactant therapy.
Bronchopulmonary dysplasia	• Late sequelae of using supplemental oxygen for > 1 month (oxygen toxicity), lung infection, and/or mechanical ventilation in neonates. • **Pathophysiology:** Disruption of lung development with abnormal pulmonary vasculature and large alveoli (uniformly dilated acini with thin septa are seen). Severe disease may lead to necrotizing bronchiolitis and scarring. • **Presentation:** Persistent requirement of supplemental oxygen for > 28 days after birth. • **Rx:** Mostly supportive.
Retinopathy of prematurity	• Another *late sequela* of using supplemental oxygen. • **Pathophysiology:** Occurs due to *disorganized retinal vascularization*, which may lead to scarring, retinal detachment, and blindness, if not treated. • **Rx:** Treat significant disease with laser photocoagulation and intravitreal injection of anti-VEGF (anti-vascular endothelial growth factor) agents (e.g., ranibizumab).
Patent ductus arteriosus	• Normally, rise in blood oxygen levels after birth signals ductus closure. In preterm or low-birth-weight infants, there is an increased risk of hypoxia, resulting in increased risk of this condition.
Necrotizing enterocolitis	• **Risk factor:** Prematurity and formula feeding. • **Pathophysiology:** Preterm babies do not have fully developed digestive system, resulting in increased bacterial fermentation and risk of bowel-wall injury. • Discussed further in pediatric Gastroenterology section.
Apnea of prematurity	• Due to immature neurorespiratory system. • **Presentation:** Apneic episodes (baby stops breathing for > 20 seconds and is associated with hypoxemia). • **Rx:** Supportive care, CPAP and methylxanthine (e.g., caffeine or theophylline).
Bile-acid deficiency diarrhea	• Preterm or low-birth-weight infants have a low pool of bile acids. • **Presentation:** Malabsorption syndrome **(poor weight gain and diarrhea).** • **Rx:** Dietary modification with a change to medium-chain-triglyceride feeds can improve this, as these do not require bile acid for absorption.
Anemia of prematurity	• **Pathophysiology:** Due to shortened RBC life span and *decreased* RBC production. • **Lab values:** Normocytic anemia with low reticulocyte count and low erythropoietin level. • **Rx:** Supportive.
Anemia of iron deficiency	**Prevention:** All preterm infants who are exclusively breastfed should be on iron supplementation till 1 year of age.

Preterm and small for gestational age infants also have increased risk of the following conditions:
- Perinatal asphyxia → Meconium aspiration
- Hypothermia
- Hypoglycemia
- Hypocalcemia
- Polycythemia → Jaundice.

22.6 Infant Feeding

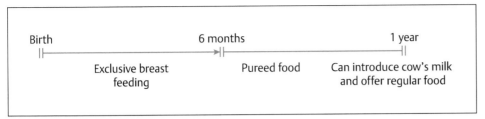

Birth   6 months   1 year

Exclusive breast feeding   Pureed food   Can introduce cow's milk and offer regular food

Human milk vs. formula feeds	• Human milk has more whey protein than formula feeds. Whey improves gastric emptying and is absorbed better.
	• Human milk has significant immunoglobulin A (IgA) content which improves gut immunity of the baby.
	• Human milk has less vitamin D. Consider vitamin D supplementation, beginning the first few weeks of life, in infants who are exclusively breastfed.[a]
Formula feeds	• A common cause of failure to thrive in infants is improper mixing of formula (e.g., mixing with too much water).
	• Usually contains supplemental vitamin D.
Cow milk	• It is usually fortified with vitamin D.
	• Exclusive cow milk feeding is associated with iron deficiency.
Goat milk	• It is low in vitamin D and folic acid.

[a]Recent studies show that maternal supplementation of vitamin D in recommended dosages will obviate the need for infant supplementation.

22.7 Normal Variants in Newborns and Children (!)

Dirty diapers (bowel movements)	• In the first few days after birth, stools can look thick dark green (meconium), then it starts becoming yellow.
	• Three to four stools per day is common in newborns (< 1–2 months). After 1–2 months, infants can go without having bowel movement for days (especially if breastfed). This does not mean constipation. In diagnosing constipation, stool consistency is important (look for thick, hard, pelleted stools).
Wet diapers	• In the first week, number of wet diapers = age in days. For example, a 4-day-old infant has on average four wet diapers/day.
	• Five to six wet diapers/day after the 5th day of life is normal.
Expected weight loss	Weight loss of < 7% in the first week of life is normal. Weight loss of > 7% is abnormal.
Effects of maternal estrogen exposure	• A female newborn can have white discharge, breast enlargement, and swollen labia due to maternal estrogen exposure.
	• Small amount of vaginal spotting (estrogen withdrawal bleeding) can also occur.
Thymic shadow in CXR	Large upper mediastinal shadow that looks like a sail of a ship. This is not seen in adults, as thymus naturally involutes. 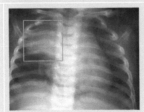 Source: Nevit Dilmen, CC BY-SA 3.0, via Wikimedia Commons.

⚠ **Caution**

(!) These are commonly used as red herrings in board questions.

💡 **MRS**

< 7% weight loss within the first 7 days of life is normal.

22.8 Sudden Infant Death Syndrome (SIDS)[2]

Background: Unexplained sudden death of an infant (i.e., < 1-year-old). Postmortem exam may reveal *unexplained* intrathoracic petechiae or mild pulmonary edema.

Risk factors: The most important risk factor is prone sleeping (sleeping on stomach). Other risk factors include siblings of infants who died from SIDS, prematurity, low birth weight, and exposure to cigarette smoke.

Best method for prevention: Sleeping in supine position (placing the infant on the back).

22.9 Primitive Reflexes in Infants

> **MRS**
>
> SMRPA: **S**he **M**akes **R**obots **P**lay **A**rrows for 6 months. The last of these reflexes generally disappear by 6 months.

Reflex	Description		Should disappear by
Step	When the sole of foot touches a hard surface, infant starts doing stepping motions		1–2 months
Moro (aka startle reflex)	Place baby on a padded floor, slightly raise him up, support the head with a hand and then release suddenly, allowing the head to fall backward for a moment, and then quickly support it again. You will see the following reflex →		2–4 months
Rooting	Stroking the infant's cheek will cause the infant to turn toward the stroked side and starts sucking.		3–4 months
Palmar grasp	Place your finger on infant's open palm and the infant's hand closes around your finger, and as you try to move the finger, the infant will tighten its grip.		5–6 months
Asymmetric tonic neck	When the infant's head is turned toward one side, the extremities on that side will extend while the extremities on the other side will flex.	\n\n*It looks like the baby is shooting an arrow or fencing.*	6 months

22.10 Developmental Milestones

The MRS in this table might sound a little too stretched out, but give it a try and see if it helps remembering this high-yield topic. If not create your own.

Age	Skills			MRS ☺
	Motor	**Language**	**Social**	
2 months	• When in prone position can lift head to 45 degrees • Tracks **to** midline	• Coos	• Looks for familiar objects and people • Social smile	
4 months (3–5 months)	• Can lift head to 90 degrees • Can roll from front to back and back to front • Can sit when trunk is supported • Tracks **past** midline	• Turns to sound of voice • Laughs	• Can mimic some facial expressions	• You must put your hand for support to help the baby sit. For = four = "4 months" • Front rolls = front = four = rolls at 4 months of age • Comedy is "FOR" laughs. FOR = four
6–8 months	• Can sit momentarily without support • Can transfer objects from one hand to other	• Responds to name • Babbles	• Can become anxious when strangers are present	• "6" looks like a picture of a baby sitting with its back arched. • "666"—baby recognizes the number of the beast = stranger anxiety in 6 months. Also recognizes its own name.
10 months	• Can pull to stand and walk by holding/supporting • Can crawl (the mobile stage where babyproofing the house is needed) • Uses three fingers for pincer grasp	• Can say mama and dada	• Can wave goodbye	• "A **decade** of **support**ing **walk**athon." Decade = 10: support walks.
12 months (1 year)	• Can walk first few steps alone • Can throw ball • Can do two-finger pincer grasp	• Responds to simple spoken requests, makes sounds with changes in tone (sounds more like speech), says "mama" and "dada" and tries to say words.	• Imitates • Separation anxiety • Can come to you when called	• 1 year: • One can walk alone for more than one steps for the first time • One can do proper finger grasp • One can throw • One can speak more than one word besides dada and mama • One becomes anxious of leaving one's parent • One can imitate

14–15 months	• Can walk backwards • Can build two-block towers	• Can understand simple commands without gesture	• Tries to get attention from adults	
18 months	• Can run and kick ball • Can feed themselves • Can build 2–4-block towers	• Points to body parts • Can speak 10–25 words	• Can play alone (pretend play)	• 18 is the age of emancipation of minors. Now think of it like this—they can run away from home, eat by themselves, and play by themselves. 18-month-old baby does the same. • 18 months can speak ≈ 18 words.
24 months = 2 years	• Can walk up and down the stairs • Can jump and climb • Can build six-block towers	• Can form two-word combinations • Can speak approximately 200 words • Half of speech is understandable by strangers	• Engages in parallel play	• Can walk two directions in stairs • Can speak two-word combinations • Can verbalize 200 words • Every second sentence is understandable—half of speech is understandable • 2 = 1 +1 = parallel play
3 years	• Can ride a tricycle • Can draw or copy a circle	• Three-word sentence • More than half of speech is understandable by strangers	• Knows age and gender	• 3 years = 3-word sentence • 3 years = TRIcycle; **cycle** can be associated with **circle** = can draw a circle • (This is the MRS method of associating one fact with another)
4 years	• Can hop on one foot • Can draw/copy a square • Can draw a man's picture with 4 parts	• Four-word sentence • Can identify colors	• Co-operative play (can play team sports like soccer)	• Square has 4 equal sides • 4 years old = 4-word sentences • Can play in a team of 4
5 years	• Can draw a triangle • Can walk backwards • Can skip	• Five-word sentences • Counts till 10	• Starts having friends	• Drawing a triangle is more complex than drawing a circle or a square. • Five guys are friends who started a hamburger business. • Five = 5-word sentences

🔍 Clinical Case Scenarios

3. A mother brings in her 13-month child for a routine check-up. The baby can say simple words like "mama" and "ta-ta." She can walk alone a few steps and is able to throw a ball. What is the likely developmental assessment in this child?
   a. Language delay, gross normal
   b. Language normal, gross delay
   c. Language delay, gross delay
   d. Normal development

4. Delia can draw a circle, Maya can draw a square, and Akbar can draw a triangle. How old are they?

22.11 Pediatric Vaccination

Vaccine	Birth	2 months	4 months	6 months	12 months	15 months	18 months	---	4–6 years
Hep B	First dose[a]	Second dose (1–2 months)		Third dose					
DTaP[b]		First dose	Second dose	Third dose		Booster dose			Booster dose
RV (rotavirus)		First dose	Second dose	Third dose[c]					
HiB (Hae-mophilus influenzae B)		First dose	Second dose	Third dose[d]	Booster dose				
IPV (inactivated polio vaccine)		First dose	Second dose	Third dose					Booster dose
PCV-13		First dose	Second dose	Third dose	Booster dose				
Chicken pox (varicella zoster)					First dose				Booster dose
Hep A virus					First dose (given between 1 and 2 years of age)[e]				
MMR					First dose				Booster dose

[a]In preterm babies, age count starts from the day of birth. Give vaccination as above, starting from birth. The only exception is to hold Hep B vaccine if baby's weight is < 2 kg or <4.4 lbs.

[b]DTaP is stronger than TDaP. DTaP is used for primary vaccination in children < 10 years of age, whereas TDaP is given as booster dose in adolescents and adults.

[c]There are two types of vaccines available for rotavirus. One type needs only two doses; the other one, three doses.

[d]There are two types of commercial vaccines available for Haemophilus. The second type does not need re-dosing at 6 months.

[e]Two doses are needed for lasting protection. The second dose can be given 6 to 18 months after the first dose.

Additional vaccination: Influenza is given yearly after 6 months of age. Children 6 months to 8 years of age who are receiving flu vaccination for the first time in their life, require 2 doses of vaccine in that single season to optimize response.

 MRS

DTaP vs. TDaP.
– **D** is given to **D**iapers.
– **T** is for **T**en years and older
– **D** is given **D**ouble boosters : i.e., 2 booster doses are given after 1st round of vaccination.

 MRS

☺ Hep B = B at birth.

☺ DR HIP is given at 2, 4, and 6 months—DTaP, RV, HiB, IPV, PCV.

☺ At 12–15 months: ☺ 1-year old CHAMP: Chicken pox, HiB, A = Hep A virus, MMR, PCV-13.

☺ Whichever alphabets of DR HIP are included in CHAMP are booster doses. That means **HP** are the booster doses given at 12–15 months.

☺ 4–6 years (5 ± 1): ☺ MeDIC is given at 5 years = MEasles–mumps–rubella, DTaP, IPV, Chicken pox. MeDIC has 5 letters.

☺ **Live** vaccines are **LIVE** CRIME = **CRIME** = Chicken pox, Rotavirus, Influenza-live-attenuated type, MMR, *and lastly for E (just a random fact that you might not need) Epidemic typhus.*

22.11.1 Contraindications to Vaccines

Pertussis-containing vaccines	Encephalopathy (e.g., coma, decreased level of consciousness, prolonged seizures) within days of vaccine administration not attributable to another identifiable cause
Any live vaccine	Severe immunodeficiency (e.g., HIV with low CD4 count < 200/mm³, severe combined immunodeficiency)
Rotavirus	Hx of intussusception
Any vaccine	Severe allergic reaction (e.g., anaphylaxis)

- Vaccinations are life-saving. Outside of the information mentioned above, it might be safe to say that there are **NO other contraindications**.
- Per CDC, even development of Guillain–Barré syndrome after vaccination is not a contraindication but requires caution in the future.

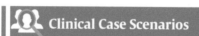 **Clinical Case Scenarios**

5. Parents refusing vaccination for their child. What is the NSIM?

6. A pediatric patient is here for vaccination. His mother reports ongoing mild illness (e.g., mild cold). What is the NSIM?

22.12 Pediatric Cardiology

Physiologic murmur	The only murmur that might be physiologic is the grade I or II ejection mid-systolic murmur that decreases with preload reduction (e.g., standing, Valsalva). – NSIM in a well-looking child is reassurance, after ruling out anemia.
Pathologic murmur	Ejection systolic murmur more than grade II, and all holosystolic or diastolic murmurs are likely pathologic. – NSIM is echocardiography.

22.12.1 Congenital Heart Disease

 MRS

ASD in **AD**ults

Acyanotic heart defects	Cyanotic heart defects
• VSD (ventricular septal defect)—MC heart defect seen in children • ASD (atrial septal defect)—MC congenital heart defect encountered in adults • PDA (patent ductus arteriosus)	• Tetralogy of Fallot (MC cyanotic congenital heart defect) • Transposition of great vessels (most common cyanotic congenital heart disease that presents *in a neonate*) • Tricuspid valve atresia • Truncus arteriosus • Tiny left ventricle (hypoplastic left ventricle) • Total anomalous pulmonary vein return, *with obstruction* (6 T of cyanotic heart disease)
As left-sided heart pressures are higher than the right-sided ones, there is only left-to-right shunt; hence, no mixing of oxygenated and deoxygenated blood in the left side of heart.	In these conditions, right-to-left shunt leads to mixing of deoxygenated and oxygenated blood in the "left side of heart" leading to cyanosis.
• NSIDx is echocardiography. • Most accurate test is cardiac catheterization.	

22.12.2 Acyanotic Congenital Heart Defects (VSD, ASD, PDA)

These conditions can have the following **common features**:

- Small defects can be asymptomatic and sometimes are detected incidentally in adults.
- Larger defects can present with heart failure (increased RR, dyspnea, and feeding difficulty), which may manifest at birth (very large defects) or few months later (moderate-sized defects).
- Development of right-to-left shunt can occur later in life, due to development of the following pathology: increased pulmonary artery blood flow → pulmonary hypertension (loud pulmonic S2) → increased right heart pressure → RV (right ventricle) hypertrophy. Pressure generated by hypertrophied right heart + increased pulmonary pressure leads to right-sided pressure becoming greater than on the left side, resulting in right-to-left shunt and development of cyanosis. This is called **Eisenmenger syndrome** and it usually develops later.[3]

[3]Presence of right-to-left shunt may lead to paradoxical emboli, i.e., DVT leading to arterial emboli (e.g., CCS: symptoms of DVT with a new stroke or acute claudication).

Specific features:

Type of acyanotic heart disease	Exam finding (all may have loud pulmonic S2)	Treatment
VSD	• Harsh holosystolic murmur over left lower sternal border	• For small and asymptomatic defect, do expectant management (may spontaneously close by 1–2 years of age). • For symptomatic or large defects, recommend surgical repair.
ASD	• Fixed wide splitting of S2	• Most close spontaneously • For symptomatic patients or who have significant left-to-right shunt, do surgical repair.
PDA	• Loud, machinery-like *continuous* murmur (the ductus never closes as it is not a valve, hence continuous murmur is heard throughout systole and diastole) • Wide pulse pressure and bounding pulse	• In *premature infants*, first try COX-2 inhibition with **ibuprofen** or indomethacin. • In preterm infants who fail COX-2 inhibition and term infants, who have audible murmurs, percutaneous PDA closure or surgery is recommended.

MRS

SAD to see it split in two.
Split in two = S2 is split.
SAD = ASD.

MRS

Ruby wears PADS =
congenital Rubella infection
is associated with PDA.
Ruby is a female, so PDA is
more common in females.
• **P**rostaglandins keep the
PDA **P**atent. Ibuprofen, by
decreasing prostaglandin
production, promotes
closure of PDA.

Few points on PDA

- Present at birth in all neonates. After birth, rise in neonatal blood oxygen levels signals ductus closure.
- Neonatal hypoxemia increases risk of PDA. Premature babies have increased risk of hypoxemia, hence premature infants have increased risk of PDA.
- It is also more common in **females** than males.
- PDA is associated with maternal rubella infection.
- When Eisenmenger syndrome develops in PDA, postductal *circulation* starts receiving mixed blood, which results in differential cyanosis (lower body is cyanotic, toes develop clubbing, whereas upper body remains unaffected).[4]

[4]**Differential cyanosis with Eisenmenger syndrome due to PDA**

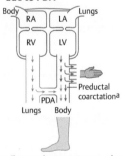

Differential cyanosis can also occur with preductal coarctation and coexistent PDA. In this case the differential cyanosis is *early-onset* as it does not require development of Eisenmenger syndrome (area distal to coarctation may have lower pressures than pulmonary circulation leading to right-to-left shunt).

	Reminder: Heart sounds
S1	Closure of mitral and tricuspid valve causes blood flow disruption leading to vibration or sound heard as S1.
S2	Due to closure of aortic and pulmonic valves • Physiologic splitting of S2 occurs during respiration.

22.12.3 Cyanotic Congenital Heart Defects

Condition	Presentation/exam	Cardiomegaly and mediastinal findings in X-ray	Pulmonary vascular markings[a]
Tetralogy of Fallot (TOF) • Pulmonic stenosis → right ventricular hypertrophy → increased right-sided heart pressures → right-to-left shunt through VSD → cyanosis • Overriding aorta • VSD	• VSD murmur (holosystolic murmur) • Pulmonic stenosis murmur (systolic ejection murmur) • Single S2 may be heard due to very little blood flowing through the pulmonary valve.	• Cardiomegaly may not be present at birth (Boot-shaped heart may take some time to develop) Source: Chatzis AC, Sofianidou J, Kousi T, Karapanagiotou O, Kanakis MA. Rare multiple bronchial abnormalities in a patient with congenital heart disease. Clin Case Rep. 2017 May; 5(5): 727–728.	Decreased (due to pulmonic stenosis)
Tricuspid valve atresia (TVA)[b] • Think of this as a condition with nonexistent tricuspid valve. • Blood goes from the right atrium to the left atrium through ASD. • All the blood flows through left ventricle (left ventricular hypertrophy and left-axis deviation) • Left ventricle maintains blood supply to pulmonary circulation through coexistent PDA (PDA dependent)[c]	• No blood flow out of right ventricle, so there is no sound of pulmonic valve closure, so there is single S2 (only aortic component) • ASD and PDA murmurs are present	Cardiomegaly is usually not present at the time of presentation. May take some time to develop.	Usually decreased (due to decreased right ventricular outflow)
TAPV (total anomalous pulmonary vein return) with obstruction • Oxygenated blood via pulmonary vein returns into the superior vena cava (SVC)/right atrium instead of left atrium. ASD, VSD, and/or PDA is present to maintain systemic circulation. • Significant problem occurs when there is obstruction, i.e., when pulmonary veins enter SVC or right atrium in an acute angle. This can present with severe cyanosis and respiratory distress in the first week of life. • If there is no obstruction, it can present similar to large ASD defects.	• High-flow murmur • If ASD is not present, the left side of heart gets little blood, so single S2 might be heard (as there is no aortic component). In this case systemic circulation is maintained by PDA.	• Right-sided heart enlargement • Large shadow just above the heart (anomalous connections which are all in one side of the heart).	• Increased (pulmonary blood flow returns to right heart which again sends it to pulmonary circulation)

Condition	Presentation/exam	Cardiomegaly and mediastinal findings in X-ray	Pulmonary vascular markings[a]
Tiny left ventricle (hypoplastic left ventricle)	• Severe cyanosis in the first week of birth • Single S2 (as there is no aortic component)	• Right-sided heart enlargement • As opposed to TAPV, there is no large shadow above the heart.	May show increased pulmonary venous congestion
Transposition of great vessels Aorta originates from the right ventricle and pulmonary artery from the left ventricle. Blood mixing occurs with VSD, ASD, and/or PDA • It is the most common cyanotic heart disease that presents in a neonate. • Common in diabetic mothers	• Big aorta is abnormally located anteriorly to pulmonary artery, hence the aortic component easily dwarfs the pulmonic component of S2, resulting in single S2 sound. • Presence of VSD/PDA or ASD murmur	"Egg-on-a-string" sign: egg = heart and string = narrow mediastinum	Increased pulmonary vascular markings
Truncus arteriosus • Pulmonary artery and aorta are abnormally merged to form a big outflow tract that gets blood from both the ventricles.	Single S2—with ejection systolic murmur due to increased flow		Increased pulmonary vascular markings. **Reason:** In the normal state, RV (right ventricle) has much lower pressure than LV (left ventricle). In this case both RV and LV have equal pressure, with more than usual blood flowing through RV.

[a]Note the conditions that have increased pulmonary vascular markings versus the ones that do not.

[b]TOF and TVA may have some common features. To differentiate TOF from TVA, look at the axis on EKG: there is **right**-axis deviation in TOF and left-axis deviation in TVA (see next page discussion on how to determine axis in EKG).

[c]To be compatible with life, most **neonatal** cyanotic heart diseases (e.g., transposition of great vessels, TAPV, TVA, hypoplastic left heart) require **PDA** or ASD (in some cases VSD) to supply systemic circulation. These conditions *may become* acutely symptomatic after 2–3 days, when ductus arteriosus normally closes.[5] Prostaglandin infusion (PGE1) can be used to keep the PDA patent until definitive surgical correction.

MRS

I misplaced my egg today. Misplaced = transposed.

[5]Exceptions are:
• TOF (already has a VSD), and
• Truncus arteriosus (mixing occurs in the trunk itself).

In a nutshell

Cyanosis presentation time

Severe defect	Cyanosis at birth, e.g., TOF with pulmonary atresia (severe pulmonary valve stenosis)
Less severe defect (ductal-dependent)	2–3 days after birth, when ductus closes
Mild to moderate defects	Late-onset cyanosis For example, cyanosis during feeding or crying

How to determine the axis?

To know the axis, look at the first and third lead
- When both are up, then 👍 thumbs up for both, meaning axis is normal.
- When only lead I is up, your left hand is up, and axis is tilted to left side = left-axis deviation. Note: when you write 1, 2, 3, 4, ..., 1 is always written in the left side, and 3 is always written in the right.
- When lead III is up, your right hand will be up = right-axis deviation.

Lead I	Lead III	Conclusion
⋀	⋀	Normal
⋀	⋁	Left axis deviation
⋁	⋀	Right axis deviation

22.12.4 Coarctation of the Aorta

Pathophysiology: Narrowing of the aorta, due to thickening of **tunica media** near the ductus arteriosus. It is often associated with other heart defects such as ASD, VSD, PDA, and/or bicuspid aortic valve.

[6]Preductal coarctation means location of coarctation is proximal to ductus arteriosus.

Preductal coarctation[6] (infantile coarctation) Associated with Turner's syndrome	Postductal coarctation
Arteries to head / Post ductal low pressure area / Coexistent PDA may or may not be present.	Pre ductal high pressure area / Post ductal coarctation / Ductus arteriosus / Descending aorta / Coexistent PDA may or may not be present.

Severe preductal coarctation	Mild preductal coarctation	
• May present with heart failure or shock, few days after birth when PDA closes. NSIM is prostaglandin infusion. • In patients with coexistent PDA, differential cyanosis can occur, as poststenotic arterial blood is mixed with venous blood through PDA. Oxygen saturation is normal in upper extremities and low in lower extremities, (upper body is pink and lower body is blue).	May present later during life • Differential cyanosis may not be seen.	• May present during later years of life • No differential cyanosis is seen, as there is no right-to-left shunt: increased pressure in the PDA area proximal to coarctation prevents right-to-left shunt.

Common features:

- Increased perfusion in the head, upper torso, and upper extremities
  - HTN in upper extremity.
  - Increased pressure in intercostal arteries, leads to pressure atrophy of posterior ribs and rib notching (it takes time to develop this, hence not seen in infants).
  - Increase risk of intracranial aneurysm and rupture.
- Decreased perfusion below the aortic arch.
- Low BP and decreased pulses in lower extremities.
- Decreased renal perfusion.
- Decreased leg perfusion (presents as claudication).

NSIDx: Transthoracic echocardiogram

Management: For significant stenosis, do surgical repair or percutaneous angioplasty.

 Clinical Case Scenarios

7. A 6-month-old male baby is brought in for a routine check-up. As soon as you put the stethoscope on the baby's chest he starts crying, breathes rapidly, and begins to turn a dusky blue color. In addition to oxygen, which of the following will rapidly alleviate these symptoms?

   a) Keep in upright position

   b) Give intramuscular epinephrine

   c) Place in lateral knee-chest position

   d) Give an infusion of PGE1 (prostaglandin)

8. You are examining a newborn male baby just after delivery. His entire trunk is blue. He has a pulse rate of 90, grimaces with some activity. His respirations are irregular with an oxygen saturation of 80%. He ends up requiring intubation. On auscultation you hear a single loud S2 and a harsh murmur in the left lower sternal border. What is the baby's APGAR score and the likely diagnosis?

   a) APGAR 6; transposition of the great vessels

   b) APGAR 4; tetralogy of Fallot

   c) APGAR 5; tetralogy of Fallot

   d) APGAR 4; transposition of the great vessels

22.13 Differential Dx of Chronic Stridor

Condition	Laryngomalacia	Vascular anomaly (ring or slings)	Choanal atresia
Etiology	• Loose upper laryngeal structures • Occurs in neonates and infants	• Abnormal development of aortic arch resulting in compression of trachea, esophagus, and/or bronchus • Associated with cardiac defects	• Failure of recanalization of nasal passage • Associated with CHARGE syndrome (**C**oloboma, **H**eart defects, **A**tresia choanae, **R**etardation of growth/development, **G**enitourinary abnormalities, and **E**ar problems, e.g., deafness)
Presentation	Noisy breathing and/or cyanosis when supine or crying[a] • Relieved by prone position	• Stridor that *improves with neck extension* • Not relieved by prone position • May have coexistent obstructive esophageal symptoms	• In bilateral atresia mouth breathing maintains oxygenation. So, cyanosis is precipitated by feeding.[a] This one goes away with crying. • Unilateral may be asymptomatic and incidentally detected.

Condition	Laryngomalacia	Vascular anomaly (ring or slings)	Choanal atresia
Diagnosis	Laryngoscopy	• CT or MRI angiography and echocardiogram • Bronchoscopy can be done, if concerns for airway obstruction.	• **Best initial step:** try to pass a catheter through the nose to posterior pharynx. • **NSIDx**—CT imaging (test of choice). *Caution: do not choose rhinoscopy.*
Management	• For mild symptoms, reassurance, as it mostly resolves on its own. • For severe symptoms (e.g., poor weight gain, rapidly worsening symptoms), laryngoplasty can be done.	For symptomatic lesions, recommend surgical correction.	Endoscopic or surgical repair

[a]Caution: may get confused with Tet spells.

22.14 Pediatric Gastroenterology

22.14.1 Congenital Abdominal Wall Defects Due to Errors in Fetal Development

	Umbilical hernia	Omphalocele (aka Exomphalos)	Gastroschisis
Definition	Protrusion covered by skin, which may contain bowel	Bowel (covered by membrane sac, but no skin) protrudes through umbilical ring.	Naked bowel (not covered by skin and membrane) protrudes through abdominal wall. Exposed bowel leads to inflammation and injury (results in matted bowel appearance)
Association	• Usually an isolated defect • May be associated with hypothyroidism	Associated with other conditions, such as neural tube defects, cardiac disease, trisomy, etc.	Usually an isolated defect
Prenatal maternal findings	None	Polyhydramnios Elevated AFP	
Treatment	Resolves spontaneously. If persists beyond 2 years, consider surgical repair.	First step: • Cover with gauze-dressing soaked with warm saline (not cold), and cover dressing with clear plastic wrap. • Use NG tube to decompress bowel and give antibiotics +IV fluids. Second step: • **Small defects**—Primary closure • **Larger defects**—A silo[a] is used for temporary cover and bowel is slowly reduced over days; and then to OR for final closure.	Second step is primary surgical closure in most case. If not successful, NSIM is closure using silo over days (similar to management of larger omphalocele).

[a] Silo bag is commonly made up of silicone

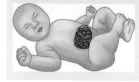

22.14.2 Causes of Gastrointestinal Obstruction in Pediatrics

Condition	Clinical presentation (Pay attention to timing of presentation, a very important clue)	Etiology/pathophysiology	Steps in management Remember: First SIM is always stabilization before diagnosis (e.g., IV fluids, electrolytes replacement, +/-nasogastric nasogastric tube for GI decompression).
Necrotizing enterocolitis	**Timing:** Within the first 2 weeks of life **Presentation:** Feeding intolerance, abdominal distension/tenderness, frank blood in stool, bilious vomiting, etc. **Specific lab findings:** Elevated lactic acid, anion gap metabolic acidosis (*Like ischemic colitis in adults*)	• Unknown • Transluminal and mucosal necrosis (equivalent of ischemic colitis in adults) • Occurs in **premature infants**	**NSIDx:** Abdominal **X-ray.** Findings include dilated bowel loops, air in bowel wall (pneumatosis intestinalis), and/or air in portal veins. **Rx:** Antibiotics and surgery.
Congenital pyloric stenosis aka Infantile hypertrophic pyloric stenosis	**Timing:** 2–4 weeks of age **Presentation:** Projectile nonbilious[a] vomiting. Physical exam may reveal palpable olive-sized mass (in RUQ, just lateral to rectus abdominis) and visible peristaltic waves. • What is the most likely acid–base disorder?[b]	• It is postulated that progressive thickening occurs after birth, hence symptoms are not present at the time of birth. • It is more common in males • Associated with transesophageal fistula	**NSIDx/NSIM:** Abdominal ultrasound (US) to confirm dx. **Rx:** Surgical pyloromyotomy.
Duodenal atresia	**Timing:** Presents at around birth **Presentation:** Bilious vomiting, abdominal distension, feeding intolerance that occurs after the *first feed*.	• Failure of the lumen to re-canalize during gestation (in utero) • Presents at birth (*as opposed to pyloric stenosis or biliary stenosis*) • Associated with Down syndrome	**NSIDx** abdominal X-ray: Double bubble sign with absent distal gas is diagnostic. Some experts recommend routine upper GI series to make sure it is not high-grade volvulus causing duodenal obstruction. **Rx:** Surgical correction. There are two gas collections in the upper abdomen, corresponding to the stomach and proximal duodenum, with no bowel gas beyond this point. Source: Pathology. In: Gunderman R, ed. Essential Radiology: Clinical Presentation, Pathophysiology, Imaging. 3rd ed. Thieme; 2014.

Condition	Clinical presentation	Etiology/pathophysiology	Steps in management	
Meconium ileus	**Timing:** First few days after birth **Presentation:** Abdominal distention and bilious vomiting.	Stool is so thick and sticky, it gets stuck in the ileocecal valve area causing obstruction (the pathology is similar to gallstone ileus). This occurs in patients with cystic fibrosis.	**NSIDx** is abdominal X-ray: "Multiple" air-fluid levels (dilated loops of small bowel) **After that NSIDx** is contrast enema—which will reveal microcolon (due to underused colon) **Rx:** Depends upon severity • If mild, hyperosmolar enema to break down the meconium. • If complicated or not responding to the above measure, do surgery.	
Jejunal or ileal atresia (intestinal atresia)	**Timing:** Within 24 hours of birth **Presentation:** Bilious vomiting and abdominal distention • Similar in presentation to meconium ileus	• Due to mesenteric vascular occlusion in utero (different etiology from duodenal atresia). • Risk factors include maternal cocaine or alcohol use	**NSIDx:** Abdominal X-ray • In jejunal atresia, large stomach, duodenum, and jejunum can be seen. **NSIDx** is upper GI series • In ileal atresia, X-ray picture may be similar to meconium ileus with "multiple" air-fluid levels, proximal to level of obstruction. In this case, **NSIDx** is contrast enema, which may show microcolon (similar to meconium ileus).[d] **Rx:** Surgery	**Contrast enema showing microcolon** Source: Sinha S, Sarin Y, Ramji S. Ileal atresia with duplication cyst of terminal ileum: a rare association. J Neonatal Surg. 2012; 1(2): 27.
Intestinal malrotation with volvulus	**Timing:** Can occur anytime in the first year of life **Presentation:** Acute vomiting, abdominal distention, and pain. Can cause bowel ischemia.	Incomplete bowel rotation during gestation can predispose to volvulus	Abdominal X-ray can rarely be normal but note that it can also have *double-bubble sign*, if malrotation occurs in the duodenal area. **NSIDx** is upper GI series (look for spiral cork-screw, or apple-peel-like patter), or abdominal ultrasound. **Rx:** Surgery	Source: Pathology. In: Gunderman R, ed. Essential Radiology: Clinical Presentation, Pathophysiology, Imaging. 3rd ed. Thieme; 2014

Hirschsprung disease	Timing: Can present anytime—from neonatal period up *until childhood or adolescence*, if the involved segment is small.	• Failure of migration of neural crest cells resulting in the absence of ganglionic cells in distal colon	NSIDx: Abdominal X-ray (look for gastric and colonic distension[c])	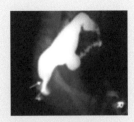
(most common cause [MCC] of obstruction in neonates)		• Associated with Down syndrome	After X-ray, NSIDx/ NSIM is *contrast enema* (narrowing is seen in the rectosigmoid area).	
	Presentation:		Gold standard for diagnosis is rectal mucosa biopsy.	Contrast enema showing narrowing in the rectosigmoid area.
	• Failure to pass meconium within 48 hours		**Rx:** Surgical repair	Source: Modified from Pratap A, Gupta DK, Tiwari A, et al. Application of a plain abdominal radiograph transition zone (PARTZ) in Hirschsprung's disease. BMC Pediatr. 2007; 7: 5.
	• Abdominal distension			
	• May have tight anal canal and rectal exam may cause explosive expulsion of flatus and stool, as it temporarily relives obstruction.			

[a]GI obstruction before ampulla of Vater (point of entry for bile duct) does not present with bilious vomiting (e.g., congenital or acquired pyloric stenosis).

[b]With increased loss of gastric acid (H^+Cl^-), there is metabolic alkalosis (high serum bicarbonate) with compensatory respiratory acidosis. Also look for low serum chloride.

[c]All other conditions listed in the table can be differentiated from Hirschsprung disease by looking at colonic air. Hirschsprung has increased colonic air. *If colonic air is absent*, it is not Hirschsprung.

[d]US of abdomen can be used to differentiate in between them. Images of dilated bowel loops in meconium ileus are filled with echogenic material, while the loops in atresia are fluid-filled.

22.14.3 Management of Neonatal Bilious Vomiting

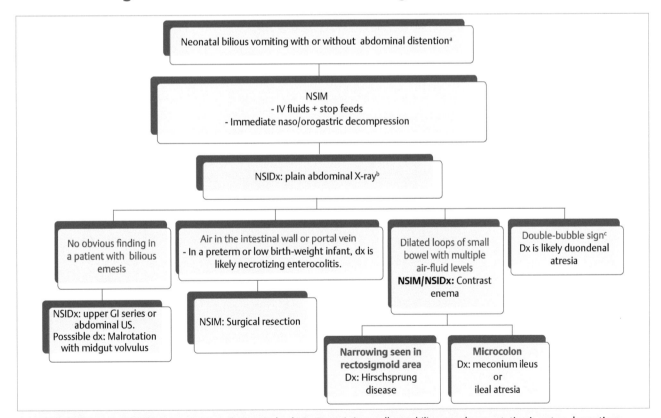

[a]Neonatal bilious vomiting is an emergency. Congenital pyloric stenosis is usually nonbilious, and presentation is not as dramatic as other cases of intestinal obstruction.

[b]If signs of perforation, NSIM is immediate exploratory laparotomy.

[c]Can also be seen in intestinal volvulus.

22.14.4 Intussusception

Definition: Telescoping of a proximal part of intestine into the lumen of a distal segment (commonly the ileojejunal part telescopes into cecum and ascending colon).

Etiology: MCC is gastroenteritis due to rotavirus. Other causes are Meckel's diverticulum, GI polyps, Henoch–Schonlein purpura, etc.

Clinical presentation:

- Early—intermittent abdominal pain.
- Late—toxic-looking child, irritable, vomiting, with severe abdominal pain and often in chest to knee position. Red currant jelly stool or bloody stool can occur due to bowel ischemia.

Physical examination: May reveal palpable tender sausage-shaped mass.

Work-up: NSIDx is abdominal US.

Treatment:

- If no evidence of bowel perforation, NSIM—air enema, i.e., pneumatic reduction (under X-ray fluoroscopy guidance) or hydrostatic enema (using saline or contrast) under US or X-ray fluoroscopy guidance. Any of these technique can be used. These essentially push back the telescoped segment.
- If evidence of bowel perforation, NSIM—surgery.

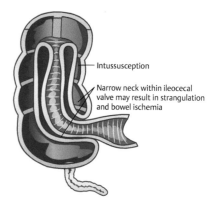

22.14.5 Meckel's Diverticulum

Pathophysiology: Failure of vitelline duct to regress and involute. The Meckel diverticulum often contains the same tissue as that of the stomach or pancreas.

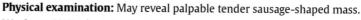

Clinical presentation: Presents commonly in 2–3-year-old babies with painless melena, iron deficiency, or intussusception.

Diagnostic test: Technetium-99m scan (aka Meckel scan), which looks for ectopic gastric tissue.

Management: Surgical excision.

MRS

Rule of 2s for Meckel's diverticulum

- 2–3 years of age at presentation
- 2% prevalence in general population (only a minority of them become symptomatic)
- 2:1 male-to-female ratio
- 2 feet proximal to ileocecal valve is the MC location
- 2 inches in length
- 2 types of ectopic tissue: gastric and pancreatic tissue

22.14.6 Differential Diagnosis of Chronic Food Regurgitation/ Vomiting in Infants

	Clinical features	Management
Physiologic GERD (gastroesophageal reflux disease)	• Small amount of regurgitation/vomiting after feeding, which may be present in infants until **1 year of age**. • Infants should have no loss of developmental milestones.	• Reassurance and frequent, small volume feeds in an upright position while feeding. *(Note that thickened feeds are not recommended.)*
Pathologic GERD	Food regurgitation/vomiting + • loss of developmental milestones or poor weight/height gain AND/OR • presence of other warning signs (e.g., wheezing, increased irritability related to regurgitation episode)	• Thickened feeds • Antacid therapy (e.g., H_2-antagonist or proton pump inhibitor)
Cow's milk or soy-protein allergy	Food regurgitation/vomiting + *eczema* *(allergic)*, poor weight gain ± colitis (bloody stool)	• Avoid dairy and soy protein • Use hydrolyzed formula (predigested proteins), if needed.

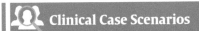

9. A full-term male infant was brought in by mother with the following history: For the last 2 weeks the baby has developed frequent episodes of vomiting, and small specks of blood in his stools. Mother started using a cow-milk based formula feed 1 month ago and then later she changed it to soy-based formula but the baby still continues to have the vomiting. Physical exam reveals no abdominal tenderness. What is the likely dx?

a) Meckel's diverticulitis
b) Feed allergy
c) Necrotizing enterocoilits
d) Infectious diarrhea

22.14.7 Esophageal Atresia with or without Tracheoesophageal Fistula

Background: abnormal fetal/embyronal development of esophagus/trachea, associated with fetal chromosomal abnormality.

Clinical presentation will depend on the type of abnormality (blind pouch vs connected to trachea), and part of esophagus involved (to better understand the clinical features depending on the type of abnormality look at the box on the right side, get a bigger picture of the different type of abnormalities and then refer to this table below for its corresponding feature/s):

The following diagram depicts different types of abnormalities. Just understand what clinical features would be present; no need to remember each type.

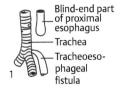
Blind-end part of proximal esophagus
Trachea
Tracheoeso-phageal fistula
1

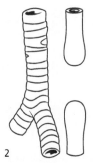
2

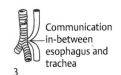
Communication in-between esophagus and trachea
3

Type of abnormality	Upper part of esophagus	Lower part of esophagus
Esophagus is a blind-end pouch, NOT connected with trachea	Drooling and infant cannot eat. No respiratory issue while attempting to feed	Abdominal X-ray shows decreased amount of air (gasless intestines).
Esophagus is connected to trachea	Respiratory issue while attempting to feed (e.g., during feeding the baby develops coughing and chocking with cyanosis)[a]	Abdominal X-ray will reveal lot of air in intestines.

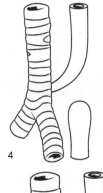
4

[a]Can present with severe respiratory distress requiring intubation in a neonate.
For example, an infant with picture 2 malformation (see right side) will have the following features: drooling, inability to eat, and gasless intestines. The infant will have no respiratory issues when fed. An infant with picture 5 malformation will have respiratory issues while attempting to feed and abdominal X-ray will reveal lot of air in intestines.

Work-up: In esophageal atresia, diagnosis can be made by attempting to insert a feeding tube into the stomach and doing a plain X-ray. Upper GI series using gastrografin can also be used. In some cases, endoscopy and bronchoscopy might be needed.

Treatment: Surgical repair.

Association: The VACTERL anomalies (**V**ertebral anomalies, **A**nal atresia, **C**ardiac defects, **T**racheoesophageal fistula and/or **E**sophageal atresia, **R**enal and **L**imb anomalies).

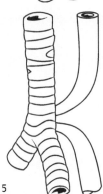
5

Clinical Case Scenarios

10. A 4-day-old male baby is brought in by his mother because she noted that he vomits each time she feeds him. The baby was diagnosed with Down syndrome prenatally. What is likely diagnosis?

    a) Pyloric stenosis

    b) Duodenal atresia

    c) Hirschsprung disease

    d) Tracheoesophageal fistula

11. A 4-month-old baby coughs up each time mother feeds him. She feeds the baby upright with no relief of symptoms. On examination, the baby is crying and irritable. She recently noticed that the baby has started to wheeze. What is the likely diagnosis?

    a) Pathologic GERD

    b) Physiologic GERD

    c) Esophageal atresia

    d) Transesophageal fistula

    e) Transposition of the great vessels

12. A 2-year-old child is brought in by her mom because she appears pale and is less playful. The child is not in distress and is actively playing around the office. He is found to have iron-deficiency anemia. His lead level is undetectable. Stool for occult blood test is positive. What is the NSIDx?

    a) Abdominal ultrasound

    b) Technetium-99m scan

    c) Colonoscopy

    d) Barium enema

    e) Abdominal CT scan

13. A 5-year-old boy is brought into the emergency room by his mother. The child has been vomiting since this morning. On exam, the child is noted to be in a flexed position lying on the exam table. The abdominal exam notes a tender mass below the umbilicus. What is the best diagnostic test?

    a) Ultrasound

    b) Air-contrast enema

    c) Flat upright abdominal X-ray

    d) Abdominal CT scan

14. A 7-month-old child presents with acute onset bilious vomiting. Abdominal exam reveals abdominal tenderness. Abdominal X-ray reveals double-bubble sign. What is the diagnosis?

    a) Duodenal atresia

    b) Intestinal malrotation with volvulus

    c) Jejunal atresia

    d) Hirschsprung disease

15. What is the NSIDx for the case number 14?

22.15 Pediatric Hepatobiliary Disorders

22.15.1 Neonatal Jaundice

Definition: in a neonate, jaundice is defined as bilirubin levels above 5 mg/dL.[7]

Physiologic jaundice	Pathologic jaundice
• Occurs due to decreased bilirubin conjugation by immature liver cells and shortened RBC life span; it should meet all the following criteria:	
Appears after >24 hours of birth	Appears within first 24 hours of life
Total bilirubin is usually low, but may reach up to 12–15 mg/dL[a]	Total bilirubin of > 15 mg/dL[a]
Unconjugated bilirubinemia	Direct **(conjugated)** bilirubin > 2 mg/dL
Peaks in 3–5 days of life	Rate of bilirubin rise > 5 mg/dL per day
Returns to normal before the end of the first week of life	Elevated bilirubin in the second week of life
If all of the above present, likely physiologic jaundice. NSIM is reassurance.	If any of the above present, think of pathologic jaundice. NSIM: address underlying cause.

[a]High total bilirubin may require phototherapy or exchange transfusion to prevent kernicterus. This is more likely to occur with pathologic jaundice.

22.15.2 Kernicterus

Background: Significantly high bilirubin level increases the risk of bilirubin deposition in neonatal brain tissue leading to brain injury. Premature infants are at a higher risk.

Clinical presentation: Lethargy, irritation, hypotonia, seizure, intellectual disability cerebral palsy.

Prevention:

Term infant with no risk factor[a]	Indication for phototherapy[b] (total bilirubin in mg/dL)	Indication for exchange transfusion (total bilirubin in mg/dL, despite aggressive phototherapy and significant neurological dysfunction)
24 hours of age	> 12	> 19
48 hours of age	> 15	> 22
72 hours of age	> 18	> 24

[a]Start therapy at lower levels for neonate born at ≤ 37 weeks' gestational age and in infants with risk factors (e.g., sepsis, acidosis, hypoalbuminemia, hemolytic anemia, etc.).
[b]Phototherapy might degrade riboflavin (vitamin B2) and lead to vitamin B2 deficiency particularly in preterm infants.

Classification of neonatal jaundice by bilirubin type

Conjugated (direct) bilirubinemia	Unconjugated (indirect)	
	Hemolysis[a]	Other causes
• Extrahepatic obstruction due to anatomic causes such as biliary atresia • Sepsis • Neonatal hepatitis • Metabolic disorders • Genetic disease • Congenital jaundice syndromes: Dubin–Johnson syndrome and Rotor syndrome	• RhD incompatibility • Drug reaction • Red cell defects • G6PD • Alpha thalassemia • Spherocytosis • Sickle cell disease • Polycythemia (due to increased number of RBC, which eventually breaks down)	• Physiologic jaundice • Breast milk jaundice • Breastfeeding failure jaundice • Congenital jaundice syndromes: Gilbert syndrome and Crigler–Najjar syndrome (type I and II)[b]

[a]Exam tip: When a CCS includes indirect bilirubinemia in a newborn, look first at hemoglobin count and peripheral blood smear.
[b]Crigler–Najjar type I is a more severe form and results in severe unconjugated hyperbilirubinemia in infants. These patients need liver transplantation.

Breast milk jaundice versus breastfeeding-failure jaundice

	Etiology	Features	NSIM
Breast milk jaundice	Inhibitor of glucuronosyltransferase, present in breast milk, causes indirect (unconjugated) hyperbilirubinemia in infants.	• Presents after 3–5 days of life, when physiologic jaundice normally resolves, and *peaks within 2 weeks of birth*. • Can go as high as 12–20 mg/dL. • To differentiate between the two, look for signs of dehydration (e.g., hyper- or hyponatremia) or lethargy that points toward breastfeeding-failure jaundice.	Temporarily hold breastfeeding and let the bilirubin decline; use alternate feeding (formula milk) in the interim. Resume breastfeeding after bilirubin levels have trended down.
Breastfeeding-failure jaundice	Inadequate caloric intake, commonly due to poor breastfeeding techniques, leads to increased enterohepatic circulation of bilirubin and unconjugated hyperbilirubinemia.		• Teach proper breastfeeding technique • Increase frequency of feeds to >10/day

Anatomic causes of jaundice in neonates

Condition	Presentation	Diagnostic test	Management
Biliary or choledochal cyst	Jaundice, palpable mass • Can cause pancreatitis	US ± ERCP (endoscopic retrograde cholangiopancreatography) • Cysts may be single or multiple	Surgery Malignant transformation can occur despite surgery
Biliary atresia	Initially the infant is well, but within 2 months of age develops severe jaundice[a]	US may show absent or abnormal gallbladder and biliary ductal dilatation. Gold standard for dx is intraoperative cholangiogram.	• Surgically a connection is created between the biliary duct and the intestine. • After surgery, start ursodeoxycholic acid. • Outcome: > 50% of patients will require liver transplantation for biliary cirrhosis even after corrective surgery.

[a]**Note that** timing of presentation is similar to pyloric stenosis and not similar to duodenal or intestinal *atresia*.

22.16 Pediatric Dermatology

Neonatal rash

Skin rash	Diagnosis and additional info	Management
Source: Zeimusu, Public domain, via Wikimedia Commons.	**Capillary hemangioma (aka strawberry or superficial infantile hemangioma)** • Lobules of capillaries separated by fibrous septa	• Reassurance • Initially grows rapidly and then regresses spontaneously.
Red-blue spongy mass Source: Hemangioma. In: Lang G, ed. Ophthalmology: A Pocket Textbook Atlas. 3rd ed. Thieme; 2015	**Cavernous hemangioma** • Formation of large cavernous vascular channel • MC benign tumor of liver/spleen	• For larger or more symptomatic lesions, consider surgical removal. • For asymptomatic lesions, observe. The lesion regresses spontaneously in greater than two-thirds of cases.

Skin rash	Diagnosis and additional info	Management
 Source: Gzzz, CC BY-SA 4.0, via Wikimedia Commons.	**Mongolian spot (aka congenital dermal melanocytosis)**	Reassurance, typically regresses spontaneously.
 Erythematous base-area with dry, white or yellow, greasy scales Source: Modified from Siegfried EC, Hebert AA. Diagnosis of Atopic Dermatitis: Mimics, Overlaps, and Complications. J Clin Med. 2015; 4(5): 884–917.	**Seborrheic dermatitis** • Occurs in infants and old adults	• Conservative approach with frequent use of emollient shampoo. • If it fails, then use low-potency topical steroids and/or topical antifungals.
• Multiple yellow or white pustules on erythematous base. • Rash can occur anywhere in the body.	**Erythema toxicum neonatorum**	Toxicum is a misnomer. The name should have been "benign self-limiting erythema toxicoid neonatorum," where toxioid = toxic appearing, but not toxic. NSIM is reassurance. It lasts about a week.

22.17 Pediatric Infections

22.17.1 TORCH Infection[8]

When a pregnant woman gets primary infection with these organisms, the infection can spread to her fetus. TORCH infection acquired in utero has entirely different presentation.

Consider TORCH infection when a newborn is found to have the following:

- Intrauterine growth restriction (IUGR), microcephaly.
- Jaundice, hepatitis, and hepatosplenomegaly ± thrombocytopenia.

Look for the following associated features to differentiate in between them.

Condition	Specific clinical features	Lab tests and management
Toxoplasmosis	Hydrocephalus, intracranial calcifications (diffuse), chorioretinitis	Serum toxoplasma antibody (IgM) and polymerase chain reaction (PCR) of cerebrospinal fluid (CSF) and other fluids (e.g., blood, urine) **Rx:** Pyrimethamine + sulfadiazine • Add folinic acid (leucovorin)

[8]TORCH
- Toxoplasmosis
- Others = syphilis, varicella zoster, Zika virus, etc.
- Rubella
- Cytomegalovirus (CMV)
- Herpes virus

MRS

Toxo CHIPS
C = chorioretinitis
H = hydrocephalus
I = intracranial calcification
P = pyrimethamine
S = sulfadiazine

MRS

Syphilis causes S's
- **S**niffles, **S**kin rash (may involve **S**oles), **S**aber shins, **S**addle nose, **S**ensorineural hearing loss, **S**ight problem (due to keratitis)

MRS

Rubella can lead to **PDA**, and involves **E**ye, **E**ar, **S**kin.
- Ruby wears PADs as she PEES a lot.
PADs = patent ductus arteriosus

MRS

- CMV PICks his ear a lot, which made him deaf.
PIC = periventricular intracranial calcifications
Deaf = hearing loss
- CMV = Calcifications Medial to Ventricles

MRS

Local HERMES
Her = HERpes simplex virus
MES = **m**outh, **e**ye, and **s**kin disease = localized herpes infection

MRS

MRS of association: *You can associate one fact with another to try to remember certain points.*
VariceLLA = AL = A-Limbia = no limbs = limb hypoplasia

Condition	Specific clinical features	Lab tests and management
Syphilis	• **Early features**: Generalized maculopapular rash or *ulcers* (involves palms/soles), rhinorrhea (sniffles) • **Late features (> 2 years of age):** Hutchinson teeth, mulberry molars, high-arched palate, saber shins, saddle nose, sensorineural hearing loss, interstitial keratitis, etc.)	First test: VDRL (Venereal Disease Research Laboratory test) or RPR (rapid plasma reagin). Confirmatory test: dark-field microscopy or FTA-ABS (fluorescent treponemal antibody absorption test). **Rx:** Parenteral penicillin (IV or IM)
Rubella	• PDA (patent ductus arteriosus) • Eye: cataracts, glaucoma, retinopathy • Ear: hearing loss • Skin: "Blueberry muffin" rash Source: CDC, Public domain, via Wikimedia Commons.	Best initial test is rubella IgM antibody. Viral culture is commonly done of nasopharyngeal secretions. **Rx:** Supportive care
CMV	Periventricular intracranial calcification, hearing loss	Test for CMV (PCR and viral culture in urine and saliva) **Rx:** Ganciclovir or valganciclovir
HSV 1 or 2	Comes in three different forms and overlaps can occur • **Localized** form affects eye (keratoconjunctivitis), skin, or mouth (vesicular lesions on erythematous base) • **CNS infection:** Meningoencephalitis • **Systemic disseminated infection:** Skin, hepatitis, CNS infection, etc.	Test for HSV PCR in mucosa, skin lesions, blood, and CSF. • Do lumbar puncture in all cases (even if clinically localized). **Rx:** IV acyclovir
Varicella	• Presentation can be similar to congenital HSV infection with vesicular skin lesions and eye lesions. Cerebral cortical atrophy and seizures can also occur. • Look for limb hypoplasia to differentiate from HSV. *More than 50% of cases have limb hypoplasia.*	**Dx:** It is a clinical diagnosis. PCR and antibody testing can be done. **Rx:** IV acyclovir

22.17.2 Viral Exanthem

Common presentation: Prodromal symptoms such as fever, malaise, lethargy, and headache can be seen in all.

	Measles (rubeola)[a]	Rubella[a]	Mumps[b]	Roseola infantum	Erythema infectiosum (fifth disease)
Viral etiology	• All are **RNA** viruses • Preventive vaccine is given together as MMR[c]			HHV (human herpesvirus) 6 and 7	Parvovirus B19 (a DNA virus)
Exathem (As you can see, the rashes can look similar, so good history and additional exam findings are important for differentiating)	Erythematous macules and papules, confluent in some areas (*Notice the confluent area around the inner thighs in the picture below*) • Can be pruritic Source: CDC, Public domain, via Wikimedia Commons.	Erythematous rash that looks like measles, except that this one is not confluent. Source: Prof. Dr. Dr. F.C. Sitzmann, Homburg/Saar Copyright: DGK, CC BY-SA 3.0, via Wikimedia Commons. • Can be pruritic	None	Discrete, rosy-pink, nonpruritic, maculopapular rash Source: Emiliano Burzagli, Public domain, via Wikimedia Commons.	Erythematous malar facial rash (looks like slapped cheek), followed by development of generalized erythematous maculopapular rash. As the rash starts to fade, it may have lacy reticular appearance. • Rash can recur, at times, for months. Source: Andrew Kerrderivative work: Berita, Public domain, via Wikimedia Commons.
Location	Spreads from *head to trunk* (centripetal spread)	–		Starts from *trunk* and spreads to extremities and head (centrifugal spread)	Starts from face and spreads to trunk and extremities
Additional clinical signs	Cough (due to pneumonitis), coryza, conjunctivitis, Koplik[d] spots (**grey-white** papules with erythemtaous background on buccal mucosa) • Koplik spots are pathognomonic (so it is important to do an oral exam) Source: CDC, Public domain, via Wikimedia Commons.	• Forchheimer spots = pinpoint or larger petechial rash (*red spot*) on the soft palate • Sore throat	Parotitis (bilateral or unilateral)	High-grade fever for few days followed by rash[e]	Joint pain (in adults can occur without rash. Look for hx of exposure to children, e.g., teachers or daycare-center workers)

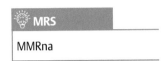

MMRna

	Measles (rubeola)[a]	Rubella[a]	Mumps[b]	Roseola infantum	Erythema infectiosum (fifth disease)
Typical lymph node involvement	Nonspecific	Posterior cervical lymphadenopathy	Enlarged parotid or submandibular glands	Lymph nodes in cervical, occipital, or auricular area	Nonspecific
Complications	• Otitis media • Pneumonia • Myocarditis • Encephalitis • Subacute sclerosing panencephalitis (rare)	• Polyarticular arthritis or arthralgia • Congenital rubella syndrome	• Orchitis (MC complication in *post-pubertal* men) • Meningitis/ Encephalitis (MC complication in *prepubertal* children)	Aseptic meningitis or encephalitis	• Aplastic crisis, or pure red cell aplasia (more likely to occur in patients with pre-existing hemolytic disease or immunosuppression) • Infection during pregnancy can lead to transplacental infection and fetal hydrops
Management	• Supportive treatment • Vitamin A supplementation • May use ribavirin in severe cases	• Supportive treatment	Supportive treatment only (e.g., Tylenol or NSAIDs as needed, and warm or cold compresses of parotid gland)	Supportive treatment	• Supportive treatment • For joint pain, use NSAIDs
Prevention of transmission	Isolation at home for 4 days after onset of rash.	Isolation at home for 7 days after onset of rash.	Isolation at home for 5 days after onset of symptoms.	No specific isolation recommended —use hand hygiene.	After onset of rash, immunocompetent patients are not contagious. They can go to school or daycare center.

[a]Caution with rubella vs. rubeola (measles): as name is similar you may lose mark. Rubella and rubeola (measles) are also similar in presentation, that is why rubella is known as 3-day measles or German measles.

[b]Mumps is not really a viral exanthem (does not usually have rash), but is included here.

[c]When is MMR first given? When is it given the second time? Remember the MRS: 1-year-old CHAMP and 5 MeDIC boosters.

[d]4 Measly C's = Cough, Coryza, Conjunctivitis, Koplik spots (Koplik also sounds like it starts with the word C) 4 days of isolation at home starting from the first day of rash.

[e]MRS- Rose is always late, means rash in roseola comes late. Rash comes after fever has resolved. This is an important pointer to dx.

Clinical Case Scenarios

16. A 3-year-old girl is brought in by her parents with concerns over a rash for the last 3 days. 6 days ago, she developed symptoms of fever, runny nose, and dry cough. Upon examination, she is *febrile* and has erythematous maculopapular skin rash all over the face and trunk. Which of the following is the likely cause of this skin lesion?

    a) Erythema infectiosum

    b) Rubella

    c) Rubeola

    d) Roseola infantum

22.17.3 Scarlet Fever

Etiology: Infection with Group A *Streptococcus* (e.g., pharyngitis, otitis media, or skin infection) that produces erythrogenic toxin.

Pathophysiology: The rash is a delayed hypersensitivity (type IV) reaction to the toxin, hence occurs in patients with prior exposure to strep.

Cutaneous findings:

Diffuse erythema with papules that can be so fine that it feels like a "sandpaper" (*spares palms and soles*).

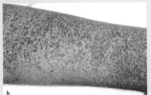

Source: Herpes Virus Diseases. In: Steffers G, Credner S, eds. General Pathology and Internal Medicine for Physical Therapists. 1st ed. Thieme; 2012

Red cheeks with sparing of circumoral area, making it look like a circumoral pallor.

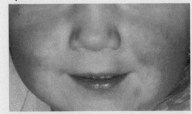

Source: Estreya at English Wikipedia, Public domain, via Wikimedia Commons.

Strawberry or raspberry tongue

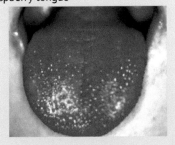

The bright red coloration and prominent papillae create a raspberry-like appearance.
Source: Diseases of the propharynx. In: Probst R, Grevers G, Iro H, eds. Basic Otorhinolaryngology: A Step-by-Step Learning Guide. 2nd ed. Thieme; 2017

Resolution phase: Skin desquamation of hands and feet (especially in face, palms, and soles)

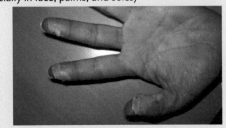

Source: Kronawitter, CC BY-SA 3.0, via Wikimedia Commons.

Management: Treat underlying streptococcal infection with penicillin or amoxicillin.

[9]Note that this is one of the few indications of aspirin in pediatric patients.

22.17.4 Kawasaki Disease (!)

Pathophysiology: Vasculitis, which is typically self-limiting.

Clinical features: Fever, bilateral conjunctivitis, mucositis (e.g., strawberry tongue, odynophagia), lymphadenopathy, and erythematous rash with extremity changes (erythema or edema of hands and feet, *affecting palms and soles*). (!)

Lab findings: Elevated ESR, CRP, ferritin ± thrombocytosis (all signifying acute inflammation).

Management: Aspirin[9] + IVIG (intravenous immunoglobulin).

Complication: Coronary artery aneurysm and myocardial infarction (screen with echocardiogram).

22.17.5 Acute Unilateral Lymphadenitis

MC causative organism is *Staph. aureus*.

Management:

Mild case (mildly tender nodes and well-appearing child)	Clinical follow-up
Moderate case (mild fever and irritability)	Oral antibiotics
Severe case (e.g., fluctuant nodes and ill-appearing child)	Incision and drainage might be required along with parenteral antibiotics[a]

[a]If coexistent periodontal disease or poor oral hygiene, empiric antibiotic therapy should cover anaerobes (e.g., clindamycin or amoxicillin-clavulanate).

22.17.6 Childhood Respiratory Illnesses

	Croup (laryngotracheobronchitis)	Bronchiolitis (infection of lower respiratory tract commonly due to virus infection)
Etiology	MCC is parainfluenza virus. **Other causes:** Respiratory syncytial virus (RSV), influenza virus, bacterial infection.	MCC is RSV (respiratory synctial virus) Other causes: rhinovirus, parainfluenza, and other viruses.
Age	Uncommon in children > 6 years of age	Uncommon in children > 2 years of age • Viral infection in children > 2 years old usually only involves the upper respiratory tract.
Clinical presentation **Both have prodromal signs of infection (fever, malaise, etc.)**	• Hoarseness (due to laryngitis) • Barking cough (due to tracheitis) ± stridor ± respiratory distress	Runny nose, dry cough (suggest upper respiratory tract infection) + wheezing (suggest bronchiolar involvement) ± respiratory distress
Diagnostic test	X-ray is not needed in a case of classical croup, which is responding to interventions. If X-ray is done, it may show the *steeple sign*[a] suggestive of subglottic narrowing.	Clinical dx. CXR might be done to rule out other conditions.

	Croup (laryngotracheobronchitis)	Bronchiolitis
Management	• **Mild (no stridor at rest)**—oral dexamethasone and supportive treatment. • **Severe (stridor at rest, or respiratory distress)**—oral, IV, or IM dexamethasone and racemic epinephrine. May need intubation if not responding to epinephrine.	Mostly supportive treatment (may use bronchodilators).[b] **Prevention:** Immunoprophylaxis with palivizumab may be indicated in the following patient groups—bronchopulmonary dysplasia, high-risk congenital heart defects, and high-risk premature infants. It is given monthly during RSV season.

[a]Tracheal air column gradually tapering toward the glottis (like a church steeple): Chest X-ray shown below.

[b]MC complication of bronchiolitis is apnea (intractable apnea may require intubation). Also, RSV infection has been implicated with development of asthma.

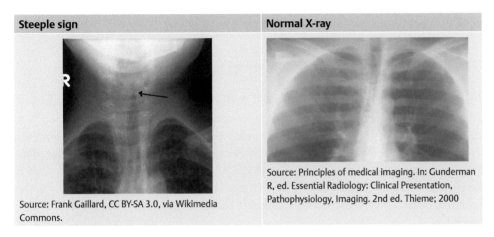

Steeple sign

Source: Frank Gaillard, CC BY-SA 3.0, via Wikimedia Commons.

Normal X-ray

Source: Principles of medical imaging. In: Gunderman R, ed. Essential Radiology: Clinical Presentation, Pathophysiology, Imaging. 2nd ed. Thieme; 2000

22.17.7 Reye Syndrome

Background: Any viral infection (e.g., flu, chicken pox) + aspirin use in children can lead to mitochondrial damage and development of fat deposition and inflammation in various organs including liver (microvesicular steatosis), kidney, brain, etc.[10]

[10]Only time aspirin is given to a child is for Kawasaki disease and rheumatic fever.

Clinical features:

Cerebral damage/edema	⟹ Delirium, seizures, and coma
Liver damage	⟹ Liver failure with elevated LFTs, serum ammonia, hypoglycemia, etc.
Renal and cardiac failure can also occur	

Management: Supportive.

22.17.8 Pertussis (Whooping Cough)

Etiology: Respiratory tract infection with *Bordetella pertussis* (a highly contagious pathogen).
Presentation: Episodes of paroxysmal nonproductive cough, which usually ends with sudden inspiration (whooping sound) or vomiting. Usually associated with rhinorrhea. Patients may develop pneumonia, apnea, and respiratory distress.
Diagnosis: Patients with the above-mentioned presentation and hx of exposure to lab-confirmed pertussis do not require diagnostic lab confirmation. If no such hx, confirm dx by doing PCR or culture of nasopharyngeal secretions or pertussis serology.

Management:
- Antibiotic treatment is recommended in all patients with symptoms of ≤3 weeks.
- If symptoms have lasted > 3 but < 6 weeks, consider treatment in health care workers, pregnant patients, and who have close contact with infants.

Post-exposure prophylaxis: Antibiotic prophylaxis is recommended for all close contacts, regardless of vaccination status.

Antibiotic choice

Age < 1 month	Azithromycin
Age 1–2 months	Azithromycin, Clarithromycin,[a] or Erythromycin[a]
Age ≥ 2 months	Azithromycin, Clarithromycin, Erythromycin, or Sulfamethoxazole-trimethoprim[b]

[a]In less than 1-month-old baby, clarithromycin safety data are unknown and erythromycin use has been associated with *pyloric stenosis*.

[b]Sulfamethoxazole-trimethoprim is contraindicated in infants < 2 months of age, because of increased risk of kernicterus.

22.18 Foreign Body Aspiration

Presentation: Sudden respiratory symptoms, distress, and/or cyanosis that usually occur after an infant was unattended for a period of time. Exam question usually does not mention a baby eating or playing with peanuts, as it would be too easy. There may be a symptom-free interval as well. Some infants may present with respiratory symptoms of **days or even weeks duration**.

Physical exam: Depending on the location of the foreign body, patients may have *localized or generalized* wheezing or stridor, e.g., if it is in the right main stem bronchus, the child will have wheezing in the right side of the lung. If lodged in trachea, the child will have stridor ± bilateral wheezing.

Management:
- In unstable patient (e.g., RR of > 30/min), NSIM is intubation.
- In stable patient, NSIM is inspiratory and expiratory CXR (chest X-ray) first. If the foreign body is radio-opaque dx becomes easy. If it is not radiopaque, it may just show nonspecific findings such as little change in thoracic cavity with inspiration.

If the foreign body is seen in chest X-ray, or there is probability of foreign body aspiration (e.g., classical hx, even if CXR unremarkable)	Rigid bronchoscopy (foreign body can be removed with rigid bronchoscope)
Medium probability of foreign body aspiration	Chest CT scan or diagnostic flexible bronchoscopy

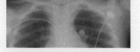

Source: Pathology.
In: Gunderman R, ed.
Essential Radiology: Clinical
Presentation, Pathophysiology,
Imaging. 2nd ed. Thieme; 2000

Clinical Case Scenarios

17. A 2-year-old boy is brought in by his mother with a fever of 103°F. He is having a seal bark cough. Physical exam reveals lymphadenopathy and stridor. X-ray image shown in left-hand side. After providing supportive care, what is the next best step in management?

    a) Intubate

    b) Oral steroids + racemic norepinephrine

    c) Nasopharyngeal swab

    d) Laryngoscopy

18. A 5-year-old child presents with few days history of lethargy and confusion. LFTs reveal high liver enzymes. 1 week ago, he had a flu-like infection and joint pain. He was staying with grandmother at that time and she had given him some over-the-counter painkillers. What is the likely dx?

22.19 Pediatric Genitourinary Conditions

22.19.1 Urinary Tract Infection (UTI)

Presentation: Infants can present with fever, increased irritability ± signs of sepsis (e.g., conjugated hyperbilirubinemia).[11]

How to obtain urine sample?

- In children wearing diapers or who are not toilet-trained, NSIM is straight catheterization of urethra to obtain sterile specimen.
- In older children, NSIDx is clean-catch urine sample.

[11]UTI is the MCC of fever in small children without obvious source.

Age	Management	
< 2 months	• Hospitalize, obtain blood-urine cultures, and give IV antibiotics (e.g., ampicillin + gentamicin).	Also, renal bladder US is indicated. If renal US is abnormal, NSIDx is voiding cystourethrogram (VCUG).
≥ 2 months and < 2 years	• Hospitalization is not indicated for uncomplicated UTI. **Oral cephalosporin** (e.g., cephalexin or cefixime) is 1st line agent.	
≥ 2 years	• **Oral cephalosporin** (e.g., cephalexin or cefixime) • Renal-bladder US is not indicated for the first episode of *uncomplicated* UTI.	

Indications for renal imaging in pediatric UTI

Clinical situation	Is renal and bladder US recommended?	Indication for VCUG[a]
Single episode of febrile UTI < 2 years of age	YES	VCUG is recommended only in patients with **abnormal** renal US.
Multiple episodes of febrile UTI in ≥ 2 years of age		VCUG is recommend **in this case along with** US
UTI in any age + family hx of renal or urologic conditions, or children with HTN or poor growth		
Additional indication	UTI not responding to antibiotic therapy	UTI due to microbe other than *Escherichia coli* and fever of ≥ 39°C (102.2°F).

[a]How VCUG (voiding cystourethrogram) is performed? Radio-contrast material is instilled into the bladder via a urinary catheter and subsequent X-rays are taken.

> ### 🔍 Clinical Case Scenarios

19. An 18-month-old child had a first episode of uncomplicated UTI 1–2 weeks ago. She is here for follow-up. She is currently asymptomatic and has no other problems. What is the NSIM?

    a) Do nothing

    b) Renal and bladder US

    c) VCUG

    d) CT scan of abdomen and pelvis

20. Renal and bladder US show mild right-sided hydronephrosis. What is the NSIM?

22.19.2 Vesicoureteral Reflux (VUR)

Definition: Backward flow of urine from bladder, ranging from mild (normal ureters with no or minimal dilation) to severe (ureters are dilated and tortuous). VUR increases risk of infection and subsequent renal scarring and can lead to chronic kidney disease and hypertension.

Diagnosis: Made with VCUG.

Management: Mild cases require observation and/or prophylactic antibiotic therapy. Surgery may be needed in severe cases or breakthrough UTIs despite prophylactic antibiotics.

Follow-up: Dimercaptosuccinic acid (DMSA) renal imaging can be used to screen for renal scarring. If new renal scarring is found despite medical treatment, surgery may be needed.

22.19.3 Enuresis (Bedwetting)

First step is to look for secondary causes. Increased urinary frequency during daytime points toward underlying pathology:

Look for the following features	Likely Dx
Polydipsia, polydipsia or polyphagia	Diabetes mellitus
Polydipsia, polyuria (but no polyphagia)	Diabetes insipidus
Dysuria, urgency, abdominal pain, hesitancy	UTI
Behavioral changes	Psychological stress

If none of the above present, look at the age of the patient:

Age < 5 years	Bedwetting can be normal in this age.
	NSIM: Reassurance and education on toilet-training methods.
Age ≥ 5 years	Further workup may include screening urinalysis and voiding diary.

Management of enuresis in patients ≥ 5 years, with no underlying secondary etiology:

First SIM	Use positive reinforcement for not wetting the bed (e.g., sweet treat like lollilops), and minimize fluid intake at evening/night time.
Second SIM	If enuresis persists despite the above, NSIM is to use enuresis alarm (a special moisture sensor placed in the child's gown which triggers an alarm to go off at the start of urination)
Third SIM	If above fails, use oral desmopressin (**drug of choice**).
	Second choice is tricyclic antidepressants (e.g., imipramine, amitriptyline)

22.19.4 Posterior Urethral Valve

Etiology: Obstructing membranous folds in the posterior urethra due to abnormal development.

Pathophysiology and clinical presentation:

- **Severe obstruction** can present as early as in utero with the following pathophysiology:

Bladder outlet obstruction → decreased urine output → severe oligohydramnios (absence of protective cushioning effect of amniotic fluid) → potter effects (flat facies, clubbed foot, pulmonary hypoplasia which may present as acute respiratory distress in newborn)
Bladder outlet obstruction → bladder distention → bilateral hydroureter and hydronephrosis → obstructive renal failure

- **Mild obstruction** can present later with bladder outlet obstructive symptoms or recurrent UTI in a young infant.

Dx: Voiding cystourethrogram.

Management: Ablation of valve or urinary diversion.

22.20 Renal Tumors and Differential Diagnosis

	Wilms' tumor (nephroblastoma)	Neuroblastoma
Background	• MC **renal or abdominal** malignancy in children • Occurs in children < 10 years of age	• Tumor arising from neural crest cells – From **adrenal** = adrenal mass – From paravertebral **sympathetic** ganglia = paraspinal mass • It is the MC malignancy in **infants** and MC extracranial solid cancer in **childhood.**[a]
Clinical presentation	Asymptomatic abdominal mass, hematuria, and/or HTN	Presentation can be different depending on the location, spread, and neuroendocrine secretion • It can present with abdominal mass. • It can present with the following paraneoplastic syndromes: – **VIP secretion:** features similar to VIPoma (watery diarrhea) – **Opsoclonus-myoclonus-ataxia syndrome:** dancing eyes, myoclonus of extremities, and/or ataxia – **Can secrete catecholamines:** usually mild HTN, but rarely can cause pheochromocytoma-like presentation
Diagnostic test	**First step:** Abdominal US **Second step:** CT or MRI of chest/abdomen (for staging purposes)	• **For abdominal mass,** the first step is usually abdominal US. Then obtain biopsy of mass. • Also test for urinary homovanillic acid (HVA) and vanillylmandelic acid (VMA)—these are typically increased. • **Staging tests**—MIBG[b] scan, CT or MRI, and bone marrow biopsy.
Treatment	Nephrectomy and chemotherapy ± radiation	Based on histology and staging
Additional points	Associated with the following conditions: • **WAGR syndrome** = **W**ilms' tumor, **A**niridia (no iris), **G**enitourinary anomalies, mental **R**etardation [MRS-2] • **Beckwith–Wiedemann syndrome.**[c, MRS-2] (In these syndromes, recommend serial abdominal US to screen for Wilms)	Pathophysiology is similar to pheochromocytoma, but notable differences are: • Neuroblastoma does not usually present with palpitations, HTN, etc. • Pheochromocytoma is more likely to be benign, and neuroblastomas are more likely to be malignant.

[a]MC malignancy in children in ALL (acute lymphoblastic leukemia).

[b]Radio-labelled MIBG is an analog of norepinephrine, so it selectively concentrates in sympathetic nerve tissue.

[c]**Beckwith–Wiedemann syndrome.**

Pathology: Mutation in a portion of chromosome 11 encoding insulin-like growth factor, which leads to increased growth and risk of neoplasm.

Clinical features: Macrosomia, macroglossia, hemihyperplasia/hemihypertrophy (one side of body is bigger than the other side), and umbilical hernia or omphalocele.

MRS

[MRS-2]In "W" we can see 11: W = 11. **W**AGR, **W**iedemann, and **W**ilms are associated with abnormalities in chromosome **11**.

22.21 Pediatric Musculoskeletal Pathology

Newborn foot deformity	Condition	Management
Note: Only the anterior part of the foot is affected (metatarsals).	**Metatarsus adductus** • MC foot deformity **Pathology:** In utero compression, due to reasons such as small primigravid uterus, breech position, oligohydramnios, etc.	• Almost all cases resolve spontaneously, so NSIM is reassurance. • Rarely splinting might be needed.
	Positional calcaneovalgus deformity **Description:** Hyperdorsiflexion of foot with hind foot (calcaneus) touching the ground (calcaneo deformity) • Valgus = outward deviation of foot	• Resolves spontaneously • Rarely splinting might be needed
Equinus deformity	**Clubfoot (talipes equinovarus)** **Description:** • Equino = horse-like, i.e., only the front part of the foot touches the ground • Talipes = twisted foot • Varus = inwardly twisted foot	NSIM: Casting and bracing. If conservative treatment fails, do surgical correction.

22.21.1 Hip Joint Exam[12]

[12]Screen for developmental dysplasia in all newborns, and up until the child walks normally.

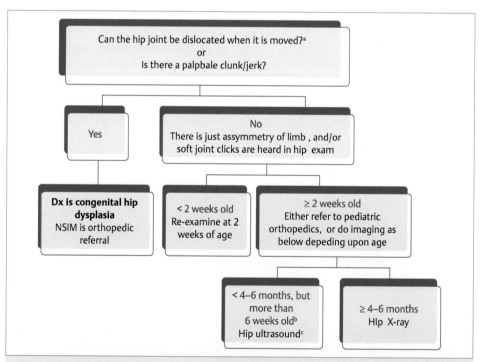

^aThat means Barlow test is positive. Ortolani maneuver is when the dislocated hip can be easily reduced.

^bIf age is < 6 weeks, schedule US at 6–8 weeks of age, as US can be false positive in < 6-week-old infant.

^cX-ray is not helpful in this age (< 4–6 months), as the ossification process is not complete yet.

22.21.2 Congenital Hip Dysplasia (Developmental Dysplasia of the Hip)

Cause: Multifactorial (laxity of ligaments, mechanical injury, etc.).
Risk factors: Female sex, breech position, tight lower-extremity swaddling, family hx, etc.
Diagnosis: Generally made by physical exam and radiological imaging (as shown on previous page).
Management:

Patient group		Management
0–1.5 years	Dislocated but reducible hip	Abduction splinting (known as Pavlik harness)
	Dislocated and nonreducible	Reduction (closed or open) and casting
> 1.5 to 4 years of age		Usually open reduction is required + casting
> 4 years old		Poor prognosis Reduction with constructive osteotomy may be needed.

22.21.3 Pediatric Diseases of Hip and Knee

	Osgood–Schlatter disease	Legg–Calve– Perthes disease	Slipped capital femoral epiphysis (SCFE)
Background	It is a benign self-limiting condition due to overuse and/or repetitive strain of quadriceps muscle, resulting in traction phenomenon at its point of insertion in tibial tubercle.	Idiopathic avascular necrosis of femoral head in children. • More common in males than females	Major risk factor is obesity. Other risk factors include growth hormone or sex hormone abnormality, and hypothyroidism.
Clinical presentation (age helps a lot in differentiating)	Age-group: adolescent male Patellar tendon • Location of pain is in the red-circle shown above (at the area of patellar tendon insertion where tibial tubercle is). This pain worsens with activity. • Edema and tenderness over that area may be present. It may also have a palpable soft-tissue mass.	• Presents in **3–12** years of age with *slowly progressive* groin pain and limping[a] • Can be *bilateral*	Presents in early adolescence and can be **bilateral** • Classic presentation: **Acute** painful limp and inability to bear weight on affected extremity ± hx of minor trauma. • Sometimes they can present with hx of months of hip or knee pain[a]
Diagnosis	Dx is made on clinical grounds. • X-ray is done in atypical symptoms such as pain at night or rest, or in acute onset after trauma.	• X-ray is first step but might be normal earlier in the disease course. • Best test is MRI or bone scan.	• Plain X-ray is often enough to see the slipped disc.
Management	Conservative measures (ice after activity, NSAIDs as needed and exercises to strengthen knee muscles)	• Non-weight bearing in affected leg. • Splinting, or surgery.	NSIM is non-weight bearing in affected leg. Definitive treatment: internal fixation (if left untreated, can lead to avascular necrosis of femoral head)

[a]Hip pathology can present with referred pain to anterior thigh or knee. Some patients with hip pathology can present *only* with knee or thigh pain.

22.21.4 Growing Pains

Background: Nonpathologic lower extremity pain of unknown etiology that occurs in children.

Presentation: Pain in thighs, calves, or knees, mostly in evenings or at night and not present in the morning and does not interfere with sleep. Patients can also have abdominal pain or headaches.[13]

Exam is normal, and activity is not affected.

Rx: Reassurance, and inquire about any source of significant stress for the child (especially in children with coexistent headaches and stomach pain).

[13]Similar to fibromyalgia or tension headaches in adults.

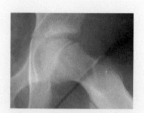

Source: Creative Commons CC0 License.

> ### Clinical Case Scenarios
>
> 21. A 12-year-old boy comes in with his mother, limping on a side. This has been going on for months. The boy reports pain in the left knee area. The pediatrician orders an X-ray of the knee and hip. X-ray of hip is shown below. What is the likely diagnosis?
>
>   a) Legg–Calve–Perthes disease
>
>   b) Slipped capital femoral epiphysis
>
>   c) Osgood–Schlatter disease
>
>   d) Developmental dysplasia of the hip

22.21.5 Acute Monoarthritis in Pediatric Population

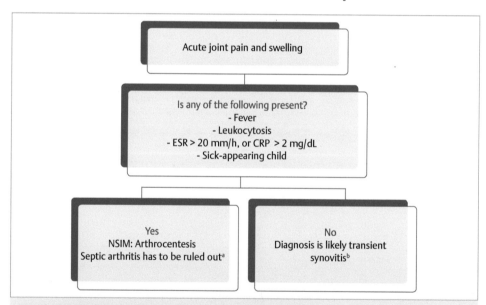

[a]See Chapter 8, section of septic arthritis for further management.

[b]**Transient synovitis** is inflammatory synovitis associated with concurrent viral infection or recent immunization. Patients can usually bear weight, but limp while walking. Treat with NSAIDs as needed. It is a benign and self-limiting condition.

22.21.6 Osteogenesis Imperfecta

Background: Autosomal dominant inheritance of connective tissue disorder with defect in type I collagen.

Clinical features: Osteopenia, recurrent fractures, blue sclera,[14] generalized hypotonia, opalescent (translucent) teeth, etc.

[14]Thinning of sclera allows underlying epithelium to show through. Other causes of thin (blue) sclera:
- Marfan syndrome
- Ehler–Danlos syndrome
- Long-term steroid use (acquired)

22.22 Pediatric Neurology

22.22.1 Febrile Seizures

Simple febrile seizure	Complex febrile seizure
Diagnostic criteria: All the following should be present	Any of the following:
• Seizure lasts < 15 minutes	• Focal onset (e.g., shaking of one side of body)
• No more than 1 seizure episode in 24 hours	• Seizure lasts > 15 minutes
• Seizure types can be generalized tonic-clonic, atonic, or tonic spells (but not focal)	• More than one episode in 24 hours
If all of the above present, no indication for any diagnostic work-up except to search for underlying cause of illness.	Consider MRI and/or EEG
• If completely asymptomatic and has concurrent viral upper respiratory tract infection (URTI)-like symptoms, may not need further testing.	
• If no foci of infection identified, do urinalysis.	

Lumbar puncture is indicated if any of the following is present:

• Meningeal signs.
• Infants 6–12 months of age, with no hx of immunization for *Haemophilus influenzae* or *Streptococcus pneumoniae.*
• Seizure while on antibiotics, which can mask signs of meningitis.
• Seizure occurring after the second day of febrile illness (simple febrile seizures usually occur in the first day of febrile illness).

22.22.2 Cerebral Palsy

Background: Abnormality in brain development due to injury in early days of life. It can result from different causes, including prematurity (most important), in utero exposure to alcohol, vascular insufficiency, toxin, infection, complicated labor, and delivery, etc.

Clinical presentation with various subtypes of cerebral palsy:

In the first few months of life, all subtypes present with *hypotonia*. The following specific features typically develop only after few months:	
Spastic type (look for upper motor neuron signs)	• Spasticity, clonus, and contractures • Diplegia (bilateral lower extremity is more affected than upper extremity), hemiplegia, or quadriplegia. • Varus and/or valgus deformities can ensue with development of orthopedic issues, such as hip dysplasia.
Dyskinetic	• Abnormal repetitive movements or dystonic episodes develop later
Ataxic	• Later ataxic movements are more apparent
Most patients have varying degrees of different brain function abnormalities, such as intellectual disability, speech–language disorder, behavioral–emotional instability, seizure disorder, and visual or hearing issues.	

Diagnostic test: MRI scan.

Management: Supportive care for activities of daily living. Antispasmodics such as botulinum toxin may help.

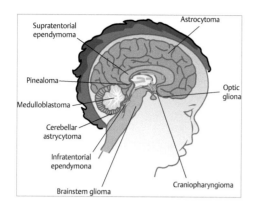

22.22.3 Pediatric Intracranial Malignancies

Posterior Fossa Tumors

MC intracranial location of brain tumor in children is posterior fossa, which includes cerebellum, brain stem, and ventricles. These tumors are more likely to cause obstructive hydrocephalus due to its proximity to ventricular outflow tract.

Benign astrocytoma (e.g., cerebellar astrocytoma)	MC intracranial tumor
Medulloblastoma	MC pediatric **malignant** intracranial tumor Typically arise from middle of cerebellum
Brain stem glioma	Can cause sudden dramatic focal neurological deficits because of its location
Infratentorial ependymoma	Commonly cause hydrocephalus

Supratentorial Tumors (area of brain above cerebellum)

MRS

Pinealoma – 3 Ps

Pinealoma (tumor of pineal gland)	**Presentation:** paralysis of upward gaze (**P**arinaud syndrome), **P**tosis, **P**recocious puberty
Craniopharyngioma	Arise from sella turcica **Presentation:** Visual defects ± hypopituitarism **Finding in imaging:** Suprasellar cystic area with calcifications

Neurocutaneous Syndromes

MRS

Sturge—**SUMs** up the price of port-wines

MRS

Tuberous **S**clerosis is associated with several types of **S**kin rash (including **S**ebaceum adenoma) and **S**everal types of intra- and extracranial tumors.

Condition	Cutaneous manifestation	Neurological issues
Sturge–Weber syndrome	"Port-wine stain" rash (due to hemangioma) in the trigeminal nerve area Source: Infectious diseases. In: Biousse V, Newman N, eds. Neuro-Ophthalmology Illustrated. 1st ed. Thieme; 2009	**S**eizures **M**ental retardation **U**nilateral focal neurological deficit may be present (hemianopia, hemisensory deficit, and/or hemiparesis)
Tuberous sclerosis (autosomal dominant)	**Adenoma sebaceum:** (Adenoma is a misnomer as these are angiofibromas). Can be misdiagnosed as noninflammatory acne Source: Phacomatoses. In: Biousse V, Newman N, eds. Neuro-Ophthalmology Illustrated. 2nd ed. Thieme; 2015 Other types of skin rash can also be present	Various kinds of tumors in multiple organs. For example, • In brain (hamartomas, subependymal tumors, astrocytomas, etc.), • In kidney (angiomyolipoma)

Condition	Cutaneous manifestation	Neurological issues
Neurofibromatosis	• Cutaneous neurofibromas • Café-au-lait spots 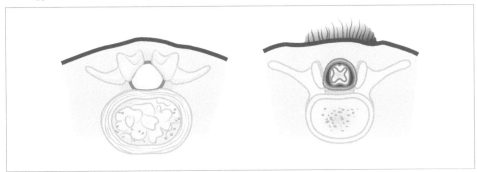 (a) Café-au-lait macule. (b) Multiple neurofibromas. Source: Neurofibromatosis 1 (NF1). In: Sterry W, Paus R, Burgdorf W, eds. Thieme Clinical Companions: Dermatology. 1st ed. Thieme; 2006	**Type I neurofibromatosis** • Optic nerve gliomas (look for papilledema and vision loss) • Lisch nodules (seen as brown spots in iris) **Type II neurofibromatosis** • Bilateral vestibular schwannomas • Meningioma or gliomas

 MRS

ONE POLAND
ONE = NF 1
Papilledema due to
PO = **OP**tic nerve glioma
Lisch nodules
AD = autosomal dominant
N - NF

MRS

Type II (2) has two-sided acoustic neuroma (i.e., bilateral)

22.22.4 Spina Bifida

Etiology: Failure of fusion of posterior vertebral arch, during fetal development.

Types	Spina bifida occulta	Meningocele	Myelomeningocele
Definition	• Without herniation • Look for tuft of hair at the back	Herniation of only meninges	Herniation of spinal cord along with meninges
Presentation	• Scoliosis • Back pain • Lower-body neurological dysfunction (e.g., bowel/bladder dysfunction, lower extremity weakness, numbness) These features tend to be more severe and frequent in higher grade spina bifida, but can also occur in occulta.		
Association	Spina bifida is associated with Arnold–Chiari type II malformation (downward shifting of brain through the bottom of the skull). This increases risk of coexistent hydrocephalus.		

Diagnosis: Often made prenatally with ultrasound. AFP is typically elevated. Amniocentesis is performed to rule out genetic disorders.

Management: Supportive+/- surgery. Myelomeningocele requires surgical correction. For high-grade spina bifida, in utero surgery to repair the baby's spinal cord can be done before birth.

22.22.5 Differential dx of Acute-Onset Flaccid Paralysis in Children

	Guillain–Barre syndrome	Foodborne botulism	Infantile botulism (< 1 year)
Etiology	Autoimmune destruction of myelinated peripheral nerves incited commonly by infection (e.g., *Campylobacter jejuni* diarrhea)	Ingestion of **preformed** *Clostridium botulinum* **toxin** • Can occur in outbreaks, due to home-canned foods[a]	Ingestion of **botulinum spore** • Can have history of ingestion of high-risk foods such as honey • Ingestion of environmental dust or soil contaminated with botulinum spores can also occur[a]
Presentation All may present with the following: • Poor muscle tone • Absent deep tendon reflexes • Floppy infant	*Ascending* flaccid paralysis (i.e., weakness begins in feet and legs)	Acute-onset weakness that initially involves small muscles of eyes and face (ptosis, poor gag reflex, etc.). Then it starts involving bigger muscles. • *Descending* flaccid paralysis	
Management	In significant disease (e.g., nonambulatory status), use IV immunoglobulin or plasmapheresis.	For severe or high-risk cases, administer botulinum antitoxin (immunoglobulin) • < 1-year-old—use human-derived antitoxin • > 1-year-old—use horse-derived antitoxin[b] Antibiotics are not recommended for foodborne botulism, because it can lead to increased lysis of bacteria and release of toxins.	

[a]In adults, additional causes include poorly prepared concentrated cosmetic Botox toxin and wound infection due to heroine injections contaminated with botulinum spores.

[b]Horse-derived antitoxin given to infants has been associated with lifelong sensitivity to equine antigens. In > 1-year-olds, horse-derived antitoxin can be safely given and is less cost-prohibitive than human-derived.

 MRS

Human infant: i.e., infants need human-derived antitoxin.

22.23 Genetic Disorders

22.23.1 Inherited Muscular Dystrophies

	Myotonic dystrophy	Duchenne muscular dystrophy	Becker dystrophy
Genetics (Gold standard of diagnosis for these disorders is genetic testing.)	Autosomal dominant transference of abnormal number of nucleotide repeats.	X-linked transference of mutation in dystrophin gene, leading to muscle degeneration and replacement by fibrous tissue.	
		Dystrophin protein is *absent*.	Dystrophin protein is *reduced*.
Clinical presentation All the following may have elevated creatine kinase (a muscle enzyme).	Can present at any point in life depending upon severity (in infants or in adults) • Progressive weakness • Myotonia (slowed relaxation)	• Pseudohypertrophy of calf muscle (due to fibrous replacement) • Proximal leg weakness (patients typically use hands to stand up; this is known as Gowers' sign)	Weakness is less severe than in Duchenne.

	Myotonic dystrophy	Duchenne muscular dystrophy	Becker dystrophy
Other notable features	• Cataract • Testicular atrophy • Receding hairline • Arrhythmias [MRS-3]	Cardiomyopathy	
Prognosis	MCC of death is due to heart failure or respiratory failure.	• Will end up being wheelchair bound *by adolescence* • Death by age of 20–30 due to heart failure or respiratory failure (diaphragmatic muscle involvement)	• Better prognosis than Duchenne • Death by age 40–50

22.23.2 Friedreich's Ataxia

Background: MC form of hereditary ataxia. It is an autosomal recessive disorder due to inheritance of abnormal number of trinucleotide repeats.[15]

Timing of presentation: Varying degrees of severity that may present anytime during life, even at 2 years of age. (!)

Presentation: Spinocerebellar degeneration with cerebellar symptoms (ataxia, dysarthria, etc.) and dorsal spinal column involvement (loss of proprioception). It is one of the many forms of spinocerebellar ataxia.[MRS-4]

Prognosis: MCC of death is heart failure, as these patients usually have associated hypertrophic cardiomyopathy.[MRS-4] There is also increased risk of diabetes.

[15]**Genetic disease due to trinucleotide repeats**
- Increased number of repeats of three nucleotides occurring in a consecutive fashion in a chromosome—e.g., (CTG-CTG-CTG-CTG)^n
- **Examples:** Friedreich's ataxia, Huntington disease, fragile-X syndrome, myotonic dystrophy, etc.
- The more the number of repeats the more severe is the disease and earlier the presentation.

22.23.3 Fragile X Syndrome

Pathology: Inherited expansion of trinucleotide repeats in X-chromosome. The X-chromosome is so long that it becomes fragile and breaks down easily during chromosome-staining preparation.

Clinical features: Large testes, large jaw, large ears, and intellectual disability.

Prognosis: Outcome depends upon degree of intellectual disability.

⚠ **Caution**

(!) if it presents at 2 years of age, you might confuse it with ataxic type of cerebral palsy.

22.23.4 Hereditary Enzyme Deficiencies[16]

Phenylketonuria (PKU)

Etiology: Autosomal recessive genetic deficiency of phenylalanine hydroxylase.

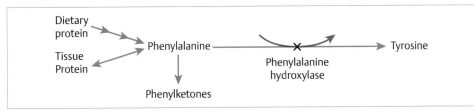

[16]Most hereditary enzyme deficiencies are autosomal recessive conditions.

Pathophysiology	Presentation
Absence of melanin (tyrosine is needed for melanin production)	Blue eyes, fair skin
Neurotoxic effect of phenylalanine	Microcephaly, seizures, cognitive impairment, developmental delay, etc.
Increased phenylketones	"Mousy" or "musty" odor of breath or urine

Diagnostic test: Serum quantitative amino acid analysis will show high phenylalanine levels.

Treatment: Omission of phenylalanine in diet.

Prevention of neurologic sequelae: All babies are routinely screened for this disorder in developed countries nowadays, along with other conditions such as hypothyroidism.

Lesch–Nyhan Syndrome

Background: Inherited deficiency of enzyme HGPRT (hypoxanthine-guanine phosphoribosyl-transferase), which is involved in purine metabolism.

Clinical features: Self-mutilation, gout, and CNS dysfunction (dystonia, choreoathetosis).

Lysosomal Storage Disorders

Disease	Enzyme deficiency	Clinical presentation
Niemann–Pick disease	Sphingomyelinase • Results in sphingomyelin accumulation in various tissues	• Hepatosplenomegaly, jaundice • Failure to thrive • Learning difficulties, intellectual disability • Cherry-red macula
Tay–Sachs disease	Hexosaminidase deficiency • Results in ganglioside accumulation	• Cherry-red spots • Mostly nervous system involvement: intellectual disability, blindness, deafness, paralysis, and seizures.
Pompe disease (this is a type of glycogen storage disease and inborn errors of carbohydrate metabolism)	Acid maltase deficiency • Acid maltase helps in breaking down glycogen	• Heart failure • Hepatomegaly (glycogen is stored in liver)
Gaucher disease	Glucocerebrosidase a.k.a. glucosylceramidase	• Hepatosplenomegaly • Anemia, thrombocytopenia • Bone loss (bone pain, pathological fractures) • A subtype of Gaucher involves CNS damage (leading to seizures and intellectual disability)
Krabbe disease (aka Globoid cell leukodystrophy)	Galactocerebrosidase	Mostly nervous system involvement: intellectual disability blindness, deafness, paralysis, and seizures.
Fabry disease (X-linked; all others are autosomal recessive)	Alpha-galactosidase	• Angiokeratomas • Burning neuropathic pain in extremities • Renal failure • Stroke in young patients

MRS

Niemann Picks a red sphinx
• Red = cherry-red macula
• Sphinx = sphingomyelinase

MRS

Niemann picks a fight with Tay–Sachs because both are wearing the same cherry-red dress.
• That means both have cherry-red spots
• Look for hepatosplenomegaly to point toward Niemann

MRS

PAM has pump failure
PAM = Pompe - acid maltase deficiency
Also, Pompe = pump failure = heart failure

MRS

Gaucher's Gluttony involves Gobbling up RBC, platelets, bone and, sometimes, even brain cells.
GLUttony = **GLU**cocerebrosidase or **GLU**cosylceramidase

MRS

Fabry is a guy's name (so X-linked)
FABRY: A = angiokeratoma, A = alpha galactosidase, B = burning neuropathic pain (paraesthesias), R = renal failure, and Y = young patient with stroke

Other Inborn Errors of Carbohydrate Metabolism (Nonlysosomal Disorders)

Condition	Enzyme deficiency	Additional info
Galactosemia[a]	Deficiency of either galactose-1-phosphate uridyltransferase or galactokinase	• Failure to thrive, jaundice, liver failure, hypoglycemia • *Bilateral* cataracts (look for bilateral white eye reflex)[b]
Hereditary fructose intolerance	Aldolase-B	**Pathophysiology:** Ingested fructose cannot get broken down and gets trapped inside cells leading to osmotic injury of cells. **Presentation:** Is like galactosemia, but symptoms only occur after infant is introduced to fructose-containing diet, e.g., formula feeds containing sucrose or fruits. (*Note, fructose is not present in milk*).
Benign fructosuria	Frucose 1-phosphate	Ingested fructose does not get trapped inside cells, as opposed to fructose intolerance. Hence, no clinical effects except that ingested fructose just get eliminated in urine.
Von Gierke's disease (a type of glycogen storage disease)	Glucose 6-phosphatase	• Liver cannot secrete glucose during fasting (fasting hypoglycemia) • Increased glucose stores in liver, kidney, and intestinal cells (hepatomegaly, renal problems, etc.)

[a]All newborns in developed countries are screened for this.

[b]White pupil (leukocoria).

Presentation: Can be detected by casual observation in obvious cases, or with a light source such as an ophthalmoscope.

Bilateral	Likely cataract, due to disorders like hereditary fructose intolerance, galactosemia, congenital infection, etc.
Unilateral	Could be retinoblastoma

Management: All children with white eye reflex or white pupil (whether bilateral or unilateral) should be referred to ophthalmologist.

MRS

Galact—Cataract

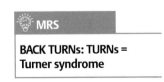

Leukocoria from a retinoblastoma | Normal red-eye reflex

Sometimes can be incidentally detected in photographs (especially when using flash).
Source: Monocular visual loss. In: Biousse V, Newman N, eds. Neuro-Ophthalmology Illustrated. 2nd ed. Thieme; 2015

22.23.5 Chromosomal Aneuploidies (Abnormal Number of Chromosomes)[17]

Condition	Chromosome abnormality	Clinical presentation	Additional information
Turner syndrome	45X	• Short stature • Cystic hygroma (neck lymphedema). In some cases, it resolves, and patients develop webbed neck. Lymphedema can occur in other body areas too. • Broad chest and wide spaced nipples • Primary hypogonadism (amenorrhea, osteoporosis) • **There is no intellectual disability**	**Association:** • **B**icuspid aortic valve (high yield) ± aortic regurgitation (look for systolic murmur of aortic stenosis and early diastolic murmur of aortic regurgitation) • **A**ortic dissection • **C**ongenital heart disease (e.g., VSD, ASD) • **C**oarctation of the aorta • Horseshoe **K**idney

[17]Best initial test for chromosomal aneuploidy is genetic testing with karyotype analysis. FISH (fluorescent in situ hybridization) is a more accurate test, and useful for equivocal cases or mosaicism.

MRS

BACK TURNs: TURNs = Turner syndrome

MRS

Kline is infertile.

MRS

ALL DOWN
- ALL Down patients end up developing early-onset Alzheimer.
- ALL males with Down syndrome are infertile.
- ALL = acute lymphocytic leukemia
- ALL = Alzheimer's

MRS

- Edward = EdEEN = eighteen no. chromosome has trisomy.
- Edward rocks heartbreak hotel.
Rocker = Rocker bottom feet
Heartbreak = heart defect

MRS

P's for Patau
Partitioned palate and lips (cleft lip/palate)
Polydactyly
Pygmy-sized everything (small head, small eye, small jaw, small body)

Condition	Chromosome abnormality	Clinical presentation	Additional information
Klinefelter syndrome	47XXY	Male with hypogonadism • Testicular atrophy, infertility, gynecomastia, and increased risk of breast cancer	Extra X chromosome appears as a dense dark staining spot near nuclei and is known as "Barr body."
Down syndrome (trisomy 21)	Extra copy of chromosome 21	Intellectual disability short stature, *atlantoaxial instability*, spasticity, white spots in iris, large single crease that traverses the whole palm (simian crease), Down facies, etc.	**Association:** • **Al**zheimer's disease • Intestinal tract abnormalities (esophageal atresia ± tracheoesophageal fistula, duodenal atresia, Hirschsprung disease, imperforate anus) • Endocardial cushion defect,[a] VSD, ASD. • **ALL** (acute lymphocytic leukemia) • All males with Down syndrome are infertile, whereas women are fertile.
Edwards syndrome (trisomy 18)	Extra copy of chromosome 18	• Profound intellectual disability • Rocker bottom feet • Micrognathia (small jaw bone) • Index finger overlapping the third finger • Anencephaly or hydrocephaly	• Intrauterine growth retardation • ASD, VSD, or PDA • Omphalocele • Poor prognosis (die within 6–12 months)
Patau syndrome (trisomy 13)	Extra copy of chromosome 13	• Cleft lip and palate • Low set ears • Extra fingers and/or toes (polydactyly) • Intellectual disability • Holoprosencephaly (brain doesn't divide in 2 halves)	

[a]Endocardial cushion defect is when the membranous defect is so large that there is a contiguous ASD–VSD and there might be a single large valve. This *is the most common heart defect* associated with Down syndrome.

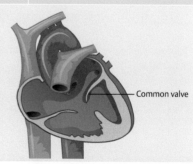

Common valve

22.23.6 Syndromes Due to Chromosomal Deletion

	Chromosome abnormality	Clinical presentation	Diagnosis
Prader–Willi syndrome	Absence of expression of paternal[a] copy of a part of chromosome 15	• Hyperphagia and obesity • Obesity-related disease—such as sleep apnea, DM • Hypogonadism and cryptorchidism (bilateral) • Hypotonia • Almond-shaped eyes	**First step:** assessment of methylation (using Southern blot hybridization or PCR)—most sensitive test.[b]
Angelman syndrome	Absence of expression of maternal[a] copy of a part of chromosome 15	• Frequent smiling and laughter • Ataxia • Seizures	**Second step:** FISH or chromosomal microarray analysis, which can detect the deletion type.
Cri-du-chat syndrome	Deletion of a portion of chromosome 5	Cri-du-chat = cries like a CAT • Looks like a CAT = look for facial deformities *(FYI—hypertelorism, wide nasal bridge, etc.)*	Karyotype • Smaller deletions may require FISH (fluorescent in situ hybridization)

MRS
- P = Prader = Paternal copy deletion
- Prader rhymes with father.

MRS
- Angels are females, so deleted gene is inherited from mother.
- Drunken happy angel syndrome: they have ataxic gait (walk like drunk people), and frequently laugh

MRS
Cri = 3 word; du = 2 word, CHAT = 4 words: 2, 3, 4,... after which comes 5 = deletion is in chromosome 5.

[a]The effects are different depending upon whether the gene deletion is inherited from mother or father. This is due to an epigenetic phenomenon known as **genomic imprinting**, where different parts of paternal and maternal copy of chromosome are silenced (through methylation).

[b]Reduced expression of maternal or paternal copy can be due to deletion, uniparental disomy, or imprinting defect. Parental specific methylation study can detect all of them, hence it is the most sensitive test.

22.23.7 McCune–Albright Syndrome

Background: Gain-of-function mutation of the gene that codes one of the trimeric G-proteins. It can lead to various effects (e.g., continuous stimulation of pituitary hormone secretion).

Clinical features:
- **P**ituitary hormonal hypersecretion and pituitary adenoma: precocious puberty, hyperthyroidism, hyperprolactinemia, etc.
- **P**igmented patches (café au lait).
- **P**olyostotic fibrous dysplasia: multiple bone lesions.

MRS

3Ps of McCune	**P**igmented patches, **P**ituitary adenomas, and **P**olyostotic fibrous dysplasia
3Ps of pinealoma	**P**aralysis of upward gaze (**P**arinaud syndrome), **P**tosis, and **P**recocious puberty
3Ps of Patau	**P**artitioned Palate and lips (cleft lip/palate), **P**olydactyly, and **P**ygmy-sized everything (small head, small eye, small jaw)

22.23.8 Marfan Syndrome

- **M** = Mitral valve prolapse
- **A** = Aortic aneurysm and dissection (can cause sudden death)
- **R** = Regurgitation of aortic valve
- **F** = FibrilliN gene defect on number FifteeN chromosome (Fibrillin rhymes with Fifteen)
- **F** = Flexible joints[20]
- **A** = Arachnodactyly (fingers that look like spiders, i.e., fingers are proportionately longer than the size of the palm)[18]
- **N** = euNuchoid proportions (unusually long arm and legs)[18]
- **S** = Subluxation of lens that is Superiorly displaced (upward displacement of lens)
- **S** = Spontaneous pneumothorax
- **S** = Skin is elastic

[18]Flexible joints and marfanoid body habitus can also occur in the following conditions:

- Hereditary homocystinuria: look for hx of stroke and *downward* dislocation of lens.
- MEN IIb: the last type of MEN syndrome
- Ehler–Danlos syndrome

⚠ **Caution**

(!) These may be confused with congenital genetic syndromes.

22.24 Drug-Induced Fetal Deformities (Teratogenesis) (!)

Background: Certain drugs when taken during pregnancy are known to cause birth defects.

Teratogen	Disease features	Additional points
Phenytoin	• Intellectual disability • Facial deformities • Cardiovascular anomalies	• Look for intellectual disability that points toward phenytoin • Look for spina bifida and absence of intellectual disability to point toward valproate/carbamazepine
Valproic acid, carbamazepine	• Spina bifida • Facial deformities (cleft palate) • Cardiovascular anomalies	
Warfarin	Nasal hypoplasia, stippling of epiphysis, laryngomalacia, congenital heart defects	
Lithium	Ebstein's anomaly = tricuspid valve is shifted downward (large right atrium but small right ventricle) and the valve is also not working properly	• **NO** craniofacial or spinal defects • Look for short PR interval
Alcohol	• Small baby (IUGR) • Small head and face (microcephaly) • Small jaw (micrognathia)[MRS-5]	
Isotretinoin	• CNS defects (hydrocephalus, microcephaly) • Facial deformity • Conotruncal abnormalities (congenital cardiovascular defects, such as truncus arteriosus, tetralogy of Fallot, etc.)[MRS-6]	

MRS

MRS-5 Nothing is large. If exam question describes macroglossia, think of something else.

MRS

MRS-6 Remember mostly face, heart, and arteries.

22.25 Lead Poisoning

Risk factor: Old house (lead-based paints), pica (pathologic craving for non-food, e.g., paint, soil, intellectual disability etc.

Clinical features: Usually nonspecific and may include poor performance in school, poor appetite, vague abdominal pain, etc.

Lab: Look for microcytic anemia with basophilic stippling (stippled RBCs). NSIDx: blood lead level.

Management depends upon blood lead level:

Blood lead level (mcg/dL)		NSIM along with evaluating for sources of lead	
10–15		Repeat level in 3 months	
15–20		Repeat level in 2 months	
20–44		Repeat level in 1 month	
45–68		Oral DMSA[a] (aka oral succimer)	
>70	With **E**ncephalopathy	EDTA[b] + BAL[c]	Immediate hospitalization
	Without encephalopathy	EDTA[b] + either DMSA or BAL[c]	

[a]DMSA = DiMERcaptoSUCCinic Acid (a.k.a. succimer)

[b]EDTA = ethylenediaminetetraacetic acid

[c]BAL is dimercaprol.

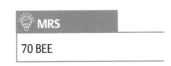

MRS

70 BEE

22.26 Vitamin Deficiencies

[19]Significant malnutrition or malabsorption syndrome can cause multiple vitamin deficiencies.

Vitamin	Risk factor[19]	Disease features
Thiamine (B1) deficiency	Diets that rely heavily on beaten rice – commonly due to alcoholism in adult patients	• Peripheral neuropathy • Heart failure (wet beriberi) • Wernicke–Korsakoff syndrome
Riboflavin (B2) deficiency	Can be due to intensive phototherapy for neonatal jaundice	Seborrheic dermatitis
Niacin (B3) deficiency results in pellagra	• Hartnup disease (hereditary defective tryptophan absorption) • Carcinoid syndrome	**4D of pellagra** • Dermatitis (photosensitive rash)—so mostly found in the neck area • Diarrhea • Dementia • Death
Pyridoxine (B6)	Isoniazid therapy	• Angular cheilosis (painful inflammation and cracking of the corners of the mouth) • Stomatitis and glossitis • Sideroblastic anemia
Vitamin C deficiency results in scurvy	Tea-and-toast diet, or eating only canned food and no fresh produce	Gingivitis, perifollicular hemorrhage, purpura, jaundice, etc.
Vitamin A deficiencya	Diets that rely heavily on beaten rice	• Night blindness or complete blindness • Keratinization of mucous membranes (corneal opacity) • Skin—follicular hyperkeratosis
Vitamin D deficiency results in rickets	Exclusively breast-fed infant	• Craniotabes (ping-pong ball like skull bones, i.e., indents when pressed and pops back to normal when released) • Bony prominences in chest (enlarged costochondral junctions) • Bowed legs (genu varum)

[a]Too much vitamin A (hypervitaminosis A) can lead to cerebral edema and intracranial HTN.

22.27 Short Stature

Definition: Height that is > 2 standard deviations (SDs) below the mean (< 2.3rd percentile) for age and gender in a given population.

22.27.1 Height–Growth Curve

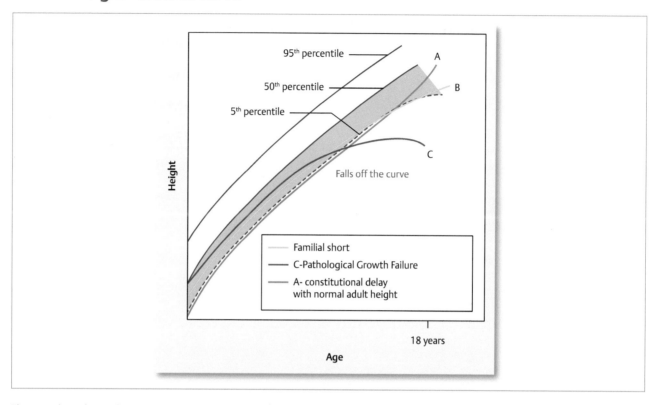

First step is to determine bone age, typically using X-ray of left hand and wrist.

	Chronological age > bone age = delayed bone development	Bone age = chronological age	Bone age > chronological age = early bone development
Normal growth velocity (tracks growth curve)	Constitutional delay of growth and puberty	Familial short stature	
Abnormal growth velocity (deviates from the normal slope of the curve)	Chronic medical diseases affecting bone development (e.g., endocrine disorder, chronic steroid therapy)	Most chromosomal abnormalities (e.g., Turner syndrome)	Precocious puberty

To make this table easy, look first at the normal growth–velocity row. These are the normal variants; learn how to differentiate between the two. Then look at the abnormal growth–velocity row and learn how to differentiate them.

Answers:

1. APGAR score is 6: heart rate of 90 (1), trunk is pink (1), coughing (2), some activity (1), and irregular respiration (1).

2. c.

3. d) Normal development.

4. Delia = 3, Maya = 4, and Akbar = 5 years.

5. Document that parents refused vaccination, despite clear-cut explanation of risk and benefit (parents **can withhold** non-life-/limb-saving treatments).

6. Patient can get the vaccination in clinic today. On the other hand, patients who are moderately to severely ill can wait until recovery to get the vaccination.

7. C. This baby is experiencing a "tet spell" due to tetralogy of Fallot, which is triggered by crying, feeding, or agitation. Placing a child in the knee–chest position or squatting will alleviate the cyanotic event. These maneuvers increase peripheral vascular resistance and left-sided heart pressure, which will decrease the right–left shunt. Note: depending on the severity of *pulmonic stenosis*, TOF can present anytime (at birth or later). Sometimes it can be detected before development of cyanosis (they are known as pink TOFs).

8. D. Based on the baby's presentation the APGAR score is 4. The MC *neonatal* cyanotic heart disease is transposition of great vessels. So statistically this is the right answer. Note that most neonatal cyanotic heart disease may have single S2. The harsh murmur may indicate coexistent VSD.

9. (b) Food allergy to cow milk and soy protein. Meckel's diverticulitis is a rare condition (look for abdominal tenderness, fevers, etc.)

10. B. Duodenal atresia is associated with Down syndrome. What will you see on abdominal X-ray?

11. A. Not likely physiologic as there is coexistent wheezing. What is the treatment?

12. B. Technetium 99m scan is the best diagnostic test to confirm Meckel's diverticulum.

13. A. Intussusception. NSIDx is abdominal ultrasound which will also help to guide the air-contrast enema.

14. B. Duodenal atresia would not present this late. Hirschsprung disease might present late but would not have double-bubble sign.

15. Upper GI series or ultrasound of abdomen can be done to diagnose malrotation with volvulus.

16. The correct answer is C. The girl has cough and coryza with ongoing fever and rash. This is rubeola (measles). It is more likely to occur in children with underlying immunodeficiency (who may have poor antibody response to vaccination), or in unvaccinated children. This is less likely roseola, as fever usually subsides when rash of roseola appears.

17. (b) This patient has croup with stridor at rest. The child's airway is not compromised to require intubation.

18. Reye's syndrome.

19. B. US is usually done after the acute episode is over (usually in few weeks), as acute inflammation may blur other findings.

20. VCUG.

21. Correct answer is b. The X-ray shows displacement of femoral epiphysis.

23. Psychiatry

One of the most powerful diagnostic tools is patient's own story of illness (history of present illness, HPI). To obtain accurate and good HPI, a physician must use open-ended questions, e.g., "What brings you in here today?" "What is bothering you today?," and "Tell me more."

Do not ask many close-ended questions, such as "Do you have headache?" "Are you here for chest pain?" With close-ended question (always of interviewer's choice), we are bound to fall into self-created cognitive traps, such as confirmation bias, availability heuristics, fast-default-mode thinking, patient-history distortions, and so on. (To learn about common cognitive traps in clinical thought process, I would recommend reading the book "How Doctors Think" by Jerome Groopman.)

23.1 Autism Spectrum Disorders (Autism, Asperger syndrome, and Childhood Disintegrative Disorder)

Background: A group of neurodevelopmental disorders, possibly of genetic etiology, seen more commonly in patients with other genetic conditions, such as fragile-X syndrome. The incidence is significantly higher in boys than in girls.

Common features:

- Problems with social communication and interaction, e.g., problems with nonverbal social cues, avoidance of socializing, not making eye contact, or hugging.
- Focused interest and repetitive pattern of activities and behavior: e.g., fixated on a toy, piano-playing, or words (repetitive use of words, phrases, grunts, or mumbles), or fixation on routines (repeats same behavior in a preset pattern).

Differentiating features:

Autism	Delay in language development and cognitive deficits
Asperger syndrome	• Like in autism, patients with Asperger exhibit repetitive behaviors, and have issues with communication and understanding social cues. • Important difference is that there is, generally, no language or cognitive impairment. Also, patients with Asperger are a bit more communicative and social.
Childhood disintegrative disorder	Unlike Asperger and autism, these patients develop normally up until at least 2 years of age, but later start developing autistic symptoms with loss of previously acquired skills.[a]

[a]Major differential diagnosis is Rett syndrome, which can have early normal-appearing development followed by loss of developmental milestones and social capabilities. Rett syndrome is due to genetic mutation and occurs only in *females*. There is also a dramatic decrease in head size and development of profound mental retardation.

Management: If physician suspects or parents raise concerns during routine visit, **NSIM** is to schedule a follow-up visit for thorough evaluation using checklist tool for screening of autism spectrum disorders. Early intervention with remedial education and behavioral therapy is recommended. In some cases, selective serotonin reuptake inhibitor (SSRIs) or stimulants are necessary, but these are not first-line therapies.

23.2 Attention Deficit Disorder aka Attention Deficit Hyperactivity Disorder (ADD/ADHD)

Background: Genetic catecholamine balance has been implicated in pathogenesis. It is more common in boys.

Clinical features: It is characterized by a lack of attention **and/or** hyperactivity. Symptoms of hyperactivity might not be present if predominantly inattentive type, or vice versa.

Inattentive features	Hyperactive features
• Difficulty concentrating on tasks or activities	• Frequent fidgeting or squirming
• Difficulty with organization	• Frequently leaving seat in classroom or at dinner table
• Often appears to not listen to peers or adults	• Impulsivity in classroom, including interruptive behaviors
• Lacks attention to detail	
• Avoids tasks that he or she dislikes or perceives as difficult	• Difficulty waiting
	• Excessive running in inappropriate settings
• Easily distractible	
• Forgetful	• Difficulty playing or maintaining play

To make the diagnosis the symptoms must be present **for at least 6 months, onset before age of 12,** and occur in more than **one setting (e.g., school and home).**

Common coexisting problems include oppositional defiant disorder, conduct disorder, emotional problems, and substance abuse.

MRS

MAD ADHD

Treatment options include the following:

● Stimulants: **M**ethylphenidate, **A**tomoxetine, **D**extroamphetamine, etc.

● Behavioral interventions which are designed to change behavior (positive reinforcement, time-out, etc.)

● Psychotherapy may be useful for adolescents but is not helpful in children. Examples include analyzing thought patterns and cognitive behavioral therapy (CBT).

Prognosis: Generally improves with age.

> For treatment of both Tourette's and ADHD, alpha agonists (guanfacine, clonidine) can also be used.

23.3 Tourette Syndrome

Background: Disorder of frequent sudden unexpected involuntary movements or vocalizations, which are referred to as tics. Tics can manifest as either motor or vocal, and patients must have both. *Onset* should be before the *age of 21.*

Clinical features:

● Motor tics usually involve the face, head, and neck.

● Vocal tics can be sudden screaming, coughing, or coprolalia (shouting profanities).

● Common coexisting problems include ADHD, obsessive compulsive disorder (OCD), etc.

● *Palilalia* (immediate repetition of one's own verbalizations) is common in Tourette syndrome.

> [1]Tetrabenazine works by inhibiting reuptake of monoamines, thereby depleting neurotransmitters, such as dopamine, serotonin, norepinephrine.

Treatment: Drug of choice for bothersome tics is tetrabenazine,[1] and other options are atypical antipsychotics. In focal motor or vocal tics, botulinum injections can be tried. Behavioral therapy can be effective, too.

23.4 Mood Disorders

23.4.1 Major Depressive Episode

Diagnostic criteria: Presence of at least 5 of the following symptoms for at least **2 weeks**, along with functional impairment. Depressed mood **or** Interest/pleasure loss should be present as one of the symptoms.

	Symptoms	Additional info
S	Sleep loss or gain	Too much or too less sleep
P[a]	Psychomotor retardation or agitation	• Motor retardation = movements are slow (patient slowly enters the room with stooped posture) • Agitation = restlessness
A	Appetite loss or gain	Significant increase or decrease in weight

C	Concentration loss or cognitive-function loss	Decrease in ability to concentrate or decrease in cognitive capabilities (pseudodementia)
E	Energy loss, or Easy fatigability	Lack of energy is the most common presenting symptom
D	Depressed mood	
I	Interest loss or pleasure loss (anhedonia)	
G	Guilt or feeling of worthlessness	
S	Suicidal thoughts, ideations, or preoccupation	Depression is a major risk factor for suicide.

^aPsychosis might be present, if depression is very severe. Mood-congruent hallucinations and delusions can develop. For example, patient can hear a voice saying, "you're worthless and you are better off dead."

Management:
- First step is
  - Review medications that can lead to depression (e.g., propranolol) and inquire regarding history of manic or hypomanic episodes. (!)
  - Screen for suicide risk.[2]
- First-line therapy:
  Psychotherapy (includes cognitive behavioral therapy **OR** interpersonal therapy) + pharmacotherapy (antidepressants).

23.4.2 Antidepressants

Drug class	Examples	Indications	Side effects
Selective serotonin reuptake inhibitors (SSRIs)	Citalopram Escitalopram Fluoxetine Fluvoxamine Sertraline Paroxetine	First-line agent for depressive and anxiety disorders	• Erectile or sexual dysfunction • May cause insomnia or anxiety • Sertraline may cause diarrhea (But generally, these are relatively safe)
Serotonin–norepinephrine reuptake inhibitors (SNRIs)	Cymbalta Venlafaxine Duloxetine	• Second-line agent for depressive and anxiety disorders. • Also useful in patients with neuropathic pain.	
Atypicals: second-line agents	Bupropion	Used for smoking cessation	• Increases seizure threshold, so avoid in patients with eating disorders and increased risk of seizures. • **No weight gain and no sexual dysfunction**
	Trazodone	Sedating, hence can be useful in insomnia	• Priapism • **Sedation**
	Mirtazapine	Useful in patients with insomnia, anxiety, or weight loss	• **Weight gain** (improves appetite)

 MRS

SPACE DIGS
- I or D needs to be present to ID depression.

⚠ **Caution**

(!) In patients with major depression, we should always ask about prior history of manic or hypomanic episodes, so we do not miss the diagnosis of bipolar disorder. Initiation of lone SSRI, in this case, may precipitate manic or hypomanic episode.

²Expression of thoughts or intent of suicide
Patient immediately loses the right of autonomy and confidentiality (harm to self).
NSIM: hospitalization (even if patient or parents refuse it).

Drug class	Examples	Indications	Side effects
Tricyclic antidepressants (TCAs)	Amitriptyline Imipramine Clomipramine	Mostly used for resistant depression	• Due to blocking effect on α1-receptors, it can cause sedation, hypotension, or orthostatic hypotension. • Also blocks M-receptors and cause urinary retention, dry mouth, etc. **TCAs have the highest risk for overdose-related toxicity.**
Monoamine oxidase inhibitors	Selegiline Phenelzine Isocarboxazid Tranylcypromine	Resistant depression	Drug–drug interaction Watch out for serotonin syndrome when taken with SSRIs Watch out for acute hypertensive crisis when taken with foods high in tyramine (wine, cheese, etc.)

Follow-up after initiating pharmacological treatment:

- Antidepressants may take at least **4 weeks** to work.[3]
- First episode of major depressive disorder: continue medication for 4–9 months.
- Second episode or very severe episode: continue for 1–3 years or indefinitely.

[3]If patient comes in after 1 week reporting that there is no change in his symptoms, NSIM is to reassess after few more weeks.

Electroconvulsive therapy (ECT)

Indications:

- Primary indication is very severe depression with immediate threat (e.g., refusal to eat or drink, immediate risk of suicide, severe psychosis).
- Severe persistent refractory depressive episode with failure of medical therapy.
- Severe depression with psychosis in pregnancy (benefits of ECT in this case outweigh the risk to fetus).

Contraindications: Recent heart attack or stroke, high-risk cardiovascular disease, unstable brain aneurysm, and intracranial space-occupying lesion.

Common side effects: Amnesia (retrograde and anterograde), muscle aches, etc.

23.4.3 Grief versus Depression after Death of a Close Family Member

	Grief (bereavement)	Depression
Common presentation	Loss of appetite, sleep and/or memory, and sadness	
Duration	<1 year	>1 year
Hallucinations	Can occur but are specific to the event and the person who died (e.g., hearing the loved one talking)	Nonspecific (e.g., hearing a voice saying that you are worthless)
Expresses "thoughts of dying"	Involves joining the deceased	Related to hopelessness (to everything)
Social and occupational function	Can usually function	Cannot function

Clinical Case Scenarios

1. Patient with hx of depression on pharmacotherapy presents with progressively worsening headache of few days duration. His BP is 190/120 mmHg. He reported going to a party and drinking red wine prior to the onset of symptoms. What is the likely mechanism?

23.4.4 Bipolar Disorder

Background: Bipolar disorders are characterized by coexistence of depressive and manic moods, which *are not attributed* to substance abuse or medical condition.

Diagnosis of manic episode: Requires persistent mood disturbance (elevated, expansive, or irritable) and increased energy or activity for at least **1 week** resulting in functional impairment

+

presence of **at least 3** of the following:

D	Distractibility (attention too easily drawn to unimportant things)
I	Irresponsibility (increased buying, gambling, foolish investments, and sexual indiscretions)
G	Grandiosity (inflated self-esteem)
F	Flight of ideas
A	Activity increased (goal-directed or purposeless)
S	Sleep requirement is decreased
T	Talkative

> **MRS**
>
> ME DIG FAST 3 graves in 1 week.
> ME are the essential symptoms.
> M = mood elevation or irritability.
> E = energy increased.

Two types:

	Bipolar I	**Bipolar II**
Criteria and definition	**Criteria:** mania ± depressive disorder	**Criteria:** Hypomania + major depressive episode **Definition of hypomania:** Irritable or elevated mood *and* increased energy/activity but does not fulfill the diagnostic criteria of mania.
Psychosis	**May or may not be present**	**Absent**
Major depressive episode required for diagnosis	NO	YES

> Major differential diagnosis is drug abuse (especially adrenergic drugs, e.g., cocaine): during drug usage patients can have features like mania/hypomania, and while not using drugs patients can have rebound depression.

Treatment of bipolar disorder:

Acute mania with agitation ± psychosis		**Mild episode:** Use a second-generation antipsychotic (e.g., risperidone, olanzapine). **Severe episode:** combination regimen (lithium or valproate + a second-generation antipsychotic)
Acute depression (!) with hx of manic or hypomanic episode		• Use a mood stabilizer (MRS) or lamotrigine. • Other option is fluoxetine + olanzapine.

> **MRS**
>
> **VAL** are mood stabilizers:
> • **V**alproate
> • **A**ntipsychotic (second generation)
> • **L**ithium

> ⚠ **Caution**
>
> (!) Initiation of lone SSRI may precipitate manic or hypomanic episode.

Adjunctive therapy: group educational sessions or CBT (cognitive behavioral therapy)

Follow-up of treatment:

• For first episode, treat for at least few years.

• For second or more episodes, do long-term therapy, or if severe, lifelong treatment.

Lithium

Pharmacology: Acts on multiple levels by decreasing dopamine/NMDA (N-methyl-D-aspartate) transmission and increasing GABAergic transmission.

Contraindications: Creatinine elevation and dehydration.

Side effects:

● Dose-dependent toxicity: Diarrhea, tremors, confusion, and/or ataxia.[4]

● Potential renal complications are nephrogenic diabetes insipidus, chronic kidney disease (due to chronic instertitial nephritis), distal (type I) renal tubular acidosis, etc.

● Thyroid dysfunction (commonly hypo- but hyperthyroidism can also occur).

● Hyperparathyroidism and hypercalcemia

[4] If patient has these symptoms, NSIDx is to check lithium levels and serum electrolytes (creatinine). After that, decrease the dose even if lithium levels are within normal limits, as these are dose-dependent side effects.

Monitoring lithium treatment: Routine lithium levels, thyroid function tests, and BMP (basic metabolic panel).

23.4.5 Pregnancy and Bipolar Disorder

Situation		Management
New diagnosis of bipolar disorder and patient is planning to conceive		Start lamotrigine
New pregnancy in a patient with bipolar disorder on these medications	Valproate or carbamazepine	Switch to other meds (risk of fetal anomalies is higher than the risk of adverse effects of switching therapy) • Lamotrigine is preferred; other drugs are quetiapine and risperidone.
	Lithium	Continue lithium • Risks associated with switching therapy are higher than risk of Ebstein anomaly.
	New-generation antipsychotics	No change

23.4.6 Milder Mood Disorders

Dysthymic disorder aka persistent depressive disorder	Cyclothymic disorder
Criteria: The following must be present for at **least 2 years**	
• Depressive symptoms that do not fulfill the criteria of major depressive disorder • Symptoms in dysthymic disorder are often milder than in major depressive disorder.	• Mood swings that alternate between baseline mild depression and period of mild hypomanic symptoms.

23.5 Schizophrenia and Other Psychotic Disorders

23.5.1 Psychosis

Definition of psychosis: Presence of delusions + hallucinations + disorganized thoughts or behavior.
- **Delusions** = Fixed, false beliefs that have no logical base (e.g., believing that your neighbor is out there scheming to kill you.)
- **Hallucinations** = Hearing voices, seeing or smelling things that are not there.

Auditory	Auditory hallucinations are more often associated with psychiatric disorders, e.g., "I hear people talking about me."
Visual	These are more often associated with delirium, dementia, substance abuse, etc.
Tactile	Very common in alcohol withdrawal syndrome, e.g., formication (sensation of insects crawling over one's skin).
Olfactory	Commonly associated with neurological disorders such as epilepsy, brain tumors, or encephalitis.

- **Disorganized thoughts**

Type of disorganized thought	What happens?	In the following example, clinician has asked the patient a question regarding topic 1 How the patient proceeds to answers this question:		
		Beginning of conversation	Middle of conversation	End of conversation
Circumstantial	Deviates from the first topic but eventually comes back to the first topic (circumstantial = circular)	Topic 1	Topic 2	Topic 1
Tangential	Does not come back to the original topic being discussed	Topic 1	Topic 2	Topic 2
Loose association	Jumps from one topic to another to another in a serially tangential fashion	Topic 1	Topic 2	Topic 3
Flight of ideas	Talkative and loosely associated thoughts with no connections (not even tangential) • Most severe	Topic 1, 2, 3	Topic 4, 5, 6	And goes on 7, 8, 9, 10, 11, 12

Other examples of disorganized thoughts:

Neologisms	Creation of new words with made-up meanings
Word salad	An incoherent collection of words, which may include neologisms.
Clang associations	Word associations based on the phonetics rather than the meaning of the word (e.g., "my spy die on a sky")
Echolalia	Immediate and uncontrolled repetition of verbalizations made by another person
Preservation	Persistent repetition of words or ideas • For example, "I love this place, place, place, place, place, place, place, place." • For example, answering "Yes" to all questions.

● **Disorganized behavior**

Echopraxia		Mimicking other person's actions
Catatonia can be of two types	Nonresponsive	No response to external stimuli in a seemingly awake person; the person can be in a weird fixed position for a long period of time and have waxy flexibility
	Hyperexcited	Excessive excited movement with no purpose

Symptoms of psychosis can be divided into the following two categories

Positive symptoms	Negative symptoms
• Hallucinations • Delusions • Disorganized thoughts, speech, and behavior • Excited or erratic mood	• Flat affect • Decreased interest • Decrease in memory and attention • Impaired executive functions such as planning or organizing • Depressed mood • Inability to socialize or pick up nonverbal cues

23.5.2 Psychosis in Various Conditions

Presentation		Likely diagnosis (given in bold)
Psychosis alone for	< 1 month	**Brief psychotic disorder**[a]
	> 1 month but < 6 months	**Schizophreniform disorder**[b]
	> 6 months	**Schizophrenia**[b]
Psychosis for 2 or more weeks + major mood disorder • Psychosis is independent of depressive or manic phase. • Either major depressive episode or bipolar disorder criteria should be fulfilled.		**Schizoaffective disorder** For example, history of severe depression and psychosis. Later depressive symptoms improve, but patient still has psychosis ("hearing voices saying that the government is spying on you").
Mood-congruent psychosis synchronous with depressive or manic phase (i.e., psychosis symptoms are only observed during major depressive or manic episode).		**Major depressive disorder or manic disorder with psychotic features** e.g., major depressive episode along with auditory hallucinations saying, "you are completely worthless." After major depressive episode resolves patient no longer has the hallucinations.

[a]Differential diagnosis of brief psychotic disorder is acute confusional states due to medical condition. These patients can have acute hallucinations, delusions, and/or agitation:

• **Sedative (alcohol or benzodiazepine) withdrawal:** Can present with hallucinations alone (alcoholic hallucinosis) or with delusions. Patients commonly have high BP, heart rate, and/or diaphoresis.

• **Delirium:** Any acute illness in old people can precipitate delirium.

• **Other causes:** Drug abuse (e.g., amphetamines—look for tachycardia, high BP, insomnia), Parkinson medications, steroids (steroid psychosis), systemic lupus erythematosus, encephalitis, etc.

[b]Differential diagnosis is **delusional disorder** (delusions alone for ≥1 month with no hallucinations. Patients are normal functioning and have no disorganized thoughts/behavior, so it does not complete the criteria for psychosis).[5]

 MRS

Brief is < 1 month. Schizophrenia is S for Six months. Schizophreniform is forming schizophrenia but not has completed the diagnostic requirement yet.

[5]At times, delusions can be shared by a group of individuals and is known as shared delusional disorder.

23.5.3 Schizophrenia

Diagnosis: Is done when patients have features of psychosis for more than 6 months without any evidence of major mood disorders.

Etiology: Is unclear and thought to be multifactorial; a result of complex interaction between genes and environment.

Prognostication:

MRS

POLiSH Females have better prognosis.

Better prognosis	Worse prognosis
Late onset	Early onset
Female	Male
Positive symptoms	Negative symptoms
History of schizophrenia in the family	No family hx
Social support is good (e.g., married)	Poor social support (e.g., single)

Antipsychotic treatment

MRS

The SAD receptors are blocked by antipsychotics.

Most antipsychotic drugs block Serotonin, Alpha(α)-1, and Dopamine receptors with varying affinity. Alpha blockade can lead to sedation and orthostatic hypotension.

MRS

Suffix +idones, +apine

		Side effects
First-line agents	**Second-generation antipsychotics:** • Risperidone, paliperidone, ziprasidone, iloperidone • Aripiprazole • Quetiapine They have better side-effect profile.[a]	• Have negative effects on metabolism (e.g., weight gain, dyslipidemia, hyperglycemia)[b] • Sedation • Lower risk of side effects related to dopamine blockade[c]
Second-line agents	**Older generation antipsychotics:** haloperidol, fluphenazine, chlorpromazine	• Higher risk of side effects related to dopamine blockade
Third-line agents	Clozapine	Risk of agranulocytopenia (neutropenia), hence only used after treatment failures with at least two other drugs.
Noncompliant patients	Long-acting depot forms of various antipsychotics are available (e.g., haloperidol, second-generation antipsychotics).	

[a]Olanzapine (a second-generation antipsychotics) is not mentioned in this list, as it has higher risk of negative metabolic effects, so not considered first line, except in cases of mild manic episode and anorexia nervosa.

[b]**Second-generation antipsychotics and metabolic side effects:**

MRS

OPQR

MRS

LIZA

Olanzapine, Paliperidone, Quetiapine, and Risperidone.	OPQR have higher risk of negative metabolic effects (e.g., weight gain, dyslipidemia, and hyperglycemia)	**Addition note:** Of the second-generation antipsychotics, PR (Paliperidone and Risperidone) have higher risk of PRolactin elevation and dopamine-related side effects.
Lurasidone, Iloperidone, Ziprasidone, Aripiprazole, etc.	They are least likely to have negative metabolic effects. However, PQR are commonly preferred due to longer clinical experience and efficacy data.	

[c]**Side effects related to dopamine blockade discussed below.**

- **Hyperprolactinemia:** Gynecomastia, menstrual dysfunction, decreased libido, erectile dysfunction, etc.
- Increased risk of neuroleptic malignant syndrome.
- Extrapyramidal symptoms (EPS) as given below:

Dystonia	**Presentation:** Sudden-onset sustained muscle contractions that may be painful and can occur in any muscle group: • Involvement of eye muscles can lead to sudden-onset extreme eye deviation. • Torticollis is a form of muscular dystonia involving the sternocleidomastoid muscle. **Rx:** Muscarinic blockers such as benztropine or diphenhydramine.
Akathisia	**Presentation:** Inner restlessness; may also present as being irritable/agitated if asked to stay put. **Rx:** Try to lower dose of antipsychotics. If not possible or still having symptoms after lowering the dose, the second step is B-blockers (propranolol) or benztropine. Benzodiazepines can be considered as the third line.
TardivE dyskinesia	May occur late *(1–6 months after therapy, or even years): tardy =late.* **Presentation:** Repetitive, involuntary, slow, purposeless movements. It usually involves face and neck muscles (e.g., repeated grimacing, tongue protruding, lip smacking, excessive eye blinking, head bobbing). It can also involve limbs, neck, or trunk. *Google video!* **Management:** If antipsychotic is required, change to clozapine or quetiapine. It **may be irreversible** despite cessation of the offending agent. • If mild and with anxiety, use benzodiazepines (e.g., clonazepam). • If focal and problematic, consider botulinum injections. • If symptoms are persistent and significant, consider tetrabenazine or valbenazine. If still problematic, deep brain stimulation of the globus pallidus can be done.
Parkinsonism	**Presentation:** Rigidity, tremors, and bradykinesia. **Rx:** First line is anticholinergics (e.g., benztropine). Second line is amantadine.

Additional meds that block dopamine receptors are antiemetics (metoclopramide, prochlorperazine, chlorpromazine, promethazine). Chronic use of these meds can also lead to side effects related to dopamine blockade.

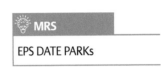

MRS

EPS DATE PARKs

MRS

+azines are antiemetics that block dopamine receptors.
I see dop of dopamine in metoclopramide, prochlorperazine, and chlorpromazine.

23.6 Acute Syndromes Associated with Psychiatric Conditions

All the following conditions may have the following presentation in common:

- **M**uscle rigidity ± muscle breakdown (elevated creatine kinase) ± myoglobinuria.
- **A**ltered mental status and agitation (patients are MAD).
- **D**ysautonomic features (e.g., high HR, high BP, diaphoresis).
- **Fever.**

MRS

MAD Fever syndrome.

Condition	Medications implemented	Scenarios of typical presentation	Treatment Discontinuation of offending medication and supportive care.
Serotonin syndrome	**Serotoninergic meds:** SSRI, SNRI, pain meds (tramadol, meperidine), dextromethorphan (over-the-counter opiate analogue used for cough suppression), drugs of abuse that increase serotonin (e.g., cocaine, MDMA), monoamine oxidase inhibitors, etc.	• Hx of depression + recent upper respiratory tract infection (implies use of over-the-counter dextromethorphan) Look for **hyperreflexia, clonus, diarrhea, and mydriasis** to differentiate from other MAD-Fever syndromes.	• Benzodiazepines • In severe cases, consider cyproheptadine (serotonin antagonist)

Condition	Medications implemented	Scenarios of typical presentation	Treatment Discontinuation of offending medication and supportive care.
Neuroleptic malignant syndrome (NMS)	Medications that block dopamine receptors, e.g., antipsychotics, antiemetics (metoclopramide).	Recent admission for psychotic features • Look for lead-pipe rigidity	**D**antrolene, **B**romocriptine, and/or **A**mantadine.
Malignant catatonia	*Not applicable*	• Look for prior few weeks hx of catatonia (nonresponsive or hyperexcited type), e.g., waxy flexibility and weird posturing • Typically occurs due to underlying affective or psychotic disorder	• First line: ECT (electroconvulsive therapy) + benzodiazepine • Do not use antipsychotics

While not a psychiatric condition, the following condition is included here, because it presents with MAD fever syndrome, and so is an important consideration in differential dx of the above:

Malignant hyperthermia **(due to genetic skeletal muscle receptor abnormality)**	Anesthetics (halothane, isoflurane, sevoflurane, etc.) with or without succinylcholine	While patient is undergoing anesthesia for surgery • *(easy scenario which gives away diagnosis)*	Dantrolene

Abbreviations: SSRI, selective serotonin reuptake inhibitor; SNRI, Serotonin–norepinephrine reuptake inhibitor.

23.7 Postpartum Psychiatric Disorders

	Postpartum blues (a form of adjustment disorder with depressed mood)	Postpartum depression	Postpartum psychosis
Timing	Resolves **within 2 weeks** of symptom onset.	Occurs within 1 year of childbirth, and symptoms should persist for at least 2 weeks.	Usually presents within weeks of childbirth.
Symptoms	Depressed mood that does not fulfill the criteria of a major depressive episode.	Same criteria as major depressive episode.	Acute psychosis + symptoms of mania or depression: • May present with waxing and waning symptoms similar to delirium.
Treatment	Clinical follow-up and support: • If it does not resolve within 2 weeks, it is considered postpartum depression and may require treatment.	• **P**sychotherapy (interpersonal or CBT) • Add SSRI (e.g., paroxetine, sertraline) if severe, or not responding to psychotherapy.	• Hospitalize • Do not leave infant and mother alone (there is risk of harm to baby) • Use atypical antipsychotics • ECT might be needed

Abbreviations: CBT, cognitive behavioral therapy; ECT, electroconvulsive therapy; SSRI, selective serotonin reuptake inhibitor.

23.8 Anxiety Disorders

23.8.1 Anxiety Attacks

Common features: All severe anxiety attacks due to underlying phobias and/or panic attacks can have the following presentation in common, which may include signs of physical **and/or** emotional distress:

- **Emotional signs: S**udden-onset intense feelings of fear/stress.
- **Physical signs** may include any of the following[6]:
  - Increased heart rate and elevated blood pressure.
  - Palpitations, tremors, sweating, dyspnea, dizziness.
  - Somatic symptoms: abdominal pain, chest pain, headaches, etc.
  - Loss of consciousness.
  - Tachypnea → hyperventilation → acute respiratory alkalosis → perioral or extremity paresthesia.
- With severe episodes, patients can also have **derealization or depersonalization** experience.[7]

Milder attacks have milder symptoms and are less likely to have derealization or depersonalization episodes.

[6]Patients can present with just the physical signs, without the emotional component of feeling of anxiety or panic.

[7]Derealization = feeling the objects around you around are unreal.
Depersonalization = out-of-body experiences.

23.8.2 Anxiety Attacks with Specific Triggers

Condition	Definition	Management
Specific phobias	• Anxiety symptoms that are unrealistic or out of proportion to an "objective" trigger. • This trigger can be an object (cars), situation (driving through a tunnel, using the elevator), or animals.	• CBT (systematic desensitization with serial exposures) • Short-acting benzodiazepines (e.g., fear of flights and impending travel)
Social anxiety disorder (social phobia)	**Duration > 6 months of the following:** • Irrational fear of exposure to unfamiliar people or scrutiny by others (talking in meetings, public speaking, presentations, etc.). Patients go through extreme measures to avoid social interactions.	• **For acute severe symptoms, use** benzodiazepines (short-term only). • **Rx:** Pharmacotherapy (SSRI or SNRI) or CBT.
Performance-only subtype of social phobia	• Anxiety symptoms only related to public speaking. • Prognosis is better than social anxiety disorder, which is more pervasive.	• If no history of substance abuse, benzodiazepines can be prescribed on a as needed basis only. • If hx of substance abuse, avoid benzos; use beta **blockers (e.g., propranolol).** These can be taken before the event to lessen some physical symptoms, which can deter a full-blown anxiety attack.
Agoraphobia	• Traditionally it was known as fear of open spaces, but a more accurate description is that this condition involves fear of being in public places where it would be difficult or embarrassing, if one has a panic attack (e.g., classroom, concert hall, park). • This might be a complication of panic attack disorder, however, may occur without history of panic attacks. • If severe, this may lead to patient being fearful and reclusive.[a]	Treatment is like panic attacks • SSRI and/or CBT • For severe symptoms that are debilitating, benzodiazepines will help.

[a]**A**goraphobia is fear of panic attacks in social places, whereas in **s**ocial anxiety disorder, fear is centered on social interactions.

23.8.3 Anxiety due to No Specific Trigger[8]

| Panic disorder | ⇒ | Severe acute anxiety episodes for no specific reason |
| Generalized anxiety disorder | ⇒ | Chronic anxiety for multiple issues |

23.8.4 Panic Disorder

Definition: Frequent severe anxiety attacks (panic attacks) with no distinguishable trigger for **at least 1 month**. This condition often causes agoraphobia, as a patient will have no foresight into when an attack would happen and therefore becomes fearful of being outside their comfort areas. Panic disorders can be subdivided into *panic disorder with and without agoraphobia*.
Rx: SSRI and/or CBT. For severe symptoms that are debilitating, consider benzodiazepines.

23.8.5 Generalized Anxiety Disorder

Definition: Excessive stress, worry, or anxiety that is hard to control for multiple issues for at least 6 months. It is often out of proportion to the stressors and leads to **functional impairment**. Women are more likely to be affected then men and it frequently coexists with other disorders such as depression, fibromyalgia, etc.
Presentation: Restlessness, loss of sleep, fatigue, inability to concentrate, irritability, and muscle tension. Acute anxiety attacks can occur, but unlike in panic disorder, the anxiety/worry about something usually heightens slowly to a peak (as opposed to panic disorder, where the attack is sudden in onset and occurs without warning).
Rx: SSRI (or SNRI) *and/or* CBT. Can combine treatment options in severe cases.

23.8.6 Obsessive Compulsive Disorder

Definition:	Examples	
Obsession = recurring and intrusive thoughts	Obsessive thoughts of needing things in the future (resulting in fear of throwing things away)	Obsession about dirty hands and germs causing disease
Compulsions = actions on the thoughts	Keeping all the things (hoarding)	Washing hands multiple times per day to relieve anxiety of obsession.

Other obsessions can be continuous thoughts and images of harm, forbidden sexual behaviors, etc.

These obsession and compulsions occur in everyday life, in a repetitive manner, and can interrupt a patient's daily life. Often the compulsions are the only way for the patient to relieve themselves of the obsessions and anxiety.

Rx:
First line: CBT of exposure and response prevention: expose to the obsessed situation and prevent the reflex compulsive behavior from occurring.
Second line: SSRI.
Third line: clomipramine or venlafaxine.

 In a nutshell

- For most anxiety conditions, treatment of choice is CBT and/or SSRI (or SNRI).
- The general rule is that if the condition is mild, we can choose in between CBT and SSRI/SNRI.
- If more severe, start treatment with a combination of CBT and SSRI (or SNRI).
- Benzodiazepines can be given for severe symptoms that are debilitating (for short-term use), or for severe disease not responsive to CBT and SSRI (or SNRI).

23.8.7 Anxiolytics

Class	Examples	Usage	Side effects
Selective serotonin reuptake inhibitors (SSRIs)	Paroxetine, escitalopram, sertraline, etc.	First-line agents for maintenance pharmacotherapy	• Erectile or sexual dysfunction • Insomnia • May cause transient worsening of anxiety in the first few weeks of initiation • Sertraline may cause diarrhea • **(But generally, SSRIs or SNRIs are relatively safe)**
Serotonin–norepinephrine reuptake inhibitors (SNRIs)	Venlafaxine, desvenlafaxine, duloxetine		
Direct serotonin agonist	Buspirone (!)	Second-line agents: typically used in patients who do **NOT** have coexistent depression.	Insomnia, agitation, nausea
Benzodiazepines	Lorazepam Alprazolam Clonazepam Diazepam	Used for short term only in: • Severe symptoms that are debilitating or • For severe attacks	• Sedation • **Paradoxical agitation, especially in elderly** • Has synergistic sedative effect with alcohol • Can cause withdrawal symptoms
Barbiturates	Phenobarbital	Not commonly used due to potential toxicity	

⚠ **Caution**

(!) Do not confuse Buspirone with antidepressant Bupropion.

23.9 Trauma and Stress-Related Disorders

The following anxiety-related conditions can occur after a traumatic event due to maladaptive response.

	Type of stressor	Duration/timing	Pathologic response	Management
Adjustment disorder	Mild: E.g., getting fired, changing school, bankruptcy.	Occurs within 3 months of initial stressor and should not last for > 6 months after termination of stressor.	**Emotional:** anxiety and/or depression that do not meet criteria for major depressive disorder or generalized-anxiety disorder[a] **AND/OR** **Behavioral changes:** E.g., misbehaving, truancy, sexual promiscuity	Psychotherapy
Acute stress disorder	Life-threatening or high-trauma event[b]	< 1month	• Distressing **F**lashbacks, memories, or nightmares. • **A**voidance of sources of reminders of trauma. • **P**ervasive depressive/anxiety symptoms associated with traumatic event. • Functional **L**imitation or impairment. **All of the above should be present.**	First line: trauma-focused CBT. Second line: SSRI or SNRI. Additionally, use prazosin with sleep disruption or nightmares.
PTSD (posttraumatic stress disorder)	Either • Experienced by patient himself, OR • Witnessed, OR • After sudden unexpected death of a loved one, even if not witnessed.	Lasts > 1 month after trauma		
PTSD with dissociative features		Lasts > 1 month after trauma	FLAP + features of dissociative disorder (see below)	

 MRS

FLAP of posttrauma.

[a]Note that criteria for generalized-anxiety disorder is pervasive anxiety symptoms for at least 6 months.
[b]Example of high-traumatic events include violent assaults, sexual assaults, witnessing or being in a bad car accident, ICU stay, terrorist attacks, etc.

23.10 Dissociative Disorders

Background: Dissociative disorders are conditions that change a person's **identity, memory, and/or perception of reality.** They are usually associated with *significant* trauma or stress (e.g., hx of childhood abuse or lethal combat).

Disorder	Clinical features	Rx
Dissociative amnesia	• Loss of memory of one's past • **Mild:** Forgetting a portion of your life (e.g., "I don't' remember going to the army.") • **Severe:** Loss of identity (forgetting who you are) • **Dissociate fugue subtype:** Loss of identity that occurs with purposeless travel. For example, family reports that the patient "just disappeared" and when patient is found, he does not know who he is. • Other working and procedural memory is typically intact; hence patient can sound very sane. • Does not fulfill criteria of PTSD or other dissociative disorders.	Treatment for these disorders can be very limited, and usually only consists of behavioral therapy (e.g., CBT) and removal of ongoing stress.
Dissociative identity disorder (aka multiple personality disorder)	Existence of two more **separate and distinct identities** within an individual. One identity typically is not aware of presence of other identities. • Inability to recall personal information of the other identity, otherwise alert and oriented.	

Depersonalization or derealization disorder	• **Isolated**ᵃ recurrent/persistent episodes of the following:
	  – Depersonalization = out-of-body experiences
	      OR
	  – Derealization = feeling the objects around you are unreal
	• During these episodes reality testing is intact
	• Does not meet criteria for other diagnosis that can have derealization or depersonalization episodes.ᵃ	

ᵃDerealization/depersonalization episodes can also occur in other dissociative disorders, acute panic disorder, PTSD, acute stress disorder, major depressive disorder, schizophrenia, and some personality disorders (**A**voidant, **B**orderline, and **S**chizotypal).

MRS

ABS of personality disorders can have depersonalization/derealization.

23.11 Defense Reactions

Definition: Unconscious processes that form to deal and/or cope with thoughts unacceptable or unpleasant to conscious mind.

Defense reaction	Description	Situation or stimuli	Response	
Reaction formation	Doing opposite of what one is **really** feeling	A recovering drug addict	Creates a campaign against drug abuse	The subconscious desire for the drug is redirected
Sublimation	Redirecting subconscious unacceptable impulse to a socially acceptable behavior	A recovering drug addict	Creates a drug-abuse support foundation	• **Against** the desire (in reaction formation) • **To a** socially acceptable behavior, but not against it (in sublimation case)

Defense reaction	Description	Situation or stimuli	Response
Denial	Denying something happened (not accepting reality)	Patient has a severe heart attack.	Patient was a body builder and after heart attack still continues to heavily exercise. (Denial that he cannot do this anymore)
Undoing	Undoing prior bad/unhealthy thoughts or behavior by doing the opposite right thing		Starts exercising in the hospital room for the first time in his life after a heart attack (patient never exercised before).
Passive-aggressive	Inner hostility is expressed in a different way (commonly by procrastination or deliberate failure)		Patient tells his wife that he would stop smoking, start exercising, and eating healthy diet but does not do it (patient agrees with her criticism, but continues to indulge in unhealthy lifestyle).
Intellectualization	Responds to a traumatic event by outlining the facts, with no emotion whatsoever.	Patient was told of diagnosis of stage IV cancer.	He talks about the treatment options, prognosis, and discusses alternative therapies in a flat-affect. (Patient is burying deep feelings with facts.)
Rationalization	Finding reasons for unacceptable behavior		He fails to follow up on scheduled oncology visits and when asked why he did not follow up, he gives multiple reasons for it.
Displacement	The redirection of negative emotions toward a new subject. It typically occurs when there is potential harm if expressed toward the original subject/object.	Boss gets angry at you; you are angry at him, but you do not show it to him.	When you come home you get angry at your wife.
Transference	The redirection of subconscious feelings, usually from the past, towards a new subject/object/group. (In this case redirection is not to avoid personal harm.)	Mother mistreated the patient all his life	He grows up to hate women.
Projection	A person has an unacceptable feeling toward someone; he/she starts thinking that this someone is having the same feeling toward them.	One is angry with his boss because of not receiving a promotion.	He starts thinking that the boss must be angry at him and that is why not giving him a promotion
Repression	Burying bad memories in the subconscious and forgetting about it	Childhood abuse	Patient does not remember anything about being abused as a child at 10 years of age.
Regression	Regressing toward earlier more child-like behavior when coping with stress	When being sick, one tends to remember their mother and sleep in a fetal position.	

23.12 Personality Disorders[9]

Background: Personality disorders are characterized by *persistent maladaptive behaviors, thoughts, and perceptions.* The patients accept these traits as intrinsic parts of their personalities and are present throughout one's adult life.

Personality disorder	Features
Paranoid	• Irrational suspicions and mistrust, often involving malicious intent from others. The patient will overinterpret many benign actions. • Unlike a delusion, the mistrust is grounded in reality and is not fantastical or overly complicated.
Histrionic	• Extreme patterns of attention-seeking behavior and excessive emotions (they often behave in overly sexual or inappropriate behavior to achieve this goal.)[10]
Narcissistic	• Patterns of grandiosity, self-admiration, and lack of empathy • These patients have inflated self-esteem and often react poorly to criticism.
Dependent	• Pervasive desire to be under the care of another person • Often end up in abusive relationships • They tend to have long-standing relationships

Borderline	• Unstable self-image and image of others
	• **Unstable self:** Emotional outburst, fears of abandonment, prone to self-injurious behavior (including suicide attempts), depressive disorder, etc.
	• **Unstable image of others:**
	  – Unstable/chaotic relationship
	  – Splitting (a type of defense reaction) is common (e.g., "You are the best doctor; the previous doctor was the worst.")

Antisocial[a]	• Disregard the rights and feelings of others • These patients **lack empathy** and often commit crime without second thoughts or regret. • They can exhibit manipulative, impulsive, and explosive behavior. • To diagnose this disorder, patient's age should be ≥ 18 and have previously diagnosed conduct disorder.

[a] Do not confuse this with intermittent explosive disorder (IED). IED is characterized by gross destruction or violence out of proportion to stimuli. However, unlike antisocial disorder, patients with IED function well in work and are not pervasive in other aspects of life.

Personality disorders which have problems with socialization:

Schizoid	⇨	• Detached from social relationships and interactions because they have **little to no interest in socializing**
Avoidant	⇨	• Unlike schizoids, these patients **have interest in socializing** but are anxious, uncomfortable, or fearful of social situations (as they have extreme sensitivity to humiliation and criticism), often to the extent that they isolate themselves.
Schizotypal	⇨	• They are withdrawn and reclusive because they have pervasive and unwarranted **mistrust of other people.** They are often paranoid. • These patients often have mystical/magical thinking and strange behaviors that fall short of delusions or hallucinations (e.g., belief in extrasensory perception such as mental telepathy)

Obsessive Compulsive personality disorder: Pervasive desire for orderliness, cleanliness, perfectionism (with excessive attention to details) and need to control their environment. These lead to *repetitive or ritualized behaviors* (e.g., hoarding and symmetry). Perfectionism may lead to problems with completing the task.

---

¹⁰**Clinical tip:** When examining patients with inappropriate behavior, a chaperone will help.

 MRS

The **C**hild who has **C**onduct disorder will grow up to become an **AD**ult with **AS**D (antisocial disorder).

MRS

Avoidant tries to avoid disappointment but wants company. Schizoid does not give a damn at all.

MRS

Schizotypals are the **weird type**s and sound almost **schizo**phrenic.

23.12.1 Treatment of All Personality Disorders

CBT is the first-line approach for any personality disorder that needs treatment. As these are innate behaviors, pharmacotherapy is often **NOT** the best approach, although SSRIs are commonly used in more severe cases.

 In a nutshell

All of the following conditions can have pathological hoarding (inability to throw away things). In board question about hoarding issues, the following differentiating points will help you.

Obsessive-compulsive personality disorder	• Lifetime and pervasive • No obsessive thoughts and anxiety (about hoarding) • Find pleasure with their task and are content with who they are
OCD	• Not pervasive • Hoarding is due to obsessive thoughts related to needing things if thrown away and these obsessive thoughts lead to anxiety. • They are also distressed by what they are doing.
Hoarding disorder	• The only issue is pathological hoarding • Unlike OCD, they do not have anxiety when they hoard. They like the hoarding process.

23.13 Eating Disorders

	Definition	BMI (look at BMI to make the diagnosis)	One's view of body shape and weight	Management
Anorexia nervosa	**Binge-purge subtype**: eating (binge) → depression or worry about having eaten a lot → purge[a] **Restricting type**: no binge/purge. They fast, diet, or do excessive exercise.	Low ≤ 18.5 Associated with pathologic features of low BMI = hypogonadism (e.g., hypo/amenorrhea), reduced bone density, etc.	Is distorted (i.e., *even though patient has low BMI*, he/she has delusions that they have high BMI and/or has continuous fear of gaining weight).	Psychotherapy (e.g., CBT) + nutritional rehabilitation. Use **olanzapine** if above fails. Hospitalize if BMI < 16, poor response to outpatient treatment, or unstable medical condition.
Bulimia nervosa	Binging → purging[a] → binging → purging, and so on	BMI > 18.5	Excessively worries about BMI	CBT + nutritional rehabilitation ± SSRI
Binge eating disorder	**No compensatory behavior** after binge eating	BMI > 18.5	Does not care about BMI	Psychotherapy (e.g., CBT) or SSRI
Even though not an eating disorder, **body dysmorphic disorder** is included here, as it is a differential diagnosis of anorexia nervosa (both have distorted body image)				
Body-dysmorphic disorder	No eating problem	BMI > 18.5	Excessive concerns about features of certain body parts (e.g., patient complains of hair loss with exam being completely normal, or has history of multiple plastic surgeries)	SSRI and/or CBT

[a]**Purge** = compensatory behavior to prevent weight gain (e.g., excessive exercise, induced vomiting, laxative or diuretic abuse, use of diet pill, compensatory caloric restriction).

 In a nutshell

Both anorexia and bulimia nervosa can present with the following features due to excessive purging behavior:

Method of purging	Associated features
Induced vomiting	• Loss of gastric acid and volume: hypochloremic metabolic alkalosis with low urine chloride • Increased risk of Mallory–Weiss tear and even esophageal rupture • Salivary gland hypertrophy and swelling (commonly parotid and submandibular glands): Recurrent damage of upper GI mucosa due to induced vomiting stimulates compensatory protective salivary hypersecretion • Damage to teeth and sometimes tongue due to gastric acid • Raw areas on the fingers or knuckles that occur with recurrent attempts to induce vomiting
Excessive laxative abuse	• Nonanion gap metabolic acidosis (chronic diarrhea) • Melanosis coli (black spots seen in colonoscopy)
Excessive diuretic abuse	• Metabolic alkalosis with high urine chloride during active diuretic use

[11]**Sleep hygiene:**
- Limiting day-time naps to 30 minutes
- Avoiding nicotine or coffee close to bedtime
- Avoiding TV or devices that emit blue light close to bedtime
- Establishing and maintaining sleep routine (e.g., reading a book in bed)

23.14 Sleep–Wake Disorders

23.14.1 Insomnia

Definition: Insomnia is diagnosed when all of the following criteria are met:

- Decreased sleep (difficulty initiating sleep, maintaining sleep, and/or waking up too early)
- Occurs despite having enough time and opportunity to sleep
- Results in daytime fatigue and functional impairment

Rx:

- First step: CBT, which includes but not limited to education regarding sleep hygiene[11] and daily exercise.
- If above fails, next step is pharmacotherapy:

MRS

Zzzzzz (sleeping)

Problem with sleep onset	Use short-acting forms: **z**aleplon, **z**olpidem, triazolam, ramelteon, lorazepam, etc.
Problem with sleep maintenance	Use long-acting forms: extended-release **z**olpidem, es**z**opiclone, tema**z**epam, doxepin, suvorexant, esta**z**olam, etc.

23.14.2 Narcolepsy

Pathogenesis: Associated with loss of hypocretin (orexin) pathway due to genetic factors. Hypocretin is an important chemical for regulating wakefulness and rapid eye movement (REM) sleep.

Clinical features: Characterized by the following tetrad:

Hypocretin is an important chemical for regulating wakefulness and rapid eye movement (REM) sleep.

MRS

- Hypnagogic hallucinations = hallucinations that occur while going to sleep.
- Hypnopompic hallucinations = hallucinations that occur while pumping out from bed.

- Excessive daytime sleepiness and when severe, patients can have sleep attacks (sudden sleep onset without warning).
- Cataplexy: Sudden loss in muscle tone and weakness, triggered by things such as laughter or emotions.
- Hypnagogic hallucinations: Hallucinations or dreams that occur just before sleep onset. ☺
- Sleep paralysis: Inability to move upon waking up, which can last for few minutes. It may be associated with hypnopompic hallucinations.

Rx:

- For excessive day-time sleepiness, use modafinil. Other stimulant options include methylphenidate or dextroamphetamine.
- For REM disorders (including cataplexy, hypnagogic hallucinations), use REM suppressing medications such as venlafaxine, fluoxetine, or atomoxetine. Second-line agents include TCAs (clomipramine, protriptyline), or sodium oxybate.

23.15 Parasomnias (Sleep Disorders)[12]

23.15.1 NREM Parasomnias

[12]Categorized into NREM or REM disorders:
NREM = non-rapid eye movement
REM = rapid eye movement

Sleep terrors	Child wakes up screaming and is visibly distressed (agitated, sweating) and inconsolable. Episodes might recur.	Child does not recall the episode the next day.
Confusional arousal	Child wakes up with mild moans, is not visibly distressed, and has mild confusion (saying "no" or "go away").	

Other condition that falls under NREM parasomnia includes sleep walking, bruxism, etc.

Management: Consider nocturnal polysomnography in children with frequent problematic NREM parasomnias, secondary enuresis, or features suggestive of sleep apnea. May use low-dose benzodiazepine at night. Also consider using scheduled nightly awakenings.

23.15.2 REM[13] Parasomnias

Nightmares	• Child can recall frightening dreams and there is full alertness upon wakening (unlike sleep terrors or confusional arousals).
	• If problematic, recommend desensitization (writing down the nightmares) and CBT.
Other REM parasomnias	• **REM sleep behavior disorder = dreams + nonparalyzed body** (e.g., kicking at night)
	• **Isolated sleep paralysis** = paralyzed body continues into wakefulness (no sleep but still paralyzed body), which is transient.
	Management: Options include melatonin, low-dose benzodiazepine (e.g., clonazepam), or REM-suppressing agents (e.g., SNRIs, TCAs, trazodone).

[13]REM sleep is associated with dreams + active eye movements and paralyzed body.

23.16 Paraphilic Disorders

Paraphilic disorders are aberrant sexual behaviors involving sexual arousal. Men are more commonly affected by these disorders than women.

Disorder	Definition
Voyeurism	Tendency to spy or peep to fulfill the desire of viewing nudity and sexual acts
Exhibitionism	Desire to reveal private parts in public
Frotteurism	• Act of rubbing genitals against another person • Considered criminal offense
Fetishistic disorder	Sexual desire toward inanimate objects (e.g., underwear, leather odors, garments, body parts)
Transvestic fetishism	Sexual desire or erotic interest in **wearing clothes** intended for the opposite gender
Sexual masochism	• Sexual activities designed to elicit pain in **partner**/s • Includes physical and verbal abuse • Can be severe enough to cause injury or death
Sexual sadism	Sexual activities designed to elicit pain in **self**.
Pedophilia	• Fantasizing about and engaging in sexual acts with children aged ≤ 13 years of age • Offenders must be 16 years or older • Is a criminal offense

MRS

Sadistic self-infliction.

Rx: First line is psychotherapy. Pharmacotherapy can be added (e.g., SSRIs).

23.17 Somatic Symptom Disorder and Other Related Disorders

Condition	Definition	Intentionally create symptoms	Underlying-motive awareness	For example, cases
Somatic symptom disorder (aka somatoform pain disorder)[a]	One more somatic symptom (e.g., fatigue, anorexia, abdominal pain) for at least 6 months with persistent worry regarding it and functional impairment. • Not explained by other psychiatric disorder	No	No	Abdominal pain of unknown origin for a long period of time with no other objective finding (no diarrhea, no weight loss)

Condition	Definition	Intentionally create symptoms	Underlying-motive awareness	For example, cases
Factitious disorder imposed on self (aka Munchausen syndrome)[a,b]	Falsified symptom generation (either medical or psychiatric symptoms) due to **subconscious motives.** Symptom generation may involve using medical instruments or medication.	Yes	No	Patient makes a cut and puts her blood in the stool and complains to doctors that she has blood in the stool. (They love taking role of a patient.)
Malingering	Falsified symptom generation (either medical or psychiatric symptoms) due to **conscious motives.**	Yes	Yes	• Prison inmate intentionally complains of chest pain to be in hospital rather than in prison. • Feigning severe back pain to get disability.

[a]**Management:** Schedule visits on a regular basis to talk about the symptoms and to develop a good relationship with the patient. As patients have no insight into their psychiatric problems, referring to a mental health clinic or CBT, before you develop a good trust relationship, will deter the patient, as he/she may feel invalidated by the doctor. If symptoms continue, after establishing trust and despite reassurance, the next step is CBT. SSRI may help, especially in patients with depressive/anxiety symptoms.

[b]Factitious disorder imposed on another (Munchausen syndrome by proxy), commonly by parents on children. If it involves child, it is considered child abuse. NSIM is consultation with child-abuse specialist and contact child protective services.

Other related disorders

Illness anxiety disorder (aka hypochondriasis)		• Preoccupation with a specific disease and the idea of having the disease, despite appropriate medical evaluation and reassurance. • Patients do not really have symptoms of the disease, or if present, are only mild. **Rx:** Same as somatic symptom disorder.
Conversion disorder (aka functional neurological symptom disorder)		• It differs from somatic symptom disorder, as this has loss of neurologic function. • Various examples of dramatic neurological presentation include sudden-onset weakness, seizures (psychogenic), cognitive dysfunction, speech and visual defects, sensation of lump in throat while swallowing, etc. **Rx:** First-line treatment is education about the condition. Second line is CBT + physical therapy.

Differential diagnosis	
Somatic symptom disorder	Abdominal **pain** + preoccupation/anxiety of symptom
Hypochondriasis	Abdominal **gurgling** + thinking **cancer** + preoccupation/ anxiety of symptom

The following categorization of psychiatric disorders is not mainstream psychiatry, but may help you to understand underlying management principles.

Psychodystonic disorders (ego-dystonic disorders)	Psychosyntonic disorder (ego-syntonic disorders)
Definition: When one is NOT aware of their own psychopathology and does not have insight into their mental illness.	**Definition:** When one is aware of one's psychopathology and has insight into their mental illness
Classic examples: Fibromyalgia,[a] somatization disorders, etc.	**Classic examples:** Depression, anxiety, OCD, etc.
First SIM is to create a trust-based relationship in these patients by scheduling frequent follow-up. If you refer them to psychiatrist immediately, they can get angry at you, saying- "Are you implying that it is all in my head?"	Patients can be referred to psychiatrist if needed; in fact, patients often request psychiatric evaluation themselves.

[a]Fibromyalgia is a distinct form of somatoform pain disorder with specific findings on physical exam (tender points). It is a maladaptive response to chronic underlying stress and commonly coexists with depressive/anxiety disorder.

23.18 Child and Elder Abuse/Neglect

23.18.1 Child Abuse

The following presentations suggest child abuse:

Unusual burn pattern	• Burns in only hands and feet or burns with sharp demarcation, which suggest deliberate immersion in hot water. • Atypical pattern of burn incongruent with history provided.
Abusive head trauma without convincing explanation	**Cause of injury:** Shaken baby syndrome, direct blunt trauma, etc. **Presentation:** Nonspecific mild symptoms (e.g., nausea and vomiting), or severe symptoms of increased intracranial pressure (e.g., altered mental status, apnea). Look for coexistent cutaneous bruising. **Workup:** When suspected, NSIDx is fundoscopy to look for retinal hemorrhages (typically seen in shaken-baby syndrome). Do CT head to look for intracranial hemorrhage and skull-bone fractures, skeletal survey and routine lab (CBC and coagulation studies)
Unusual fractures	• Long-bone fracture in a nonambulatory child • Fracture in bones that are usually hard to fracture (e.g., sternum, scapula) • Multiple fractures in various stages of healing
Other features	• Malnourished children (child-neglect) • Frequent injuries or bruises, including defensive bruising • A frightened child • Any STD in a child should raise high suspicion of sexual abuse

General management:
- The examiner may separate the child and the parent or guardian during the visit, as the child may not be comfortable answering sensitive questions in their presence.
- When suspicion of child abuse is strong, it is required by law to report it to child-protective services. Health care providers with the help of social services should assess risk of the child returning home.

23.18.2 Elder Abuse

Elder abuse is also common and serious, and often has different motivations. Aspects of elder abuse include the following:
- Physical harm to elder
- Neglect
- Financial gain for the abuser

Management: Report to department of elderly affairs.

23.19 Practice questions

In each CCS, what is the first-line therapy?

CCS	Treatment of choice (first-line therapy)
Major depressive episode	Psychotherapy + SSRI
Major depressive disorder and patient reports that he wants medication with minimal risk of sexual dysfunction.	Psychotherapy + bupropion
Major depressive disorder with significant insomnia or restlessness	Trazodone or mirtazapine
Major depressive episode with refusal to eat or drink and/or immediate risk of suicide	Electroconvulsive therapy
Bipolar disorder presenting with major depression	Any of MRS ☺ VAL = **V**alproate, second-generation **A**ntipsychotic (e.g., quetiapine, lurasidone), **L**ithium, OR lamotrigine.[a]
Bipolar disorder presenting with acute mania	Mild episode	Second-generation antipsychotics (e.g., risperidone, olanzapine)
	Severe episode	Combination regimen of lithium or valproate + second-generation antipsychotics.[a]
Acute psychosis	Second-generation antipsychotics (risperidone, quetiapine, etc.)

[a]Lamotrigine has not been shown to be effective in acute mania.

23.20 Psychotherapy

Type of psychotherapy	Methodology	Used for
Cognitive behavioral therapy (CBT)	• Identify maladaptive thoughts and responses • And then, try to change the response to a more adaptive one.	First step in maladaptive conditions such as depressive/anxiety disorders, bipolar disorder, phobias, hoarding, personality disorders, OCD, etc.
Exposure and response prevention (a type of CBT)	Expose patient to the obsessed situation and prevent the reflex compulsive behavior from occurring	OCD
Systemic desensitization with serial exposure (a type of CBT)	Patient is exposed/simulated to incremental phobic stimuli and is taught relaxation techniques during the exposure.	Phobias, nightmare disorders, PTSD
Biofeedback	Stressful situation → HR /BP increases → patient is notified of increased HR or BP → patient recognizes and learns to control the stress	Used for anxiety disorders, tension headaches, hypertension, etc.
Psychodynamic psychotherapy	Explore past relationship and conflicts and break it down	Defense mechanism disorders such as transference, etc.
Interpersonal psychotherapy	Focuses on patient's interactions with other people (friends, family, colleagues, etc.)	Depression

Abbreviations: PSTD, posttraumatic stress disorder; OCD, obsessive–compulsive disorder.

Answer:

1. Monoamine oxidase inhibitors (phenelzine or tranylcypromine) can interact with tyramine-containing foods (e.g., aged cheese, red wine), leading to excessive release of norepinephrine and acute hypertensive crisis.

24. Biostatistics

*"Lies, damned lies, **and statistics with biases.**"*

24.1 Incidence and Prevalence

	Incidence	Prevalence
Definition	Number of "new" cases/number of people **at risk** of acquiring that disease • During a specified period of time	Total number of cases (new + old)/whole population • Over a specified period of time = **period prevalence** • At any particular point in time = **point prevalence**
Use	Acute cases, e.g., incidence of Zika virus infection in August	Chronic cases only,[a] e.g., prevalence of diabetes in United States
Gives an idea of	Risk of getting the disease	How widespread is the disease.

[a]It does not make sense to calculate prevalence of acute disease.

Attack rate

● Attack rate is a special type of incidence rate helpful in outbreaks.

● Attack rate = Number of new cases in a population at risk/number of population at risk.

● For example, 100 people were eating at a Chinese buffet, and 25 people got diarrhea = the attack rate is 25%.

24.1.1 The Incidence to Prevalence Pool for Chronic Diseases

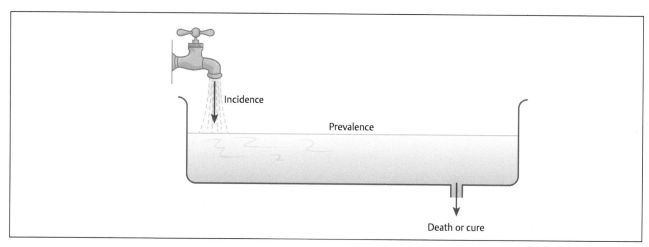

24.1.2 What May Affect this Pool?

Cause	Effect
Improved diagnostic tool	Increases prevalence as well as incidence
• A new treatment that controls the disease better, or • Improved care for chronic diseases	Over time prevalence increases with an increase in survival
A new treatment that cures the disease	Decreases prevalence by increasing cure rate

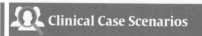 **Clinical Case Scenarios**

In the beginning of 2016, 20 out of 100 people in a small town had diabetes. By the end of 2016, 10 more people were diagnosed with diabetes.

1. What is the incidence of DM in 2016 in the small town?

2. What is the prevalence at the end of 2016?

24.2 Defining Characteristics of a New Diagnostic Test[1]

Reliability (how reliable is this test?)	Test should give the same values "REPEATEDLY."	For example, a new finger-stick device, created to measure low-density lipoprotein (LDL), gives values of 100, 123, and 145, when tested repeatedly on the same patient on the same day. **This test is not reliable.**
Validity (how valid is this test?)	Test result is compared with a gold standard test.	After some adjustment, the test reliably gives LDL values of 123 mg/dL in the same patient. However, when LDL is checked with the "gold standard method of LDL testing" it comes back as 150 mg/dL for the same patient. **This test has an issue with validity.**

[1]Reliability, validity, sensitivity, specificity, positive predictive value (PPV), negative predictive value (NPV), accuracy.

Reliably repeatedly gives the same value.

Validity is checked by comparing it with a gold standard

24.2.1 Sensitivity, Specificity, Positive Predictive Value (PPV), and Negative Predictive Value (NPV)

		Patients with true disease[a]	Patients without disease[a]	
Results of a new diagnostic test	Positive	True positive (TP)	False positive (FP)	TP/(TP + FP) = TP/(total number of patients with positive result) = PPV[b]
	Negative	False negative (FN)	True negative (TN)	TN/(TN + FN) = TN/(total number of patients with negative result) = NPV[c]
		TP/(TP + FN) = TP/(total number of patients with disease) = sensitivity[d]	TN/(TN + FP) = TN/(total number of patients without disease) = specificity[e]	

[a]Typically, new diagnostic tests are compared with gold standard tests, which have the highest sensitivity and specificity.

[b]Test question commonly asks PPV in this manner: "If the test is positive, how likely does the patient truly has the disease?"[2]

[c]If the test is negative, how likely is that the patient does not have the disease?[2]

[d]MRS: Truly sick people are sensitive. So, sensitivity is a ratio that involves only the patients with the disease (true positive and false negative).

[e]MRS: Truly healthy minds are very specific in what they want to do.

For all the following calculations, the "TRUE" value is always the numerator, and the denominator is the sum of "TRUE" and "FALSE" values.

[2]**PPV and NPV:** statistical measures of a test's ability to identify truly positive (PPV) and truly negative (NPV) states.

Tests with	High sensitivity	High specificity
	Identifies all patients with the disease, and if negative, can virtually rule out the diagnosis.	If the test is positive, it is likely to be truly positive.
Good for	• Screening purposes. • Ruling out the diagnosis	Confirming the diagnosis
Example test	Antinuclear antibody (ANA) has high sensitivity for SLE (systemic lupus erythematosus), so if ANA is negative SLE is very unlikely. But, if ANA is positive it does not confirm the dx, as healthy old people might have positive ANA, but may not have underlying connective tissue disease.	Anti-dsDNA or anti-Smith antibodies are tests with high specificity for SLE, which means if they are positive, SLE is very likely. However, if negative there is still a possibility of SLE, as these tests have low sensitivity.

Clinical Case Scenarios

To answer most of the following questions, we recommend drawing the two by two table given on previous page. Practice creating the table again and again until you are very good at it.

3. A test developed for diagnosing lung cancer has a sensitivity of 80%. There are 100 patients who actually have lung cancer in the study and 300 who do not. Calculate the total number of false negatives?

4. A 60-year-old man requests fecal occult blood (FOB) testing for colon cancer screening as he does not want to do colonoscopy. He reports that he has been eating barbecued meat, processed food, and bacon at least two times per day all his life. A detailed artificial intelligence software analysis reveals that patients with similar baseline characteristics have a 10% prevalence of colon cancer. FOB comes back positive. Studies have reported that FOB has a sensitivity of 80% and a specificity of 70%. What is the likelihood that this patient really has colon cancer?
   a. 82%
   b. 46%
   c. 23%
   d. 55%
   e. 96%
   f. 81%

5. If FOB had come back negative, what is the likelihood that the patient does not have colon cancer?

6. What is the accuracy of FOB in patients with these baseline characteristics?

7. What happens to NPV of a test as prevalence increases?

8. When a test with 12% NPV comes back negative, what are the chances that the patient truly has the disease?

24.2.2 Effects of Using Different Cut-Off Values

Let's say that we have created a test for diagnosis and that the test result has a numerical value. When we plot the frequency distribution of results obtained from general population, this will generally produce a bell-shaped (symmetric) distribution curve. Examples of such tests include fasting blood glucose, HbA1C, serum cholesterol, etc.

In the following graphs, fasting blood sugar cut-off is set at 126: > 126 mg/dL is diabetes and < 126 is not diabetes.

Imagine a scenario (graph on the right) where two frequency distribution curves do not overlap. It would have made our statistical life much easier.

Hypothetical graph:

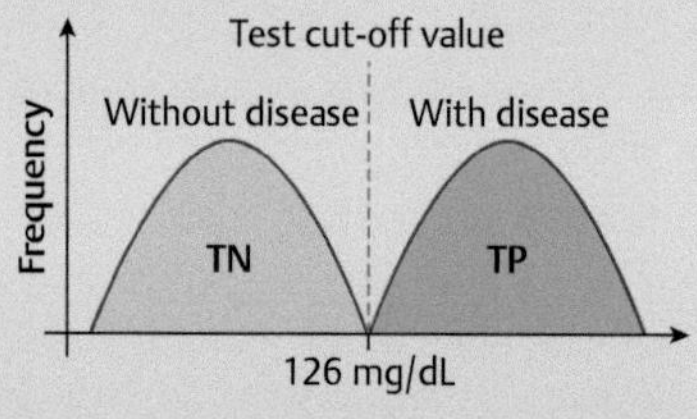

This type of distribution does not happen in real life.

In real life, the frequency-distribution curves "overlap":

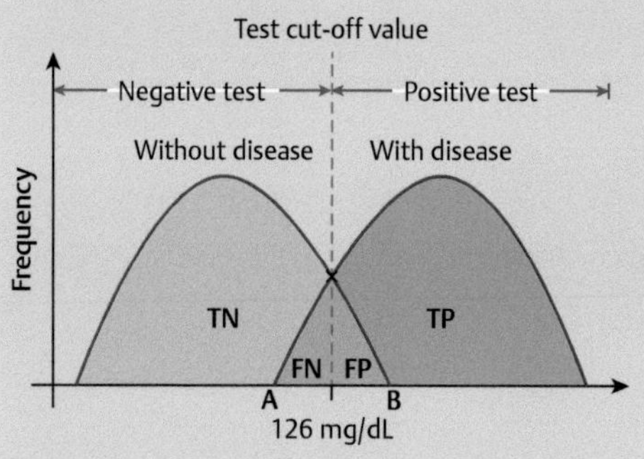

To help you understand the graph on the left, let's separate these into two:

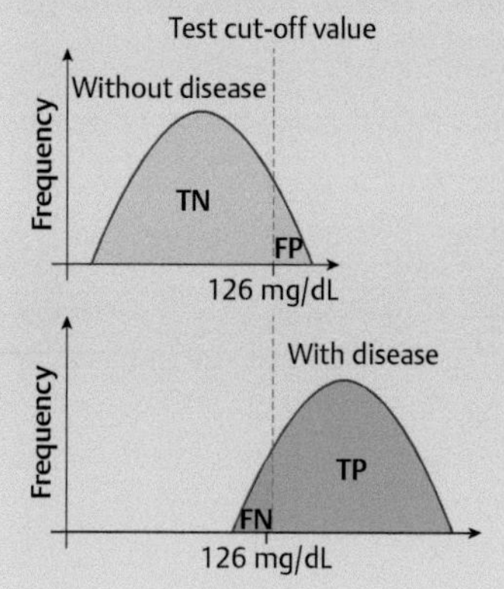

Fig. 24.1

We can use different cut-offs for the test to serve different purposes, but we need to know what happens to test characteristics when we change the cut-off:

In the Fig. 24.1 on previous page, what happens if the cut-off is shifted:	From X to A (left shift): e.g., the cut-off value of fasting blood sugar to diagnose diabetes is decreased from 126 to 100 mg/dL	From X to B (right shift): e.g., the cut-off value of fasting blood sugar to diagnose diabetes is increased from 126 to 140 mg/dL
Sensitivity and Negative predictive value	Increases	Decreases
Specificity and positive predictive value	Decreases	Increases

24.2.3 The ROC Curve (Receiver Operating Characteristic Curve)

- In this graph the true positive fraction/rate (TP/TP+FN= sensitivity) is plotted against the false positive rate (**100-Specificity**).

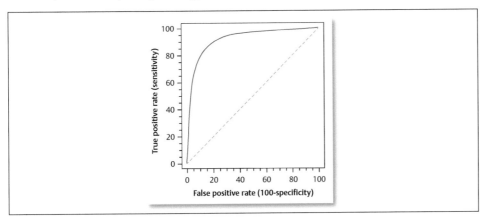

- The best test is plotted in the upper left corner (100% sensitivity and 100% specificity). Note, the horizontal axis is not specificity but 100-specificity.
- Accuracy of the test is measured by the area under the curve. The closer the ROC curve is to the upper left corner, the higher is the overall accuracy of the test.
- In the above example the red-line test has better accuracy than the dotted-line test.

Clinical Case Scenarios

9. What is the specificity/sensitivity of points A, B, and C in the following ROC curve?

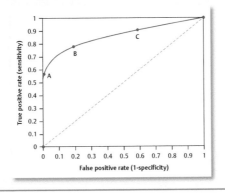

24.3 Different Types of Statistical Studies

Study designs	Observational studies				Higher standard studies		
	Case report	**Cross-sectional**	**Cohort**	**Case–control**	**Controlled trial**	**Systematic review**	**Meta-analysis**
Timing and/or type	Anecdotal	Usually surveys • Snapshot of present time	Prospective, or retrospective	Retrospective	Interventional	Overview of literature to date	
Study design and purpose	• Rare disease reporting • Case history with illustrative images, treatment, and follow-up	• Thorough surveys to identify current health problems • Typically measures prevalence and can also identify associations	• Starts with risk factor and identifies diseases • Two cohorts: one group that is exposed and the other group that is not (both cohorts are considered to be **free of a given disease**) • Identifies various effects due to risk factor exposure and natural history	Starts with disease and identifies risk factors • Case = with disease Control = without disease • Identifies risk factor/s, or source/s of exposure	• Comparison of interventions • Is the intervention effective and what are adverse effects?	Compilation of studies	Statistical analyses of data gathered from systematic review. *(All meta-analyses are derived from systematic review but not all systematic reviews are meta-analyses).*
Question posed	What happened to this person?	What is happening now?	What will happen when you have certain risk factors or exposure? (prospective cohort study)	What happened?	Which is better?	What has been published so far?	How we can merge all the data (gathered from previous studies) to create a single data?
Examples	A case report of a newly reported autoimmune condition that does not fit into other known diagnosis.	How many people have diabetes and how many of them are obese and eat refined carbohydrates?	• Framingham Trial • Hormonal replacement study of Women's Health Initiative	A cholera outbreak in United States was identified to be due to mangoes from Mexico.	• Randomized, double-blind placebo-controlled study (this design is considered to be the highest quality of evidence)		
Weaknesses (see below in the bias section of this chapter)	It is not conclusive, but helps in hypothesis generation	Cannot determine cause and effect relationship	• Attrition (loss of study participants) or migration • Selection bias is built in • Confounding bias	• Recall bias • Confounding bias	Usually expensive and time-consuming	• Publication bias (studies have shown that statistically significant papers are more likely to be put up for publishing than nonsignificant ones) • Selection bias (publishing only the outcomes with statistically significant results)	

24.4 Analysis of Data

24.4.1 Measures of Central Tendency

Measure	Description	Example data: height of 11 Martians in inches: 1, 1, 2, 2, 3, 4, 5, 5, 5, 6, 7	When to use
Mean	Average	(1 + 1 + 2 + 2 + 3 + 4 + 5 + 5 + 5 + 6 + 7)/ number of observations = 41/ 11 = 3.72	• Typically used with a standard bell-shaped distribution curve (middle picture below) • Affected by fat tails and outliers
Median	Half of the values lie above the median and half of the values lie below the median	**1, 1, 2, 2, 3, 4, 5, 5, 5, 6, 7** **Median = 4**	Use this measure when there are significant fat tails or outliers (in the left and right images below)
Mode	The most common variable/s	5 • Some data might have two modes, called *bimodal distribution* (e.g., 1, 1, 1, 2, 3, 3, 3)	• Typically used when data are not numerical

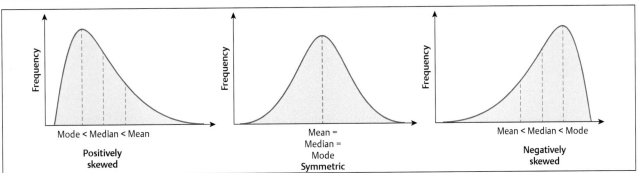

Mode < Median < Mean
Positively skewed

Mean = Median = Mode
Symmetric

Mean < Median < Mode
Negatively skewed

👥 Clinical Case Scenarios

10. Which of the following correctly describes the height of Martians?
    a. Normal distribution (symmetric distribution)
    b. Positively skewed
    c. Negatively skewed

11. What is the best measure of central tendency for height of Martians?

24.4.2 Bell-Shaped (Normal) Distribution Curve and Standard Deviation

The following curve is known as bell-shaped, Gaussian, normal, or symmetric distribution curve. Frequency distribution is plotted on the *Y*-axis and numerical values on the *X*-axis. This reflects the usual and expected distribution of values in the real world (e.g., USMLE-exam score, height of males, IQ of general population, fasting blood sugar). In this curve, mean = median = mode.

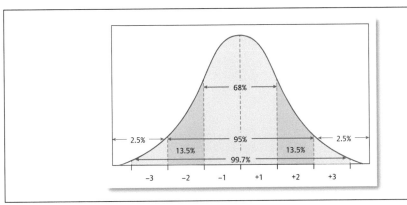

💡 MRS

Positively skewed graph looks like a arrow-head pointing in positive direction (to be exact-upper half of an arrow head) =>.
Negatively skewed graph looks like a arrow-head pointing in negative direction.
MRS: Fat mode- Mode is the nearest to the fat portion of the graph.

Remember the following numbers:

• 68% fall within 1 SD (standard deviation)
• 95% fall within 2 SD
• 99.7% fall within 3 SD

🔍 Clinical Case Scenarios

12. Assuming a normal (Gaussian) distribution, a study of 1,000 participants found the mean serum cholesterol value to be 210 with SD of 10. What number of people in that study had serum cholesterol > 230?

13. Assuming a normal (Gaussian) distribution, a study of 1,000 people found the mean height to be 170 cm with SD of 5. What number of people in that study had height in between 165 and 180 cm?

24.4.3 What Statistical Test to Use to Interpret Study Data?

What are you comparing?	Example	Test
Only nominal (categorical) variables	"This or that" category (e.g., male or female, old or young, risk factor or without risk factor, disease and without disease)	**Chi-square** (see below for two examples)
2 nominals with 1 numerical	Comparing mean height of male and female (male and female are 2 nominal variables)	**T-test or Z-test**
More than 2 nominals with one numerical	Comparing mean height of male, female, and aliens.	**ANOVA**
Two numerical variables	Comparing correlation of height with income	**Pearson correlation**

Chi-Square

Example 1

	Disease (e.g., chronic obstructive pulmonary disease [COPD])	No disease
Risk factor (tobacco abuse)	10 A	100 B
No risk factors	1 C	100 D

Example 2

Study duration: 6 months	Developed myocardial infarction (MI)	No MI
Aspirin (exposed)	5 A	95 B
No aspirin (placebo)	20 C	80 D

MRS

When you create this table, make it a habit to place disease or event (e.g., MI) on top of box "A" and the risk factor or intervention to the left of box "A."
Just like that, for the sensitivity/specificity table, always put disease on top of box "A" and positive test to the left of box "A."

Odds ratio	Relative risk	Absolute risk reduction (ARR)
Examples: • Odds of getting the disease when one has risk factors, compared to those who do not (**cohort study**). • Odds of having been exposed to risk factors when one has the disease, compared to those without the disease (**case–control studies**).	Chance/risk/probability of event occurrence in the treatment group vs. control group	Measures the size of difference between incidence rate in treatment group minus the control group.
Look at example 1 of chi-square in previous page: • Odds of a person with risk factor developing the disease = A/B • Odds of a person without risk factor developing the disease = C/D • **Odds ratio** is A/B divided by C/D. It is easier to calculate the ratio with above information then to remember the formula given below: $= \dfrac{(A/B)}{(C/D)} = \dfrac{(AD)}{(BC)}$	Incidence rate in exposed divided by incidence rate in nonexposed = (A/total patient in treatment group) divided by (B/total patient in control group) $= \dfrac{A/(A+B)}{C/(C+D)}$	Difference of incidence or event rate in the groups $= A/(A + B) - C/(C + D)$
• Odds ratio > 1.0 = event is MORE likely to occur • Odds ratio < 1.0 = event is LESS likely to occur (protective effect) • Odds ratio of 1 = no effect	Similar to odds ratio, RR < 1 is protective and RR > 1 means higher risk. • Relative risk of 1 = no effect.	0 = no effect

 Clinical Case Scenarios

14. In example 1, of chi-square on previous page the sample was derived from a cohort study. What are the odds of getting COPD in a smoker when compared to a nonsmoker?

15. In example 2, what is the relative risk of getting MI on placebo in comparison to aspirin?

16. What is the ARR in example 2?

Number Needed to Treat/Harm

- Number needed to treat (NNT) = 1/ARR. In example 2 of chi-square on previous page NNT = 1/0.15 = 6.6. This means that approximately six people need to be treated with aspirin *for 6 months (study duration)* to prevent one MI event.
- Number needed to harm (NNH) = 1/ARI. ARI = absolute risk increase = Adverse event rate in treatment group – Adverse event rate in placebo group.

24.4.4 Determining Statistical Significance of the Results

Null Hypothesis and p-Value

- **Null hypothesis** says that "whatever one is trying to prove with the study" is not found in real world. Examples of null hypothesis include:
  - The treatment has no effect on the outcome studied.
  - The risk factor being studied does not increase risk of the disease.
  - Even if correlation is found in the study, it is by random chance only. When the study is repeated, the effect will not be there.
- *p*-**Value** = the of probability of null hypothesis being true. If a study has *p*-value of < 0.05, it means there is < 5% chance that null hypothesis might be true. Traditionally, *p*-value of < 0.05 has been used to consider the study to be statistically significant and to be able to reject the null hypothesis (!). This criterion is called the alpha (α) criterion.

⚠️ **Caution**

(!) In statistics we either reject null hypothesis or fail to reject it. We do not say null hypothesis is found to be false.
The parallel of this is found in the judicial process: defendant is either found to be guilty or not guilty. They do not say, "defendant was found to be innocent."

Take the following example of an observational study

- A study postulated that smoking increases risk of skin cancer.
- In this case the null hypothesis would be that smoking is not related to skin cancer or does not increase the risk of skin cancer.
- After analyzing data, the p-value was found to be 0.2, which means that there is a 20% chance that null hypothesis might be true. Here we fail to reject null hypothesis.
- In this study, we found no sufficient evidence to accept that smoking is related to skin cancer.[3]

[3]Absence of evidence of harm from smoking does not equate to evidence of absence of harm of smoking.

Confidence Interval

Studies can include only a sample of population and they cannot involve the whole population of the world. So, we must extrapolate the data gathered from the sample to try to reflect the real world. To do that, statisticians have created the confidence interval.

Take the following example: A studied effect had odds ratio of 1.68 with 95 % confidence interval (1.13–2.17). In this example, the odds ratio of the study was 1.68. The statistical analysis is 95% confident that the real-world number lies within this range of 1.13 to 2.17.

This confidence interval is affected by:

Sample size	The bigger the sample size, the more likely it is to represent the true world population and have a smaller range of confidence interval.
SD (standard deviation)	Smaller SD gives narrower confidence interval: (e.g., if all world population had the same height, a small sample for study of height could represent the true world.)

Another important point is that confidence interval has a *flat distribution* curve (the real-world value can be any specific number within that range and with equal probabilities). So, if we are dealing with a ratio (e.g., relative risk, odds ratio) and the confidence interval includes the number 1 (which implies no effect), the study is not statistically significant.

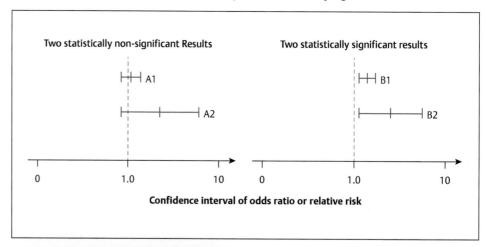

Clinical Case Scenarios

17. If A1 and A2 studies both have the same sample size, what can you infer about the difference of SD (standard deviation) in between them?

18. If B1 and B2 studies both have the same SD, what can you infer about the difference in the sample size between them?

19. If p-value of A1 is 0.02, is the study statistically significant?

2

Types of Error

Type I = falsely rejecting the null hypothesis	• The study conclusion shows a difference, but in reality, there is none.[a] • This error can only occur when null hypothesis is rejected.[b]	• p-Value = probability of making type I error. • α[c] is a preset cut-off for p-value (0.05 or 5%). • When p-value is less than α, null hypothesis is rejected, and the study is considered statistically significant. • Another way to look at it is that a p-value of 0.05 (5%) means there is 95% probability of statistical significance (1 − probability of null hypothesis = 1 − 0.05).
Type II = failing to reject null hypothesis when it should have been rejected	• When the conclusion does not show a difference, but in reality, there is a difference. • This error can only occur when we fail to reject null hypothesis.	• β = probability of type II error = 1 − statistical power of the study.[d] • Studies with greater sample size have greater statistical power.

[a]This is the number one (I) error which we should not make, when the study shows a difference, but in reality, there is none. Such conclusion can lead us to recommending patients drugs/interventions that have no benefit at all. As all drugs/interventions have adverse effect, it might actually cause harm. This would go against our Hippocratic dictum of Primum non nocere (Do no harm).

[b]Take an example of a study with p-value of >0.05. This study is **NOT** considered statistically significant, and the null hypothesis is not rejected. So, probability of type I error is zero in this case.

[c]alPha: p-value.

[d]Exam question will provide statistical power to calculate β-error (it will not ask you to compute statistical power, as it is out of scope for medical exams).

Clinical Case Scenarios

20. A study has postulated that smoking increases risk of skin cancer. p-Value is found to be 0.1. Which of the following represents the chance of error that this study does not reflect the real world?

α-error

β-error

21. How can you decrease the chance of β-error?

24.5 Types of Biases[4,5]

Bias can occur in each step of the study	Examples
How did we take the sample (what population are we studying?)	Selection bias
At which point during the disease course are we starting the study?	Length time bias, lead time bias
How are we collecting the data?	Recall bias, observer bias, Hawthorne effect, instruction/procedural bias
How long we are going to continue the study for?	Latency bias
Are we adjusting the data for appropriate confounding variables?	Confounding bias (it can come from unknown confounding variable/s)
Are we going to publish these data?	Publication bias occurs when • We push to publish only the positive findings, or • Journals accept publication only for studies with significant results. This will affect findings of meta-analysis.

[4]"Errors" in statistics are from numbers and math.
[5]"Biases" are source of mistakes from design and method of the study.

24.5.1 Biases Defined

Selection bias	⇨	Participants chosen are not representative of the target population due to poor randomization or poor planning with regard to choosing study participants.
		• For example, healthy 20-year-old college students versus hospital population.
		• Respondent bias is a type of a selection bias: e.g., a study done in a local radio station will more likely include strongly opinionated respondents than the moderates.
Sponsorship effect	⇨	Knowing that the pharmacy company is paying for the study may lead to unintentional preferences to that intervention and its effect.
Hawthorne effect	⇨	Knowledge of being observed may change the observed behavior or responses (subtly or without intent).
Instruction or procedural bias	⇨	Allowing unclear definitions or instructions may give leeway for investigator discretion and subjectivity.

Type of bias	Definition	Examples of biases in raw statistical data	How to counteract this bias?[a]
Confounding bias	Variables that may affect the outcome are more prevalent in one study group	An observational study found that smokers have lower risk of Alzheimer's disease (Is smoking protective for Alzheimer's disease?) • Confounding variable might be decreased life span. Smokers die before they get Alzheimer's disease.	Randomization: a method of assigning subjects to different arms of a study in a random manner. Successful randomization results in groups with similar baseline patient characteristics. It is meant to automatically adjust for known or unknown confounding factors.
Lead-time bias		A study compares survival of cancer patients using a new screening test in one group vs. without screening in another group. The study claims that the new screening test for cancer improves disease survival, but in reality, it does not, because they failed to consider the lead-time bias.	• The research should start with the point of origin, not with the point of diagnosis. • Randomization
Length bias		More aggressive cancers spend less time in the asymptomatic detectable preclinical phase (less likely to be diagnosed with screening tests). Indolent cancers that spend more time in asymptomatic phase are more likely to be diagnosed with the help of screening test. This will create an underlying selection bias.	
Recall bias	• More recent events are remembered more clearly, or • Participants may not be able to recall important events, or • They may have more incentives to think harder when they have the disease in comparison to control subjects	Occurs typically in case–control or retrospective cohort studies	

Type of bias	Definition	Examples of biases in raw statistical data	How to counteract this bias?[a]
Observer bias (experimenter effect)	• Able to relate or elicit more response from certain types of participants (observer expectancy) • Technical skills between investigators	If an observer who gathers data knows that the researcher hypothesized that males have more mannerisms when they speak, they may pick up more mannerisms from males during interview even if it is not really true.	**Blind trial:** The researcher who is gathering data from participants **does not know** who is in the treatment group or placebo group and be unfamiliar with study hypothesis.
Latency bias	• When the duration of study is not enough for the studied outcome to show up, the study might not detect any difference	• A 2-week study of thiamine supplementation in alcoholic shows no effect. • After a 2-year follow-up, a statistically significant decreased risk of cognitive dysfunction is found in the study participants in the thiamine group. (The 2-week study result has the latency bias.)	Adequate study duration

[a]Randomized double-blind placebo-controlled trial counteracts almost all biases, that is why it is the "holy grail" of studies. Double-blind = both participants and researchers gathering data do NOT **know** who are in the treatment group and the placebo group.

Clinical Case Scenarios

The following data are taken from a 6-months study.

Table 1:

	Gout attack	No gout attack
Allopurinol	2 A	98 B
Placebo	10 C	90 D

Adverse event: Table 2

	Rash	No rash
Allopurinol	5 A	95 B
Placebo	1 C	99 D

Calculate-the following with the above data?

22. Relative risk in Table 1?

23. Absolute risk reduction (ARR) in Table 1?

24. Number needed to treat (NNT) in Table 1?

25. Number needed to harm (NNH) in Table 2?

Answers

1. Define denominator first: How many people in the small town are at risk of acquiring diabetes? 100 – 20 (who already have diabetes) = 80 are at risk. So, incidence = 10/80 = 12.5 %.

2. (20 + 10)/100 = 30%. **Note:** For prevalence, the denominator is the whole population.

3. Create the table first:
   - **Sensitivity** = TP/Total number of patients with disease. So, 80% = TP/100; so, TP = 80.
   - TP + FN = Total number of patients with the disease: TP + FN = 100 → 80 + FN = 100: so, FN = 20.

4. We have to find out the PPV in this case. Create another table, collect all the information given in the question (estimated prevalence = 10%, sensitivity = 80%, and specificity = 70%), and step by step fill in the table.
   - First step in these types of question which involves calculating PPV or NPV is to work with prevalence: **Prevalence** = Patients with disease/Total number of patients.
   - Now pick an easy number like 100; we can start with 100 people who truly have the disease. Now as the given prevalence is 10%, and as we have assumed that 100 people have the disease, we can compute the following:
     - 10% = 100/Total number of individuals.
     - Total number of individuals = 1,000.
     - 100 (who truly have the disease) + who do not have the disease = 1,000.
     - There are 900 people who truly do not have the disease.
   - Now we must use the given sensitivity of 80% and specificity of 70% to try to complete the table:

     Sensitivity = True positive (TP)/Total number of patients who truly have the disease

     80% = TP/100: so, TP = 80.

     Specificity = True negative (TN)/Total number of patients who do not have the disease

     70% = TN/900; so, TN = 630.

TEST		Patients with disease (total 100)	Patients without disease (total 900)	
	Positive	True positive (TP) = **80**	False positive (FP) 630 + FP = 900 So, FP = 270	TP/TP + FP = positive predictive value (PPV)
	Negative	False negative (FN) 80 + FN = 100 so, FN = 20	True negative (TN) = **630**	TN/TN + FN = negative predictive value (NPV)
		TP/TP + FN = sensitivity = 80%	TN/TN + FP = specificity = 70%	

   Answer is C: PPV turns out to be = 80/(80 + 270) = ~23%.

5. NPV = 630/630 + 20 ≅ 97%.

6. **Accuracy (!)** = $\dfrac{\text{(All true values)}}{\text{(All values)}}$ = $\dfrac{\text{(TP+TN)}}{\text{(TP+FP+FN+TN)}}$ = 71%. = 71%.

7. With increased prevalence, sensitivity and specificity ratio of the test does not change due to equal impact on both the numerator and denominator. However, NPV and PPV change with prevalence. Increased prevalence will increase the PPV and decrease the NPV.

8. 1 – NPV = 88%.

⚠ **Caution**

(!) Do not confuse with validity, reliability, and accuracy (it is important to remember what each stand for).

9.

	Sensitivity (approx.)	Specificity (approx.)
A	57	99
B	80	80
C	90	40

10. Negatively skewed, as the mean is less than the mode. In exam, easy way to do deal with this kind of questions is to calculate the median and mode. You always need to **remember** that if mode is in the **right**-hand side of the mean, then it is **negatively skewed**.

11. For skewed graphs (be it positively or negatively skewed), median is the right answer for central tendency (as you can see from the graphs, the median is always in the center.)

12. 230 is 2 SD above mean = 2.5% are 2 SD above mean. So, 2.5% of 1,000 = 25.

13. For this type of question, it is easier to draw the graph. Start with only 68 and 95% part and see if this will suffice. Starting from mean use the SD to create the graph as below.

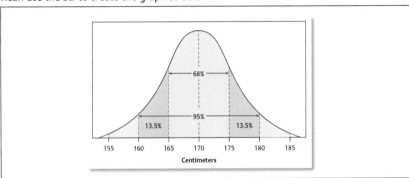

165 cm is 1 SD below mean and 180 cm is 2 SD above mean. By looking at the graph above, we can see that 68% + 13.5% is within this height range. So, 81.5% of 1,000 = 815 people.

14. • Odds of a person with tobacco abuse developing COPD = 10/100.

   • Odds of a person who does not smoke developing COPD = 1/100.

   • Odds ratio = 10.

   Interpretation: A smoker is 10 times more likely to get COPD than a nonsmoker. Note that if the same data were taken from a case–control study it would be interpreted differently: "a person who has COPD is 10 times more likely to be a smoker than a person who does not have COPD."

15. To answer this, it might be easier to calculate the incidence rate in each group first:

Study duration: 6 months	Developed MI (event)	No MI	Total number of patients in each group	Incidence rate
Aspirin (exposed)	5 A	95 B	A + B = 100	5/100 = 5%
No aspirin/ placebo	20 C	80 D	C + D = 100	20/100 = 20%

Now, relative risk = 20/5 = 4. Conclusion: Those who are not on aspirin have *four times the risk* of MI compared to those who are taking aspirin.

16. ARR = 20% − 5% = 15% = 0.15. (Note to calculate ARR, we just have to calculate the difference. If the value comes back as negative integer, we can just remove the negative sign. Example: if you calculate ARR as 5%−20%=−15%, you can just remove the negative sign. Either way the ARR is 15%, or 0.15)

17. SD is lower in A1.

18. Sample size in B1 is greater.

19. No. For statistical significance always look at the following:

   • *p*-value < 0.05, **AND**

   • The confidence interval for comparative ratios (odds ratio, relative risk, etc.) should not include number 1.

We have to weigh NNT with NNH in all our treatment decisions: the type of treatment benefit (mortality benefit vs. cosmetic improvement), and the type of harm (non-life-threatening rash vs. toxic epidermal necrolysis).

20. We have not rejected null hypothesis in this case, so the change of type I error is zero. β-error is the answer.

21. Increase sample size.

22. Incidence rate of acute gout on allopurinol = 2/Total number of patients on allopurinol = 2/2 + 98 = 2/100 = 0.02. Incidence rate in placebo = 10/100 = 0.1. So, relative risk = 0.02/0.1 = 0.2.

    Conclusion = those who take allopurinol have 0.2 times the risk of gout attack compared to those who do not take allopurinol.

23. ARR = 0.02 − 0.1 = 0.08.

24. NNT = 1/ARR = 1/0.08 = 12.

    Conclusion of NNT = 12 patients with gout need to be treated with allopurinol for 6 months to prevent one acute gout episode.

25. Computation is similar to NNT. What ARR is to NNT, absolute risk increase (ARI) is to NNH.

    - NNT = 1/ARR and NNH = 1/ARI

    - ARI = Adverse event rate in the allopurinol group (5/100) − adverse event rate in the placebo group
      (1/100) = 0.05 − 0.01 = 0.04.
      So NNH = 1/0.04 = 25.

    - Conclusion of NNH = we will get one event of rash due to allopurinol, if we treat 25 people with allopurinol for 6 months.

25. General Surgery

Wounds that have no gap separating the boundaries (e.g., clean surgical wounds) will undergo "primary healing," from the apposed edges of the tissue. Wounds that have a large gap (e.g., large debridement of infected ulcer) will undergo "secondary healing healing" which involves production of excess extra-cellular matrix to fill up the wound (this excess extraceullar matrix looks granular hence called granulation tissue), neo-vascularization and eventual formation of scars.

25.1 Preoperative Evaluation

	Indication
Baseline electrocardiogram (EKG)	EKG is needed in most cases, except in healthy patients undergoing low-risk surgery
Preoperative **pharmacologic** cardiac stress testing	Usually not needed, but can be considered for a patient with poor functional status (inability to complete a flight of steps without resting), in whom preoperative angiography followed by intervention can possibly improve surgical outcome.
Chest X-ray (CXR)	Patients with cardiopulmonary disease or undergoing high-risk surgery
PFT (pulmonary function testing)	No need for routine pre-op PFTs in patients with stable lung disease. PFTs are indicated in lung resection candidates, or when it is uncertain if respiratory status is at baseline in patients with chronic lung disease.

25.2 Cardiac Risk Factor and Surgery

Situation		NSIM	
Recent myocardial infarction (MI) without percutaneous coronary intervention (PCI)		At least 2 months should lapse before considering elective noncardiac surgery	
Recent MI with PCI	Angioplasty alone	Elective noncardiac surgery should be delayed for at least:	2 weeks
	Bare metal stent		1 month
	DES (drug-eluting stent)		>6 months[a]
Congestive heart failure		Surgery should be performed when the patient is euvolemic.	

[a]If risk of further delay of elective surgery is higher than cardiac risk, elective surgery can be considered earlier (after at least 3 months of DES placement, but not less than 1 month).

Additional info: Perioperatively, continuing dual-antiplatelet therapy, or discontinuing platelet-receptor blocker and giving ASA (acetylsalicylic acid) alone, is determined on a case-by-case basis. If surgery *needs* to be done within 4 to 6 weeks of stent placement, dual-antiplatelet therapy needs to be continued preoperatively unless the risk of bleeding is considered higher than the risk of stent thrombosis.

25.3 Neck Mass

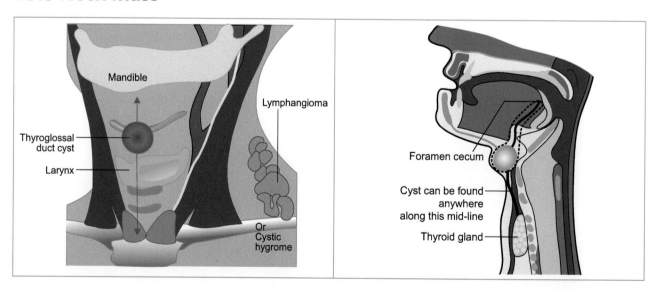

Congenital cysts[a]	Additional points	Management
Thyroglossal cysts (remnant of the thyroglossal duct)	**Location:** midline • Moves with swallowing	Surgical removal
Dermoid cysts	**Location:** midline • Does not move with swallowing	Surgical removal
Branchial cysts	**Location:** Anywhere anterior to the sternocleidomastoid muscle (*yellow line* in the picture)	May be harder to excise and may recur
Cystic hygroma	**Location:** posterior lateral neck • Associated with Turner syndrome	Surgery or sclerosing agents • As it can extend into the chest, do CT scan prior to surgery. There is a chance of recurrence.

[a]Usually found in children and young adults. All of them can also become infected and present with red, hot, tender cystic mass.

25.4 Inguinal and Femoral Hernias

Risk factors:

- White male
- Increased abdominal pressure: Obesity, chronic cough, constipation, etc.
- Poor connective tissue strength: Smoking, diabetes, unhealthy diet, etc.

Hernia anatomy:

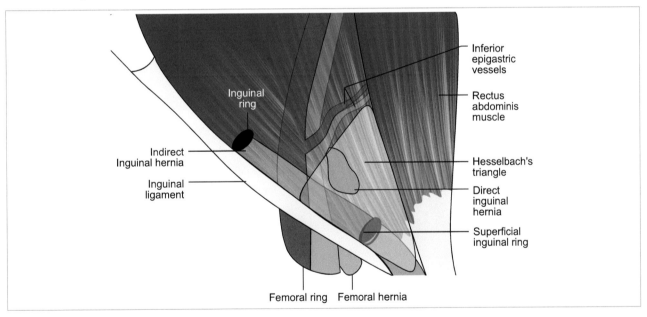

Inguinal triangle is bordered by inguinal ligament, inferior epigastric vessels, and lateral border of rectus abdominis muscle.

Types:

Indirect inguinal hernia	Defect in the deep inguinal ring (entry to the inguinal canal)[a] • Hernia may completely traverse the inguinal canal and descend into the scrotum.
Direct inguinal hernia	Defect in fascia transversalis of the abdominal wall, which acts as the posterior wall of the inguinal canal
Femoral hernia	Defect in the femoral ring (entry to the femoral canal)[a]

[a]Neurovascular structures pass through femoral and inguinal canals. Due to the above risk factors, the ring and canal may get bigger and weaker, which allow intra-abdominal contents like mesentery or intestines to pass through.

Management:

- For **reducible** inguinal or femoral hernias, elective repair is usually offered. These are usually asymptomatic or can be mildly tender in some cases.

- **Irreducible hernias** are incarcerated hernias, which can be complicated by strangulation[1]:

	Pathophysiology	Management
Incarcerated hernia	• Trapped hernia • May lead to bowel obstruction with or without strangulation	Longstanding incarcerated hernias need to be repaired electively.
		For acutely incarcerated hernia, NSIM is urgent surgery. In uncomplicated acutely incarcerated hernia, manual reduction may be attempted followed by elective repair.
Strangulated hernia	Trapped hernia → increased venous congestion → edema → increased inflammation → more edema → decreased arterial blood supply and strangulation. • Commonly associated with bowel obstruction • May lead to intestinal necrosis • This usually has severe pain and signs of sepsis.	Emergent surgery

 In a nutshell

As a rule in, explorative laparotomy is indicated if any of the following is present:

Signs of peritonitis	Generalized abdominal guarding, rigidity, or rebound tenderness
Signs of intestinal ischemia	Air in the bowel wall (pneumatosis intestinalis)
Signs of perforation	Free air under the diaphragm
Hemodynamic instability with high suspicion for intra-abdominal source	

For this chapter, these are called "abdominal danger signs." Looking out for these during any patient encounter is very important, so remember these danger signs.

25.5 Gastrointestinal Tract

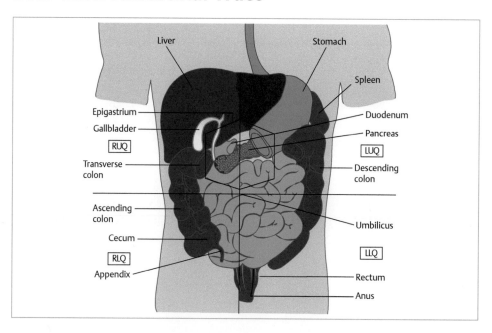

[1]Irreducible hernia that is tender but shows no signs of obstruction or sepsis can be omental- or mesentery-only hernia.

LLQ, left lower quadrant; LUQ, left upper quadrant; RLQ, right lower quadrant; RUQ, right upper quadrant.

Localized tenderness in the following region	Think of the following
Epigastric tenderness	Gastric pathology, pancreatitis, duodenitis, etc.
RUQ tenderness	Cholecystitis, cholangitis, hepatitis, etc.
RLQ tenderness	Appendicitis, ileitis (Crohn's disease), etc.
LUQ tenderness	Splenic rupture, inflammation of descending colon, etc.
LLQ tenderness	Diverticulitis, sigmoiditis, etc.

Abbreviations: LLQ, left lower quadrant; LUQ, left upper quadrant; RLQ, right lower quadrant; RUQ, right upper quadrant.

25.5.1 Bowel Obstruction

	Paralytic (adynamic) ileus	Mechanical small bowel obstruction
Etiology	• Postoperative (most common within 1 week of surgery) • Peritonitis, pancreatitis, local abdominal wound infection, dyselectrolytemia, etc.	**H**ernia, **A**dhesions,[a] **V**olvulus (cecal),[b] **I**ntussusception,[c] **N**eoplasm, and **G**allstone ileus
Bowel sounds	Hypoactive	Hyperactive or borborygmic in early stages; hypoactive in late phase
Work-up	First initial diagnostic step is X-ray. CT may be done if further information is needed.	
Radiologic findings	Both small and large bowels are involved (air in the distal colon and rectum typically signals a diffuse pathology) 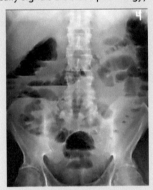 An upright view of the abdomen showing multiple air-fluid levels in nondilated small and large bowels including the rectum (*red arrow*) indicating ileus. Abdominal X-ray. Source: Abdominal pathologies and findings. In: Shi Y, Sohani Z, Tang B et al., eds. Essentials of Clinical Examination Handbook. 8th ed. Thieme; 2018.	Usually small-bowel involvement (and distal-bowel collapse) 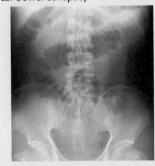 A supine X-ray demonstrating dilated small bowel. To differentiate small bowel gas from colonic distention, look at the folds that extend all the way across the lumen, indicating that it is the small bowel. Also, the large bowel only has four parts: ascending, transverse, descending, and sigmoid (a square on the edges ⊓). Source: Pathology. In: Gunderman R, ed. Essential Radiology. Clinical Presentation, Pathophysiology, Imaging. 2nd ed. Thieme; 2000.
Rx	• NPO + IV (intravenous) fluids + NG (nasogastric) tube decompression[d] • If any of the "abdominal danger signs" is present, NSIM is explorative laparotomy.	
	Avoid opiates and immobility (encourage ambulation)	Surgical exploration, if not improving

MRS

I am **HAVING** mechanical bowel obstruction.

[2]**Sigmoid volvulus**

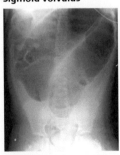

Source: Mont4nha, CC0, via Wikimedia Commons.

[a]Postoperative adhesions can occur as early as within 1 week of surgery.

[b]Volvulus of sigmoid colon can cause large bowel obstruction. It typically occurs in an elderly patient when the sigmoid colon gets twisted on its axis. It has a "coffee bean" appearance on X-ray.[2] NSIM is flexible sigmoidoscopy (to untwist the bowel) and a rectal tube.

[c]For intussusception, see Chapter 22 (Pediatrics). Do you remember what is the treatment?

[d]NG tube is most helpful in patients with pain due to stomach distention and frequent or large-volume vomiting.

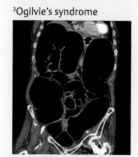

[3]Ogilvie's syndrome

Source: Milliways, CC BY-SA 3.0, via Wikimedia Commons.

> ⚠ **Caution**
>
> (!) One potential side effect of neostigmine is life-threatening bradyarrhythmia.

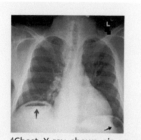

[4]Chest X-ray shows air under the right diaphragm (red-arrow). Black arrow is the normal omnipresent gastric shadow.
Source: Modified from Clinical_Cases: I made the photo myself, licensed under Creative Commons license., CC BY-SA 2.5 , via Wikimedia Commons.

25.5.2 Ogilvie's Syndrome (Colonic Pseudo-obstruction)

Background: Acute or subacute nonobstructive dilation of large bowel due to impairment of the enteric autonomic nervous system.

Risk factors: Typically occurs in *older patients* after hospitalization, surgery, etc.

Presentation: Look for large-bowel distention with minimal involvement of small bowel. Patients usually appear comfortable despite significant abdominal distention. Some patients can have nausea, vomiting, and *even diarrhea.*

Best SIDx: CT abdomen[3] or water-soluble contrast enema (to rule out obstructive lesions). Plain abdominal X-ray is helpful in follow-up.

Management: Conservative, NPO + IV fluids + NG tube decompression as needed. If cecal diameter is > 12 cm or if conservative management fails, consider neostigmine. (!) If neostigmine fails, NSIM is colonoscopic decompression. If this fails, next is surgical management with cecostomy.

Complication: Ischemia and perforation (If any of the abdominal danger sign develops, NSIM is explorative laparotomy with colonic resection and ileostomy).

25.5.3 Intestinal and Gastric Perforation

Etiology: Any severe gastric or intestinal pathologycan cause perforation.

Presentation: *Generalized* guarding, rigidity, and/or rebound tenderness. In generalized peritonitis, even a little movement can cause significant pain.

Management:

- In suspected visceral perforation, first SIM is to start IV fluids and antibiotics.
- First SIDx is upright abdominal/CXR. Look for air under the diaphragm.[4] Do not choose CT scan as the best initial test.
- NSIM—immediate explorative laparotomy.

25.5.4 Abdominal Compartment Syndrome

Background: Complicated abdominal surgery, especially requiring administration of large volume of fluids, can lead to severe edema of the abdomen and its contents, resulting in increased intra-abdominal pressure. Other risk factors include early closure of abdominal wound, severe burns, liver transplantation, etc.

Clinical pathophysiology:

Increased abdominal pressure can cause compression of	Presentation
Lung	Shortness of breath
Vena cava and renal vein	Renal failure
Vena cava	Decreased cardiac preload/output and hypotension

Work-up: Intra-abdominal pressure can be measured by different methods. Most commonly used is intrabladder pressure measurement (look for pressure of ≥ 20–25 mmHg).

Treatment: Surgical decompression and temporary abdominal closure with mesh or plastic to protect the bowel. Primary closure is done after 48 to 72 hours.

25.5.5 Appendicitis

Pathophysiology: Obstruction of appendiceal lumen can lead to inflammation ± infection. Causes of obstruction include lymphoid hyperplasia (due to viral infection), fecalith, parasites, etc.

Presentation: Classic sequence of symptom development: anorexia → vague periumbilical pain → RLQ (right upper quadrant) sharp and severe pain (localized signs of peritonitis, such as rebound tenderness and guarding in RLQ, are usually present at this stage). Other symptoms are nausea, vomiting, low-grade fever, and elevated white blood cells (WBCs).

Clinical signs of appendicitis:

Rovsing's sign	Deep palpation in LLQ elicits pain in RLQ (increased pressure in the colon is felt in the inflamed appendix)
Psoas sign	Extension of hip causes pain in RLQ
Obturator sign	Internal rotation of hip elicits pain in RLQ

Abbreviations: LLQ, left lower quadrant; RLQ, right lower quadrant.

These signs may or may not be present. Presence of obturator and psoas sign depends on the location of the appendix.

Management:

- No need for radiologic imaging in classic presentation. NSIM—IV antibiotics directed against GI (gastrointestinal) pathogens, followed by laparoscopic appendectomy.
- In atypical presentation, abdominal CT scan can confirm the diagnosis.

During surgery, even if appendix looks grossly normal, it should be removed (microscopic appendicitis might be present).

> **Complication:** Appendiceal abscess can develop if patient presents late (e.g., > 5 days of hx suggestive of appendicitis):
> - In an ill-appearing patient, NSIM is appendectomy.
> - In a well-appearing patient, either early appendectomy OR conservative management followed by late appendectomy can be done (antibiotics ± percutaneous drain, followed by appendectomy after approximately 6 weeks).

25.5.6 Hemorrhoids

Background: Enlarged anorectal veins that commonly occur due to prolonged history of constipation and straining during defecation. Other causes include pregnancy and increased portal pressure in cirrhosis (cirrhosis patients have mostly internal hemorrhoids).

Classification:

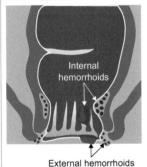

Presentation: Usually painless bleeding associated with defecation. (!) *External* hemorrhoids may be painful (somatic innervation), whereas *internal* hemorrhoids are typically painless (even when they cause bleeding).

⚠ **Caution**

(!) Bleeding independent of bowel movement is likely not due to hemorrhoids.

Rx: Initial step is to prevent constipation with high-fiber diet, adequate fluid intake ± sitz baths. Use oral or topical analgesics for pain. For refractory cases, refer to colorectal surgery (rubber band ligation or surgical hemorrhoidectomy may be needed).

Complication: Vein thrombosis can cause severe pain. Management is immediate hemorrhoidectomy (simple clot removal is not recommended due to a high chance of recurrence).

25.5.7 Other Anorectal Conditions

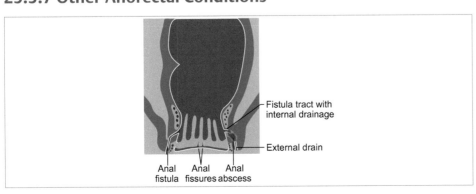

Condition[a]	Additional info	Management
Anorectal abscesses	Fever + perineal pain. Look for "fluctuant mass"[b]	Surgical drainage. Antibiotics are indicated in **all cases**. (use antibiotics that cover gram +ve, gram −ve, and anaerobes, e.g., amoxicillin-clavulanate).
Fistula in ano (anorectal fistula)	Most fistulas form as a result of anorectal abscess. They have internal and external openings.	Surgical excision
Anal fissures	**Etiology:** Local trauma, infection, inflammatory bowel disease, malignancy, etc. **Feature:** These anal tears occur distal to the dentate line, hence are very painful. Anal area exam may require anesthesia. MC location is midline posterior wall.	First step is conservative treatment with topical vasodilators (nifedipine or nitroglycerin), topical analgesic, stool softener, sitz bath, and fiber diet. Surgical correction is done if conservative management fails.
Pilonidal cysts	• When hair or debris gets trapped in the pores of skin in the cleft of buttock, this can lead to "foreign-body"-mediated nonhealing and development of cysts ± abscess. • Usually occurs in midline sacrococcygeal area. • Can present as a painless pit or painful cystic mass with fluctuation ± bloody or purulent discharge.	Abscess needs to be incised and drained. In recurrent or chronic cases, excision of cyst and sinus tract is done.

[a]New-onset anorectal lesions in elderly or high-risk patients, or in atypical location (e.g., multiple anal fissures that are not in the midline), or all nonhealing lesions should be evaluated for anal cancer by proctosigmoidoscopy ± biopsy.

[b]"Fluctuant mass" is almost always an abscess.

25.5.8 Anorectal Mass

Condition	Morphology	Additional points	Management
Squamous cell carcinoma of anus	Look for *chronic, nonhealing* fungating mass with ulceration/s and irregular surface (+ enlarged inguinal nodes).	• Common in patients with HIV • Related to human papilloma virus infection (the same virus that causes cervical cancer)	NSIDx: Biopsy. **Rx:** Chemoradiation even in localized disease is preferred over surgery, to preserve anal sphincter. (Surgery can be done for recurrent or persistent disease.)
Condylomata lata (secondary syphilis)[MRS-1]	These warty lesions have *moist surfaces* and no ulcerations, but multiple superficial erosions may be present.	Look for other features of secondary syphilis (e.g., systemic symptoms, generalized lymphadenopathy)	**NSIDx:** Serologic testing for syphilis **Rx:** Penicillin IM.
Condylomata acuminata (anogenital warts)[MRS-1]	These warty lesions have *dry surfaces* and no ulceration.	Primary HPV infection. Extensive disease can occur in immunosuppressed patients.	**Rx:** Topical imiquimod or podophyllotoxin, cryotherapy, etc.

MRS

[MRS-1]Condylomata lata vs acuminata: **Later** manifestation of syphilis is **Lata**. Papilloma virus is **accumulated** in **acuminata**.

25.6 Trauma

Blunt Trauma (e.g., Motor Vehicle Accident, Skiing Accident)

25.6.1 Blunt Head Trauma

Head CT in blunt head trauma is indicated if any of the following is present:
- Altered level of consciousness
- Open or depressed skull fracture
- Any sign of basilar skull fracture: e.g., periorbital bruise (raccoon-eyes sign), retroauricular bruise (battle sign), cerebrospinal fluid (CSF) leak, hemotympanum.[5]
- Age ≥ 65 years
- Retrograde amnesia of ≥ 30 minutes prior to injury
- Two or more episodes of vomiting
- Headache
- High-risk trauma (e.g., occupant ejected from vehicle)
- High risk for bleeding (anticoagulant therapy or hx of bleeding disorder)
- Seizure

25.6.2 Complications of Blunt Head Trauma

Traumatically amputated digits or extremities need to be wrapped in a saline-moistened gauze, put in a plastic bag, and then placed on ice.

[5]CT cervical spine also needs to be done in this case.

Dx is primarily made by radiological findings in a patient with blunt-head trauma	Epidural hematoma	Subdural hematoma	Diffuse axonal injury	Cerebral contusion
Pathology	Bleeding of middle meningeal **artery**	Tearing of bridging **veins**	• It is primarily due to mechanical damage from rapid acceleration/ deceleration which results in damage to axons, leading to diffuse axonal swelling and cerebral edema.	Regions of **hemorrhagic necrosis** due to direct impact and acceleration/ deceleration injury
Classical presentation All of these can present with focal neurological deficits, seizures, and features of increased intracranial pressure[a] or coma.	**Classic presentation:** Immediately after head trauma, there is LOC (loss of consciousness), followed by a period of awareness and followed by LOC again.	**Acute:** May have hx of transient LOC followed by "lucid interval" after which there is worsening of mental status (similar to epidural hematoma). **Chronic presentation:** Fall, followed by progressive (over few weeks of) neurological deterioration (e.g., increasing memory loss, falls ± seizures).	• Varying level of consciousness or CNS (central nervous system) dysfunction can occur depending on the severity; comatose state signals poor outcome. • Look for signs of increased intracranial pressure[a]	

	Epidural hematoma	Subdural hematoma	Diffuse axonal injury	Cerebral contusion
CT scan findings (main differentiating factor)[b]	() Biconvex-shaped (lens-shaped) hematoma 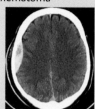 Source: Epidural Hematoma. In: Sartor K, Hähnel S, Kress B, ed. Direct Diagnosis in Radiology. Brain Imaging. 1st ed. Thieme; 2007.	Crescent-shaped hematoma 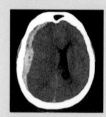 Source: Pathology. In: Gunderman R, ed. Essential Radiology: Clinical Presentation, Pathophysiology, Imaging. 3rd ed. Thieme; 2014.	Difficult to detect in CT scan because of microscopic nature of injury; radiologically visible signs may include • Blurring of gray–white matter interface • Diffuse areas of punctate hemorrhages These pathologic findings are better seen on magnetic resonance imaging (MRI). 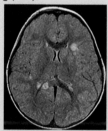 This axial FLAIR MR image in a patient unconscious after a high-speed motor vehicle accident demonstrates multiple bilateral foci of increased signal intensity in the corpus callosum and at gray matter–white matter junctions, indicating diffuse axonal injury. Source: Pathology. In: Gunderman R, ed. Essential Radiology: Clinical Presentation, Pathophysiology, Imaging. 2nd ed. Thieme; 2000.	• Areas of hemorrhage, localized particularly in basal *frontal and temporal* areas (typically near to skull bones) • Sometimes the areas of hemorrhage can coalesce later to become a large hematoma. 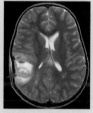 MRI scan Source: Pathology. In: Gunderman R, ed. Essential Radiology: Clinical Presentation, Pathophysiology, Imaging. 3rd ed. Thieme; 2014.
Management	\multicolumn{4}{l}{• Prevent hypoxia and hypotension}			

Management

• Prevent hypoxia and hypotension

• If impending herniation is suspected, recommend head of bed elevation + IV mannitol prior to imaging.

• Surgical evacuation for patients with neurological deterioration and big hematoma. • Small uncomplicated hematomas can be managed expectantly with close monitoring.	Large hematomas causing mass effect might need to be evacuated.

ICU supportive care: In patients with severe brain trauma and evidence of mass effect on imaging, ventriculostomy for more accurate monitoring of ICP (intracranial pressure) is needed, and CSF drainage can be done.

In patients with severe brain injury, give seizure prophylaxis for a week (e.g., levetiracetam).

[a]Signs of increased intracranial pressure:

• Hypertension (HTN) and bradycardia.

• Unilateral oculomotor nerve palsy (unilateral pupillary dilatation and nonreactive pupils): it is one of the early signs of uncal herniation.

• Late sign of herniation: hemiplegia (not explained by primary lesion) and respiratory arrest.

[b]Patients with unremarkable neuroimaging and who have hx of transient LOC or transient neurological dysfunction (such as confusion or memory loss) are diagnosed with *concussion*. NSIM: Avoid contact sport for the next 24 hours.

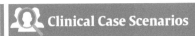

Clinical Case Scenarios

1. A 40-year-old female with no past medical history and not taking any medication slipped and fell while walking and was "out cold" for 1 minute. Currently patient does not have any symptoms. She does report that she cannot remember what she was doing for approximately 15 minutes prior to the fall. Physical exam is unremarkable except an area of mild scalp laceration that was sutured. Is CT scan indicated?

25.6.3 Blunt Thoracic Trauma

First SIDx is CXR, EKG, and FAST (focused assessment with sonography in trauma).

Flail chest syndrome 	**Definition:** Blunt chest trauma resulting in fracture of three or more adjacent ribs in two or more places. **Clinical findings:** • Paradoxical motion of the flail segment (chest moves inward during inspiration and outward during expiration). • Coexistent lung contusion and hemothorax might be present. **NSIDx:** CT chest angiography to rule out aortic injury. **Rx:** Supportive treatment only (e.g., intubation or noninvasive positive pressure ventilation as needed).
Pulmonary contusion	**Background:** MC injury found in blunt thoracic trauma. **Clinical findings:** Localized chest tenderness, shortness of breath, and hypoxia may be present. CXR may reveal localized infiltrate. **Rx:** Supportive treatment.
Hemothorax	**Work-up:** Bedside chest US can diagnose this accurately. **Rx:** Tube thoracotomy. Indications for surgical thoracotomy: • Immediate bloody drainage of ≥ 20 mL/kg (or ≥ 1,500 mL) • Ongoing bleeding > 3 mL/kg/h (or 600 mL in the next 6 hours) Hemodynamic instability due to hemothorax may require surgical ligation of the bleeding vessel.
Aortic injury or rupture[a]	• Majority of patients die immediately following trauma. • If the rupture is contained, patient may present with left-sided hemothorax, widened mediastinum, and resistant hypovolemic shock. • **NSIDx:** CT scan or transesophageal echocardiography (Note that management is similar to aortic dissection). • **Rx:** Surgical repair.
Esophageal rupture	**Presentation:** Severe retrosternal chest pain, no hemodynamic compromise; if shock is present it is usually responsive to IV fluids. **Clinical findings:** Widened mediastinum, pneumomediastinum, subcutaneous emphysema (crepitus on chest palpation), and/or pleural effusion.[b] **NSIDx:** Flexible esophagoscopy, or water-soluble contrast (gastrografin[c]) swallow study. **Rx:** Surgical repair.
Myocardial rupture[a]	Patients usually die immediately after trauma, or present with signs of cardiac tamponade. The heart shadow on CXR in acute tamponade may not be big and globular, as there is no time for pericardium to stretch and adapt to fluid accumulation (similar to myocardial rupture in acute MI). **NSIDx:** Bedside US or echocardiography. If patient is crashing and no immediate bedside imaging available, blind pericardiocentesis is done. **Rx:** Surgical repair.
Myocardial contusion[a]	Injury can occur in valves, septal wall, or myocardium. Usually presents with arrhythmias (e.g., bundle branch block, AV blocks, tachycardia), heart failure, and/or cardiogenic shock.

Diaphragmatic rupture	More common on the left side, as liver protects the right diaphragm.
	Presentation: Epigastric or abdominal pain or referred pain to shoulder + shortness of breath. Can present late, even months to years after trauma (especially in children).
	NSIDx: CT chest and abdomen.
	Rx: Explorative laparotomy with surgical repair of diaphragm.
Bronchial rupture	**Presentation:** Pneumothorax that does not resolve with chest tube. May cause tension pneumothorax. CXR shows air in mediastinum and subcutaneous tissue.
	NSIDx: CT thorax and bronchoscopy.
	Rx: Surgical repair.

[a]In patients with flail chest or fracture of the first rib/scapula/or sternum, which suggests severe chest trauma, CT scan with contrast is recommended to look for aortic injury. Myocardial injury is more likely to have also occurred in these cases.

[b]Similar presentation occurs in esophageal perforation due to iatrogenic cause (e.g., after endoscopy), or due to forceful vomiting.[6]

[c]Non-water soluble contrast (e.g. barium swallow) can cause chemical mediastinitis in patients with esophageal perforation.

[6]Esophageal perforation due to repetitive vomiting is known as Boerhaave syndrome.

 In a nutshell

Findings associated with injury of various mediastinal structures

	Hypotension	Widened mediastinum	Pneumomediastinum/ subcutaneous emphysema	Chest percussion
Aortic injury	Yes Hypovolemic shock not responsive to IV fluids	Yes	No	Dullness if hemothorax present (usually on left side)
Esophageal rupture	Yes, but usually responsive to fluids	Yes	Yes	Dullness (elevated amylase in pleural fluid will be found in thoracentesis)
Myocardial rupture	Yes (cardiogenic shock)	No	No	–
Myocardial contusion				
Diaphragmatic rupture	No	No	No	May be tympanic
Bronchial rupture	Yes (obstructive shock due to tension pneumothorax)	May occur with rupture of the main bronchi or trachea		Tympanic (pneumothorax)

25.6.4 Blunt Abdominal Trauma[7]

Initial Assessment

[7]Majority of the blunt head, thoracic, and abdominal traumas occur as a result of motor vehicle accidents.

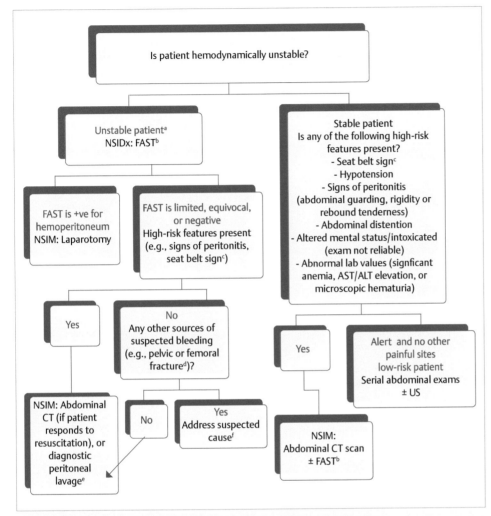

Is patient hemodynamically unstable?

Unstable patient[a]
NSIDx: FAST[b]

FAST is +ve for hemoperitoneum
NSIM: Laparotomy

FAST is limited, equivocal, or negative
High-risk features present (e.g., signs of peritonitis, seat belt sign[c])

Yes

No
Any other sources of suspected bleeding (e.g., pelvic or femoral fracture[d])?

NSIM: Abdominal CT (if patient responds to resuscitation), or diagnostic peritoneal lavage[e]

No

Yes
Address suspected cause[f]

Stable patient
Is any of the following high-risk features present?
- Seat belt sign[c]
- Hypotension
- Signs of peritonitis (abdominal guarding, rigidity or rebound tenderness)
- Abdominal distention
- Altered mental status/intoxicated (exam not reliable)
- Abnormal lab values (signficant anemia, AST/ALT elevation, or microscopic hematuria)

Yes

Alert and no other painful sites
low-risk patient
Serial abdominal exams ± US

NSIM:
Abdominal CT scan ± FAST[b]

[a]Most likely cause is significant bleeding from splenic or hepatic laceration.

[b]FAST = focused assessment with sonography in trauma. In hemodynamically stable patient, as there might not be enough intraperitoneal blood to be detected by US, FAST is not used as first line for diagnosis.

[c]"Seat belt sign" is ecchymosis over abdomen where it contacts with seat belt.[8]

[d]Sources of significant bleeding that can cause hemodynamic instability and not be clinically obvious, can be in pelvis, femur, or abdomen.

[e]Diagnostic peritoneal lavage is not commonly used nowadays, since US and CT are readily available.

[f]In pelvic fractures with significant bleeding, NSIM is pelvic binder and IR-guided angiographic embolization. (These bleeding sites are often NOT surgically accessible.)

Abbreviation: US, = ultrasound

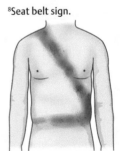

[8]Seat belt sign.

25.6.5 Blunt Abdominal Trauma and Visceral Organ Injury

	Presentation	Additional points
Duodenal hematoma	Epigastric pain, nausea, and vomiting	• Commonly seen in children • Usually presents 24–48 hours after trauma with abdominal symptoms (e.g., vomiting), as enlarging hematoma starts causing obstruction. **NSIDx:** CT scan of abdomen. **Rx:** Supportive (it is usually self-resolving). If severe, surgical management with decompression may be needed.
Pancreatic injury		Supportive treatment as per acute pancreatitis (see gastroenterology chapter). Patients also may go on to develop pancreatic pseudocysts > 1 week after trauma.
Liver lacerations	Intraperitoneal free fluid ± hemodynamic instability	• Associated with right lower rib fractures • RUQ tenderness + referred pain to right shoulder
Splenic rupture or laceration (MC source of significant bleeding in abdominal trauma)		• Associated with left lower rib fractures • LUQ tenderness + referred pain to left shoulder • Ecchymosis in left flank (indicates **retroperitoneal** hemorrhage) **Rx:** Repair is attempted, but if not possible (e.g., smashed spleen), splenectomy is done. Vaccinations after splenectomy are administered 2 weeks post-op.
Mesenteric vessel injury can lead to bowel ischemia and perforation	Signs of bowel ischemia ± perforation	Ischemia leading to perforation can present in a delayed manner (12–24 hours after the event).

25.6.6 Urologic and Perineal Trauma

Management of asymptomatic hematuria after blunt trauma.

Asymptomatic microhematuria without pelvic fracture	Follow-up only
Asymptomatic gross hematuria	Requires further investigation; see below
Asymptomatic microscopic hematuria (≥ 25 WBC/hpf) with pelvic fracture	

Examine in a retrograde fashion (genitals, urethra, bladder, ureter, kidneys)	Additional points *(Local bone fractures can point toward damage of internal organ, e.g., in lower rib fractures + hematuria, think of renal damage; in pelvic fracture + hematuria, think of urethral injury)*
Urethral injury	**Findings:** Urge to void but cannot urinate or feels like one is urinating but nothing comes out. Look for perineal area hematoma and high-riding prostate. **Clinical clue:** If there is resistance with urinary catheter insertion, think of urethral injury. **NSIDx:** Retrograde urethrogram. **Rx:** Suprapubic catheter for temporary urinary diversion and delayed repair.
Extraperitoneal (lower) bladder injury	Usually associated with pelvic fracture. **Findings:** Gross hematuria and urinary retention. Extraperitoneal bladder injury will have no chemical peritonitis. **NSIDx:** Retrograde cystogram. **Rx:** In majority of cases, isolated extraperitoneal bladder injury is managed conservatively with catheter drainage alone. Surgical repair is needed in complicated cases (e.g., injuries involving bladder neck or associated rectal or vaginal injury).
Rupture of dome of bladder	May be associated with pelvic fracture. **Findings:** Chemical peritonitis (abdominal guarding, rigidity, rebound tenderness, etc.) **Rx:** Surgical repair.
Renal laceration	Associated with lower rib fractures. **Findings:** Hematuria and no bladder symptoms. Hemodynamically instability might occur due to significant bleeding. **NSIDx:** CT abdomen with IV contrast. IV pyelography may be done if patient is unstable for transfer to CT scan. **Rx:** Surgery is indicated if renal pedicle is avulsed or in patients with hemodynamic instability. **Complication:** AV fistula (look for late development of high output heart failure) and renal artery stenosis (can lead to renovascular HTN).
Ureteral injury	Ureteral injury is rare with blunt trauma. If there is gross hematuria, but all imaging studies are unrevealing (including CT abdomen), obtain delayed CT images (images are taken minutes after contrast injection).
Scrotal or testicular injury	In all patients with scrotal hematoma and/or tenderness, **NSIDx is** US of scrotum with Doppler to assess vascular compromise.

25.7 Penetrating Injuries

25.7.1 Penetrating Injury to Head and Neck

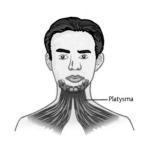

Definition of penetrating neck injury: Injury that penetrates the platysma muscle (otherwise it is a "superficial" injury and not penetrating).

Indications for surgical exploration in all penetrating neck injuries:

- Hemodynamic instability
- Expanding hematoma
- Signs of esophageal or tracheal injury (coughing or spitting up blood)

If above-mentioned dangers signs are not present, management depends upon area of neck injured and the type of penetrating injury (as shown below):

Zones		Gunshot wound (GSW)	Stab wound
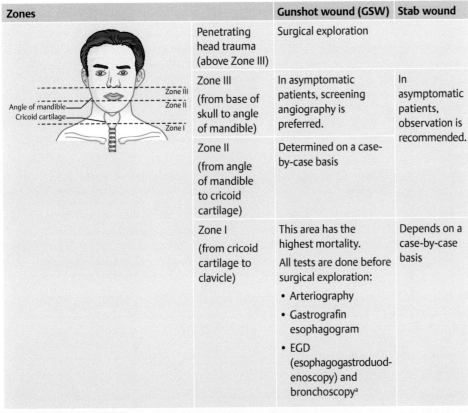	Penetrating head trauma (above Zone III)	Surgical exploration	
	Zone III (from base of skull to angle of mandible)	In asymptomatic patients, screening angiography is preferred.	In asymptomatic patients, observation is recommended.
	Zone II (from angle of mandible to cricoid cartilage)	Determined on a case-by-case basis	
	Zone I (from cricoid cartilage to clavicle)	This area has the highest mortality. All tests are done before surgical exploration: • Arteriography • Gastrografin esophagogram • EGD (esophagogastroduodenoscopy) and bronchoscopy[a]	Depends on a case-by-case basis

[a]Damage to lung (pneumothorax) and lung vessels may also occur.

25.7.2 Penetrating Injury to Abdomen (Gunshot Wound and Stab Wound)

Area: Any penetrating injury below the level of nipple is considered to involve abdomen.

Management

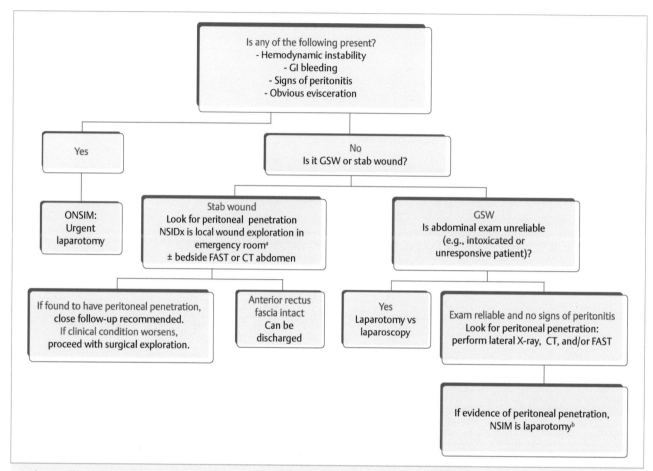

^aStab wounds can be examined by local exploration. For GSW, local wound exploration is unreliable.
^bAll GSWs that penetrate the peritoneum require explorative laparotomy, except in select cases. For example, low-caliber bullet wound with isolated solid organ injury (usually liver) can be conservatively managed.
Abbreviations: FAST, focused assessment with sonography in trauma; GSW, gunshot wound.

Clinical Case Scenarios

CCS of **abdominal trauma**—cover the second column and try to answer the NSIDx.

CCS	NSIDx
MVA (motor vehicle accident) patient with ecchymosis over abdomen + hemodynamic instability	FAST
Above patient's FAST is negative. Patient responds to IV fluid resuscitation.	CT abdomen and pelvis with IV contrast
MVA patient with ecchymosis over abdomen + hemodynamic instability + diffuse abdominal tenderness	Explorative laparotomy
MVA patient with diffuse abdominal tenderness, guarding, and rigidity. Patient is hemodynamically stable.	CT abdomen and pelvis with IV contrast
GSW patient with diffuse abdominal tenderness, guarding, and rigidity	Explorative laparotomy
Stab wound with NO hemodynamic instability, GI bleeding, signs of peritonitis, or evisceration.	Local wound exploration in ER
GSW in intoxicated patient with NO hemodynamic instability, GI bleeding, signs of peritonitis, or evisceration.	Laparoscopy

Abbreviations: FAST, focused assessment with sonography in trauma; MVA, motor vehicle accident; GSW, gunshot wound.

25.7.3 Penetrating Wound to Thighs

Zone	Management
Lateral thigh	Safe zone. No large arteries.
Medial upper thigh	Danger zone • Asymptomatic patients also get CT angiography
High-velocity GSW (military and big-game rifles) in lateral or medial thigh	Usually require surgical exploration

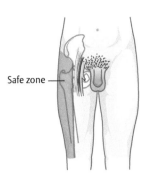

Safe zone

25.7.4 Arterial Injury due to Penetrating Trauma of Extremities

High probability signs of arterial injury (100% predictive in penetrating injury) due to penetrating trauma[a]	Signs of POSSIBLE arterial injury
Expanding or pulsatile hematoma	Stable hematoma
5Ps (pulselessness, pain, pallor paresthesia, paralysis)	Decreased pulses
Bruit or thrill over the wound	Proximity to great vessels
Active hemorrhage	Nerve deficit
NSIM: Directly send patient for surgical exploration ± intraoperative angiography.	**NSIDx:** CT or MR angiography.

[a]Note that these signs are less reliable in blunt trauma or fracture. Repeat exam after resuscitation, rewarming, fracture repositioning (if displaced or angulated fractures), and assess for compartment syndrome.

25.7.5 Compartment Syndrome

Etiology: Long-bone fractures, overly constrictive cast, reperfusion injury (e.g., postarterial embolectomy of extremity), circumferential burns, etc. Fascia prevents expansion of compartment under pressure resulting in ischemia.

Clinical features: Severe pain out of proportion to injury, painful passive stretching of muscles. Late signs include loss of motor function.

Management: Remove any dressing, splint, or cast, keep limb at the torso level, maintain blood pressure, and do emergency fasciotomy.

🗨️ Clinical Case Scenarios

2. Patient presents with displaced and angulated arm fracture. Exam reveals arterial bruit and reduced pulse distal to the fracture area. What is the immediate NSIM?
   a. Emergent surgery
   b. Reduction of dislocation and angulation
   c. CT angiography

3. After intervention, distal pulses have returned back to normal and bruit is no longer heard. What is the immediate NSIM?
   a. Send patient to operating room now.
   b. Fracture stabilization
   c. CT angiography

25.8 Fractures and Other Musculoskeletal Injuries after Trauma

25.8.1 General Management of Fractures

Small fractures without significant displacement or angulation	⟹ Closed reduction + casting[a]
With significant displacement, angulation, or comminuted fracture	⟹ ORIF (open reduction and internal fixation)
Open fracture (orthopedic emergency)	⟹ Clean and debride the wound. There is increased risk of bone infection; wound closure should be done within 6 hours.
Fracture with coexistent second-structure injury (e.g., fracture + joint dislocation or instability, or fracture + another bone fracture)[b]	⟹ These are considered unstable fractures and surgical management with orthopedic referral is recommended.

[a]Exceptions: Uncomplicated fractures that may not need casting are fracture of rib, clavicle, pelvic rami, proximal humerus fracture in adults, etc.

[b]For example, radioulnar fractures, or ulnar fracture associated with dislocation of radial head.

25.8.2 Pediatric Growth Plate Fractures (Salter–Harris Classification)

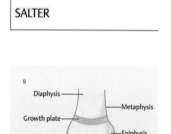

9

Diaphysis
Metaphysis
Growth plate
Epiphysis
Normal

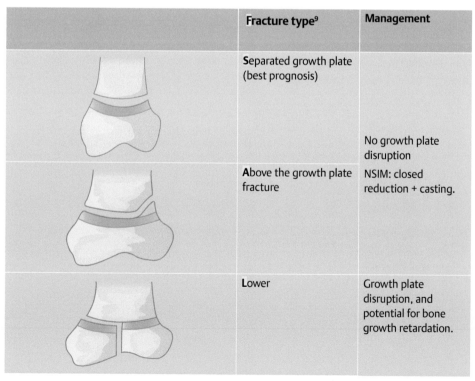

	Fracture type[9]	Management
	Separated growth plate (best prognosis)	No growth plate disruption NSIM: closed reduction + casting.
	Above the growth plate fracture	
	Lower	Growth plate disruption, and potential for bone growth retardation.

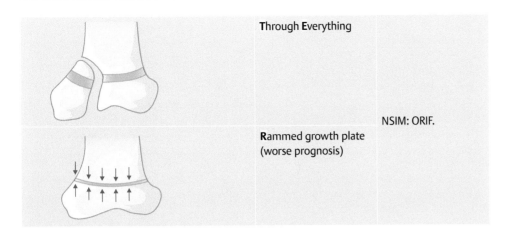

	Through Everything
	NSIM: ORIF.
	Rammed growth plate (worse prognosis)

25.8.3 Skull Fracture (!)

Type of skull fracture	Management
Linear closed fracture	Conservative management
Comminuted or depressed skull fractures	Prophylactic antibiotic + antiepileptic and surgical management.
Basilar skull fracture[a]	Conservative management. CT cervical spine is indicated to look for cervical spine injury.

[a]Look for periorbital ecchymosis (raccoon sign),[10] ecchymosis behind ear (battle sign), or clear-fluid dripping from nose or ear (CSF leak). MC location of basilar skull fracture is the temporal bone.

In a nutshell

Basilar Skull or Facial Bone Fractures and Associated Nerve Injury

Temporal bone fracture	⟹	Facial nerve
Maxillary fracture or orbital blowout fracture	⟹	Second branch of trigeminal nerve (decreased sensation in the midface area)
Mandibular fracture	⟹	Third branch of trigeminal nerve (decreased sensation in the lower face area)

⚠ **Caution**

(!) For all skull fractures, test of choice is CT scan (not X-ray).

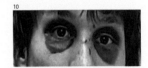

Source: Marion County Sheriff's Office, Public domain, via Wikimedia Commons.

25.8.4 Fractures in Upper Torso and Extremities

	Additional points	Management
Clavicular fracture	Typically occurs in the junction of middle and distal third of the clavicle	Shoulder sling
Supracondylar fracture of humerus	**Typical injury pattern:** Child falling on an outstretched hand, with resulting hyperextension of elbow. This can be complicated by neurovascular injury: most commonly injured structures are brachial artery and median nerve. Brachial artery injury can lead to ischemic necrosis resulting in fibrosis of flexor muscles of upper extremities.	Casting (refer to the Salter–Harris classification)

Source: James Heilman, MD, CC BY-SA 3.0, via Wikimedia Commons.

Galeazzi fracture	Radial midshaft fracture associated with distal radioulnar joint instability	Splint + referral to orthopedic surgery (needs surgical stabilization and repair)[a]
Monteggia fracture	Proximal third ulnar fracture associated with dislocation of radial head	Splint + referral to orthopedic surgery (ORIF)[a]
Distal radial fracture with dorsal displacement (Colles' fracture)	**Typical injury pattern:** Old patient with underlying osteoporosis or young athlete with high-velocity fall on an outstretched hand. • This results in dinner-fork deformity of hand	Closed reduction + casting
Distal radial fracture with palmar displacement (Smith's fracture)	**Typical injury pattern:** Old patient with underlying osteoporosis or young athlete with high-velocity fall on hand inwardly.	Higher risk of neurovascular injury. Refer to orthopedic surgeon after reduction and casting.
Scaphoid bone (carpal navicular) fracture	**Typical injury pattern:** Fall on an outstretched hand **Presentation:** Pain/tenderness in the anatomical snuff box (base of first metacarpal). **Work-up:** Scaphoid X-ray (it may be negative in initial stages). If negative, MRI can be done to confirm dx. **Complication:** Avascular necrosis of head (osteonecrosis)	• Nondisplaced fracture (≤1 mm): thumb-spica cast and repeat X-ray in 1–2 weeks. • Displaced fracture: ORIF

[a]The general rule: A fracture with coexistent injury of second structure (e.g., fracture + joint dislocation or instability) requires surgical management (orthopedic referral).

25.8.5 Shoulder Dislocation

Anterior shoulder dislocation (MC dislocation)	• Can cause axillary nerve injury, which presents as weakened shoulder abduction (deltoid muscle) and decreased sensation over shoulder. • Dislocation can be recurrent. **Rx:** Reduction followed by immobilization in **ad**ducted and **i**nternal **r**otated positions, using a commercially available shoulder immobilizer.
Posterior shoulder dislocation	• Can occur after seizures or electrocution. • May be missed on regular-view X-rays; special views are required. **Rx:** May require closed reduction under anesthesia or open reduction, followed by immobilization.

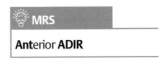

MRS

Anterior **ADIR**

25.8.6 Hip Fracture

Presentation: Hip pain after fall.

Work-up: First SIDx is hip X-ray. CT hip can be done, if X-ray is equivocal.

Type of fracture	Management[a]
Femoral neck fracture	Hip hemiarthroplasty (placement of femoral head prosthesis[b]; the socket does not need to be replaced)
Femoral neck + acetabular fracture	Ball and socket replacement (i.e., complete hip replacement or hip arthroplasty)
Intertrochanteric fracture	ORIF
Femoral shaft fracture[c]	Intramedullary rod fixation

[a]Surgery is done ASAP (usually within 24–48 hours).

[b]Femoral head will likely not survive due to disruption of blood supply.

[c]Bilateral fractures can cause severe blood loss leading to hemodynamic instability. It can also cause fat emboli.

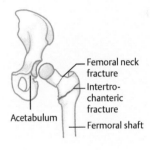

25.8.7 Knee Injury

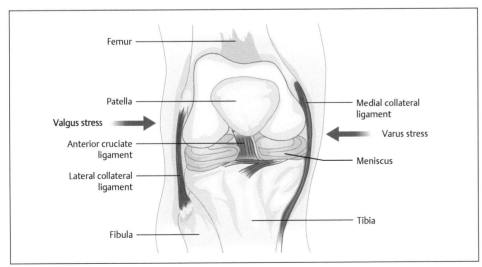

Patients undergoing major orthopedic surgery (total hip arthroplasty, total knee arthroplasty, or hip fracture surgery) should received DVT prophylaxis for 4–5 weeks. Use either low-molecular weight heparin, DOACs, warfarin, aspirin or intermittent pneumatic compression devices.

	Typical injury pattern	Clinical findings	Management[a]
Collateral ligament injury	Blow from sides • Blow from the medial side (varus force) can cause lateral collateral ligament injury (as in the picture above) • Blow from the **L**ateral side (va**L**gus force) can cause medial collateral ligament injury	• Varus joint laxity in lateral collateral ligament injury • Valgus laxity in medial collateral ligament injury	Physical therapy and exercise program in uncomplicated cases In refractory cases, gross knee instability, or complicated injury, consider arthroscopic or surgical knee repair
Meniscal tear	Rotational stress (due to twisting force with feet fixed)	• Might present with late swelling after injury • Sensation of *catching, locking*, and/or knees giving out	
Anterior cruciate ligament (MC knee ligament injury)	Sudden deceleration and direction change (e.g., while playing tennis or badminton)	Anterior drawer sign (leg can be pulled anteriorly, when knees flexed)[b]	Athletes or young patients who want to maintain active life, or severe cases may need arthroscopic evaluation and reconstruction

Injury of medial meniscus, medial collateral, and ACL (anterior cruciate ligament) can occur together.

[a]MRI is needed to diagnose and exclude other injuries in these cases.

[b]Posterior cruciate ligament injury has opposite findings and is less common.

25.8.8 Ankle Fracture

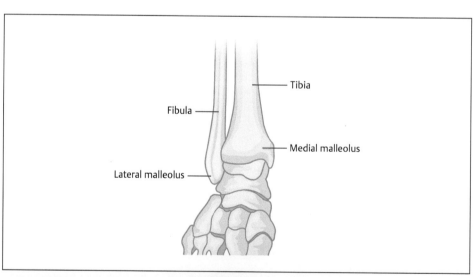

Fracture type	Management
Nondisplaced isolated *medial or posterior malleolar* fracture[a]	Splint, non-weight bearing, and re-evaluation after 1 week to ensure no other fracture/injury is missed. Walking cast is placed with weight-bearing as tolerated after that.
Lateral malleolar fracture + deltoid ligament injury	Splint, non-weight bearing, and follow-up with orthopedic surgery in few days. These require operative fixation.
Bimalleolar or trimalleolar fracture	If significant swelling is present, delayed ORIF is done.

[a]Lateral malleolar fractures tend to be more complicated.

25.8.9 Stress Fracture

Typical patient profile: Athletes, dancers, and avid runners with risk factors for decreased bone density (e.g., low BMI).
Presentation: Slowly progressive and insidious-onset bone pain. Look for point tenderness.
Diagnosis: First SIDx is plain X-ray. If negative, NSIDx is MRI scan.

Management:
High-risk stress fracture occurs in the following bones: pars interarticularis of the lumbar spine, femoral head/neck, patella, anterior tibial cortex, medial malleolus, *talus, tarsal navicular, proximal fourth or fifth metatarsal, base of the second metatarsal, and great toe sesamoids.* Common complication of the high-risk fracture is malunion.

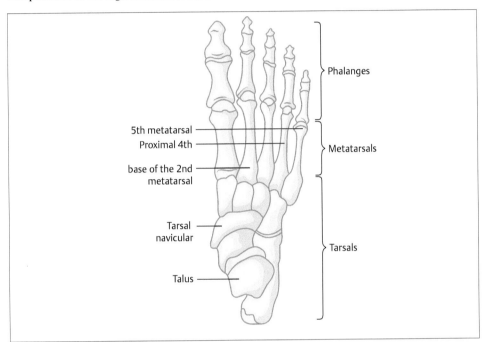

Phalanges

5th metatarsal
Proximal 4th
base of the 2nd metatarsal
Metatarsals

Tarsal navicular

Talus
Tarsals

High-risk stress fracture	Non-high-risk fractures
Orthopedic consultation (casting or internal fixation might be needed)	• Reduced weight-bearing ± splinting and physical therapy • Patients with stress fractures should avoid running

Differential diagnosis of anterior tibial stress fracture is medial tibial stress syndrome (aka shin splints): Both can occur in runners. Differentiating feature is that in medial tibial stress syndrome there is diffuse, rather than point, tenderness.[11] Patients may continue running but shorter distance run is recommended.

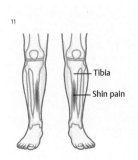

[11]

Tibia

Shin pain

25.8.10 Achilles Tendon Rupture

Presentation: While playing sports one hears a loud pop and starts having Achilles area pain. Palpation can reveal a gap in tendon.
Rx: Surgical repair. For inactive patients, casting in plantar-flexed position can be done.

25.8.11 Penile Fracture

Background: Traumatic rupture of corpus cavernosum, which typically occurs due to trauma, commonly during sex.

Management: For any urinary symptom, retrograde urethrogram to rule out coexistent urethral injury should be done. Emergent surgical repair is recommended.

25.9 Postoperative Complications

25.9.1 Post-op Fever

Timing	Etiology	Management
Immediate (during or within few hours of surgery)	• Febrile transfusion reaction • Prior infection, or • Malignant hyperthermia due to anesthetics (drugs ending in "+ ane"—e.g., halothane, desflurane, or "+ thonium"—e.g., suxamethonium). Look for muscle rigidity and elevated CK (creatine kinase).	For malignant hyperthermia, use IV dantrolene.
Day 1–3	Atelectasis	Incentive spirometry is the best prevention.
Day 3–5	UTI	NSIDx is urinalysis.
Day 5–7	Thrombophlebitis or deep venous thrombosis	NSIDx is duplex US.
Day 7–10	Surgical wound infection or dehiscence	Wound gram stain culture and antibiotics, usually followed by late reclosure.
10–15 days after abdominal procedure	• Deep abscess (subphrenic, pelvic, or subhepatic) • Bowel anastomosis issues (e.g., leakage into the peritoneal cavity)	NSIDx is CT scan. Abscess needs percutaneous drain. Surgery may be required in complex abscesses or to address underlying issue.

> **MRS**
> Wind = Atelectasis
> Water = UTI
> Walking = Thrombotic complications due to immobility
> Wound = Wound infection

> Other causes of postoperative fever include iatrogenic bowel injury during abdominal surgery (presents within 24 hours), drug allergy (few days), etc.

25.9.2 Postsurgical Complications

Case scenario	Additional points	
Immediate postoperative urinary retention	NSIDx is bedside bladder scan. Urinary catheterization is done to relieve retention (straight catheterization one to two times, followed by indwelling catheter placement, if recurrent).	
Decreased urinary output in the immediate postoperative period	Zero Foley catheter output	Catheter is either kinked or blocked. NSIM is to check the catheter.
	Minimal Foley output	NSIM is IV fluids.
Postsurgical abdominal distention, nausea, and vomiting suggestive of bowel obstruction	**Etiology:** Paralytic ileus, mechanical obstruction (due to early development of adhesions which can occur as early as 1 week), or Ogilvie's syndrome (in old patients)	
AAA repair (abdominal aortic aneurysm repair)	Bowel ischemia (inferior mesenteric artery occlusion due to aortic graft)	**Presentation:** Bloody diarrhea and abdominal tenderness.
	Aortoenteric fistula	Late complication due to fistula formation between the duodenum and aortic graft. **Presentation:** Upper GI bleeding.
Thoracic aortic repair	It is the MCC of spinal-cord infarction (look for flaccid paralysis after surgery).	
Thoracic surgery (e.g., coronary artery bypass grafting)	Acute mediastinitis due to surgical contamination, or local extension from surgical wound infection. Usually occurs within 2 weeks. **Presentation:** Fever, chest pain, and widened mediastinum. **Rx:** Surgical drainage/debridement + IV antibiotics.	

Answers

1. No need for imaging, if there are no risk factors and no signs of neurological compromise or headache, in a patient with minor head trauma and scalp injury.

2. (b) Reduction of dislocation and angulation. Note: Hard signs are less reliable in blunt trauma.

3. (b) Fracture stabilization.

Index